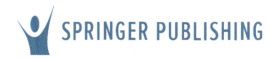

SPRINGER PUBLISHING

GET THE MOST FROM YOUR BOOK

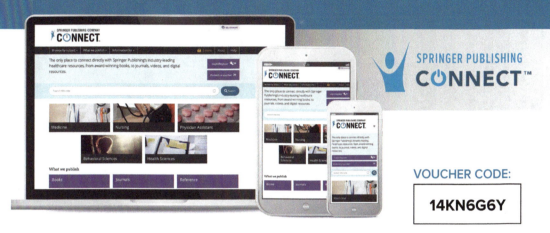

VOUCHER CODE:

14KN6G6Y

Online Access

Your print purchase of *Environmental Health: Foundations for Public Health* includes **online access via Springer Publishing Connect**™ to increase accessibility, portability, and searchability.

Insert the code at http://connect.springerpub.com/content/book/978-0-8261-8353-8 or scan the QR code and insert the voucher code today!

Having trouble? Contact our customer service department at **cs@springerpub.com**

Instructor Resource Access for Adopters

Let us do some of the heavy lifting to create an engaging classroom experience with a variety of instructor resources included in most textbooks SUCH AS:

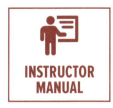
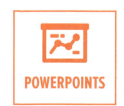
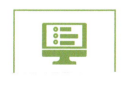

Visit **https://connect.springerpub.com/** and look for the **"Show Supplementary"** what is available to instructors! First time using Springer Publishing Connect?

Email **textbook@springerpub.com** to create an account and start unlocking valuable resources.

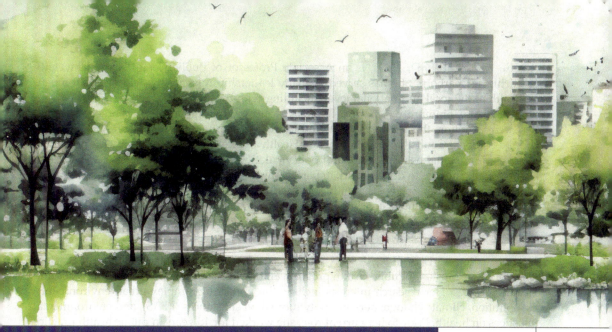

ENVIRONMENTAL HEALTH

Natalie Sampson, PhD, MPH, is an Associate Professor of Public Health at the University of Michigan-Dearborn. She has served in many leadership roles in the field of environmental health at the local and national level, including with the American Public Health Association (APHA), Community Action to Promote Healthy Environments, Environmental Health Research-to-Action, the Michigan Center on Lifestage Environmental Exposures and Disease, and the National Council for Environmental Health and Equity. Dr. Sampson works to democratize environmental health science and policymaking in an effort to improve environmental health for all. She gets to do this work in partnership with brilliant leaders, including longtime community organizers, activists, youth, students, agency partners, educators, and researchers. As a faculty member, she primarily teaches courses on environmental health and community organizing and enjoys engaging in active, practice-based learning with her students throughout Metro Detroit.

Lindsay Tallon, PhD, MSPH, CPH, is an Associate Professor of Public Health and Assistant Director of the Master of Public Health program at the Massachusetts College of Pharmacy and Health Sciences. Her research interests include the impact of complex urban environments, air pollution, climate change, per- and polyfluoroalkyl substances (PFAS), and environmental injustices on health. Prior to her current role, she worked for 15 years in public health practice in the fields of emergency preparedness, medical marijuana, and volunteer programs such as the Medical Reserve Corps and Americorps. Her national service and leadership roles include working with the American Public Health Association (APHA), the Association for Prevention Teaching and Research, and the Council on Education in Public Health. As a faculty member, she teaches classes in environmental health, public health emergency preparedness, and research methods while focusing on anti-oppressive teaching methods and enhancing the connection between public health education and practice.

Natasha DeJarnett, PhD, MPH, BCES, is an Assistant Professor in the Christina Lee Brown Envirome Institute at the University of Louisville Division of Environmental Medicine researching the health impacts of extreme heat exposure and environmental health disparities. She is also a professorial lecturer in Environmental and Occupational Health at the George Washington University Milken Institute School of Public Health. In addition, Dr. DeJarnett is the Deputy Director for Environmental Justice Data and Evaluation at the White House Council on Environmental Quality. Previously, she was interim associate director of Program and Partnership Development at the National Environmental Health Association, leading the areas of research, climate and health, and children's environmental health. She also previously served as a policy analyst at the American Public Health Association (APHA), where she led the Natural Environment portfolio, including air and water exposures, along with climate change. Her previous service leadership included: Member, Children's Health Protection Advisory Committee, U.S. Environmental Protection Agency; Chair, Governing Board, Citizens' Climate Education; President-Elect, Board of Directors, Physicians for Social Responsibility; Chair-Elect, Environment Section, APHA; Member, Advisory Board, APHA Center for Climate, Health and Equity; Member, Board of Trustees, for the BTS Center; Special Advisor, Environmental Health and Equity Collaborative; and Member, Steering Committee, International Transformational Resilience Coalition.

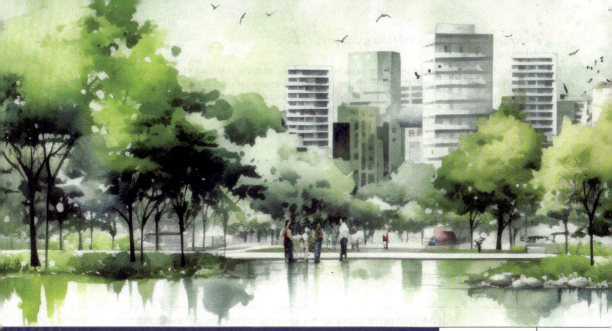

ENVIRONMENTAL HEALTH

Foundations for Public Health

Natalie Sampson, PhD, MPH
Lindsay Tallon, PhD, MSPH, CPH
Natasha DeJarnett, PhD, MPH, BCES

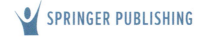

Copyright © 2025 Springer Publishing Company, LLC
All rights reserved.

No part of this publication may be reproduced, stored in a retrieval system, or transmitted in any form or by any means, electronic, mechanical, photocopying, recording, or otherwise, without the prior permission of Springer Publishing Company, LLC, or authorization through payment of the appropriate fees to the Copyright Clearance Center, Inc., 222 Rosewood Drive, Danvers, MA 01923, 978-750-8400, fax 978-646-8600, info@copyright.com or at www.copyright.com.

Springer Publishing Company, LLC
902 Carnegie Center, Suite 140, Princeton, NJ 08540
www.springerpub.com
connect.springerpub.com

Senior Acquisitions Editor: David D'Addona
Senior Director, Content Development: Taylor Ball
Compositor: Amnet
Production Editor: Rachel Haines

ISBN: 978-0-8261-8352-1
e-book ISBN: 978-0-8261-8353-8
DOI: 10.1891/9780826183538

SUPPLEMENTS:

 A robust set of instructor resources designed to supplement this text is located at http://connect.springerpub.com/content/book/978-0-8261-8353-8. Qualifying instructors may request access by emailing textbook@springerpub.com.

Instructor Materials:
LMS Common Cartridge–All Instructor Resources: 978-0-8261-9197-7
Instructor Manual: 978-0-8261-8354-5
Instructor Test Bank: 978-0-8261-8355-2
Instructor Chapter PowerPoint slides: 978-0-8261-8356-9
Sample Syllabus: 978-0-8261-6876-4

Student Materials:
Podcasts: See the List of Podcasts for more information.
Podcast Transcripts: 978-0-8261-8865-6

24 25 26 27 / 5 4 3 2 1

The author and the publisher of this Work have made every effort to use sources believed to be reliable to provide information that is accurate and compatible with the standards generally accepted at the time of publication. Because medical science is continually advancing, our knowledge base continues to expand. Therefore, as new information becomes available, changes in procedures become necessary. We recommend that the reader always consult current research and specific institutional policies before performing any clinical procedure or delivering any medication. The author and publisher shall not be liable for any special, consequential, or exemplary damages resulting, in whole or in part, from the readers' use of, or reliance on, the information contained in this book. The publisher has no responsibility for the persistence or accuracy of URLs for external or third-party Internet websites referred to in this publication and does not guarantee that any content on such websites is, or will remain, accurate or appropriate.

Library of Congress Cataloging-in-Publication Data
Names: Sampson, Natalie, editor. | Tallon, Lindsay, editor. | DeJarnett, Natasha, editor.
Title: Environmental health : foundations for public health / [edited by]
    Natalie Sampson, Lindsay Tallon, Natasha DeJarnett.
Other titles: Environmental health (Sampson)
Description: New York, NY : Springer Publishing Company, [2025] | Includes
    bibliographical references and index.
Identifiers: LCCN 2024013924 (print) | LCCN 2024013925 (ebook) | ISBN
    9780826183521 (paperback) | ISBN 9780826183538 (ebook)
Subjects: MESH: Environmental Health | Environmental Justice | Climate
    Change | Environmental Policy | Public Health | United States
Classification: LCC RA566 (print) | LCC RA566 (ebook) | NLM WA 30 | DDC 362.1--dc23/eng/20240517
LC record available at https://lccn.loc.gov/2024013924
LC ebook record available at https://lccn.loc.gov/2024013925

Contact sales@springerpub.com to receive discount rates on bulk purchases.

Publisher's Note: **New and used products purchased from third-party sellers are not guaranteed for quality, authenticity, or access to any included digital components.**

Printed in the United States of America.

We dedicate this book to our families.

CONTENTS

Contributors *ix*
Foreword *Charles Lee* *xiii*
Preface *xv*
Acknowledgments *xix*
List of Podcasts *xxi*
Resources *xxiii*

SECTION I: FOUNDATIONS OF ENVIRONMENTAL HEALTH

🎙 **Podcast: History of Per- and Polyfluoroalkyl Substances (PFAS)** 1

1. Fundamentals of Environmental Health and Justice   3
   Natalie Sampson, Lindsay Tallon, Natalie Conti, and Anchal Malh

2. Environmental Health in Practice   23
   Ali Abazeed and Samir Deshpande

3. Confronting the Realities of Climate Change   43
   Natasha DeJarnett, Viniece Jennings, and Neha Pathak

4. Environmental Health Policies and Protections: Successes and Failures   72
   Adrienne L. Hollis, Vernice Miller-Travis, and Daria E. Neal

SECTION II: THE ENVIRONMENTAL HEALTH SCIENCE TOOLKIT

🎙 **Podcast: The Science of PFAS Detection**   95

5. Environmental Health Science for the People   97
   Monica Unseld and Omega Wilson

6. Understanding (Unequal and Cumulative) Risks in Our Daily Environment   117
   Cielo A. Sharkus, Tatiana C. Height, April M. Ballard, Ami Zota, Wilma Subra, and Lariah Edwards

7. Understanding the Environment and How It Relates to Health Using Toxicology and Epidemiology Research Methods   139
   Chanese A. Forté, Aurora B. Le, Dana C. Dolinoy, and Jaclyn M. Goodrich

8. Mapping Environmental Health and Justice Issues   163
   Juliana Maantay and Mozhgon Rajaee

SECTION III: INTERCONNECTED: ENERGY, AIR, WATER, FOOD, AND WASTE

🎙 **Podcast: PFAS Where We Live, Work, and Play**   191

9. **Energy and Health**   193
   Carina J. Gronlund, Anchal Malh, Parth Vaishnav, Gibran Washington,
   Bruce Tonn, Amy J. Schulz, and Marie S. O'Neill

10. **The Air We Breathe**   214
    Beto Lugo Martinez and Shir Lerman Ginzburg

11. **Clean Water for All**   235
    Margaret J. Eggers, Mary Grant, Marcela González Rivas, Anne K. Camper,
    James Olson, John Doyle, and Monica Lewis-Patrick

12. **Food Safety, Security, and Sovereignty**   272
    Sara El-Sayed, Sandra M. Long, and Benjamin Ryan

13. **Waste and Sustainability**   291
    Denise Patel and Neil Tangri

SECTION IV: REIMAGINING ENVIRONMENTAL HEALTH FOR ALL

🎙 **Podcast: Firefighters and Forever Chemicals: Occupational Exposure to PFAS and Health-Related Consequences**   319

🎙 **Podcast: Halting the PFAS Cycle and Its Costs on Individuals, Communities, and Society**   319

14. **Healthy Communities for All**   321
    Kate Robb and Sandra F. Whitehead

15. **Preparing for and Recovering From Disasters in Our Changing Climate**   344
    Mitch Stripling

16. **Ensuring Occupational Health**   369
    Eric Persaud and Devan Hawkins

17. **Ensuring Children's Environmental Health and Justice**   397
    Nsedu Obot Witherspoon and Leyla Erk McCurdy

18. **Integrating Environmental Health and Justice Into Healthcare**   419
    Maida P. Galvez, Emma N. Chang, Perry E. Sheffield,
    Hannah M. Thompson, Blair J. Wylie, and Tatiana C. Height

19. **Organizing for Environmental Health and Justice: Lessons From #StopGeneralIron**   445
    Jim Bloyd

Glossary of Key Terms   471
Index   483

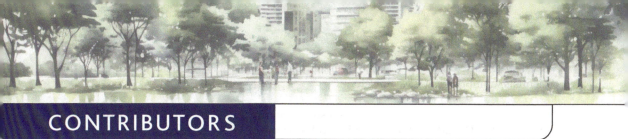

CONTRIBUTORS

Ali Abazeed, MPH, MPP, Chief Public Health Officer, Founding Director of Public Health, City of Dearborn Department of Public Health, Dearborn, Michigan

April M. Ballard, PhD, MPH, Assistant Professor of Environmental Health, Department of Population Health Sciences, School of Public Health, Georgia State University, Atlanta, Georgia

Jim Bloyd, DrPH, MPH, Coordinator, Collaborative for Health Equity Cook County, Adjunct Instructor, School of Public Health, University of Illinois at Chicago, Chicago, Illinois

Anne K. Camper, MS, PhD, Regents Professor Ermerita, Norm Asbjornson College of Engineering, Montana State University, Bozeman, Montana

Emma N. Chang, MPH, BSN, RN, Fellow, Department of Environmental Medicine and Public Health, Icahn School of Medicine at Mount Sinai, New York, New York

Natalie Conti, MLS(ASCP)CM, MS, Graduate Student, Environmental Health Sciences–Industrial Hygiene, University of Michigan School of Public Health, Ann Arbor, Michigan

Natasha DeJarnett, PhD, MPH, BCES, Assistant Professor, Department of Medicine, University of Louisville, Louisville, Kentucky

Samir Deshpande, MPP, Environmental Health Manager, City of Dearborn Department of Public Health, Dearborn, Michigan

Dana C. Dolinoy, PhD, MSc, Professor, Departments of Environmental Health Sciences and Nutritional Sciences, University of Michigan School of Public Health, Ann Arbor, Michigan

John Doyle, Crow Water Quality Project Director and Crow Environmental Health Steering Committee, Little Big Horn College, Crow Agency, Montana; Member, National Environmental Justice Advisory Council, Environmental Protection Agency, Washington, D.C.

Lariah Edwards, PhD, Associate Research Scientist, Department of Environmental Health Sciences, Mailman School of Public Health, Columbia University, New York, New York

Margaret J. Eggers, MA, MS, PhD, Associate Research Professor and Associate Director, Environmental Health Program, Microbiology and Cell Biology Department, Montana State University, Bozeman, Montana; Crow Environmental Health Steering Committee, Little Big Horn College, Crow Agency, Montana

Sara El-Sayed, PhD, Director of The Biomimicry Center, Assistant Research Professor, Swette Center for Sustainable Food Systems, Julie Ann Wrigley Global Futures Laboratory™, Arizona State University, Tempe, Arizona

Chanese A. Forté, PhD-PhD, MPH, Scientist, Global Security Program, Union of Concerned Scientists, Cambridge, Massachusetts

Maida P. Galvez, MD, MPH, FAAP, Professor, Department of Environmental Medicine and Public Health, Department of Pediatrics, Icahn School of Medicine at Mount Sinai, New York, New York

Shir Lerman Ginzburg, PhD, MPH, Assistant Professor of Public Health, School of Arts and Sciences, Massachusetts College of Pharmacy and Health Sciences, Boston, Massachusetts

Marcela González Rivas, MSc, PhD, Associate Professor, Graduate School of Public and International Affairs, University of Pittsburgh, Pittsburgh, Pennsylvania

Jaclyn M. Goodrich, PhD, Research Associate Professor, Department of Environmental Health Sciences, University of Michigan School of Public Health, Ann Arbor, Michigan

Mary Grant, Public Water For All Campaign Director, Food & Water Watch, Baltimore, Maryland

Carina J. Gronlund, PhD, MPH, Research Assistant Professor, Social Environment and Health Program, Survey Research Center, University of Michigan Institute for Social Research, Ann Arbor, Michigan

Devan Hawkins, ScD, Assistant Professor of Public Health, Director of Bachelor of Public Health Program, School of Arts and Sciences, Massachusetts College of Pharmacy and Health Sciences, Boston, Massachusetts

Tatiana C. Height, EdD, Assistant Professor, Alcorn State University, Lorman, Mississippi

Adrienne L. Hollis, PhD, JD, Vice President, Environmental Justice, Climate and Community Revitalization, Conservation, National Wildlife Federation, Bowie, Maryland

Viniece Jennings, PhD, Deputy Director, National Oceanic and Atmospheric Administration Center for Coastal and Marine Ecosystems, Florida A&M University, Tallahassee, Florida

Aurora B. Le, PhD, MPH, CSP, CPH, John G. Searle Assistant Professor, Department of Environmental Health Sciences, University of Michigan School of Public Health, Ann Arbor, Michigan

Monica Lewis-Patrick, Chief Executive Officer, We the People of Detroit, Detroit, Michigan

Sandra M. Long, BS, REHS, RS, CP-FS, Environmental Health Manager, Town of Addison, Development Services Department, Addison, Texas

Juliana Maantay, MUP, PhD, Professor, Department of Earth, Environmental, and Geospatial Sciences, Lehman College, City University of New York, Bronx, New York

Anchal Malh, MS, Graduate Student, Science Researcher and Writer, University of Michigan-Ann Arbor, Ann Arbor, Michigan

Beto Lugo Martinez, Executive Director, SciCAN.org, California Environmental Justice Coalition, RISE4EJ, Kansas City, Missouri

Leyla Erk McCurdy, MPhil, Environmental Health Consultant, Arlington, Virginia

Vernice Miller-Travis, BA, Executive Vice President, Metropolitan Group, Cofounder, WEACT for Environmental Justice, Bowie, Maryland

Daria E. Neal, BA, JD, Adjunct Instructor, Howard University School of Law, Washington, D.C.

James Olson, JD, LLM, Of Counsel, Olson, Bzdok & Howard, P.C., Founder and Sr. Legal Advisor, For Love of Water (FLOW), Adjunct Professor, Great Lakes Water Studies Institute, Northwestern Michigan College, Traverse City, Michigan

Marie S. O'Neill, MS, PhD, Professor, School of Public Health, University of Michigan, Ann Arbor, Michigan

Denise Patel, MPH, Environmental Health Consultant, New York, New York

Neha Pathak, MD, FACP, DipABLM, Chief Physician Editor for Health and Lifestyle Medicine at WebMD, Chair, American College of Lifestyle Medicine Global Sustainability Committee, Atlanta, Georgia

Eric Persaud, DrPH, MEA, Occupational Health Specialist, South Richmond Hill, New York

Mozhgon Rajaee, PhD, MPH, MS, Associate Professor, Department of Public and Environmental Wellness, Oakland University, Rochester, Michigan

Kate Robb, MSPH, Deputy Director, Center for Public Health Policy, American Public Health Association, Washington, D.C.

Benjamin Ryan, PhD, MPH, REHS, Professor of Public Health and Global Initiatives, Frist College of Medicine, Belmont University, Nashville, Tennessee

Natalie Sampson, PhD, MPH, Associate Professor of Public Health, College of Education, Health, and Human Services, University of Michigan–Dearborn, Dearborn, Michigan

Amy J. Schulz, PhD, MPH, MSW, Professor, Department of Health Behavior and Health Education, School of Public Health, University Diversity and Social Transformation Professor, University of Michigan, Ann Arbor, Michigan

Cielo A. Sharkus, PhD, Department of Civil and Environmental Engineering, University of Massachusetts Amherst, Amherst, Massachusetts

Perry E. Sheffield, MD, MPH, FAAP, Associate Professor, Department of Environmental Medicine and Public Health, Department of Pediatrics, Icahn School of Medicine at Mount Sinai, New York, New York

Mitch Stripling, MPA, Director, Pandemic Response Institute, Lecturer, Mailman School of Public Health, Columbia University, New York, New York

Wilma Subra, MS, Technical Director, Louisiana Environmental Action Network, New Iberia, Louisiana

Lindsay Tallon, PhD, MSPH, CPH, Associate Professor of Public Health, Assistant Director MPH Program, School of Arts and Sciences, Massachusetts College of Pharmacy and Health Sciences, Boston, Massachusetts

Neil Tangri, PhD, Science and Policy Director, Global Alliance for Incinerator Alternatives, San Francisco, California

Hannah M. Thompson, MD, MPH, Assistant Professor, Department of Environmental Medicine and Public Health, Icahn School of Medicine at Mount Sinai, New York, New York

Bruce Tonn, PhD, President, Three³, Inc., Knoxville, Tennessee

Monica Unseld, PhD, MPH, Until Justice Data Partners, Louisville, Kentucky

Parth Vaishnav, PhD, Assistant Professor, School for Environment and Sustainability, University of Michigan, Ann Arbor, Michigan

Gibran Washington, MS, Program Manager, EcoWorks Detroit, Detroit, Michigan

Sandra F. Whitehead, PhD, Associate Professor and Program Director, Sustainable Urban Planning Program, George Washington University, Washington, D.C.

Omega Wilson, West End Revitalization Association, Mebane, North Carolina

Nsedu Obot Witherspoon, MPH, Children's Environmental Health Network, Washington, D.C.

Blair J. Wylie, MD, MPH, Founding Director of The Collaborative for Women's Environmental Health at Columbia University, Virgil G. Damon Professor of Obstetrics and Gynecology, Vagelos College of Physicians and Surgeons, Columbia University, New York, New York

Ami Zota, ScD, MS, Associate Professor, Department of Environmental Health Sciences, Mailman School of Public Health, Columbia University, New York, New York

FOREWORD

This book is a comprehensive and engaging introduction to environmental health written for persons entering the field. It is my privilege to provide a perspective regarding the historical impact of environmental justice on the environmental health field based on my nearly half-century of work in the area. When I started to work on issues related to the confluence of race, class, and the environment, the field did not even have a name. Today, these issues animate just about every aspect of environmental health, as evidenced by the chapters in this book. Why? Because virtually everything has an environmental dimension. In the words of trailblazing environmental justice activist Jeanne Gauna, the environment is the place where we live, work, play, and learn. For this reason, justice-seeking persons entering the environmental health field will find it to be inextricably linked to the great challenges facing society locally, nationally, and globally—and therefore profoundly relevant, challenging, full of opportunity, and exciting.

My own perspective can be viewed through the lens of a theory of change that speaks to a cyclical series of successive actions, including community activism and capacity building, research and bringing evidence to bear, policy change, and systems transformation. By "systems" I mean systemic racism; environmental, economic, and social marginalization; and policy, science, and governance. Some of this is aspirational and will be accomplished by those who are entering the field and will grow to be leaders of the future.

In a remarkably short period of time, the environmental justice movement has reached a level of practice where advocates have brought about important policy advances, including the passage of legislation. Sometimes this has involved years, if not decades, of tenacious advocacy on the part of community leaders and their allies for issues that go against the grain of entrenched values, policies, and practices that serve as structural barriers to equity and justice.

These policy changes often involve new research, data sources, and analytic methods. For example, the issue of environmental justice may have never emerged without the advent of two things: mapping tools such as geographic information systems and large-scale environmental databases. In combination, they made it possible to visualize the inequitable distribution of environmental burdens and lack of benefits. These now form the basis for prioritizing billions of dollars of resources to benefit communities in which the most egregious concentration of environmental burdens and lack of benefits are located.

These developments played a major role in shaping the policy thread that runs through the four Executive Orders (EOs) that focus on environmental justice (EOs 12898, 13985, 14091, and 14096). They span nearly 30 years, reflect much of the growth and maturation of the environmental justice issue, and identify issues that will be key challenges for the foreseeable future. For me, this policy thread is epitomized by the connection between the legacy of racism and other structural drivers of inequity, cumulative impacts, and the climate crisis, as articulated in EO 14096. In this EO, President Biden also articulates a definition of environmental justice that includes "full protection" and calls for "whole-of-government" approaches.

I am proud of having contributed to this formulation. Now, it is up to you—the environmental health researchers, teachers, practitioners, and leaders of the future—to move us substantially toward fulfilling the vision that President Biden articulated. There is no better time to enter the field of environmental health. To paraphrase Environmental Protection Agency Administrator Michael Regan, now is the time to make environmental justice part of the DNA of the environmental health field. The environmental health challenges of the foreseeable future demand it, and there has never been a time when you could make more important contributions to the field.

Charles Lee
Principal Author of *Toxic Wastes and Race in the United States*
Lead Organizer of the First National People of Color Leadership Summit

PREFACE

"The only way to survive is by taking care of one another."

—Grace Lee Boggs

As we prepared this textbook over the past few years, a lot has happened. Historian Heather Cox Richardson says about the United States today, "A country that once stood as the global symbol of democracy has been teetering on the brink of authoritarianism."[1(p2)] Just as the textbook went to print, we learned that the Supreme Court of the United States was making decisions that gravely endanger our democracy further. They overturned the Chevron doctrine, established by the Supreme Court in *Chevron U.S.A., Inc. v. Natural Resources Defense Council, Inc.* (1984)[2], and they lifted the statute of limitations on legal challenges to regulations indefinitely. In simple terms, they gave judges greater power in policymaking, and they did so in ways that will likely favor corporate interests and undermine public health. One might think: But isn't this an environmental health textbook? Shouldn't the focus be on exposure science and chemicals? On air and water quality and strategies to protect human health? Yes, it should be, and we do cover these topics.

Yet, while writing this textbook, we saw ongoing threats to democracy on the news and all around us, and we were reminded time and time again of the ways environmental health and justice are fragile. In a truly democratic society, voting is a right, and governments are accountable to the people. Policies regarding environmental protection are influenced by public opinion, allowing space for meaningful input from all, particularly those most affected by the issues under discussion. In theory, democracies have transparent systems where information is accessible. Informed people can find and use science to protect themselves and their communities, and to inform their advocacy in improving society toward environmental health for all.

We have also seen environmental health recede into the shadows in public health, despite the pressing need for it, especially during times when environmental public health crises dominate the headlines. These crises range from the COVID-19 pandemic, which originated from a zoonotic source, to extreme weather events caused by global climate change. In 2016, the Council on Education for Public Health, the leading public health accrediting body, made the decision to remove environmental health competencies from the requirements for graduate schools and programs of public health. This decision puts the already burdened public health workforce at risk of not comprehending the significant connection between health and the environment, as well as the immense public health challenges we face today. If you are an instructor, a student, and/or an environmental health professional, we hope you will recognize the importance of including environmental health in public health curricula.

As you embark on reading this book, you will see that *Environmental Health: Foundations for Public Health* is organized into four sections: Foundations of Environmental Health (Chapters 1–4); The Environmental Health Science Toolkit (Chapters 5–8); Interconnected: Energy, Air, Water, Food, and Waste (Chapters 9–13); and Reimagining Environmental Health for All (Chapters 14–19). In the first section, we offer a context for the breadth and depth of this field and help readers understand basic concepts, frameworks, and our most pressing issues. Among them are climate change, environmental racism, and the chemicals in our daily lives. We include a primer on policy and regulatory science, which is often left out of environmental health training. The content shared in Sections II and III is all about the inner workings of the scientific field—where it has been and where it is going with regards to methods and tools and core issues. Finally, we believe that we must reimagine environmental health for all, which is the goal of the last section of the book. We want readers to see exactly how and where they can plug in to protect the health of their family, coworkers, community members, patients, or constituents no matter where their personal and professional paths take them.

Everyone comes to environmental health with their own lived experiences—whether they think about their experiences with this lens or not. As such, we aimed for this textbook to humanize the realities of pressing environmental health issues confronting society. Some chapters, for instance, include interviews and first-person accounts or notes about the realities of environmental health in our authors' lives. The features in each chapter are opportunities to ground these lessons in your own daily life too. The "In Real Life" feature offers ways you may investigate the topics more deeply. For instance, how do you find out about the quality of your drinking water? The "Time is Now" feature hopefully inspires you to act with a variety of resources and tools. We encourage you to engage in each chapter's topics in new ways and adapt the lessons and activities as you see fit.

With each new author we invited to contribute to this book, we grew increasingly excited about the project and what it could offer readers. Their diverse perspectives are invaluable, and several themes quickly emerged:

- We are part of our environments, and our environments are part of us. Environmental health is shaped by our built, natural, and social environments. Arguably, every physical and mental health outcome has an environmental component.
- The authors push us to rethink the concept of risk that has long been central to environmental health. Although characterizing and managing risks remain a vital component of the field, we must continue to conceive ways to understand our complex realities. The concept of risk is explored in depth in Chapters 6 and 7.
- Climate change (and society's overreliance on fossil fuels) is relevant to every chapter in this book. Chapter 3 provides a foundation for a discussion about how climate change affects health. In Section IV, we explore how climate adaptation will be necessary for disaster preparedness efforts and for protecting children, as well as in our occupational and healthcare settings and communities.
- We need solutions at all levels that are achievable through equitable partnerships. These solutions can become resources for local, state, and federal governments to take coordinated action on environmental health and justice. Solutions also involve intergenerational coalitions that advance science and policy. Prioritizing profit over people does not result in real solutions, as discussed in Chapter 19, among others.

Another inherent theme of this book is that the field of environmental health cannot be understood or advanced without grounding these lessons in the past. In Chapter 4, we learn about historical events that led to major environmental protections in the United States, such as the Clean Air Act and the Superfund program. In Chapter 5, we learn about the harms perpetrated by public health and healthcare systems—from the experiences of DES daughters to the nonconsensual gynecological research by Dr. J. Marion Sims on enslaved Black women. In several chapters, we discuss the role of redlining, a harmful, racist housing policy that has shaped many environmental injustices we see today, particularly for communities frontline to expansive industrial sites and countless environmental exposures. In Chapter 16, we learn about the role of labor organizing in improving occupational health, in just one more example of how the study of environmental health requires the study of history.

This book is rooted in the premise that the goal of environmental health science, policy, and practice should be environmental justice for all. Environmental justice is an intentional theme in this book. It entails upholding environmental justice principles, which include the commitment to refrain from speaking on behalf of others. We worked hard to respectfully share case studies, and you will read the direct words of many people who experience environmental injustice. Chapter 5 reminds us about why we engage in the work of environmental health science (*If not for the greater good, then why?*), as well as the many forms this work can take.

Chapter 19 gives us a powerful example of what happens when the power structure shifts and community concerns are heard.

Please take care as you read, especially if much of what is discussed is new to you or the book restates inequities you know all too well from your own life. Although this is a textbook, we wrote it for a wide audience; whether you are a student taking a university environmental health course, or pursuing a career in environmental health, or a global citizen concerned about the future of our planet, this book most likely relates to you, your loved ones, your communities, and your work.

At this moment, some of us are seeking deeper lessons about environmental health. Some of us crave more tools, perspectives, and resources. Some of us need healing or hope. Most of us crave solutions. It is a lofty goal for a textbook to achieve all of this, and we accept that we likely did not do so fully. Yet, as we wrote and edited, we tried. As Marianne Kaba explains, we attempted to practice "hope as a discipline."[3(p26)]

Natalie Sampson
Lindsay Tallon
Natasha DeJarnett

REFERENCES

1. Richardson HC. The fight for our America. *The New Republic*; September 26, 2023. https://newrepublic.com/article/175736/heather-cox-richardson-democracy-awaken
2. *Chevron U.S.A., Inc. v Natural Resources Defense Council*, 467 US 837 (1984).
3. Kaba M. *We Do This 'Til We Free Us: Abolitionist Organizing and Transforming Justice*. Haymarket Press; 2021.

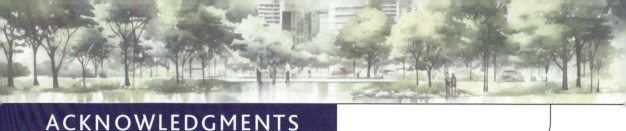

ACKNOWLEDGMENTS

We would like to extend our deepest appreciation to Natalie Conti and Anchal Malh, whose brilliant contributions are evident throughout this textbook. You came on board to assist but stepped all in as partners. We have learned so much from both of you and appreciate your commitment to ensuring this textbook is engaging for other students. Thank you also for making this a fun process. The field of environmental health is lucky to have you.

Of course, we must thank Taylor Ball, David D'Addona, and the team at Springer for trusting and supporting our vision for this textbook. Taylor, you have helped us grow as editors, and we deeply value your perspectives and skills. David, your excitement and support for this project from the beginning has been inspiring.

Thanks also to our families for bearing with us, as this work took us away from you for hours on end. Dylan, Bryce, Cam, Ruby, and Zeke, we love you more than words can express. Matt, Emma, and Steve, thank you for your assistance and encouragement. Lise, John, and Mike, thanks for being you. Melanie Sampson, your support and editing skills remain unmatched.

Our friends and colleagues offered invaluable support as well. Beth Doyle and Carly Levy, this book would not have happened without you. Paul Erwin, thank you for your expert guidance in the field of public health, from your early days at the East Tennessee Regional Health Office, and for your advice on textbooks. We also owe a debt of gratitude to our institutions, colleagues, and students at the University of Michigan-Dearborn and the Massachusetts College of Pharmacy and Health Sciences.

Finally, we must acknowledge the contributing authors in this text. We know that many of you are on the ground doing the work every day, striving toward environmental health and justice. Your work is inspiring, and we are grateful that you took the time to share your wisdom so that the next generation of environmental practitioners, researchers, regulators, and advocates can learn from you.

LIST OF PODCASTS

These five podcast episodes in *The PFAS Chronicles* discuss the history of per- and polyfluoroalkyl substances (PFAS) and their effects on the environment and human health. The speakers also touch on the science of detection, the interconnectedness of PFAS in the environment, possible solutions for the problem of PFAS, and lessons we can learn from PFAS.

Access the podcasts via the QR code or http://connect.springerpub.com/content/book/978-0-8261-8353-8/chapter/ch00

ABOUT THE PODCAST HOSTS

Natalie Conti is a current Master of Science student in Environmental Health Sciences with specialization in Industrial Hygiene at the University of Michigan School of Public Health. She is interested in the impact of industries on worker health (including physical and psychosocial factors) and the health of the surrounding environment and communities. Working previously as a medical laboratory scientist, Natalie is passionate about health advocacy and communication. Natalie is currently funded by the National Institute for Occupational Safety and Health (NIOSH).

Anchal Malh is an alumna of the University of Michigan School of Public Health, where she received her Master of Science in Environmental Health Sciences. Previously, she held internships at *The New York Times* and the National Center for Institutional Diversity where she conducted editorial research and specialized in science communications. Anchal is passionate about making science education and research accessible to marginalized populations. Anchal is a former Kessler Scholar and Rackham Merit Fellow at the University of Michigan and recipient of the 2019 New York Times College Scholarship.

THE PFAS CHRONICLES

History of Per- and Polyfluoroalkyl Substances (PFAS)

In this introductory episode on PFAS—also known as per- and polyfluoroalkyl substances—hosts Natalie Conti and Anchal Malh meet with Phil Brown, the Director of the Social Science Environmental Health Research Institute and Codirector of the PFAS Project Lab at Northeastern University. During their conversation they explore the history of PFAS. They trace PFAS's origins to household products and discuss how these chemicals are ever-present in our bodies and environment today. Tune in to uncover more about these "forever chemicals."

The Science of PFAS Detection

Hosts Natalie Conti and Anchal Malh are back for another educational episode on PFAS. This time, they investigate how PFAS are studied and monitored. In this conversation with Dr. Katherine Manz, Assistant Professor of Environmental Sciences at the University of Michigan School of Public Health, they begin to explore how PFAS contaminate water and soil with implications for environmental health and justice. Tune in to explore how the human body responds to PFAS exposure.

PFAS Where We Live, Work, and Play

In this episode, hosts Natalie Conti and Anchal Malh meet with Sandy Wynn-Stelt of the Great Lakes PFAS Action Network to discuss where PFAS show up in our everyday life and how they impact human health. During their conversation, they discuss PFAS in the places we live, work, and play, and what solutions scientists are coming up with to remediate the presence of these forever chemicals in our environment. Tune in to unearth where PFAS may be lurking in your environment and the steps you can take to reduce your exposure.

Firefighters and Forever Chemicals: Occupational Exposure to PFAS and Health-Related Consequences

In this second-to-last episode on PFAS in our environment, hosts Natalie Conti and Anchal Malh sit with advocates Ayesha Khan and Jamie Honkawa of the Nantucket PFAS Action Group. During their conversation, they discuss exposure to PFAS in firefighting communities and ways to improve protections for community members. Tune in to learn how certain occupations can lead to increases in exposure to PFAS and related health effects.

Halting the PFAS Cycle and Its Costs on Individuals, Communities, and Society

In this final episode, hosts Natalie Conti and Anchal Malh wrap up their conversation on PFAS in the environment with Kristin Mello and Christopher Clark of Westfield Residents Advocating for Themselves (WRAFT). They discuss the ways research, policies, and technology can help us to reduce PFAS exposures for all, highlighting the work of current advocacy groups. They also remind us about environmental justice issues related to PFAS. Listeners are left with final takeaways on what the field of environmental health—and all of society—can learn from PFAS. Finally, there is a call-to-action: How can we ensure marginalized communities, particularly communities of color and low-wealth communities, are not experiencing disproportionate impacts from PFAS? Tune in to conclude our case study on PFAS.

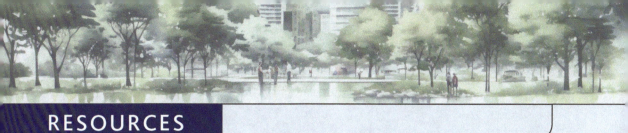

RESOURCES

STUDENT RESOURCES

The five podcast episodes in *The PFAS Chronicles* discuss the history of per- and polyfluoroalkyl substances (PFAS) and their effects on the environment, the science of detection, the interconnectedness of PFAS in the environment, possible solutions for the problem of PFAS, and lessons we can learn from PFAS. Access the podcasts via the QR code or http://connect.springerpub.com/content/book/978-0-8261-8353-8/chapter/ch00

INSTRUCTOR RESOURCES

 A robust set of instructor resources designed to supplement this text is located at http://connect.springerpub.com/content/book/978-0-8261-8353-8. Qualifying instructors may request access by emailing textbook@springerpub.com.

- **LMS Common Cartridge–All Instructor Resources**
- **Instructor Manual**
  - Learning Objectives, Key Terms, Case Studies and Reflection Questions, Discussion Questions, Learning Activities
- **Instructor Test Bank**
  - Approximately 300 multiple-choice, true/false, and short-answer questions with rationales and sample answers
- **Instructor Chapter PowerPoint slides**
- **Sample Syllabus**

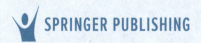

Visit https://connect.springerpub.com/ and look for the "**Show Supplementary**" button on the **book homepage**.

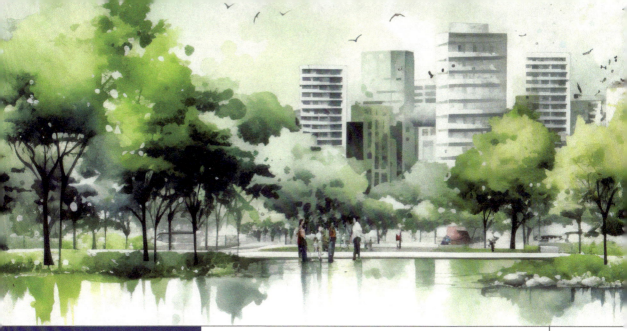

SECTION I

Foundations of Environmental Health

HISTORY OF PER- AND POLYFLUOROALKYL SUBSTANCES (PFAS)

In this introductory episode on PFAS—also known as per- and polyfluoroalkyl substances—hosts Natalie Conti and Anchal Malh meet with Phil Brown, the Director of the Social Science Environmental Health Research Institute and Codirector of the PFAS Project Lab at Northeastern University. During their conversation they explore the history of PFAS. They trace PFAS's origins to household products and discuss how these chemicals are ever-present in our bodies and environment today. Tune in to uncover more about these "forever chemicals."

Access the podcast via the QR code or http://connect.springerpub.com/content/book/978-0-8261-8353-8/chapter/ch00

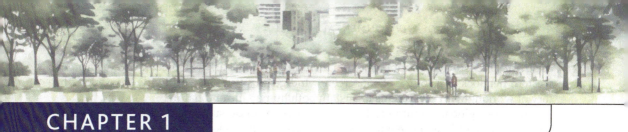

CHAPTER 1

Fundamentals of Environmental Health and Justice

Natalie Sampson, Lindsay Tallon, Natalie Conti, and Anchal Malh

LEARNING OBJECTIVES

- Explore the past, present, and future of environmental health.
- Evaluate the pivotal role of environmental health science, policy, and communication in promoting public health.
- Begin to explain how federal environmental protections work in the United States, along with their limitations.
- Acquire foundational knowledge and familiarity with the essential tools of environmental health science.
- Honor and appreciate the significant contributions of various fenceline communities in mobilizing to improve environmental health and justice throughout history.

KEY TERMS

- cancer cluster
- climate change
- commercial determinants of health
- cumulative risk
- ecosystem
- endocrine disruption
- environmental health
- environmental justice
- environmental racism
- exposome
- One Health
- Planetary Health
- political determinants of health
- precautionary principle
- public health
- risk
- social determinants of health (SDOH)
- toxicants

OVERVIEW

Even in ancient times—before people knew about pollution and infectious diseases—people recognized the relationship between their surroundings and health. The Code of Hammurabi in ancient Babylon had provisions related to public health, including rules for water usage. Early civilizations in Greece and Rome understood the importance of clean water and sanitation in preventing diseases. Ancient Rome created a system of aqueducts and sewage systems around 2,300 years ago that supplied clean water to cities and reduced the risk of waterborne illness. However, this clean water was delivered and often drunk from lead-based pipes and cups.[1] Around the same time, the book *On Airs, Waters, and Places* by Hippocrates, an ancient Greek physician, is thought to be the first book to connect human diseases to the environment. In the Islamic Golden Age, beginning in the seventh century C.E., the practice of obstetrics was developed, and practitioners noted the influence of healthy lifestyle, air, and climate on the health of offspring.[2] Centuries ago, Indigenous Peoples in the Americas identified a variety of botanical resources to support health, including willow bark as a precursor to aspirin and western hemlock as a source of sunscreen.[3,4] Indigenous Peoples worldwide have a long history of working with ecosystems to sustain both human life and nature.

Today, our global community has a much deeper understanding of how we impact our environment and how our environment impacts us. For millennia, humans have developed within **ecosystems**, the biological communities of organisms working together that provide us with essential resources such as clean air and water, food, and shelter. Healthy ecosystems also regulate the environment by purifying air, breaking down waste, and adapting to change. However, we have a significant impact on ecosystems through our interactions with them. Human control over the natural world has resulted in significant consequences, including deforestation, pollution, habitat and biodiversity loss, and overconsumption of resources. Many people may not enjoy being reminded of the impacts that humans have caused, but it is crucial to acknowledge and appreciate the interdependence between all living beings and the ecosystems that support us.

Our connection to the environment has both positive and negative impacts on our health, and the study of these ingrained connections is the focus of the field of environmental health (Box 1.1). Positive impacts include those beneficial products of our ecosystems, such as access to clean air and water, healthy food, and opportunities for physical activity. Negative impacts can include exposure to pollutants and hazards from industrial processes and nature itself, as well as lack of access to healthy resources. Poor environmental conditions lead to a multitude of health issues, from cancer and respiratory disease to poor mental health and reduced life expectancy. These issues are compounded for many through environmental racism and injustice.

This chapter sets the stage for the textbook. We examine the history of the field of environmental health, including many notable events, scientific advances, major policy milestones, and underlying concepts and frameworks. We begin to examine the many ways that humans

---

BOX 1.1. DEFINITIONS OF ENVIRONMENTAL HEALTH

American Public Health Association (APHA): Environmental health is the branch of public health that: focuses on the relationships between people and their environment; promotes human health and well-being; and fosters healthy and safe communities. Environmental health is a key part of any comprehensive public health system. The field works to advance policies and programs to reduce chemical and other environmental exposures in air, water, soil, and food to protect people and provide communities with healthier environments."[a]

National Environmental Health Association (NEHA): "Environmental health is the science and practice of preventing human injury and illness and promoting well-being by: identifying and evaluating environmental sources and hazardous agents; and limiting exposures to hazardous physical, chemical, and biological agents in air, water, soil, food, and other environmental media or settings that may adversely affect human health."[b(para1)]

World Health Organization (WHO): Environmental health involves "aspects of human health and diseases that are determined by environmental factors. Environmental health also refers to the assessment and control of environmental factors that can potentially affect health. Environmental health focuses on the direct pathological effects of chemicals, radiation, and certain biological agents in dwellings, in urban, agricultural, or natural environments, as well as their indirect effects on well-being. It connects the social and cultural environments, as well as genetic components."[c(p9)]

Sources: [a]Environmental health. American Public Health Association. 2019. https://www.apha.org/topics-and-issues/environmental-health; [b]About. National Environmental Health Association. https://www.neha.org/about; [c]Morand S, Lajaunie C. A brief history on the links between health and biodiversity. *Biodiversity and Health*. 2018:1–14. doi:10.1016/b978-1-78548-115-4.50001-9.

interact with their social and physical environment, and we introduce some of the most pressing environmental health issues today related to climate change and chemical exposures. In this chapter, we also begin to share case studies that highlight the environmental harms that the field of environmental health must work to prevent and address. Before embarking on a deeper dive into science and policy in later chapters, we introduce the concepts of environmental racism and justice that must be confronted to achieve health equity. Ultimately, this chapter emphasizes the value of environmental health as a central component of public health.

RECENT HISTORY OF ENVIRONMENTAL HEALTH

As a profession, the roots of environmental health have always been central to the field of public health due to the major impact that the environment has on our health. For example, in the 1800s, the emergence of the Sanitary Movement led to the creation of the first health departments in the United States and a reliance on civil engineers to design healthier cities. With advancements in the development of epidemiology, John Snow helped to stop a cholera outbreak by connecting it to contaminated water in London, highlighting the importance of environmental factors in disease prevention. Some of the first environmental research and eventual protections occurred in workplaces with the Labor Movement working to address unsafe labor conditions and the field of occupational health becoming more established at the turn of the 20th century. Table 1.1 provides a glimpse of select environmental health events, milestones, and advances throughout history in the United States.

TABLE 1.1. MILESTONES IN RECENT U.S. ENVIRONMENT PUBLIC HEALTH HISTORY

1800s TO EARLY 1900s
• The Sanitary Movement launches to improve living conditions, sanitation, and hygiene practices during the Industrial Revolution.
• Governmental health departments and organizations are formally established, beginning efforts for disease surveillance, vaccination programs, sanitation improvements, and health education.
• 1902: Maryland develops the first workplace safety and workers' compensation program, and momentum for federal workers' compensation continues to grow over the next century.
• 1905: Upton Sinclair publishes *The Jungle*, a novel that exposes the harsh conditions and exploitation faced by immigrant workers in the meatpacking industry in Chicago during the early 20th century.
• The Dust Bowl occurs in the Great Plains region of the United States during the 1930s, an environmental disaster worsened by poor farming practices and characterized by prolonged drought, severe dust storms, and erosion.
• 1937: The National Association of Sanitarians is established in the United States, shaping the sanitarian profession as experts who specialize in inspection and assessment of environments such as restaurants, food production facilities, water supplies, sewage systems, and public spaces.

1940s
• 1948: The Donora Smog occurs with the combination of high levels of air pollution and the stagnant atmospheric conditions, killing 20 people and causing respiratory problems for 6,000 of the 14,000 people living in Donora, Pennsylvania.
• Continuing for more than 40 years, uranium mining begins on Navajo lands during the mid-20th century, resulting in miner and resident exposure to radioactive materials and increased rates of cancer and other health problems (see Case Study 7.1).
• Chemical production ramps up following a heavy use mid-century during World War II and then by various industries increasing use of chemicals in agriculture, pharmaceuticals, and consumer goods.

(continued)

TABLE 1.1. MILESTONES IN RECENT U.S. ENVIRONMENT PUBLIC HEALTH HISTORY (*continued*)

1950s

- The Toms River Chemical Corporation (later known as Ciba-Geigy and then Novartis) dumps waste materials, including carcinogenic compounds, into unlined lagoons and landfills in Toms River, New Jersey, over the decade, which results in a childhood cancer cluster and other health issues for residents for decades to follow (see Case Study 1.2).
- Many major dam construction projects are underway in the United States, including Glen Canyon Dam in northern Arizona, to provide hydroelectric power and manage water resources; they raise many concerns about ecosystem impacts.
- Los Angeles begins experiencing extreme smog events that make it unsafe to be outside for extended periods of time, leading to new regulations to manage vehicle emissions and industrial pollution that eventually influence federal regulations.

1960s

- 1962: Rachel Carson publishes *Silent Spring* about the dangers of widespread pesticide use and its impacts on ecosystems and human health, catalyzing the environmental movement.
- Support grows for scientific research linking asbestos exposure and mesothelioma, a rare and aggressive cancer.
- 1969: The Cuyahoga River in Ohio catches on fire (again, having done so several times in the last century) and gains national attention as a symbol of water pollution during the early years of the environmental movement.

1970s

- 1970: With bipartisan support in Congress, President Nixon establishes the Environmental Protection Agency (EPA), and several landmark policies follow, including the National Environmental Policy Act (1970), major amendments to the 1963 Clean Air Act (1970, 1977), the Clean Water Act (1972), the Safe Drinking Water Act (1974), and the Toxic Substances Control Act (1976).
- 1971: The National Association of Sanitarians becomes the National Environmental Health Association (NEHA), reflecting a broader focus on environmental health issues beyond traditional sanitation practices.
- 1972: DDT, or dichlorodiphenyltrichloroethane, a synthetic pesticide, is banned under the Federal Insecticide, Fungicide, and Rodenticide Act.
- The prescription of diethylstilbestrol (DES), a synthetic estrogen, to pregnant people is discontinued in the early 1970s, raising awareness about the potential dangers of exposing fetuses to certain drugs during pregnancy.
- 1978: A state of emergency is declared in Niagara Falls, New York, due to chemical waste dumping in the Love Canal community, prompting national attention to chemical disposal and health (see Case Study 13.2).
- 1979: The Toxic Substances Control Act is used to ban polychlorinated biphenyls (PCBs), a group of synthetic organic chemicals that were widely used in various industrial applications, including electrical equipment, coolants, and hydraulic fluids.

1980s

- 1980: The Centers for Disease Control and Prevention (CDC) establishes the National Center for Environmental Health to promote health and prevent diseases related to environmental factors.
- 1980: The Comprehensive Environmental Response, Compensation, and Liability Act (CERCLA), commonly known as Superfund, is established to support cleanup of hazardous waste sites by holding responsible parties financially accountable for costs.
- 1984: One of the world's worst industrial disasters occurs in Bhopal, India, when the Union Carbide Corporation experiences a gas leak, releasing toxic methyl isocyanate gas, resulting in thousands of immediate deaths and long-term health effects for many nearby residents.

(*continued*)

TABLE 1.1. MILESTONES IN RECENT U.S. ENVIRONMENT PUBLIC HEALTH HISTORY *(continued)*

1980s

- 1987: The Montreal Protocol, an international treaty, is signed to phase out the production and use of ozone-depleting substances such as chlorofluorocarbons (CFCs); it is relatively effective in addressing this issue over the next decade.
- 1989: The Dineh-Navajo Water Rights Settlement Act, also known as the Colorado River Water Rights Settlement Act, is passed to ensure a more secure water supply for the Navajo Nation and the Hopi Tribe.
- The WHO begins publishing guidelines on community noise in the 1980s, recognizing noise as an environmental health concern.
- Scientists and legislators begin acknowledging scientific evidence that secondhand smoke is linked to cancer and methylmercury in seafood is linked to developmental delays.
- The EPA begins using a risk-assessment framework, a systematic process for evaluating potential risks to human health from environmental hazards.

1990s

- 1990: The Clean Air Act is amended, and new regulations lead to phasing out municipal waste incinerators, but many still operate today.
- 1991: The National People of Color Environmental Leadership Summit is held in Washington, D.C. as a groundbreaking moment in the Environmental Justice Movement, where the 17 Principles of Environmental Justice are drafted.
- 1993: The groundbreaking Six Cities study reveals a strong link between air pollution and mortality risk.
- 1994: President Clinton signs Executive Order 12898: Federal Actions to Address Environmental Justice in Minority Populations and Low-Income Populations as a first federal action to address environmental injustice.
- 1996: The book *Our Stolen Future* is published, introducing theories about ways that pesticides and industrial pollutants may lead to endocrine disruption.
- Body burden studies become common as a research approach using biomonitoring (e.g., blood or urine samples) to measure the levels of many chemicals in the human body.

2000s

- 2003: The Human Epigenome Project begins to map the epigenetic modifications present in the human genome.
- 2005: The exposome takes off as a guiding framework in the field after the publication of *Complementing the Genome with an "Exposome": The Outstanding Challenge of Environmental Exposure Measurement in Molecular Epidemiology*.
- 2009: The EPA launches an action plan to address per- and polyfluoroalkyl substances (PFAS) in the environment, including studying their occurrence, toxicity, and potential regulation.
- In the early 2000s, the phrase *big data* is coined alongside the rise of the internet and technological advancements, and this concept leads to the development of informatics to help manage the variety and volume of data.

2010s

- 2010: The Deepwater Horizon oil spill happens in the Gulf of Mexico, highlighting a greater need for disaster research and response.
- 2014: The Flint Water crisis unfolds in Flint, Michigan, where many local, state, and federal officials are negligent in preventing and addressing lead contamination in the public water supply, and resulting in increased national awareness of the concept of environmental racism (see Case Study 15.2).
- 2015: As an international treaty, the Paris Agreement is adopted and aims to limit global warming to below 2 degrees Celsius above preindustrial levels through global climate action.
- 2016: The Standing Rock Sioux Tribe protests the construction of the Dakota Access Pipeline, which posed a threat to their water source and sacred sites.

(continued)

TABLE 1.1. MILESTONES IN RECENT U.S. ENVIRONMENT PUBLIC HEALTH HISTORY (*continued*)

2010s
• 2018: California bans the use of flame retardants in furniture, mattresses, and children's products over a range of health concerns, including endocrine disruption, cancer, and respiratory issues (see Case Study 17.2). • Public acceptance of climate change increases with increasingly severe and frequent extreme weather events, ongoing scientific research, and expanding global advocacy, particularly among youth.
2020s
• 2021: President Biden signs Executive Order 14008, Tackling the Climate Crisis at Home and Abroad, which establishes the Justice40 Initiative to direct at least 40% of overall benefits from certain federal investments in climate and clean energy programs to disadvantaged communities. • 2022: In response to a powerful community organizing campaign by residents of the Southeast Side of Chicago, the City of Chicago denies a permit to Reserve Management Group (parent company to General Iron) to relocate its metal recycling operation, indicating the potential local governments have in promoting environmental justice (see Chapter 19, "Organizing for Environmental Health and Justice: Lessons From #StopGeneralIron"). • 2023: After the introduction of ChatGPT in 2022, many artificial intelligence platforms launch, which create new opportunities for studying environmental health issues but raise many concerns related to underlying bias, ethics, and security. • With concerns about indoor air pollution, there are increased efforts to phase out gas appliances, with several states incentivizing electrification of cooking and heating appliances. • Movement is growing to ensure equitable access to nature after decades of research investigating the benefits of outdoor activities, green space, and contact with nature on physical and mental health. • Precision medicine is evolving rapidly; it takes into account individual differences in genes, environment, and lifestyle, but more work is needed to address ethical issues and equitable access.

When reviewing the history of environmental health, we cannot minimize the role that structural racism and, particularly, **environmental racism** has played in shaping environmental health. **Structural racism** describes the way in which society fosters racial discrimination through reinforcing systems of oppression.[5] Infrastructure, education, employment, housing, and public health have long been structured to advantage the majority, primarily White populations, and disadvantage communities of color.[6] According to Dr. Robert Bullard, environmental racism refers to any environmentally-related policy, practice, or directive that differentially affects or disadvantages (whether intended or unintended) individuals, groups, or communities based on race or color. It involves the placing of landfills, hazardous waste sites, transportation infrastructure, and other polluting facilities in communities that predominantly consist of people of color and residents with low wealth.[7] Environmental racism can also involve disproportionate impacts from unequal hazards in consumer products, as discussed in Chapter 6, "Understanding (Unequal and Cumulative) Risks in Our Daily Environment," among others. The result is notable health inequities by race, income, and other factors.

ENVIRONMENTAL HEALTH TODAY

Today, society recognizes the ways environmental health is relevant to most public health issues. For instance, there is growing evidence of the ways that environmental health affects reproductive health. Exposure to pollutants, **endocrine disruption** (i.e., chemicals harming the regulation of hormones), and climate change can impact fertility, contribute to pregnancy complications, and lead to reproductive disorders.[8,9] In another example, violence and environmental health are interconnected. Studies show that climate change, particularly extreme heat events, are linked to increased incidence of domestic violence.[10] Globally, competition for natural resources, such as water and arable land, may increase with climate change and escalate into armed conflicts.

Environmental health works to address a range of health outcomes, as we know that pathways between exposures and health are complex. When we think of environmental health, many people may think about respiratory issues, such as asthma or cancer associated with various carcinogens (i.e., known cancer-causing substances). Yet, toxic substances can cause a wide range of harms on various developmental and organ systems, including neurological, reproductive, immune, and nervous systems. A single exposure can lead to a variety of health outcomes, and multiple exposures can contribute to a single health concern. These are the complex relationships that toxicology and epidemiology allow us to study, as discussed in Chapter 7. More recently, we have also recognized the mental health aspects of environmental health. For instance, do people have access to green space, such as parks, to help cope with stress? Could individuals be experiencing anxiety due to climate change? Moreover, are events like wildfires impacting cultural or economic well-being, which are often associated with stress, depression, and anxiety?

New frameworks and ways of thinking about environmental health have emerged in the past few decades. In particular, there has been a move away from primarily managing environmental exposures as a relationship between one exposure and one health outcome toward new approaches to our complex realities. We have recognized the scientific and policy challenges of **cumulative impacts** for many decades. Yet we have only more recently begun strategizing how to study and account for the many outside factors—both chemical and nonchemical stressors—that may harm us. In 2005, Dr. Christopher Paul Wild proposed the concept of an **exposome** that called for epidemiologists to recognize the totality of our external exposures, including chemical, biological, and psychosocial, and other cumulative and interactive factors.[11]

One Health and **Planetary Health** are important frameworks in our changing climate that are important to understand as a part of environmental health. Beginning in the 1970s and 1980s, there has been increased attention to the interconnectedness of human and animal health, as science advanced and the occurrence of many zoonotic diseases (e.g., avian flu, hantavirus, Lyme disease) persisted with shifting global patterns. One Health is a collaborative approach in which many disciplines work together with a goal of improving health while recognizing the interconnectedness of people, animals, plants, and the environment (Figure 1.1). After the widespread introduction of antibiotics in the 1940s and 1950s, we also saw the beginnings of antibiotic resistance and misuse, which has complicated the treatment of zoonotic infections and poses challenges in controlling their spread today. More recently, the World Organisation for Animal Health and the Food and Agriculture Organization of the United Nations started endorsing and promoting the One Health approach. The One Health framework can apply to environmental health efforts to navigate food systems, land use, and global climate change.

ACCORDING TO THE CDC, ONE HEALTH IS:

A collaborative, multisectoral, and transdisciplinary approach—working at the local, regional, national, and global levels—with the goal of achieving optimal health outcomes recognizing the interconnection between people, animals, plants, and their shared environment.

(continued)

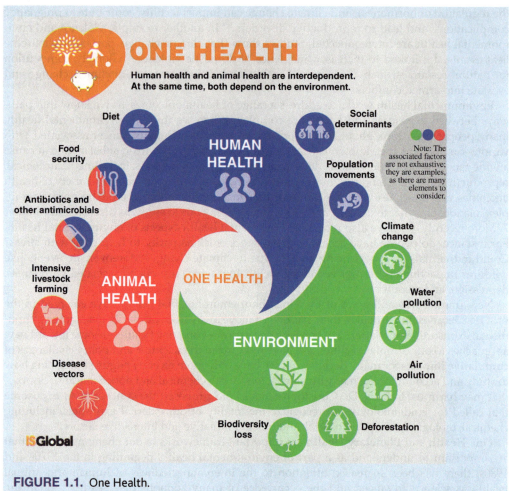

FIGURE 1.1. One Health.
Source: González SS. One Health: How to achieve optimal health for people, animals, and our planet. ISGlobal. April 6, 2021. https://www.isglobal.org/en/healthisglobal/-/custom-blog-portlet/one-health-una-sola-salud-o-como-lograr-a-la-vez-una-salud-optima-para-las-personas-los-animales-y-nuestro-planeta

Similar in some ways to One Health, Planetary Health is a transdisciplinary field that emphasizes the interconnections between human health and the health of the planet. It recognizes that human well-being is closely connected to sustainability, biodiversity, and ecosystem health. Planetary Health requires systems thinking in recognizing that everything is connected and as our environment changes, so does our health.

CASE STUDY 1.1: Train Derailment in East Palestine

On February 3, 2023, a Norfolk Southern Railway train derailed in East Palestine, Ohio, a town of about 4,800 people. A total of 38 cars derailed, including 11 of the 20 total hazardous material cars, carrying chemicals utilized in plastics fabrication like butyl acrylates and vinyl chloride.[12] Specifically, vinyl chloride is a chemical found in polyvinyl chloride (PVC) products. These products are used daily in home building and infrastructure projects and also utilized in certain medical equipment.

Local authorities worked quickly, as they were worried that rising temperatures in one of the railcars could lead to an explosion and send shrapnel up to a mile from the site.[12] Due to this concern, they opted to do a controlled release and burn of the vinyl chloride after evacuating 2,500 nearby residents.[12] The Environmental Protection Agency (EPA) did not order the controlled burn. The decision was made by the local fire chief and Ohio Governor Mike Dewine

(continued)

CASE STUDY 1.1: Train Derailment in East Palestine (*continued*)

after consultation with Norfolk Southern, local law enforcement, and emergency response personnel in Ohio. Governor Dewine explained that officials had two "bad options."[13]

The controlled burn of 150,000 gallons of these chemicals took place on February 6.[14] A black plume of smoke filled the air and left residents to wonder what it would mean for their outdoor and indoor air and water quality in the days and months that followed the derailment. There were many conflicting opinions among responders and community members about the immediate health impacts and potential health effects that may appear months or years later.

On March 31, 2023, the response team announced that, "[the] EPA's review of preliminary data indicated levels of semi-volatile organic chemicals (VOCs) ... [to be] similar to typical background levels."[15] This implied that the risk of harm from these VOCs was no greater than before the incident. Yet, despite this information, some residents' experiences did not line up with this risk assessment. They experienced symptoms like headaches, rash, coughs, vomiting, and eye irritation. There is also concern that residents and first responders will experience health issues in the decades to come. Vinyl chloride is linked to various cancers, including liver, brain, and lung cancers, lymphoma and leukemia, diabetes, and immune disorders.[16] As with other environmental health disasters, stress and concerns about property values and overall community well-being emerged.

The EPA has responded to the derailment and subsequent events with air monitors and soil and water sampling. The cleanup and monitoring efforts are ongoing, and updates are made frequently through the EPA's website. Norfolk Southern Railway has conducted soil remediation and funded various initiatives, including a new park, a training center for first responders, and improvements to water infrastructure. In partnership with the East Liverpool City Hospital and the Ohio Health Department, the East Palestine Health Clinic opened in spring 2023 with resources to provide screening and specialized care to residents living near the derailment. Even so, much more work is needed to understand and address short- and long-term community health concerns and identify strategies to prevent such devastating events in the future.

For information on the sampling strategy and updates from the EPA about this event go to: www.epa.gov/east-palestine-oh-train-derailment

REFLECTION QUESTIONS

1. When decisions have to be made quickly in emergency situations, what strategies can decision makers use to ensure effective communication for impacted communities?

2. There is a difference in risk perception from decision makers and the people of East Palestine. How can we consider these potential differences in our pursuit of environmental justice?

THE PLACES WE LIVE, LEARN, WORK, AND PLAY

Our social environments and our physical (both built and natural) environments play an important role in our overall well-being. In the 1970s and 1980s environmental health engaged in a push for healthier homes. Federal and state agencies started paying closer attention to indoor air quality, lead exposure prevention, pest control, and overall home safety. Chapters 14, 16, 17, and 18 look closely at the ways our communities, schools, workplaces, and healthcare system can be designed to promote rather than hinder environmental health for all. In public health, we often use the term **social determinants of health (SDOH)** to recognize the upstream factors that shape the environments where we are born, live, learn, work, play, worship, and age and how we experience them. These determinants are often grouped into five broad categories, which we revisit throughout this textbook many times:

- economic stability,
- education access and quality,
- social and community context,
- healthcare access and quality, and
- neighborhood and built environment.

More recently, others have proposed complementary determinants of health frameworks—structural, political, and commercial.[17,18] Structural determinants of health include the power relations and formal and informal rules in society that shape and maintain health inequities.[19] **Political determinants of health** consider the many ways that policies and politics influence health. **Commercial determinants of health** consider the role of the private sector in influencing health. These interacting factors that impact health mean that those working in public health and healthcare cannot work alone and must recognize that other sectors have an important role to play in promoting environmental health equity.

CLIMATE CHANGE AND HEALTH

Climate change is one of public health's greatest modern threats. In her essay, *How to Talk About Climate Change So People Will Listen*, climate scientist Katharine Hayhoe explains, "We've known since the 1850s that digging up and then burning coal—and, later, oil and gas—produces heat-trapping gasses that are wrapping an extra blanket around the planet."[20] Indeed, in 1856, Eunice Newton Foote introduced this concept when she presented her research at the American Association for the Advancement of Science meeting. She discussed how sunlight could pass through the atmosphere and warm the Earth's surface, but heat radiation emitted from the surface could be trapped by certain gasses, leading to higher temperatures. Foote's experiments involved exposing various gasses to sunlight and measuring their temperature changes, with carbonic acid gas (carbon dioxide) exhibiting the most significant temperature increase.[21]

Today, climate change is very much underway. Inarguably, human activities have caused the Earth's global surface temperature to increase about 2 degrees Fahrenheit or 1 degree Celsius since the preindustrial era (1850–1900).[22] Public health has a key role to play in helping communities prepare for and adapt to extreme events, as well as in efforts to slow further climate change. Globally, this means ongoing global climate migrations, primarily within but also across nations. Disasters including floods, storms, wildfires, and droughts caused a record 32.6 million within-nation displacements globally in 2022.[23]

CHEMICALS AND HEALTH

Everyone is exposed to chemicals in their daily lives. Exposure to chemicals can result in an increased risk of acute and chronic diseases based on the quantities, length of exposure, and toxicity of the chemicals one is exposed to, as described in Chapters 6 and 7. Exposure to chemicals can range from toxic chemicals released from industrial facilities and household cleaning products to chemicals in drinking water and food. We also know that polluting industries are more likely to be in low-wealth communities, particularly communities of color who also experience greater social stressors that may make them more likely than others to experience the health impacts of toxic chemical exposures.[24] Some industrial facilities that commonly release toxic chemicals into the environment include:

- drinking water and wastewater treatment plants;
- oil and gas drilling and production facilities, refineries, storage tanks, and injection wells;
- gasoline service stations;
- dry cleaners;
- solid, industrial, and hazardous waste landfills and incinerators; and
- agricultural, mining, industrial, and a host of other facilities releasing toxic chemicals into the environment.[25]

Of course, chemicals make our daily lives possible in many ways, and we cannot walk through life afraid to ingest foods, breathe the air, or touch the world around us. We rely on water, glucose, amino and fatty acids, minerals, and other trace elements for our bodies to function. We rely on chemicals to create safe cars, communication devices, medical devices, and so much more. Yet some are **toxicants**, natural substances or human-made chemicals that may have toxic effects on humans, animals, plants, or the environment and require regulation. Science has confirmed that lead, mercury, bisphenol A (BPA), phthalates, and per- and polyfluoroalkyl substances (PFAS), among many other chemicals, have great potential to harm human health. Many of these chemicals are discussed throughout this textbook. In particular, the persistent and growing reliance on plastics in society is posing great threats to public health, as plastics rely on fossil fuels for production, are often laden with chemicals and additives, and are ever present in our bodies and ecosystems.

NATURAL HAZARDS TRIGGERING TECHNOLOGICAL DISASTERS EVENTS

Natural Hazards Triggering Technological Disasters (NATECH) events happen when a natural disaster (e.g. floods, winter storms, wildfires, and hurricanes) and an industrial accident occur together.[26] Extreme weather events can cause significant damage to facilities or industries that house hazardous substances. This damage can include technical failures from pressure and extreme temperatures, which can cause pollution events that have the ability to travel widely through air or water systems.[26] These events can impact both environmental and human health.

For instance, in 2017, 19 trillion gallons of rain fell upon the Houston region of Texas when Hurricane Harvey passed through.[27] The floodwaters covered most of the city and surrounding facilities, and industries were not equipped to deal with the torrent.[27] According to the Chemical Safety and Hazard Investigation Board report, flooding from the hurricane disabled the refrigeration system at the Arkana chemical plant in Crosby, Texas. This plant largely manufactured organic peroxides, and the rising temperature caused spontaneous combustion.[28] The rising waters made it difficult for members of the Crosby community to evacuate, leaving many susceptible to the air pollution and chemical runoff into the water from the explosion.

To ensure environmental health and justice, agencies, communities, and industries must consider the possibility of NATECH events in disaster-preparedness planning efforts, particularly given our changing climate.[29]

CASE STUDY 1.2: Toms River, New Jersey

Contributions by Margaret J. Eggers

In the 1960s, it was discovered that the water supply for Toms River, New Jersey, was contaminated with industrial chemicals. The contamination was traced back to waste from the Ciba-Geigy Chemical Corporation site, which manufactured dyes, pigments, resins, and epoxy additives. This contamination was documented by the Agency for Toxic Substances and Disease Registry (ATSDR) in the 1970s.[30,31]

In 1995, reports from community members raised concerns about an apparent childhood cancer cluster in Toms River. The state of New Jersey conducted an analysis of its cancer registry data for the town and found a significant increase in childhood leukemia, as well as brain and central nervous system cancers, between 1979 and 1995.[32] A comprehensive epidemiologic study, completed in 2001, confirmed that there were significant associations between exposure to polluted drinking water and air and leukemia in girls.[33] However, doubt remained. Some sources noted that the cluster could just be a random result of chance due to the lack of significant correlation found for boys.[34]

Despite the discovery of some answers, the community continued to suffer immense pain for decades. Tireless activism by concerned community members led to a cleanup and more accountability by those managing the site. Residents, public health officials and researchers joined forces to develop and implement a Public Health Response Plan.[35] A major focus was understanding toxicological exposures. For example, the ATSDR used computer modeling to track the sources and levels of exposure over a 34-year period.[34,36]

Although the chemical plant closed in 1996, extensive monitoring is still underway and challenges persist. Remediation of the site as well as decision-making regarding use of the land are ongoing. Nonprofit organizations, such as Save Barnegat Bay, are leading discussions with the

(continued)

> **CASE STUDY 1.2: Toms River, New Jersey** (*continued*)
>
> New Jersey Department of Environmental Protection and BASF (who bought the Ciba Specialty Chemicals site in 2008). The organizations' goals are to ensure full transparency and accessibility to information about the site, as well as environmental justice for all affected families.
>
> **REFLECTION QUESTIONS**
>
> 1. A **cancer cluster** occurs when a specific geographic area or population experiences a higher-than-expected number of cancer cases in a specific timeframe. Even though there was a study that showed a significant increase in childhood leukemia in Toms River, why do you think doubt remained that this cancer was caused by exposure to industrial waste?
>
> 2. What role did residents, researchers, industry, and government each play in this series of events? What responsibility do you think each had in addressing the harmful impacts that played out for nearly approximately 35 years?

ENVIRONMENTAL HEALTH SCIENCE AND POLICY

Much of environmental health science and policy focuses on risk management, which is covered in more detail in Chapter 6. The EPA considers **risk** to be the likelihood of harmful effects on human health or ecological systems resulting from exposure to environmental stressors. A stressor is any physical, chemical, radiological, or biological entity that can induce an adverse effect in humans or ecosystems. These stressors may adversely affect specific natural resources or entire ecosystems, including flora and fauna, as well as the environments with which they react and where we live.

Understanding risk poses several challenges. One major challenge in understanding risk is addressing the **cumulative impacts** of multiple chemical and nonchemical environmental stressors on health, considering that there are complex interactions between various pollutants. Another challenge is understanding the life course and early life exposures and recognizing the connections between exposures during critical developmental periods and long-lasting impacts on health. Furthermore, disparities in exposures lead to unequal risks and impacts, highlighting the importance of adopting equitable policies and interventions designed with the **precautionary principle** in mind, where preventative action is taken to protect all people, even in the face of uncertainty.

These challenges may be daunting, but opportunities exist and are expanding every day for environmental health research. In Chapter 7, "Understanding the Environment and How It Relates to Health Using Toxicology and Epidemiology Research Methods," where key concepts in environmental toxicology and epidemiology are discussed, topics such as big data and epigenetics are covered. The integration of big data and analytics enables researchers to harness large amounts of environmental, clinical, and genetic data to better understand the complex relationships between environmental exposures and health outcomes. Additionally, the field of epigenetics offers new insights into how exposures can modify gene expression, shedding light into the many pathways and mechanisms through which exposures can influence health across generations. By embracing these and other approaches, environmental health researchers are poised to unravel the intricate ways that environmental factors influence health, leading to more effective interventions and policies to mitigate risk and harmful impacts.

However, researchers cannot and should not work alone in their pursuits. As discussed in Chapter 5, "Environmental Health Science for the People," environmental health is and should be for the people, and working with communities is paramount in effective research and policymaking. Collaborating with communities leads to a deeper understanding of environmental issues. True community-engaged research not only enhances the relevance and effectiveness of research and policy, but also promotes trust, transparency, and inclusivity in cocreating solutions to address environmental injustices. Furthermore, to address the complex issues that exist today, from climate change to environmental racism, solutions should be built from both the ground up with collective action from communities, as well as from the top down with policies and regulations that enact long-term change.

WORKING IN ENVIRONMENTAL HEALTH

Working in the field of environmental health is both rewarding and challenging, requiring a multidisciplinary approach that draws upon expertise in public health, environmental science, policy development, and community engagement, among other topics. The field encompasses a wide range of skills and activities, and there are many different personal and professional ways that one can contribute. Chapter 2, "Environmental Health in Practice," explains the roles and responsibilities, as well as the challenges and opportunities, of working in environmental health, particularly from the perspective of local government, but there are many career paths one can take to move society toward environmental health and justice for all. One can work in government, community, academic, nonprofit, or private settings. Some potential professional pathways include:

- advocate or community organizer
- emergency preparedness and disaster response specialist
- environmental educator
- environmental engineer
- environmental epidemiologist
- environmental journalist
- environmental lawyer
- environmental regulator
- environmental sociologist
- food safety and inspection specialist
- grant writer or grant maker
- industrial hygienist
- occupational health and safety manager
- policy analyst or expert
- sanitarian/health inspector
- toxicologist
- urban and regional planner

Of course, this list is not exhaustive, and people in many other careers can influence environmental health, including working as an elected official or in other related sectors, such agriculture, business, housing, or transportation.

The Public Health Core Values as defined by APHA and shown in Table 1.2, can serve as guiding principles for practitioners in the field of environmental health. These values

TABLE 1.2. CORE VALUES OF THE PUBLIC HEALTH CODE OF ETHICS, AMERICAN PUBLIC HEALTH ASSOCIATION (2019)[37]

CORE VALUES	DESCRIPTION
Professionalism and Trust	Work to prevent, minimize, and mitigate health harms whenever possible
Health and Safety	Promote and protect safety, health, and well-being to the maximum ability
Health Justice and Equity	Dismantle inequitable health systems and work toward equitable health systems
Interdependence and Solidarity	Recognize the connections of all beings and environments in the work
Human Rights and Civil Liberties	Recognize the autonomy, self-determination, and rights of community members in all aspects of this work
Inclusivity and Engagement	Bring together, engage with diverse communities in transparent and culturally relevant ways

Source: American Public Health Association. *Public Health Code of Ethics.* American Public Health Association. 2019. https://www.apha.org/-/media/files/pdf/membergroups/ethics/code_of_ethics.ashx

encompass social justice, equity, sustainability, scientific integrity, and the idea of flourishing or well-being. This idea goes beyond even physical and mental health. As APHA notes, the idea of flourishing refers to positive experiences both individuals and communities have when they are enabled to fulfill their inherent potential capabilities with self-determination, like creativity, intelligence, understanding, and a host of other positive qualities. The opposite of flourishing is experiencing discrimination, exploitation, and suffering. Environmental health and public health practitioners should ultimately serve society and promote flourishing by focusing on the equally important core ethical values of professionalism and trust, health and safety, health justice and equity, interdependence and solidarity, human rights and civil liberties, and inclusivity and engagement (Table 1.2).[37]

IN OTHER WORDS: COMMUNICATING ABOUT ENVIRONMENTAL HEALTH AND JUSTICE ISSUES

Many researchers have studied how best to communicate about environmental health and justice issues to different audiences. Not everyone has a deep understanding of how environments and health are connected. Throughout this text, we share many tips. A good place to begin is with the FrameWorks Institute[38] recommendations on how to communicate about issues to build support and effect change:

- Make messages relatable to real people and their health or the health of their loved ones.
- Recognize the preventable "upstream" factors that influence health.
- Distinguish environmental health and justice from merely "being green." Emphasize the need to shift blame from individual consumer actions with a call for policy and planning solutions.
- There is much uncertainty and despair related to many environmental health issues. Offer specific solutions: policies, programs, practices, or initiatives that foster environmental health.
- Challenge scarcity or "zero-sum" framing. Everyone deserves a healthy environment.

WORKING TOWARD ENVIRONMENTAL HEALTH AND JUSTICE

The field of environmental health has continued to evolve over the past few centuries, and more work is needed to improve how we study, regulate, and communicate about environmental health risks and impacts. Environmental health practice must be proactive and reactive, as the work entails daily risks and impacts, slow moving disasters, and extreme events. Much of environmental health is managing daily risks, like ensuring that businesses are following safety protocols or that hazardous products are labeled clearly for consumers. We see some environmental issues emerge slowly over time, such as ongoing exposure in our neighborhood or workplace to a specific hazard. We also see some sudden events or disasters that call for immediate response, such as a chemical spill or hurricane.

This book focuses heavily on the U.S. environmental health "system." This system is responsible for ensuring safe drinking water, clean air, vector control, food safety, chemical safety, healthy housing and community design, and emergency preparedness and disaster response in the context of climate change. In the United States, this system remains largely fragmented, but work is underway to strengthen it. Nearly a decade ago, the National Council for Environmental Health and Equity, a coalition of national environmental and public health organizations, made the following suggestions for strengthening the environmental health system that remain relevant today:

- creating an integrated infrastructure to collect and track crucial information,
- developing a well-trained and highly skilled workforce,
- providing ample and sustainable funding from diverse sources,

- ensuring that policy and programs are grounded in existing and up-to-date evidence-based research,
- encouraging and incentivizing cross-sectoral partnerships to support consideration of health impacts, and
- assuring environmental health services are equitably accessible.[39]

Many of these environmental health functions and responsibilities are discussed in Chapter 2, "Environmental Health in Practice," among other chapters.

Environmental health practitioners have a role to play in addressing **environmental justice (EJ)**. Although there are many formal definitions, EJ is both a social movement and the belief that EJ impact our everyday lives, and people of all races, incomes, and backgrounds deserve access to clean air, clean water, and a healthy community in which to thrive. It also entails recognition of intergenerational justice, which is threatened by unequal distributions of burdens between generations.[40] In 2019, the APHA passed a policy statement, *Addressing Environmental Justice to Achieve Health Equity*, that provides 15 recommended action steps for the field, including:

- Public health practitioners should advocate for sustained health coverage for EJ communities, as well as expanded healthcare and support in the face of environmental disasters, including but not limited to those resulting from climate change.
- Institutions and organizations, including government, academia, nonprofits, and advocacy groups, should join environmental communities in their response to climate change mitigation and adaptation.
- Public health agencies should form partnerships with social justice actors and organizations.
- Academic institutions should create EJ curricula, from course work to department majors, and should engage community members directly in that work by sharing institutional resources.

THE BEGINNINGS OF THE ENVIRONMENTAL JUSTICE MOVEMENT

The Environmental Justice Movement has its origins in both the environmental and civil rights movements. Many consider the Memphis Sanitation Strike of 1968 as a pivotal moment in its history. In April 1968, 1,300 Black workers from the Memphis Department of Public Works, led by Dr. Martin Luther King Jr., united to demand fair wages and safer working conditions.[41] This significant campaign marked the occasion when Dr. King delivered his famous "I've Been to the Mountaintop" speech, just a day before his tragic assassination.

Fast forward to 1982, and another significant event unfolded in Warren County, North Carolina. The Ward Transformer Company of Raleigh, North Carolina, leaked 31,000 gallons of polychlorinated biphenyls (PCBs) along 240 miles of state highways in order to avoid costly and safe chemical disposal regulations. Residents opposed the construction of a landfill intended for disposing of 60,000 tons of PCB-contaminated soil in their community. This resistance became a landmark moment in the early stages of the U.S. Environmental Justice Movement. Despite protests lasting several days, gaining national news coverage, and resulting in numerous arrests, the landfill development persisted. Subsequently, the EPA approved a PCB landfill site in Warren County, which was predominantly home to a Black and poor community. After years of legal battles, the state of North Carolina spent over $25 million to remediate the site.[41]

In October 1991, the First National People of Color Environmental Leadership Summit convened in Washington, D.C., drawing over 1,000 participants from all 50 states and around the world. This landmark event focused on elevating the leadership and voices of communities of color, sharing action strategies and developing common plans, and addressing the oversight of environmental racism by traditional environmental organizations. It urged mainstream

(continued)

environmentalists to broaden their scope beyond wilderness conservation and to actively engage with environmental health and justice issues in communities.[42] The Summit culminated in the adoption of the 17 Principles of Environmental Justice, a foundational document guiding the movement. These principles underscore the necessity for public policy that is devoid of discrimination and rooted in mutual respect and political, economic, cultural, and environmental self-determination. Additionally, they emphasize equal participation in decision-making processes and highlight the importance of educating present and future generations on social and environmental issues. Furthermore, the principles insist on the protection of victims' rights to full compensation, reparations, and quality healthcare in the face of environmental injustice.[42] These principles should shape the work of environmental health practitioners in advancing environmental justice.

Given our globalized society, environmental health and justice efforts must also consider both local and global exposures and protections, as well as how they address or perpetuate disparities between populations and places. Although air pollution is often a localized issue, for instance, it knows no political boundaries. Pollution generated in one state or nation may affect public health in another. This textbook notes the many ways wealthier nations, like the United States, may perpetuate environmental inequities through transport of waste to or extraction of resources from lower wealth nations or communities. At this moment, the Earth's climate is undergoing significant changes, and an international response that centers those most affected is necessary to ensure environmental health for all.

MAIN TAKEAWAYS

In this chapter, we learned that:

- Humans have been engaging in environmental health practice long before public health departments were established.
- The places where we live, learn, play, and work greatly affect our well-being and, as such, every sector is an environmental health sector—from transportation to agriculture to education to housing.
- There are many different personal and professional ways to contribute to environmental health in community, healthcare, academic, agency, and business settings.
- Climate change is one of the most urgent public health issues society faces today, and it is crucial to develop strategies to ensure climate justice.
- Everyone is exposed to chemicals in their daily lives, and environmental health plays a vital role in understanding and reducing the associated health risks and impacts.
- As a field, environmental health is grappling with how to comprehend and address the complex realities of human–environmental interactions with many emerging frameworks and methods.

SUMMARY

The field of environmental health has a long history and is a wide-reaching and central piece of public health. From its historical roots in the Sanitary Movement of the 1800s to the contemporary focus on topics like climate change, environmental health seeks to understand the intricate relationship between environmental exposures and health outcomes. This chapter touches on a variety of topics, such as the interconnectedness of our world, captured in frameworks like One Health and Planetary Health, and the intersection of environmental health science and policy. The importance of risk management, the challenges posed by cumulative impacts, and the diverse career paths the field offers are also addressed. Importantly, the chapter discusses the pervasive influence of environmental racism in shaping environmental health disparities, emphasizing the need for equitable interventions and a comprehensive approach. It underscores the importance of collaborative action across sectors to achieve environmental health for all and ensure the well-being of present and future generations in the face of evolving environmental challenges.

ACKNOWLEDGMENT

We wish to acknowledge Wilma Subra for her contributions. She helped us to think about how we conceptualize risk and exposure science in this chapter and throughout the text.

END-OF-CHAPTER RESOURCES

DISCUSSION QUESTIONS

1. Before reading this chapter, what were your assumptions about the field of environmental health?
2. Why is it important to understand history before we can fully understand environmental health and justice issues?
3. When did you first learn about climate change? Did you learn about the science, the politics, or the health effects?
4. What do you love about the social, natural, or built environments where you live, work, play, pray, and learn? What are the biggest environmental health threats in your community?
5. The Multisolving Institution, founded by Dr. Elizabeth Sawin, aims to "help people see and create conditions" to "improv[e] health, well-being, equity, and economic vitality."[43(para5)] This entails seeing connections across issues and working across sectors in a comprehensive way. In what ways can we look to multisolving in the context of NATECH events and climate change?

LEARNING ACTIVITIES

THE TIME IS NOW

What environmental issues affect your community or region? What is being done to address them? You may have a sense of what issues need addressing from your own experiences, or it may take a bit of internet searching. Some questions you might explore include the following:

- What issues is your EPA region working on? (The EPA is divided into 10 regions, as shown in Figure 1.2.) Go to your region's webpage and scan to learn some of the latest news.
- If you want to identify sources of contamination, the EPA's **Toxic Release Inventory (TRI)** can provide valuable information. By accessing the TRI database, you can look up facilities in your local area and learn more about how they are managing toxic chemicals that cause cancer or other chronic human health effects, notable adverse acute human health effects, and significant adverse environmental effects. Go to www.epa.gov/toxics-release-inventory-tri-program. The EPA offers another search tool to investigate contaminated sites near where you live with the Superfund program at www.epa.gov/superfund/search-superfund-sites-where-you-live.
- What environmental organizations have chapters or are based in your state? Are there chapters of any of the national long-standing organizations like the Sierra Club or the Natural Resources Defense Council? Are there grassroots organizations working in specific communities or on specific issues? Are there issue-specific organizations like watershed councils or groups focused on transition to renewable energy. Are there any

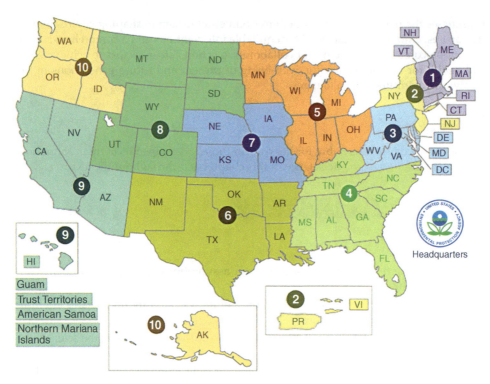

FIGURE 1.2. The Environmental Protection Agency's 10 regions.
Source: Regional and geographic offices. United States Environmental Protection Agency. Updated January 18, 2024. https://www.epa.gov/aboutepa/regional-and-geographic-offices

coalitions—groups of environmentally related organizations working together? You might sign up for e-newsletters or follow some of these organizations on social media to get updates on local issues, how you can learn more, and how you can engage.

IN REAL LIFE

The topics of this textbook can bring up a variety of emotions—fear, anxiety, grief, hopelessness, hopefulness, passion, helplessness, anger, apathy, and many others. Research shows some ways to work through these climate-related negative emotions may include connecting with others, connecting with nature, taking actions (even small ones), and taking breaks. Specific strategies to deal with specific emotions may include:

- fear/anxiety: deep breathing, mindfulness
- anger: emotional release activities (e.g., exercise, art, music, writing) and taking time to cool down before acting on emotions
- grief: emotional release (e.g., crying), support, and validation from others
- hopelessness/helplessness: focus on what you *can* do and what you *can* change

Take a minute to journal in response to the following prompts (or discuss with a trusted friend):

1. What emotions often come up for you after reading this chapter or others in this textbook?
2. What strategies do you typically use to cope with anxiety, grief, anger, or hopelessness? (Or, if you don't have many coping strategies, what coping strategies might work for you?)
3. Who or where do you go to when you need a safe or rejuvenating space?
4. What actions (small or big) are you already taking or do you want to take to address the issues you are learning about?

A robust set of instructor resources designed to supplement this text is located at http://connect.springerpub.com/content/book/978-0-8261-8353-8. Qualifying instructors may request access by emailing textbook@springerpub.com.

REFERENCES

1. Delile H, Blichert-Toft J, Goiran JP, Keay S, Albarède F. Lead in ancient Rome's city waters. *Proc Natl Acad Sci U S A*. 2014;111(18):6594–6599. doi:10.1073/pnas.1400097111
2. Fadel HE, Al-Hendy A. Development of obstetric practice during the early Islamic era. *Reprod Sci*. 2022;29(9):2587–2592. doi:10.1007/s43032-022-00887-1
3. Kimmerer R. *Braiding Sweetgrass: Indigenous Wisdom, Scientific Knowledge and the Teachings of Plants*. Milkweed Editions; 2013.
4. Aldahan AS, Shah VV, Mlacker S, Nouri K. The history of sunscreen. *JAMA Dermatol*. 2015;151:1316. doi:10.1001/jamadermatol.2015.3011
5. Bailey ZD, Krieger N, Agénor M, Graves J, Linos N, Bassett MT. Structural racism and health inequities in the USA: evidence and interventions. *Lancet*. 2017;389(10077):1453–1463. doi:10.1016/S0140-6736(17)30569-X
6. Yearby R. Structural racism and health disparities: reconfiguring the social determinants of health framework to include the root cause. *J Law Med Ethics*. 2020;48(3):518–526. doi:10.1177/1073110520958876
7. Bullard RD. The threat of environmental racism. *Nat Resour Environ*. 1993;7(3):23–56.
8. Pettoello-Mantovani M, Indrio F, Francavilla R, Giardino I. The effects of climate change and exposure to endocrine disrupting chemicals on children's health: a challenge for pediatricians. *Glob Pediatr*. 2023;4:100047. doi:10.1016/j.gpeds.2023.100047
9. Anderko L, Chalupka S, Du M, Hauptman M. Climate changes reproductive and children's health: a review of risks, exposures, and impacts. *Pediatr Res*. 2020;87(2):414–419. doi:10.1038/s41390-019-0654-7
10. Allen EM, Munala L, Henderson JR. Kenyan women bearing the cost of climate change. *Int J Environ Res Public Health*. 2021;18(23):12697. doi:10.3390/ijerph182312697
11. Wild CP. The exposome: from concept to utility. *Int J Epidemiol*. 2012;41(1):24–32. doi:10.1093/ije/dyr236
12. Sullivan B. What to know about the train derailment in East Palestine, Ohio. National Public Radio. February 16, 2023. https://www.npr.org/2023/02/16/1157333630/east-palestine-ohio-train-derailment
13. Salcedo A, Dance S, Phillips A. Officials burned off toxic chemicals from Ohio train. Was it the right move? *Washington Post*. February 17, 2023. https://www.washingtonpost.com/climate-environment/2023/02/17/ohio-derailment-controlled-burning-toxic/
14. Rogers J. Timeline leading to the controlled burn of derailed train cars in East Palestine. WFMJ. January 24, 2024. Updated January 31, 2024. https://www.wfmj.com/story/50401272/timeline-leading-to-the-controlled-burn-of-derailed-train-cars-in-east-palestine
15. Operational updates. U.S. Environmental Protection Agency. February 18, 2023. Updated May 15, 2024. https://www.epa.gov/east-palestine-oh-train-derailment/operational-updates#apr23
16. Medical management guidelines for vinyl chloride. Agency for Toxic Substances and Disease Registry. Updated October 21, 2014. https://wwwn.cdc.gov/TSP/MMG/MMGDetails.aspx?mmgid=278&toxid=51#:~:text=Vinyl%20chloride%20can%20irritate%20the,and%20bones%20of%20the%20hand
17. Dawes DE. *The Political Determinants of Health*. Johns Hopkins University Press; 2020.
18. Gilmore AB, Fabbri A, Baum F, et al. Defining and conceptualising the commercial determinants of health. *Lancet*. 2023;401(10383):1194–1213. doi:10.1016/S0140-6736(23)00013-2
19. Heller JC, Givens ML, Johnson SP, Kindig DA. Keeping it political and powerful: defining the structural determinants of health. *Milbank Q*. 2024. doi:10.1111/1468-0009.12695
20. Hayhoe K. How to talk about climate change so people will listen. *Chatelaine*. January 26, 2024. https://chatelaine.com/living/how-to-talk-about-climate-change/
21. Kurland Z, Hafner K, Feder E. The woman who demonstrated the greenhouse effect. *Scientific American*. November 9, 2023. https://www.scientificamerican.com/article/the-woman-who-demonstrated-the-greenhouse-effect/

22. Lindsey R, Dahlman L. Climate change: global temperature. Climate.gov. January 18, 2024. https://www.climate.gov/news-features/understanding-climate/climate-change-global-temperature
23. Sigfried K. Climate change and displacement: the myths and facts. United Nations Refugee Agency. November 15, 2023. https://www.unhcr.org/us/news/stories/climate-change-and-displacement-myths-and-facts
24. Johnson J, Cushing L. Chemical exposures, health and environmental justice in communities living on the fenceline of industry. *Curr Environ Health Rep.* 2020;7(1):48–57. doi:10.1007/s40572-020-00263-8
25. Toxic Release Inventory (TRI) program. U.S. Evironmental Protection Agency. Updated April 24, 2024. https://www.epa.gov/toxics-release-inventory-tri-program
26. The Industrial Accidents Convention and natural disasters: Natech. United Nations Economic Commission for Europe. Accessed June 13, 2024. https://unece.org/industrial-accidents-convention-and-natural-disasters-natech
27. Wendee N. A different kind of storm: Natech events in Houston's fenceline communities. *Environ Health Perspect.* 2021;129(5):052001. doi:10.1289/EHP8391
28. Arkema Inc. chemical plant fire. U.S. Chemical Safety Board. 2017. Accessed June 13, 2024. https://www.csb.gov/arkema-inc-chemical-plant-fire-/
29. Brown M. Harvey's flooding blamed in major gasoline spill in Texas. *AP News.* September 12, 2017. https://apnews.com/general-news-9d6ed228c32d407cb2034c4ac26d3297
30. Agency for Toxic Substances and Disease Registry. *Health Consultation, Drinking Water Quality Analyses, March 1996 to June 1999.* United Water Toms River; 2001.
31. Richardson SD, Collette TW, Price PC, et al. Identification of drinking water contaminants in the course of a childhood cancer investigation in Toms River, New Jersey. *J Expo Anal Environ Epidemiol.* 1999;9(3):200–216. doi:10.1038/sj.jea.7500020
32. Berry, MK, Haltmeier P. Childhood cancer incidence health consultation: a review and analysis of cancer registry data, 1979–1995, for Dover Township (Ocean County), New Jersey. Final Technical Report. New Jersey Department of Health and Senior Services. 1997. Accessed June 13, 2024. www.nj.gov/health/ceohs/documents/eohap/haz_sites/ocean/toms_river/toms_river_dover_twp/cansumm.pdf
33. New Jersey Department of Health and Senior Services. *Case–Control Study of Childhood Cancers in Dover Township (Ocean County), New Jersey.* Division of Epidemiology, Environmental and Occupational Health, New Jersey Department of Health and Senior Services; 2003.
34. Sucato K. What's wrong in Toms River? *The New York Times.* December 16, 2001. https://www.nytimes.com/2001/12/16/nyregion/what-s-wrong-in-toms-river.html
35. Maslia, ML, Reyes JJ, Gillig RE, et al. Public health partnerships addressing childhood cancer investigations: case study of Toms River, Dover Township, New Jersey, USA. *Int J Hyg Environ Health.* 2005;208(1–2):45–54. doi:10.1016/j.ijheh.2005.01.007
36. Fagin D. *Toms River: A Story of Science and Salvation.* Island Press; 2013.
37. American Public Health Association. Public health code of ethics. 2019. https://www.apha.org/-/media/files/pdf/membergroups/ethics/code_of_ethics.ashx?la=en&hash=3D6643946AE1DF9EF05334E7DF6AF89471FA14EC pP5-6
38. FrameWorks Institute. You say...they think (environmental health). 2014. https://www.frameworksinstitute.org/wp-content/uploads/2020/05/eh_yousaytheythink.pdf
39. Investing in a robust environmental health system. American Public Health Association. 2017. https://apha.org/-/media/Files/PDF/topics/environment/Partners/Robust_EH_System.ashx
40. Breil M, Downing C, Kazmierczak A, et al. Social vulnerability to climate change in European cities—state of play in policy and practice. European Topic Centre on Climate Change impacts, Vulnerability and Adaptation (ETC/CCA) Technical paper. 2018. https://www.eionet.europa.eu/etcs/etc-cca/products/etc-cca-reports/tp_1-2018/@@download/file/TP_1-2018.pdf
41. Bullard RD. Environmental justice in the 21st century: race still matters. *Phylon.* 2001;49(3/4):151–171. doi:10.2307/3132626
42. First National People of Color Environmental Leadership Summit. The principles of environmental justice (EJ). 1991. https://www.ejnet.org/ej/principles.pdf
43. *Multisolving: Protecting the climate while improving health, equity, biodiversity, and well-being: Friends of the Lehigh Libraries talk, Wed., May 24.* Lehigh University: Library and Technology Services. May 8, 2023. https://lts.lehigh.edu/news/multisolving-protecting-climate-while-improving-health-equity-biodiversity-and-well-being-friends

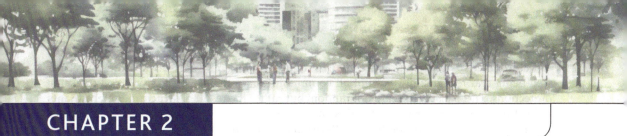

CHAPTER 2

Environmental Health in Practice

Ali Abazeed and Samir Deshpande

LEARNING OBJECTIVES

- Begin to understand the structural determinants of environmental health disparities, which are largely shaped by historic and present-day systems of structural racism and discrimination.
- Identify the roles and responsibilities of environmental health agencies and how they vary across jurisdictions.
- Rethink environmental health "surveillance" and present vital considerations for how environmental health practitioners use data.
- Examine how environmental health practitioners can facilitate public participation in meaningful ways that interrogate underlying power dynamics.
- Present an Environmental Public Health in All Policies approach with examples of what this approach may look like in practice.

KEY TERMS

- community organizing
- cumulative impact
- environmental health disparities
- environmental justice (EJ)
- environmental public health
- environmental racism
- fenceline communities
- Health in All Policies (HiAP)
- public health
- structural determinants of health
- structural racism
- White supremacy

"Nations reel and stagger on their way; they make hideous mistakes; they commit frightful wrongs; they do great and beautiful things. And shall we not best guide humanity by telling the truth about all this, so far as the truth is ascertainable?"

—W. E. B. Du Bois, *Black Reconstruction in America* (1935)

OVERVIEW

To understand environmental public health, we first need to situate it within the broader context of public health. Public health is a field whose mission and work have long been relegated to the periphery but, due to the COVID-19 pandemic, now enjoys unprecedented awareness by the general public.[1] Public health is what we as a society do collectively to assure the conditions for people to be healthy.[2] It extends beyond the confines of hospitals and clinics, encompassing a wide range of activities, from ensuring that the air we breathe and the water we drink are clean, to making our workplaces and roads safer, and to halting the spread of infectious diseases. In each of these areas, the focus is not just on avoiding harm but also on creating conditions that allow communities to thrive. **Environmental public health** is a crucial subset of this field, focusing on how our natural, built, and social environments impact our health.

Environmental health in practice involves understanding how our surroundings affect our well-being and recognizing that not all communities face the same risks or enjoy the same protections. These disparities are not random but rather the result of **structural determinants of health**, or the complex interplay of economic, political, cultural, and social forces. Policies and programs that determine these patterns are not ordained by supernatural phenomena. Whether made overtly or through the silent assent of inaction, these decisions reflect a broader pattern of environmental inequity—a theme central to this chapter and textbook.

As we delve into the subject of environmental health today, this textbook examines how historical and recent decisions continue to shape the present landscape of the field. From the Industrial Revolution to the rise of modern zoning laws, certain populations have borne the brunt of environmental neglect. Have you ever wondered why towering factory stacks and industry polluters rarely exist in affluent, White neighborhoods but seem to litter the skyline in communities of color? Have you ever noticed that warehouses are being built within feet of existing homes and schools in underresourced communities, but are rarely ever built in resourced communities? Is it concerning to you that as the Black population increases in a particular ZIP code in the United States, so too does the concentration of air pollutants, while the opposite is true for ZIP codes with high-density White populations?[3]

In this chapter, we discuss the roles and responsibilities of environmental health practitioners in tackling these inequities, in uprooting systems of structural racism and White supremacy, and in working toward thriving communities for all. In doing so, we also call on a broad array of actors to work together to this end. We acknowledge the challenges of those working in the field as well—from underfunding to the hard work of countering corporate interests. We will share and interrogate the power of data and how we use it to uplift the experiences of people closest to harm. A central value in this work is that ordinary people are the experts of their own experiences, and we explore the ways that environmental health practitioners can intentionally engage with communities. As we describe key environmental health functions, we will be laying down the foundation for an informed, empowered, and proactive approach to environmental health in practice. This chapter's introduction to environmental health practice is not just academic; it is an invitation to each reader to become an agent of change. We invite you to adopt public health not merely as a field of study or professional practice but as a critical lens for examining the world. This lens, when used with intention and care, has the power to elevate communities.

RACISM AS AN ENVIRONMENTAL PUBLIC HEALTH ISSUE

Structural racism is embedded across society, in policies, and in institutional practices that perpetuate racial and ethnic disparities.[4] It intersects with other forms of discrimination and oppression based on gender, sexuality, income, education, and other factors.[5] It is present in systems far and wide, from criminal justice to the job market, from access to credit and housing to the educational sector, and is deeply embedded within the healthcare system itself. While some people prefer to call this discrimination structural racism, many call it **White supremacy**, a term that refers to how our long-held operating systems consistently disadvantage people of color and reinforce a racial hierarchy.

Understanding historic and present-day structural racism is crucial for all of us. It is not just a topic for environmental scientists or public health professionals. It is relevant to everyone who desires a just and healthy world. In the United States, the segregation and disenfranchisement laws known as "Jim Crow" represented a formal, codified system of racial apartheid that dominated the American South for three quarters of a century beginning in the 1890s. The laws affected almost every aspect of daily life, mandating the segregation of schools, parks, libraries, drinking fountains, restrooms, buses, trains, and restaurants. "Whites Only" and "Colored" signs were constant reminders of the enforced racial order.[6] These laws spawned, among other things, local racial covenants that segregated White individuals from other communities, resulting in systemic environmental injustices that we see today. Many activists and frontline communities call environmental racism "The New Jim Crow" because of its devastating subjugation of communities of color to inequitable living conditions.[7]

Environmental racism and racial segregation are closely intertwined. The root cause of related disparities can be traced back to federal housing agencies, bankers, and insurers who discriminated through redlining. This practice often forced Black residents into crowded cities, while facilitating the migration of White residents to the suburbs. From 1935 to 1940, the Home Owners' Loan Corporation (HOLC) graded investment risk in over 200 U.S. communities.[8] Communities classified as high risk received a "D" score and were marked in red on HOLC maps. Over the next three decades, regardless of their creditworthiness, certain applicants, mainly Black applicants and some immigrants, were often limited to loans in redlined communities.[8] These communities often lacked the resources and political influence to shape land-use planning decisions, targeting them as sites for oil refineries, gas compressor stations, factories, and waste facilities.

Today, environmental racism goes beyond the cumulative effects of co-occurring exposures. Though Black communities and communities of color bear disproportionate hardships of the environmental crisis, they historically have been left out of the environmental movement. Of the nearly 2,000 environmental nonprofits that exist across the country, White people make up 85% of the staff and 80% of the boards.[9] People of color make up only 20% of the staff of 40 environmental nongovernmental organizations.[10] These disparities in representation are not merely abstractions. They create a vicious cycle wherein the concerns of those communities bearing the brunt of environmental degradation are not often heard nor prioritized.

CASE STUDY 2.1: Disparities in Government Response to Air Quality Concerns in Two Los Angeles Neighborhoods

The government's response to environmental hazards often reveals striking disparities among communities of different races and ethnicities, particularly in their handling of air quality concerns. A compelling example is seen in the contrasting responses to incidents in two Los Angeles neighborhoods: Porter Ranch and Jefferson Park.

From October 2015 to February 2016, Porter Ranch, an affluent, predominantly White, suburban community with home values starting at $400,000, suffered the largest methane leak ever recorded in the United States. The leak swiftly prompted a state of emergency declaration, leading to the evacuation of over 4,000 homes. The city of Los Angeles mandated the responsible gas company to arrange temporary housing for those displaced by this environmental crisis.[11]

In stark contrast is Jefferson Park, a neighborhood in south Los Angeles where the majority of residents are Black or Hispanic or Latino. Here, the community lived in the shadow of the AllenCo oil drilling site, which was associated with a plethora of health complaints. Despite the ongoing concerns, it was not until Environmental Protection Agency (EPA) officials fell ill during a site visit that the drilling site was closed in 2013. Astonishingly, from the site's inception in 2010 until its closure, residents lodged 251 complaints to the South Coast Air Quality Management regarding the site's impact on air quality. Yet the regulatory body issued a mere 15 citations against AllenCo.[12]

The tale of two neighborhoods—Porter Ranch and Jefferson Park—provides a stark illustration of environmental racism in action. The differing levels of urgency and response highlight how predominantly White communities often receive swift and decisive action to mitigate environmental hazards, while communities of color experience prolonged exposure and neglect. This disparity not only endangers the health of the residents but also signals a deeper issue of inequality that is systemic and pervasive.

REFLECTION QUESTIONS

1. How do the disparities in government responses to Porter Ranch and Jefferson Park reflect environmental racism?

2. What strategies could promote equitable environmental governance?

ZIP CODE AND GENETIC CODE: PLACE MATTERS

Environmental public health has a crucial role in investigating the structural forces that drive health inequalities by focusing on "place," which encompasses the majority of our environmental exposures. Your ZIP code is often a better predictor of your health outcomes than your genetic code.[13] One of the most striking examples of how environments shape health can be seen in a short journey from Detroit, Michigan, to Ann Arbor, Michigan. This trip, covering a distance of just under 40 miles, astonishingly represents a journey through six years of human life expectancy.[14]

This stark contrast highlights the profound impact our surroundings have on health. While Detroit and Ann Arbor are geographically close, their environmental, economic, and social landscapes differ significantly. These differences paint a vivid picture of how factors like air quality, access to healthcare, green spaces, and socioeconomic conditions can dramatically influence the health and longevity of communities.

But it is more than that. In Detroit, a series of deep-rooted challenges contribute to a lower life expectancy. They include the enduring effects of systemic racism and environmental injustices. For decades, the city has been home to heavy industries like automobile manufacturing, steel production, and oil refining, which have disproportionately affected the health of communities of color. Housing policies, particularly in the practice of redlining, combined with the exodus of White populations to the suburbs in the post-1950s era, further entrenched racial divides and health disparities. The subsequent decline of industrialization also played a role, leaving economic and health voids in its wake.[15]

In contrast, Ann Arbor, with its higher average income, better access to healthcare services, and plentiful green spaces, offers its residents a setting that supports a longer and healthier life. This contrast underscores the essence of environmental public health: it is not just about the presence of specific health risks in our environment, but also about the broader context in which we live our lives. It is not just about the quality of air and water or the availability of healthy food and healthcare, but also about the socioeconomic status of an area and the historical antecedents that preceded the health outcomes we see today.

ENVIRONMENTAL HEALTH IN PRACTICE

Public health is often oversimplified as a field and discipline concerned with preventing "bad stuff" from happening, but it is so much more than that. There are many groups working across the United States and globally to achieve environmental health and justice for all. This work entails a web of federal, state, and local government agencies, nonprofit organizations, grassroots community groups, consulting firms, businesses, and many others. As explained in the Environmental Health Playbook, "No single agency is responsible for resolving environmental health issues, which can limit and confound accountability. At the national level, federal policies and regulations are not comprehensive, and so provide limited or no guidance for states to take action."[16] There are some key professional associations that support and guide the field across this complex web, including the American Public Health Association, the Association of State and Territorial Health Officials, the National Environmental Health Association, and the National Association of County and City Health Officials.

FEDERALISM: THE ROLE OF FEDERAL, STATE, AND LOCAL GOVERNMENTS

In the public eye in the United States, the vast majority of attention is often paid to environmental decisions made at the federal level. This makes sense, as laws passed by Congress and regulations promulgated by the U.S. EPA and other federal agencies affect hundreds of millions of people across the country and often set the standard. At the federal level, public health research and practice are centralized within the Department of Health and Human Services (HHS). Within the HHS are the National Institutes of Health, including the National Institute of Environmental Health Sciences, the Centers for Disease Control and Prevention (CDC), and the Agency for Toxic Substances and Disease Registry (ATSDR), among others. However, these agencies are only one part of the picture. Other federal agencies (e.g., Department of Labor, Department of Housing and Urban Development) have a role to play in shaping our environments. Also other levels of government, including local, county, and state governments, can have significant influence on the policy landscape we live in, and these local actors are typically much more accessible to communities.

As described in Chapter 4, "Environmental Health Policies and Protections: Successes and Failures," most environmental laws in the United States are managed through a system of environmental federalism, whereby the federal government sets the standards and state governments enforce them. For example, the Clean Air Act, a landmark environmental law enacted in 1970, authorizes the EPA to set National Ambient Air Quality Standards "to protect public health and public welfare and to regulate emissions of hazardous air pollutants." The law also directs states to develop state implementation plans to achieve these standards.[17] This system allows the federal government to use health and safety data based on the available science, and grants states the flexibility to meet those standards with the policies and regulations that best suit their needs. These state institutions, typically state environmental agencies, regulate important issues like air quality, water quality, energy efficiency, and more.

Local mayors, city council members, or county executives are responsible for many of the services that matter in our daily lives, like roads, public transit, water infrastructure, and zoning laws. The structure of local governments can vary dramatically depending on a city's size and its priorities at the time of its founding. Some cities have strong mayor–council systems in which mayors have substantial control over administrative matters and can veto city council decisions. Others use weak mayor–council systems, in which mayors have a largely ceremonial role with less direct control over administrative matters and limited veto power over city council decisions. Some smaller towns and cities do not have mayors, relying instead on a council–management form of government. They Maybe just the elected city council or board hires the manager to manage the day-to-day operations. An elected city council or board of selectmen or aldermen hires the manager, passes legislation, and oversees performance.[18] They may serve as a board of health, or there may be a separate board of health. Boards of health may be present in other forms of government and are a good way to get involved in local environmental health matters. People working in these positions may also be much more accessible than state or federal officials. Understanding the structural power centers of your city is a critical step toward pursuing better policies.

In most cases, regulations made by state and federal governments have commenting periods, where anyone can provide public feedback on the proposed or final rule. Individuals and interest groups (ranging from environmental justice [EJ] advocates to corporate polluters) often use these opportunities to formally make their voice heard on forthcoming regulations or settlements. In some cases, the regulatory agency is required to respond to comments, forcing agencies to at minimum provide a rationale for why particular feedback is or is not considered. Chapter 4 discusses strategies for writing effective comments on environmental decisions.

Sometimes, regulatory agencies will solicit feedback through a Request for Information (RFI), often when they seek to understand public opinion around a specific program, policy, or issue area; they sometimes have specific questions or allow respondents to comment in whatever format they desire. For example, Michigan's Department of Environment, Great Lakes, and Energy utilized an RFI to "solicit initial feedback on the potential use of state funds from a State Energy Financing Institution (SEFI) to implement the priorities outlined in the MI Healthy Climate Plan (MHCP) and the Clean Energy and Jobs Act and Clean Energy Future package."[19(p1)] The RFI included specific questions about the focus of the program, funding for the program, and opportunities for economic development.

ENVIRONMENTAL PUBLIC HEALTH 10 ESSENTIAL SERVICES AND FUNDAMENTAL ACTIVITIES

Within the field of public health lies a vital resource known as the 10 Essential Public Health Services (shown in Figure 2.1).[20] These services form a comprehensive framework that outlines the necessary actions public health officials must take to maintain and improve the public's health. Within this framework, environmental public health is not just a component—it is a fundamental aspect deeply embedded in each function. By addressing the direct and indirect impacts of our environment on health, it becomes clear that anyone in public health can adopt an environmental public health lens in executing the following essential services, ensuring that the places where people live, work, and play do not become sources of illness.

1. **Assess and monitor population health status, factors that influence health, and community needs and assets.**
   - Environmental public health tracks air and water quality, exposure to hazardous substances, and community compliance with health regulations to identify potential health risks.
2. **Investigate, diagnose, and address health problems and hazards affecting the population.**
   - Specialists in environmental health are on the front line, identifying sources of environmental contamination and outbreaks of diseases related to environmental factors, such as asthma or lead poisoning.
3. **Communicate effectively to inform and educate people about health, the factors that influence it, and how to improve it.**
   - This service involves educating the public about environmental risks and how to reduce them, such as providing information on reducing exposure to pollutants or safely disposing of hazardous waste.

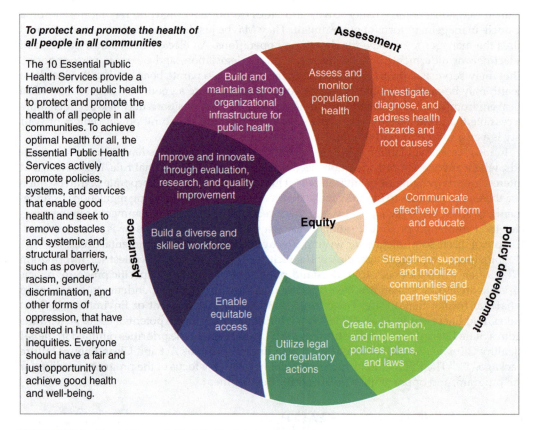

FIGURE 2.1. The 10 Essential Public Health Services.
Source: 10 Essential Public Health Services. Centers for Disease Control and Prevention. Created 2020. Published 2021. Updated September 18, 2023. https://www.cdc.gov/publichealthgateway/publichealthservices/essentialhealthservices.html

4. **Strengthen, support, and mobilize communities and partnerships to improve health.**
   - Collaboration is key in environmental health, bringing together community groups, businesses, and policy makers to tackle environmental health challenges, from cleaning up polluted sites to promoting healthy homes and workplaces.
5. **Create, champion, and implement policies, plans, and laws that impact health.**
   - Policymaking in environmental health includes regulations to control pollution; land-use planning to prevent exposure to harmful substances; and ensuring access to safe food, water, and opportunities for recreation and joy.
6. **Utilize legal and regulatory actions designed to improve and protect the public's health.**
   - Environmental health is deeply involved in enforcing clean air and water laws, safe chemical use, and building codes that protect health.
7. **Ensure an effective system that enables equitable access to the individual services and care needed to be healthy.**
   - Environmental health professionals help connect individuals with health services to address environmental exposures, and work to ensure that these services are available, especially in underserved communities.
8. **Build and support a diverse and skilled public health workforce.**
   - Training and ensuring the competency of environmental health workers are vital to effectively monitor, diagnose, and address environmental health issues.
9. **Improve and innovate public health functions through ongoing evaluation, research, and continuous quality improvement.**
   - Evaluation in environmental health assesses the impact of interventions and services aimed at reducing environmental risks to health.
10. **Build and maintain a strong organizational infrastructure for public health.**
    - Research in environmental health seeks to understand the complex interactions between environmental exposures and health outcomes and to develop innovative solutions to reduce risks.

Environmental public health clearly intersects with each of these essential services, playing a pivotal role in addressing the root causes of health problems and in implementing solutions. The field emphasizes the importance of the environment in public health and the need for integrated approaches to promote healthy, sustainable communities, highlighting the critical contributions of this field to the broader public health mission.

Environmental public health is a thread woven through the fabric of public health. While environmental health practice may differ depending on local and state jurisdictions, its core functions are crucial to the holistic practice of public health. Although local and state environmental health departments have diverse, specific roles and responsibilities, they engage in a suite of fundamental activities that safeguard community health. These functions, while variable, form the backbone of environmental public health across different jurisdictions.

- **Water quality monitoring:** Ensuring the safety and cleanliness of public water supplies is a primary concern. Routine surveillance and testing of water sources help prevent contamination that can lead to outbreaks of waterborne diseases.
- **Food-safety inspections:** By inspecting restaurants, food trucks, and markets, environmental health professionals protect the public from foodborne illnesses, ensuring that food service establishments adhere to the highest safety standards.
- **Vector control:** Departments actively work to manage and reduce populations of vectors, such as mosquitoes and rodents, that can transmit diseases to humans, a task that is becoming increasingly important in the face of climate change.
- **Air quality management:** Monitoring pollutants and managing air quality are essential, especially in areas with high industrial activity. These efforts are vital for preventing respiratory conditions and fostering a healthier living environment.

- **Inspections and licensing:** Environmental health departments conduct inspections and issue licenses for various facilities, from swimming pools to septic systems, ensuring that they operate in a manner that does not pose a risk to public health.
- **Lead-poisoning prevention:** Preventative programs aimed at mitigating lead exposure, particularly in older housing stock, are critical for protecting children from the detrimental health effects associated with lead poisoning.
- **Emergency preparedness and disaster response:** In the event of environmental disasters or emergencies, departments are on the frontline, coordinating responses to protect public health, from managing shelters to conducting hazard cleanups.
- **Outreach:** Education and community outreach are indispensable for raising awareness about environmental risks and promoting behaviors that contribute to a healthier environment, as well as learning from various constituents.
- **Assessments:** Environmental health assessments analyze the potential health impacts of various community developments and industrial projects, influencing planning and decision-making processes.
- **Enforcement of regulations:** One of the most critical roles is the enforcement of health and safety regulations, a task that ensures compliance and protects the public from environmental health hazards.

Of course, for a variety of reasons, gaps exist in the ability of local and state governments to do this work. Funding and resources vary by region, which can greatly affect capacity to effectively monitor, assess, and address environmental health issues. Implementation and enforcement of environmental protections can vary depending on local laws, as well as on political and community priorities. For communities that are fenceline to polluting industries, local governments may struggle to hold these industries accountable, because they often have extensive financial resources and legal expertise on staff to protect their economic interests. Also, some local or state governments may have more or less robust data systems needed to accurately assess the extent of environmental risk and harm.

> In the United States, Tribes are sovereign nations and have public health authority. However, as is the case with city, county, and state jurisdictions, this work varies greatly in terms of the ability to implement environmental public health services. Today, there are approximately 574 federally recognized Tribes and 326 reservations with over half of the Indigenous population living in five states, including Oklahoma, Arizona, California, Texas, and New Mexico.[21] In 2020, over nine million people identified as American Indian/Alaskan Native in the United States Census.
>
> Before we can understand the current Tribal public health infrastructure, we must acknowledge the harms of colonialism and how this has disrupted traditional ways of living and shaped health for generations. American colonialism has resulted in extensive resource extraction and barriers to food sovereignty on Tribal lands. As a result, colonialism has contributed to conditions of unsafe and inadequate housing, persistent poverty, and deeply rooted trauma for many Tribal communities.
>
> It was not until after centuries of racist practices of relocation and attempts at forced assimilation that self-determination rights were established during the Civil Rights era. At this time, Congress passed the Indian Civil Rights Act of 1968 to ensure that Indigenous Peoples were afforded the same constitutional rights of other Americans. Since reauthorized and amended several times, the Indian Health Care Improvement Act authorized provision of healthcare services to Indigenous individuals through the Indian Health Service (IHS), Tribal health programs, and urban Indian health programs with funding and support for healthcare delivery, health promotion, and traditional healing practices. In 1975, the Indian Self-Determination and Education Assistance Act made it possible for Tribes to enter contracts and make grants to federally recognized Tribes, which also helped to establish a Tribal public health infrastructure.
>
> Today, the IHS within the federal Department of Health and Human Services plays a major role in supporting Indigenous public health infrastructure, but much of this work also takes

(continued)

place in other ways within and across Tribal communities. The IHS operates a system of hospitals, clinics, and healthcare centers that serve eligible American Indian and Alaska Native individuals. Additionally, many Tribal governments have their own health department responsible for public health functions. For instance, the Ho-Chunk Nation has departments of health and natural resources based in Wisconsin that monitor and address environmental health issues affecting Tribal health. Their Division of Environmental Health works on issues related to asbestos, mold and radon inspections, and water and sewer emergencies; it also supports private wells and septic systems and helps Tribal members navigate other environmental hazards.[22]

By fostering the capability of local Tribal health departments to address environmental issues, this work is more likely to be rooted in the traditional ways of knowing, such as honoring the Seven Generations Principles, which emphasizes making environmental decisions that consider the impact beyond the present to that felt by the next seven generations. As an example, the White Earth Nation in partnership with the Centers for Disease Control and Prevention (CDC) adapted the Anishinaabe Medicine Wheel to use in the context of the COVID-19 response. As seen in Figure 2.2, the philosophies that shape the Anishinaabe way of life also shaped the White Earth Nation's pandemic response.[23]

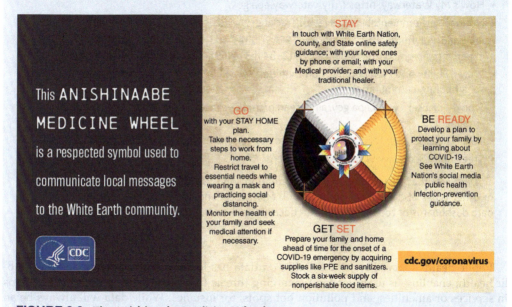

FIGURE 2.2. The Anishinaabe Medicine Wheel.

Source: Henry J, Kushwaha A, Lico A. Stories from the field: The White Earth Nation. *Centers for Disease Control and Prevention Conversations in Equity blog.* March 17, 2022. https://blogs.cdc.gov/healthequity/2022/03/17/stories-from-the-field-the-white-earth-nation

TRACKING ENVIRONMENTAL HEALTH

Data are quickly becoming one of the most valuable commodities in the world, and environmental health practitioners must engage deeply in our increasingly data-centric world as part of their work. Data help to carry out their responsibility to assess conditions and evaluate interventions. Data are coveted by governments, businesses, and individuals alike for understanding and safeguarding people, or for selling them things. Most individuals utilize data frequently as they research a product's reviews before making a big purchase or check the weather forecast before heading out for the day. Environmental health practitioners rely on all sorts of data to understand the world around us and its impacts on the people who live in it. Sophisticated sensors collect air and meteorological data to measure pollution. Satellites track forest cover and land use across the world. Cities test drinking water to ensure that it is free of contaminants.

> **DATA, DATA EVERYWHERE**
>
> There are many data sets referenced throughout this textbook and many more that can be used by community and agencies to characterize environmental health issues. Here are some of them:
>
> - Air Tracker: https://globalcleanair.org/air-tracker/
> - Environmental Justice Dashboard Centers for Disease Control and Prevention (CDC)/Agency for Toxic Substances and Disease Registry (ATSDR) Social Vulnerability Index: www.atsdr.cdc.gov/placeandhealth/svi/index.html
> - CompTox Chemicals Dashboard: www.epa.gov/comptox-tools/comptox-chemicals-dashboard
> - Cyanobacteria Assessment Network: www.epa.gov/water-research/cyanobacteria-assessment-network-cyan
> - EJSCREEN: Environmental Justice Screening and Mapping Tool: www.epa.gov/ejscreen
> - EnviroAtlas: www.epa.gov/enviroatlas
> - Freshwater Explorer: www.epa.gov/water-research/freshwater-explorer
> - Global Change Explorer: https://coast.noaa.gov/digitalcoast/tools/globalchange.html
> - How's My Waterway: https://mywaterway.epa.gov/
> - National Environmental Public Health Tracking: www.cdc.gov/nceh/tracking/index.html
> - Per- and Polyfluoroalkyl Substances (PFAS) Sites and Community Resources Map: https://experience.arcgis.com/experience/12412ab41b3141598e0bb48523a7c940/
> - Power Plants and Neighboring Communities: www.epa.gov/power-sector/power-plants-and-neighboring-communities
> - Smoke Sense: www.epa.gov/air-research/smoke-sense-study-citizen-science-project-using-mobile-app
> - Toxics Release Inventory: www.epa.gov/toxics-release-inventory-tri-program
> - Tree Equity Score: www.treeequityscore.org/
>
> Data sets that share demographic information, land-use information, or health information or other types of data may also be useful. Many local and state agencies also have their own data dashboards or tools that allow for decision-making based on more localized data.

Public health "surveillance" that relies on data has long been a vital component of public health, enabling us to understand emerging threats to health, healthcare disparities, gaps in services or amenities, and pollution hot spots, for instance. While data will always be an important element of this work for agencies and communities, Kassler and Bowman take into account our current realities and remind public health practitioners and researchers that words matter. The term *surveillance* originates from French, meaning *to watch over*, which in the context of public health refers to the practice of epidemiology. Yet for many people, surveillance carries negative associations, such as being monitored by security cameras or the police or having data collected for profit by big tech companies; authoritarian regimes especially have tools to both track and coerce behavior.[24] As such, environmental health practitioners and researchers must carefully navigate the promise of evidence-based decision-making, while ensuring public trust and respect for privacy and civil liberties.

With all of the available data in circulation today, a critical lens is necessary to evaluate and interpret it, of course. As a reminder, all models, and data that underlie them, rely on assumptions as a matter of necessity. Some of these assumptions are stronger than others, and some matter more than others. For example, as a methodological decision, the U.S. Census historically categorized people who identify as of Middle East and North African (MENA) descent as White; a decision contrary to the fact that many MENA Americans identify as people of color.[25] This means that any model that utilizes demographic data from the census may undercount people of color. Another concern is the time of day when data are collected: An engineer counting traffic at an intersection will get radically different numbers if they are counting during rush hour or at midnight, or during a weekend versus a weekday. Most models and data sources are up front about their assumptions and methodologies, and understanding these decisions are critical to evaluating data and deciding if they will work for you.

Data are ostensibly a representation of real life, but often there is a wide gap between lived experience and how data are used to inform policy and program interventions by environmental health practitioners. (Read more about regulatory science in Chapter 4.) Sometimes, inadequate data (or its collectors) are to blame when a critical variable is omitted, when an important question is not asked, or when a methodological assumption fails. For example, the U.S. EPA sets maximum safe thresholds for exposure to certain pollutants. However, when these standards are considered individually, they ignore cumulative impact or the impact of chemical stressors over time, generating a negative impact even when no individual pollutant rises above a level of concern. For decades, this has created a situation in which communities—most often communities of color or those with low wealth—are overburdened by pollution and experience higher healthcare costs, lower property values, and lower educational attainment. A recent example is the aftermath of the 2023 train derailment in East Palestine, Ohio, described in Chapter 1, which led to excessive amounts of toxic chemicals being expelled into the air and water; federal regulators claimed the danger had passed and conditions were safe, but many residents disagree, citing a litany of unexplained physical symptoms, including growths, gastrointestinal issues, and nosebleeds.[26] The EPA is now studying how to utilize cumulative impact assessments to better serve historically marginalized communities.[27]

Although many public health practitioners are eager to rely on data with good reason, we must also ask if more data are needed. Research studies that collect more data can be costly and time intensive but may be requested or conducted by communities themselves. A new study or more data may or may not actually address the questions that fenceline communities have.[28] Dr. Robert Bullard, who is widely recognized as the "father of EJ," highlights that communities of color in the United States can readily identify the sources of their environmental challenges, including highways, chemical plants, refineries, and long-standing pollution in their living spaces, air, water, and play areas. He points out that scientific research is beginning to acknowledge the intertwined nature of racial segregation and environmental pollution in America.[29] Even so, communities and agencies are still often tasked with "proving" environmental harm with statistical analyses before harms are addressed.

IN OTHER WORDS: DON'T FALL FOR IT . . .

These days environmental health practitioners have the added responsibility of countering misinformation and disinformation. There can even be what is known as an *infodemic*, which the World Health Organization defines as false or misleading information during the middle of an epidemic. This information can cause confusion and behaviors that can harm health and undermine public health efforts.

- **Infodemic:** A situation in which there is too much information, potentially including misinformation and disinformation, which leads to confusion about what protective actions to take.[30]
- **Misinformation:** The dissemination of inaccurate or misleading information that can change perceptions, influence behavior, and ultimately jeopardize the well-being of individuals and communities
- **Disinformation:** The intentional creation and spread of false or misleading information with the purpose of changing public opinion, often intentionally in order to trick people. Disinformation is different from misinformation because disinformation is created with the intention of deceiving others and not just by accident.

What can you do both as an individual and as an environmental health practitioner?[31]

- Individually:
  - look for red flags,
  - develop your media literacy skills, and
  - check your sources.

(continued)

> **IN OTHER WORDS: DON'T FALL FOR IT . . . (continued)**
> - As an environmental health practitioner:
>   - listen to individual and community concerns and questions,
>   - promote an understanding of correct health advice, and
>   - engage and empower individuals and communities to take positive action.

WORKING WITH COMMUNITIES

As mentioned earlier, a central value in this work is that people are the experts of their own experiences, which means that environmental public health must engage with communities, especially those most harmed by environmental exposures. In the face of these harms, communities often band together to advocate for shared interests. Groups can be formal or informal—ranging from a 501(c)(3) nonprofit organization to a Facebook group. They can be nation- or even planet-wide or hyperlocal, focusing on a particular city block. Sometimes they organize around ethnic or religious identity or simply a shared concern about a common resource. Ultimately, these groups, implicitly or explicitly, recognize that nobody will care about a neighborhood or community more than the people who live there. In fact, much of the work by government entities to address environmental injustice has happened because communities organized to demand it. Chapter 19, "Organizing for Environmental Health and Justice: Lessons From #StopGeneralIron," introduces the concept of community organizing in much greater detail using the story of #StopGeneralIron to illustrate the power of community.

In a representative democracy, policy makers are (at least theoretically) responsible to the electorate. But understanding their needs and desires is not always easy, particularly for larger constituencies. Although a city councillor may represent a few thousand or hundred thousand voters (already a large number), a senator may represent many millions. Furthermore, varying levels of government can have dramatically different capabilities to deal with particular issues. A state government will have a specific department tasked with environmental protection; that department will have hundreds or even thousands of employees with particular expertise; conversely, a local government may only have one employee responsible for sustainability or environmental protection, if any.

Regardless of the capabilities and resources of the agency where they work, many government-based environmental health practitioners have responsibility for facilitating public participation in their work. Public participation can produce more responsive, effective, and equitable policies and programs by identifying potential blindspots, pitfalls, and loopholes. It can even provide agencies the public backing to pursue interventions that may not be preferred by elected officials or those with conflicting interests.[32] We have seen this time and again when well-resourced corporate interests have denied the harms of tobacco or climate change, for instance, and science and public pressure enable or push agencies to act.

Public participation may take many different forms, for instance, such as engaging in zoning decisions or soliciting comments or feedback on policy or programmatic decisions. Many cities also maintain commissions or boards as opportunities for the general public to advise, participate in, and sometimes oversee priorities, projects, and policies. For example, Ann Arbor, Michigan, has maintained an environmental commission since 2001; the body is composed of 15 members of the public with two seats reserved specifically for youth members.[33]

The production, implementation, and evaluation of public policy can often be bureaucratic and confusing, even for those who have a role in influencing it, and environmental health practitioners can work with community leaders to demystify the policy process. Engaged and well-meaning residents may understandably face difficulties in understanding the responsibilities of various entities. For instance, it may be unclear whether a particular roadway is maintained by the city, county, or state or who issues permits required for a specific activity. It may not be clear who, if anyone, is responsible for keeping track of the data needed to understand a particular issue. Furthermore, most people have commitments to their jobs, communities, and families, which may limit their ability or time to actively pursue an issue.

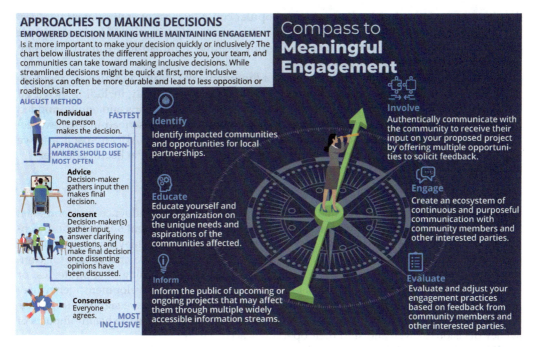

FIGURE 2.3. Approaches to making decisions and compass to meaningful engagement.
Source: U.S. Environmental Protection Agency. *Capacity building through effective meaningful engagement: a tool for local and state governments.* EPA 440B23001. September 21, 2023. https://www.epa.gov/system/files/documents/2023-09/epa-capacity-building-through-effective-meaningful-engagement-booklet_0.pdf. August Method from August Inc. *Empowered decision making.* https://www.aug.co/decision-making

Frameworks, tools, and resources are increasingly available to support environmental health practitioners in working toward meaningful public participation practices. This means government and community leaders must recognize and navigate underlying power dynamics or imbalances. Drawing from frameworks like Arnstein's "Ladder of Citizen Participation"[34] and the International Association of Public Participation (IAP2) spectrum,[35] environmental health practitioners can engage in meaningful ways that are not tokenistic or manipulative. Many governments have also moved beyond a consultative framework and incorporate community groups directly into the policy recommendation and creation process. For example, San Francisco organized the Blue Greenway Taskforce, a group of 16 public agencies and over 30 organizations and community groups in the San Francisco area, to develop a long-term vision and road map for implementing the "Blue Greenway," a 13-mile network of trails across San Francisco.[36] For any given decision, the group must be transparent and accountable about where the power lies and whether agency leaders are saying, "We will keep you informed," "We will consider your input," or "We will implement your decision." Chapter 14, "Healthy Communities for All," revisits this spectrum in a discussion of how we design healthy communities for all. Relatedly, in its efforts toward EJ, the EPA recently published guidance in *Capacity Building Through Effective Meaningful Engagement: A Tool for Local and State Governments.*[37] In it, they offer approaches to decision-making, strategies for relationship and trust building, and many examples (Figure 2.3).

WORKING TOWARD ENVIRONMENTAL HEALTH AND JUSTICE

Enormous progress has been made toward building a healthier, more equitable environment, particularly in the past 50 years. Landmark legislation like the Clean Air Act (1963) and the Clean Water Act (1972) created new, unprecedented tools for governments to clean up the world around us. Rivers catching fire were a common occurrence, such as in 1969 when the Cuyahoga River in Ohio, choked with debris and oil, ignited. This event caught the attention of the nation, leading to a new popular consciousness of environmental issues; but notably, this fire was not even the first one to occur in this specific river.[38] Federal support dramatically improved sewer systems, expanding treatment infrastructure and decreasing untreated discharges into waterways.[39]

As discussed in Chapter 1, "Fundamentals of Environmental Health and Justice," there are many ways we must strengthen our environmental health system today, including increased funding and a prepared workforce, as well as cross-sectoral partnerships and equity-minded policies and programs designed with fenceline communities.[35] As described in the next section, we can also continue to work toward a Health in All Policies (HiAP) approach, and we must continue to strive for anti-racist and anti-oppressive environmental health practice.

HEALTH IN ALL POLICIES

By this point, you probably know that the policies and practices that influence environmental health are not always explicitly packaged as such. A local government's information technology department may not perceive that it played a critical role in achieving environmental and climate justice. However, an updated, functional website can be a critical tool for communicating information about heating and cooling centers, flood mitigation strategies, or energy assistance programs to residents. Likewise, a state economic development agency may not perceive that prioritizing one type of business over another can have significant impacts on health and sustainability. Many governments are starting to realize the health impacts of agency decisions as well and shift their operations accordingly.

HiAP is an approach that seeks to identify and influence the health and equity impacts of policy decisions, to enhance health benefits, and to avoid harm.[40] While the scope of activities varies across jurisdictions, the integration of environmental public health into all operations is fundamental. Traditional barriers between different public health domains are becoming increasingly permeable as the interconnectedness between environmental factors and overall health is recognized. Whether it is through direct actions, like inspections and monitoring, or through indirect means, such as policy influence and community education, environmental public health functions are integral to the operations of public health. By adopting an Environmental Public Health in All Policies approach, we can ensure a cohesive and comprehensive public health strategy. This approach calls for the incorporation of environmental health considerations into all areas of governmental policy and practice, recognizing that a healthy environment is foundational to a healthy population. This view is multisectoral and recognizes that every government agency—be it economic development, public works, or finance—has a role to play in promoting health.

CASE STUDY 2.2: A New Health Department for Dearborn

In the 1950s, Dearborn, Michigan, began a campaign to expel the predominantly Arab immigrant population of the city's Southend neighborhood in favor of further industrial development. Weaponizing the language of public health, city hall criticized the poor-quality housing, significant air and water pollution, and proximity to industrial interests as a reason to move the residents, rather than to contain or further regulate the factories. It withheld building permits, then condemned homes in need of repair. In response, residents harnessed the experience of autoworkers who had fought long and sometimes bloody battles against car manufacturers; intent on protecting their neighborhoods, residents blocked streets frequented by heavy trucks, sued the city, and pressured businesses to clean up municipal spaces. Though it took years of litigation and came at the cost of dozens of homes, courts finally sided with residents, ordering the city to stop seizing properties, enforce air quality regulations, and reimburse homeowners.[41]

Today, Dearborn is a midsized city of approximately 110,000 residents and rich cultural diversity, with more than half of residents identifying as Middle Eastern or North African. As the hometown of Henry Ford and the Ford Motor Company, over the last century, the city has benefited from economic opportunities provided through automobile manufacturing and related

(continued)

> **CASE STUDY 2.2: A New Health Department for Dearborn** (*continued*)
>
> industries. However, with this legacy comes air, water, and noise pollution that greatly impacts environmental health for residents, particularly in the city's Southend, which is home to a large Yemeni population. Community groups have continuously advocated for environmental justice (EJ), and much more work is needed to address environmental health inequities.
>
> In 2022, Dearborn, Michigan, created a Department of Public Health with the goal of addressing the structural determinants of health and Health in All Policies (HiAP). This development has led to several new initiatives, including:
>
> - **Placement of 10 air quality monitors in partnership with JustAir, a Michigan-based startup:** Using a publicly available dashboard that is available in English and Arabic, residents can monitor air quality in realtime and sign up for alerts when the air quality reaches levels of concern.
> - **Increasing tree equity:** With various community and academic partners, the department is assessing gaps in tree equity across the city. They are working to identify policies, funding, and strategies for ensuring tree canopy that aligns with community priorities, while also supporting climate mitigation and adaptation efforts.
> - **Supporting enforcement of city ordinances:** With support from the department, the city of Dearborn sought legal action and reached a settlement with a local scrapyard over their excessive air pollution that violated the local fugitive dust ordinance. As a result, the company was required to invest more than $1 million in improved control measures.
> - **Participation in the Policy and Systems Change Academy:** Beginning in 2023, the department began working with the National League of Cities and the Urban Institute in their inaugural Policy and Systems Change Academy to accelerate work toward EJ. This work entails the identification and the root-cause analysis of the key environmental health challenges and work toward identifying promising and feasible policy solutions.
>
> More work is needed, but leaders in Dearborn know that a HiAP framework can help the city begin to address historic and systemic environmental injustice in a way that centers people and fosters cooperation across municipal departments and with the community.
>
> **REFLECTION QUESTIONS**
>
> *1. How did the historical struggle of Dearborn's Southend residents against industrial pollution and housing condemnation inform the city's current EJ initiatives?*
>
> *2. Evaluate the effectiveness of Dearborn's new Department of Public Health initiatives in addressing environmental health inequities, considering the historical context and current challenges.*

ANTI-RACISM AND ANTI-OPPRESSION IN ENVIRONMENTAL PUBLIC HEALTH PRACTICE

Acknowledging racism as a public health crisis should be more than a contemporary catchphrase, and environmental health practitioners have a role to play in addressing it. As discussed in Chapter 5, "Environmental Health Science for the People," many local agencies have made public declarations to address racism, and some have allocated resources, developed policies, and implemented interventions aimed at combating the root causes of racial disparities. Still more work is needed to acknowledge and confront the ingrained racism and White supremacy within the foundations of public health, healthcare research, and institutional practices, as well as other oppressive structures, such as ableism and sexism. This work entails:

- recognition of intersecting forms of discrimination and oppression based on race, ethnicity, gender, socioeconomic status, (dis)ability, and other factors;
- ongoing education of environmental health practitioners about structural determinants of health and how we can address them;
- supporting and amplifying leadership from fenceline communities; and
- critical examination of decision-making processes and resource distribution.[42]

Of course, we recognize that ongoing structural racism and many political factors may hinder these efforts, and in some states or communities this work may be more challenging. In particular, many parts of the United States have witnessed a sweeping movement to pass legislation that opposes use of public funds for diversity, equity, and inclusion initiatives.[43] This may mean, for instance, that state tax dollars cannot be used for related staff training or programming. In any case, environmental health practitioners can commit to an ongoing practice of learning, self-reflection, and accountability that reflects anti-racist and anti-oppressive values.

MAIN TAKEAWAYS

In this chapter, we learned that:

- Environmental health disparities are deeply rooted in historical discrimination and political neglect, not random or accidental occurrences.
- Structural racism in environmental public health manifests in disproportionate pollution burdens on communities of color, leading to unequal health outcomes.
- "Place" is a significant determinant of health, with ZIP codes often predicting health outcomes more accurately than genetic codes, especially in the context of environmental exposures.
- Effective environmental public health practice requires an interdisciplinary approach that includes addressing structural determinants of health.
- Environmental public health must be practiced with communities, recognizing that people are the experts of their own experiences.
- Data are essential in environmental public health, but data collection, analysis, and interpretation must be done with a critical lens.
- The integration of environmental health considerations into all public health policies is vital for a comprehensive and equitable approach to population health.

SUMMARY

This chapter examines how environmental public health works in practice, including the many opportunities and challenges that practitioners face in our current system. In particular, we examine governmental roles and responsibilities and note the many others involved in environmental health practice. In this chapter we begin by recognizing historical and systemic roots of current environmental health disparities before we learn about the field's essential services and functions that may be used to address these disparities. We also discuss the ways that data matter, but data are not the "be all and end all" of this work if we do not approach the data intentionally and with respect for different ways of knowing. Whether pursuing a career in environmental public health or a completely different field, we hope you can begin to see how environmental health is relevant across sectors and communities. As we confront climate change and the layers of environmental injustice present in modern society, we urge readers to recognize that we all have a role to play in ensuring environmental health and justice for all.

END-OF-CHAPTER RESOURCES

DISCUSSION QUESTIONS

1. Pick an environmental health or justice issue affecting a specific community. (You could consider some of the case studies you have already read in this textbook.) Using your example, explain how the 11 essential environmental public health functions are relevant to addressing this issue.

2. What is environmental federalism? What does it look like in the United States? What do you think are the advantages and disadvantages of this approach to protecting the environment?
3. How can environmental health practitioners in local government work with community members to promote environmental health? How might different approaches to public participation affect the outcomes?
4. As the authors state in this chapter, "Data are quickly becoming one of the most valuable commodities in the world." What does this mean in the context of environmental health? As knowledge production and dissemination grow exponentially and sharing of misinformation and disinformation continues, how can environmental health practitioners navigate these complexities?
5. In your own words, what is a HiAP approach? Use examples to explain what this approach might look like in practice.

LEARNING ACTIVITIES

THE TIME IS NOW

Make a list of all of your local elected officials. Do some research to see if they are leading any work to address local environmental health or justice issues. You might research the topics they campaigned on, review their social media, or look at meeting minutes for council meetings, for instance. Your research might address these questions:

- Are they working to address climate change?
- Are they proposing or implementing policies that could benefit from a HiAP approach?
- Are they working on the environment issues that concern you or your neighbors?

Once you have done this work, engage! This might look like:

- an email to thank them for the climate actions they are leading;
- public testimony to encourage local leaders to consider the health effects of infrastructure, zoning, or public works decisions (i.e., a HiAP approach); or
- a sign-on letter from you and other constituents asking them to adopt an issue you care about with specific proposed recommendations.

IN REAL LIFE

Funding for local environmental health programs varies greatly across the United States For instance, some state health agencies have programs to address climate change, and some do not. Many local health departments have programs to test for lead or radon in homes, and some do not. Do you know what environmental health resources or services exist to serve your community? Find out!

1. Go to your city, county, or regional health department website. (Note: Cities with large populations often have their own health department. Smaller communities may be supported by a county or regional department). Do they track and share environmental health data? Do they address:
   - climate change and health?
   - lead testing for children?
   - screening for child asthma or other environmentally-related illnesses?
   - restaurant inspections?
   - healthy childcare and school environments?
   - healthy homes?

- vector-borne diseases?
- occupational health?
- consumer products?
- contaminated land?
- other environmental health issues?

2. Go to your state health department website. Does it track and share environmental health data? Does it address:
   - climate change and health?
   - lead testing for children?
   - screening for child asthma or other environmentally related illnesses?
   - restaurant inspections?
   - healthy child care and school environments?
   - healthy homes?
   - vector-borne diseases?
   - occupational health?
   - consumer products?
   - contaminated land?
   - other environmental health issues?

A robust set of instructor resources designed to supplement this text is located at http://connect.springerpub.com/content/book/978-0-8261-8353-8. Qualifying instructors may request access by emailing textbook@springerpub.com.

REFERENCES

1. DeSalvo KB, Kadakia KT. Public health 3.0 after COVID-19—reboot or upgrade? *A J Public Health*. 2021;111(S3):S179–S181. doi:10.2105/ajph.2021.306501
2. Institute of Medicine (US) Committee on Assuring the Health of the Public in the 21st Century. Assuring America's Health. In *The Future of the Public's Health in the 21st Century*. National Academies Press; 2002. https://www.ncbi.nlm.nih.gov/books/NBK221233/
3. Jbaily A, Zhou X, Liu J, et al. Air pollution exposure disparities across US population and income groups. *Nature*. 2022;601(7892):228–233. doi:10.1038/s41586-021-04190-y
4. Gee GC, Ford CL. Structural racism and health inequities. *Du Bois Rev*. 2011;8(1):115–132. doi:10.1017/s1742058x11000130
5. Crenshaw K. Mapping the margins: intersectionality, identity politics, and violence against women of color. *Stanford Law Rev*. 1991;43(6):1241–1299. https://www.jstor.org/stable/1229039
6. Capatosto V. A brief history of civil rights in the United States: Jim Crow era. Howard University School of Law. June 3, 2020. Updated January 6, 2023. https://library.law.howard.edu/civilrightshistory/blackrights/jimcrow
7. Newkirk VR II. Environmental racism is the new Jim Crow. *The Atlantic*. June 5, 2017. https://www.theatlantic.com/video/index/529137/environmental-racism-is-the-new-jim-crow/
8. Nelson RK, Winling L, et al. Mapping inequality: redlining in New Deal America. Digital Scholarship Lab. 2023. Accessed June 14, 2024. https://dsl.richmond.edu/panorama/redlining
9. Taylor D. The state of diversity in environmental organizations mainstream NGOs foundations government agencies. July 2014. https://orgs.law.harvard.edu/els/files/2014/02/FullReport_Green2.0_FINALReducedSize.pdf
10. Green 2.0. 2023 NGO & foundation transparency report. 2023. Accessed June 14, 2024. https://diversegreen.org/wp-content/uploads/green2.0-2023-report-card.pdf
11. Sahagun L. EPA officers sickened by fumes at South L.A. oil field. *Los Angeles Times*. November 9, 2013. https://www.latimes.com/local/la-me-1109-fumes-20131109-story.html
12. Patnaik A, Son J, Feng A, Ade C. Racial disparities and climate change. Princeton Student Climate Initiative. August 15, 2020. https://psci.princeton.edu/tips/2020/8/15/racial-disparities-and-climate-change

13. Graham GN. Why your ZIP code matters more than your genetic code: promoting healthy outcomes from mother to child. *Breastfeed Med*. 2016;11(8):396–397. doi:10.1089/bfm.2016.0113
14. Life expectancy: could where you live influence how long you live? Robert Wood Johnson Foundation. 2023. Accessed June 14, 2024. https://www.rwjf.org/en/insights/our-research/interactives/whereyouliveaffectshowlongyoulive.html
15. Shkembi A, Smith LM, Neitzel RL. Linking environmental injustices in Detroit, MI to institutional racial segregation through historical federal redlining. *J Expo Sci Environ Epidemiol*. Published online December 21, 2022. doi:10.1038/s41370-022-00512-y
16. Environmental health playbook: investing in a robust environmental health system. Executive Summary: Background and Need for Action. APHA. Accessed June 14, 2024. https://apha.org/-/media/Files/PDF/topics/environment/EH_Playbook.ashx
17. Summary of the Clean Air Act. U.S. Environmental Protection Agency. September 12, 2022. Updated September 6, 2023. https://www.epa.gov/laws-regulations/summary-clean-air-act
18. City of Minneapolis. Models of city government. Accessed June 14, 2024. https://lims.minneapolismn.gov/Download/FileV2/23033/ModelsofCityGovernment.pdf
19. EGLE, Michigan Department of Environment, Great Lakes, and Energy. Request for Information on using State Energy Financing Institution (SEFI) Funds to leverage federal loans for clean energy. 2023. https://www.michigan.gov/egle/-/media/Project/Websites/egle/Documents/Forms/EXE/OCE/EQP1157-RFI-on-using-SEFI-Funds-to-Leverage-Federal-Loans-for-Clean-Energy.pdf
20. 10 Essential Public Health Services. Centers for Disease Control and Prevention. 2021. Updated September 18, 2023. https://www.cdc.gov/publichealthgateway/publichealthservices/essentialhealthservices.html
21. Sánchez-Rivera A I, Jacobs P, Spence C. A look at the largest American Indian and Alaska Native Tribes and villages in the Nation, Tribal areas and states. U.S. Census Bureau. October 3, 2023. Accessed June 14, 2024. https://www.census.gov/library/stories/2023/10/2020-census-dhc-a-aian-population.html
22. Environmental health. Ho-Chunk Nation | Department of Health. Accessed June 14, 2024. https://health.ho-chunk.com/EnvironmentalHealth/index.html
23. Henry J, Kushwaha A, Lico A. Stories from the field: The White Earth Nation. *Centers for Disease Control and Prevention Conversations in Equity blog*. March 17, 2022. https://blogs.cdc.gov/healthequity/2022/03/17/stories-from-the-field-the-white-earth-nation
24. Kassler WJ, Bowman C. Overcoming public health "surveillance": when words matter. *Am J Public Health*. 2023;113(10):1102–1105. doi:10.2105/ajph.2023.307348
25. Office of Management and Budget. Revisions to the standards for the classification of federal data on race and ethnicity. *Federal Register*. 1997;62(210):58782–58790. https://www.govinfo.gov/content/pkg/FR-1997-10-30/pdf/97-28653.pdf
26. Andrews E. 1 year after the toxic train derailment, is East Palestine safe? Depends on whom you ask. *Grist*. January 18, 2024. https://grist.org/accountability/is-east-palestine-safe-depends-who-you-ask
27. Cumulative impacts research. US EPA. January 27, 2022. Updated January 11, 2024. https://www.epa.gov/healthresearch/cumulative-impacts-research#Agency%20Directive
28. Scammell M, Howard G, Ames J, et al. Is a health study the answer for your community? A guide for making informed decisions with contributions from. HSG Guide Version 1.2. 2015. http://www.bu.edu/sph/files/2015/03/HSG_5-14-2015_nocover.pdf
29. Tabuchi H, Popovich N. People of color breathe more hazardous air. The sources are everywhere. *The New York Times*. April 28, 2021. https://www.nytimes.com/2021/04/28/climate/air-pollution-minorities.html
30. Infodemic. World Health Organization. 2021. Accessed June 14, 2024. https://www.who.int/health-topics/infodemic#tab=tab_1
31. UCSF Health. Evaluating health information. March 14, 2019. https://www.ucsfhealth.org/education/evaluating-health-information
32. Office of Management and Budget. Memorandum for the heads of executive departments and agencies. July 19, 2023. https://www.whitehouse.gov/wp-content/uploads/2023/07/Broadening-Public-Participation-and-Community-Engagement-in-the-Regulatory-Process.pdf
33. Sustainability-related boards and commissions. City of Ann Arbor. Accessed June 14, 2024. https://www.a2gov.org/departments/sustainability/about/Pages/Sustainability-Related-Boards-and-Commissions-.aspx

34. Arnstein SR. A ladder of citizen participation. *J Am Inst Planners*. 1969;35(4):216–224. doi:10.1080/01944366908977225
35. IAP2 spectrum of public participation. Involve. Accessed June 14, 2024. https://www.involve.org.uk/resources/knowledge-base/what/what-public-participation
36. Office of the Mayor: City and County of San Francisco. Blue Greenway task force: vision and roadmap to implementation. July 26, 2006. https://www.sfparksalliance.org/sites/default/files/Blue-Greenway-Vision-and-Roadmap-to-Implementation.pdf
37. U.S. Environmental Protection Agency. Capacity building through effective meaningful engagement: a tool for local and state governments. EPA 440B23001. 2023. https://www.epa.gov/system/files/documents/2023-09/epa-capacity-building-through-effective-meaningful-engagement-booklet_0.pdf
38. The 1969 Cuyahoga River fire. National Park Service. Updated May 3, 2022. https://www.nps.gov/articles/story-of-the-fire.htm
39. U.S. Environmental Protection Agency. Report to congress on impacts and control of combined sewer overflows and sanitary sewer overflows. Fact Sheet. August 2004. https://www.epa.gov/sites/default/files/2015-10/documents/csossortc2004_full.pdf
40. Green L, Ashton K, Bellis MA, Clemens T, Douglas M. "Health in all policies"—a key driver for health and well-being in a post-COVID-19 pandemic world. *Int J Environ Res Public Health*. 2021;18(18):9468. doi:10.3390/ijerph18189468
41. Howell S. Southend struggles: converging narratives of an Arab/Muslim American enclave. *Mashriq & Mahjar*. 2015;3(1):66–105. https://muse.jhu.edu/article/779789/pdf
42. Wilkins D, Schulz AJ. Antiracist research and practice for environmental health: implications for community engagement. *Environ Health Perspect*. 2023;131(5). doi:10.1289/ehp11384
43. Jackson A, Yerena A, Lee CA, et al. Anti-racist futures: disrupting racist planning practices in workplaces, institutions, and communities. *J Am Plan Assoc*. 2023;89(4):411–422. doi:10.1080/01944363.2023.2244850

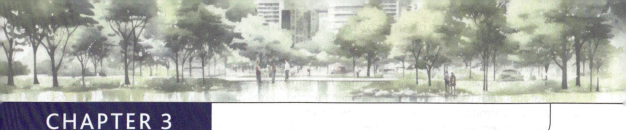

CHAPTER 3

Confronting the Realities of Climate Change

Natasha DeJarnett, Viniece Jennings, and Neha Pathak

LEARNING OBJECTIVES

- Describe the science of climate change.
- Describe current climate realities and the environmental impacts of climate change.
- Identify the physical and mental health impacts of climate change.
- Determine injustice in the environmental and health burdens of climate change.
- Consider many ways to protect health and equity in the reality of climate change.
- Identify climate interventions with population-health and community-resilience benefits.

KEY TERMS

- climate change
- climate and health adaptation
- climate justice
- climate mitigation
- climate resilience
- urban heat island effect

OVERVIEW

The science on **climate change** demonstrates that the issue is clear and well established.[1] An increase in the atmospheric concentration of greenhouse gasses (e.g., carbon dioxide) and aerosols are factors involved in changes in the climate system.[2] As a result, climate models project that a continued increase in temperature variability, particularly in tropical locations, is concerning for the coming decades.[3] Although often referred to as global warming, the impacts of climate change include consequences such as impaired air quality, extreme heat, extreme flooding, sea level rise, drought, and wildfires.[1,4] Although climate change is experienced globally, the impacts are felt differently by region and even by community.

Climate change has been defined as the *greatest global health challenge of this century*.[5] This designation implies that climate change not only degrades the environment, but it also compromises the economy, harms health, and worsens inequities. For example, the link between climate change and the intensity of extreme heat events is a major public health concern.[6] The **urban heat island effect** occurs when impervious surfaces and other infrastructure (e.g., buildings) absorb and reemit solar energy, leading to higher temperatures.[7] The urban heat island effect, an aging population, and a warming climate are future drivers of heat-related mortality.[6] During a large-scale study on heat-related mortality and climate, scholars observed that over 30% of heat-related deaths could be attributed to climate change on every continent.[8] Climate change also poses a risk to water sanitation services through reduced water resources, decreased rainfall, flooding, damage to infrastructure, as well as changes in water quality.[9] Climate change negatively impacts the amount or quantity of water that is available in different locations. To illustrate, climate change can negatively impact the sources of groundwater, the treatment of surface water, sanitation, and the water supply.[9]

The climate system has significant impacts with major economic implications on various sectors of society, including agriculture, tourism, healthcare, and real estate.[10] Projections suggest that each 1°C increase in global mean temperatures can cost approximately 1.2% of gross domestic product.[11] These temperature increases affect the processes and mediators within different sectors. For example, climate change directly affects agricultural production, as it is susceptible to weather. Climate change can alter crop yields, land area, international trade, and consumption.[12] Sea level rise also has economic effects, such as damage to coastal areas, incurring direct costs and impacting landscapes.[13] The impacts of climate change extend to potential costs from infrastructure damage caused by severe flooding, degradation of paved surfaces, increased maintenance, and limited aircraft performance.[14] Moreover, the unequal distribution of the economic burden of climate change further exacerbates economic inequality, impacting health, overall quality of life, and financial stability.[11]

This chapter aims to provide a scientific understanding of climate change and its impacts on the environment, physical and mental health, and justice. It will explore the many ways that specific populations are currently being affected or are likely to be affected in the future. In particular, it examines the systemic factors that contribute to increased vulnerability, impacts, and disparities, highlighting the need for programmatic and policy interventions. The chapter also analyzes case studies of communities impacted by fossil fuel extraction, displacement, and extreme events. Finally, the chapter provides examples of solutions that promote both health and equity.

CLIMATE CHANGES HEALTH

Climate change harms physical and mental health by decreasing the quality of the air we breathe and increasing the frequency and intensity of extreme heat events, extreme weather, precipitation extremes (flooding and drought), and wildfires, along with increasing our exposure to disease-carrying vectors (insects and ticks). In addition to the direct impacts on physical health, climate change also poses significant threats to mental well-being. The psychological toll of witnessing and experiencing extreme weather events, along with the disruption of communities and livelihoods, can lead to a variety of mental health issues. As climate change continues to unfold, understanding its complex interplay with both physical and mental health is essential for developing holistic strategies to mitigate the adverse effects.

AIR QUALITY

The burning of fossil fuels releases harmful air toxins and climate-harming greenhouse gasses into the atmosphere. Greenhouse gasses are the drivers of climate change, a global phenomenon that can further decrease air quality locally and globally. Greenhouse gasses in the atmosphere can lead to increasing and longer periods of heat, similar to how a blanket traps heat. Toxic pollutants in the air can undergo further chemical reactions in the presence of this heat to worsen air quality. Climate change also facilitates conditions that enhance the likelihood of exposure to wildfire smoke, elevated pollen levels, extreme heat, and flood conditions that produce mold—all further decreasing the quality of the air we breathe.[15-18]

Exposure to fossil-fuel-related air pollution is associated with adverse effects to every major organ system in the human body, leading to a number of health conditions, especially those related to respiratory and cardiovascular disease.[19,20] However, these health conditions are not the only impacts of exposure to air pollution. Air pollution increases the risk of diabetes, chronic kidney disease, early onset Crohn's and ulcerative colitis, fatty liver disease, and gastric and liver cancers. Low birth weight, preterm birth, stillbirth, and congenital heart disease are among the reproductive and developmental impacts of exposure to fossil-fuel-related air pollution.[19,20] Neurologic and psychiatric outcomes linked with climate-harming air pollutants include stroke, dementia, Parkinson disease, anxiety, depression, suicide, and adverse sleep effects.[19,20] See Chapter 10, "The Air We Breathe," for more discussion of the health effects of air pollution.

EXTREME HEAT

Longer seasons of warmer temperatures contribute to heat waves that occur with increased frequency and intensity. In the United States, decades of long-increased temperatures correlate with increases in heat-related health impacts.[15] Heat is associated with more deaths than any other natural weather-related disasters in the United States.[21] The immediate impacts of extreme heat can include heat-related illnesses, such as heat stress, heat exhaustion, and heat stroke. Extreme heat is also linked with adverse respiratory, cardiovascular, diabetic and renal, reproductive, and mental health outcomes.[15] In addition, heat health risks can be exacerbated when using medications that manage certain cardiovascular and mental health conditions.[15]

> **DIG DEEPER: CLIMATE CHANGE AND HEAT STROKE**
>
> Climate change is increasing exposure to extreme heat events, which can heighten the likelihood of heat-related illness. Heat stroke occurs when the body is unable to control its temperature and is the most serious heat-related illness. Heat stroke can be deadly if emergency attention is not received promptly.

CASE STUDY 3.1: 1995 Chicago Heat Wave

In July 1995, the residents of Chicago, Illinois, experienced a heat wave with temperatures soaring above 100°F (37.8°C) for five consecutive days. During and immediately following this extreme heat event, local authorities estimated that almost 700 people lost their lives owing to the extreme heat.[22] However, it is important to note that the exact number of deaths is an estimate, as the records at the time may not have specified heat as a cause or related cause of death. For example, heat stress could have led to respiratory distress or a heart attack, which would have been noted on a death certificate.

Although heat-related deaths are often less visible than other extreme weather events, they are among the most deadly. Media coverage highlighted this horrific reality. The Cook County Medical Examiner's Office was overwhelmed and used temporary refrigerated storage to manage the increased demands on their office.[23]

There were several lessons learned from this experience. In hindsight, many people criticized the mayor and city officials for delayed recognition of the severity of the events and their failure to establish proper infrastructure to address power outages and provide safe cooling centers.[22] Later analyses of the event revealed the disproportionate impacts on certain individuals and neighborhoods, particularly African Americans, older adults, socially isolated individuals, and those facing economic disadvantages.[23]

The Chicago Heat Wave of 1995 was a significant public health event as it motivated the city and many others to rethink their extreme heat preparedness and response plans. At that time, few cities had such plans in place, and even fewer had climate action plans that addressed heat.[24] Cities have increased their preparedness and response plans since 1995, but heat waves are becoming more common and intense in both duration and in temperature extremes. In 2022, around 1,700 deaths in the United States were due to heat-related causes.[25]

Several articles, books, and films have been developed to document the Chicago Heat Wave and its significance, including:

- Klinenberg E. *Heat Wave: A Social Autopsy of Disaster in Chicago.* 2nd ed. University of Chicago Press; 2015.
- Helfand J, Dir. *Cooked: Survival by Zip Code* [Documentary]. 2018.

REFLECTION QUESTIONS

1. Extreme heat is associated with many acute and chronic health issues. Why do many overlook the potential severity of extreme heat's health effects?

2. How might cities ensure that their response to extreme weather events is equitable and just, considering the health disparities revealed by the 1995 Chicago Heat Wave?

EXTREME WEATHER

Climate change is increasing the frequency and intensity of extreme weather events. Warmer water can increase the intensity of hurricanes. Further, warmer air, which holds more water, can intensify precipitation and flooding,[26] thus exacerbating extreme weather impacts. Extreme weather puts communities in direct threat of physical danger and can also harm mental wellness. Injuries can result from encounters with projectiles and debris during hurricanes and coastal storms.[26] Extreme weather can also disrupt access to needed medical services through impacted infrastructure (e.g., roads and transportation systems, power systems, and telecommunications services). Further, experiences with extreme weather are associated with an increased risk of stress, anxiety, depression, and posttraumatic stress disorder (PTSD).[27] In addition, extreme weather can displace populations, disrupting social ties and community cohesion needed to support mental health.

FLOODING

Heavy precipitation events have increased in the United States over recent decades. Floods are second to heat in deadly weather-related hazards in the United States.[28–31] Flooding can harm well-being in many ways:

- Similar to extreme weather, flooding poses physical health risks related to drowning, exposure to debris, and injury and death due to trauma.[32]
- Flooding can further compound hazardous exposures caused by drinking water contamination through stormwater overflows, where untreated sewer water can breach the drinking water supply and recreational waters. This contamination can expose populations to harmful bacteria, increasing the risk of gastrointestinal illness from norovirus, *Escherichia coli*, salmonella, and shigella.[20] Contaminated waters can also reach agricultural lands, and toxic water from flooded industrial sources can reach residential areas.
- Flooding events can also increase the risk of vector-borne infectious diseases. Floodwaters can provide breeding grounds for vectors, such as mosquitoes, increasing the risk of exposure to vector-borne illness.[32]
- Flooding that reaches indoor spaces can result in indoor mold growth, which can exacerbate asthma, trigger allergic reactions, and irritate the upper respiratory tract.[32]
- Flooding can cause the loss or destruction of property. This destruction can result in financial hardship and related stress, as well as displacement. Particularly for areas with recurrent or catastrophic floods, displacement disrupts social ties, social cohesion, and social capital. These consequences are often linked to negative mental health consequences, such as increased stress and anxiety.[32]

IN OTHER WORDS: DEFINING "PSYCHOTERRATIC" TERMS

The awareness and internalization of climate change can lead to *psychoterratic syndromes* linked with hopelessness and despair.[33,34]

Eco-Anxiety: prolonged fear of the irreversible environmental consequences of climate change for current and future generations.[35]

Eco-Paralysis: emotional distress characterized by feelings of hopelessness, apathy, and powerlessness to effectively mitigate climate harms.[36]

Solastalgia: distress related to the observable environmental consequences of climate change in or near one's home environment.[37,38]

SEA LEVEL RISE

Coastal communities face the threat of sea level rise, a slow-onset disaster that can compound risks to physical and mental health.[15] In addition to coastal erosion, sea level rise can render areas uninhabitable, causing the forced permanent displacement of communities.[20] Coastal sea rise causes increased salt content in groundwater and well water.[32] Increased salt levels in drinking water are associated with increased blood pressure,[39] increased risk of kidney disease,[40] and preeclampsia.[32,41] Sea level rise can also contribute to food insecurity through increased salt content in soil and poor agricultural production, including decreased crop yield.[32] Agricultural risks also pose an economic burden to agricultural communities and other groups with close economic ties to the land.[32] Communities with livelihoods tied to the land may experience mental health burdens associated with the gradual threat of sea level rise, and the impacts may be exacerbated by lost jobs, economic difficulties, and the inability to meet basic needs.[33] Further, due to the gradual nature of sea level rise, populations facing this existential threat can experience eco-anxiety, eco-paralysis, and solastalgia,[33] thus adding to the mental health burden of sea level rise.

Sea level rise can disrupt access to critical infrastructure through causing damage or destruction to buildings, roads, and public services. Among many impacts to health and safety, infrastructure destruction to roadway and transportation systems can hinder access to medical services in emergencies.[20,32] Storm surges exacerbated by sea level rise can overwhelm water management systems, including drinking water and wastewater treatment facilities.[42] Flooding from sea level rise and storm surges can contaminate drinking water supplies, increase the risk of vector-borne and waterborne diseases, and lead to mold growth.[32]

DROUGHT

According to the U.S. Global Change Research Program, over the last four decades, drought has contributed to the second-highest number of climate-related deaths in the United States among weather and climate disasters and has resulted in over one billion dollars in economic losses.[15] Further, drought facilitates conditions conducive to wildfires that cause community destruction, worsen air quality, and increase the likelihood of morbidity and mortality. Drought increases the risk of heat-related deaths, exacerbations of cardiovascular and respiratory diseases, and premature death. Drought also impacts the agricultural sector affecting food access, safety, and security. Drought can impair water security due to decreased water quantity, quality, and safety. Water insecurity can result in increased exposure to harmful bacteria, toxic heavy metals, and other contaminants.[15] Further, communities with close economic ties to the land can experience a heavy mental toll from drought. For example, suicide rates doubled during a record drought in the Midwest in the 1980s, including among many farmers.[43]

WILDFIRES

Climate conditions, particularly that of rising temperatures and hotter, drier summers, increase the occurrence, prevalence, and future projections of wildfires.[42] Over recent decades, the wildfire season has expanded and is producing wildfires that have more intensity, are larger in geographic size, and have longer durations.[44] In fact, the wildfire season has grown 20 to 40 days longer over the last four decades.[45] Wildfires pose critical risks to infrastructure (including energy transmission and transportation systems); can destroy the built[46] environment (including buildings and community features); threaten water supplies; enhance risks to ecosystems through vector, habitat, and vegetation changes[15]; disrupt cultural practices tied to the land; and displace populations.[42] Wildfires can also significantly contribute to greenhouse gas emissions, further exacerbating the risk of future fires in a vicious feedback loop.[46] The health threats of wildfires include smoke inhalation, burns and other traumatic injuries, respiratory exacerbations, and mental health impacts.[42]

Wildfires decrease air quality, including releasing particulate matter (PM), ozone, volatile organic compounds (VOCs), carbon monoxide (CO), nitrogen dioxide, polycyclic aromatic hydrocarbons (PAHs), and toxic chemicals into the air. These air pollutants can travel far from the actual wildfire. Smoke from Canadian wildfires in Quebec in 2002 were linked with a 30-fold increase in fine PM ($PM_{2.5}$) nearly 1,000 miles away in Baltimore, Maryland.[42] The long-range transport of wildfire smoke was also demonstrated in 2021 and 2023, when smoke from western U.S. and Canadian wildfires significantly elevated fine PM (PM$_{2.5}$) levels across the northeastern United States.[47,48] The pollutants of smoke burning from wildfires in North America have even been detected as far as Europe and China.[48,49] Wildfires are associated with cardiovascular[50] and respiratory exacerbations like asthma and chronic obstructive pulmonary disease (COPD),[16] adverse birth outcomes, and premature death.

VECTOR CHANGES

Climate change is expanding the geographic distribution and location of disease-carrying vectors, including mosquitoes and ticks. Warmer temperatures, longer warm seasons, and shorter cold seasons are creating environments more conducive to the growth and proliferation of vectors, and thereby vector-borne diseases. Vectors are organisms that can transmit a pathogen from one host to another. In the United States, vector-borne diseases related to climate change are increasing, including increases in Lyme disease transmission from ticks and West Nile virus from mosquitoes.[20] Malaria, which has not been seen as a locally acquired disease in the United States for over 20 years, also reemerged in 2023 with nine cases in Florida, Texas, and Maryland.[51]

ZOONOTIC DISEASES

Due to climate change, animal habitats are experiencing significant changes, leading to increased interactions between humans and wildlife as well as between different types of wildlife. This interaction can raise both the incidence of vector-borne diseases with animal hosts as well as zoonotic disease spillover, which occurs when there is transmission of infectious diseases from animals to humans. Examples of past spillover events include simian immunodeficiency virus making a jump to humans in the form of HIV, the Ebola virus that is believed to have originated in bats, the monkeypox virus thought to have originated in small mammals, and a variety of coronaviruses, including SARS-CoV-2, that are believed to also have a reservoir in bats.[52] These zoonotic transmissions are only going to increase in the future with a changing climate. An estimated 4,000 cross-species transmission events are projected for the year 2070 based on climate change and geographic shifts in mammal habitats.[52] As discussed in more detail in Chapter 1, "Fundamentals of Environmental Health and Justice," a One Health approach is necessary for mitigating zoonotic disease threats.

MENTAL HEALTH

Mental health and well-being are adversely affected by climate change. Anxiety, depression, grief, PTSD, stress, and substance use are associated with exposure to poor air quality, extreme heat, extreme weather, flooding, sea level rise, drought, wildfires, and vector changes. Factors that contribute to the mental health burden can include displacement, discrimination, and economic insecurity that can result from climate impacts. Further, specific populations may be at a higher risk, including children, older adults, and people of color. The mental health impacts associated with climate exposures are shown in Figure 3.1.[20]

IN OTHER WORDS: ECO-ANXIETY

Eco-anxiety means that someone may feel worry, fear, or stress from environmental issues related to climate change. The feelings can be caused by how big the problems are and by how they lead to unknowns and to uncertainty about the future. *Eco-paralysis*, a feeling of being overwhelmed and powerless to take action, can occur as a result of eco-anxiety. Finally, *solastalgia* is the emotional pain caused by seeing one's home environment destroyed through changes in the land, by the loss of plant and animal diversity, and by changes in ecosystems. These terms all highlight the human connection to the environment and the mental toll of climate change and degradation.

Effects of Climate Changes on Mental Health

Air Quality
- ADHD (children), adverse sleep effects, anxiety, autism, dementia (including Alzheimer disease), depression, long-term intellectual disabilities (children), Parkinson disease, reduced cognition (children), suicide,[20] and anxiety and depressive outcomes of asthma and cardiovascular disease[53]
- Contributing factors: Air pollution and inflammatory cell damage, discrimination, physical illness

Extreme Heat
- Aggressive behaviors, anxiety, dementia, mood disorders, medication interaction, suicide[27]
- Contributing factors: discrimination, economic instability, physical illness

Extreme Weather
- Anxiety, depression, grief, PTSD, stress, substance use, suicidal ideation and suicide, violence[27]
- Contributing factors: Discrimination, displacement; loss of loved ones, property, and social structures; social capital; trauma

Flooding
- Behavioral problems (children), depression, anxiety, grief, PTSD, stress[27]
- Contributing factors: Discrimination, displacement, economic insecurity, social cohesion

Sea Level Rise
- Helplessness, eco-anxiety, eco-paralysis, persistent worry, solastalgia[33,54]
- Contributing factors: Displacement, economic insecurity, landscape changes

Drought
- Anxiety, depression, stress, suicide[54]
- Contributing factors: Displacement, economic insecurity, landscape changes

Wildfires
- Adverse sleep effects (children), anxiety (children), behavioral problems, depression, grief, panic attacks (children), psychotic disorders (children), PTSD, stress, substance abuse[54]
- Contributing factors: Displacement, economic insecurity

Vector-Borne Disease
- Mental health outcomes related to Lyme disease (anorexia nervosa, bipolar disorder, dementia, depression, paranoia, obsessive-compulsive disorder, panic attacks, schizophrenia),[55] encephalitis (aggression, anxiety, depression),[56,57] hantavirus (memory impairment),[58] and chikungunya (depression, mood disorders[59])[53]
- Contributing factors: Healthcare access, disease progression

FIGURE 3.1. Mental health impacts associated with climate exposures.
ADHD, attention deficit hyperactivity disorder; PTSD, posttraumatic stress disorder.

CLIMATE CHANGES VULNERABILITY

All people are at risk for the health threats of climate change; however, some populations can be more susceptible, whether by biology (children, pregnant people, older adults, and people with preexisting illness), due to disproportionate exposures (communities of color, Indigenous Peoples, and certain occupational groups), or through societal factors that can hinder adaptation (people living with disabilities, rural communities, LGBTQIA2S+ people, and people experiencing homelessness).[20]

CHILDREN

Children's health is especially sensitive to climate impacts. Data from the World Health Organization reveals that 88% of the global burden of climate change falls on children under age five.[60] As discussed in more detail in Chapter 17, "Ensuring Children's Environmental Health and Justice," children bear added susceptibility to environmental hazards, including climate change, owing to a number of factors related to their size, behaviors, and development.

Poor air quality increases children's risk of asthma incidence and exacerbations. Children are also more susceptible to the increasing incidence of vector-borne and other diseases due to climate change. One such disease is La Crosse encephalitis, which is transmitted by mosquitoes and primarily affects children under the age of 16. With longer, hotter warm seasons, climate change also increases the risk of heat-related illness, including heat exhaustion and heat stroke, due in part to their physiology as well as behaviors. Children under age two have underdeveloped thermoregulatory controls.[61] Children's reliance on adults to make decisions in the best interest of their well-being could leave them at risk of dehydration and overexposure to heat without being provided water or a cool environment.[61] Adolescents and young athletes risk overexerting themselves during extreme heat events. In fact, heat stroke is the third-highest cause of death among high school athletes.[61] Further, children depend on adults for their safety and well-being during exposure to extreme weather and flooding, and these events can also affect their health due to displacement and injury.[20]

PREGNANT PEOPLE

Pregnant people bear a unique burden from poor air quality, extreme heat, extreme weather, flooding, drought, and vector-borne disease that result from climate change. These climate impacts increase the likelihood of respiratory disease, heat-related illness, undernutrition, infectious disease, maternal stress, and poverty among pregnant people.[62] These adverse impacts also affect children in utero, and are associated with preterm delivery, gestational hypertension, intrauterine growth retardation, and low birth weight.[62] Climate change increases exposure to infectious disease-carrying vectors, which can increase the risk of congenital defects.[62] For example, infants born to pregnant people who contracted the Zika virus during pregnancy are at risk of microcephaly, central nervous system abnormalities, and impaired cognitive function.[62,63] Consider also the severity of disease in pregnant people exposed to disease-carrying vectors, where pregnant people are three times more likely to have severe malaria when compared to those who are not pregnant.[63] Climate-harming air pollutants, like carbon dioxide, can cross the placental barrier and impact fetal health.[62] In utero exposure to climate impacts is also associated with long-term effects in children, including allergic rhinitis, attention deficit hyperactivity disorder (ADHD), asthma, autism spectrum disorder, cardiovascular diseases, congenital heart diseases, diabetes mellitus, eczema, impaired cognitive function, metabolic diseases, and mood disorders.[63]

OLDER ADULTS

Older adults are more susceptible to extreme heat exposure due to impaired thermoregulatory control. Additionally, they are at a higher risk of experiencing weakened immune system responses, making them more susceptible to bacterial infections such as *Vibrio*, which thrives in warmer water. Furthermore, weakened immune systems make exposure to contaminated water due to flooding and exposure to vector-borne diseases riskier. Various social factors, such as limited mobility, social isolation, and economic insecurity, further increase their susceptibility. Older adults also are more likely to have a preexisting illness, which can compound their sensitivity to climate hazards.[20]

PEOPLE LIVING WITH PREEXISTING ILLNESS

People living with a preexisting illness bear heightened sensitivity to the health impacts of climate change, including cardiovascular disease,[64] diabetes,[65] and respiratory ailments.[19] Medications for hypertension and depression are associated with an increased risk of heat-related illness and dehydration. As such, people with certain psychiatric conditions may have impaired thermoregulation, putting them at increased risk of complications during extreme heat events.[20,66,67]

COMMUNITIES OF COLOR

Communities of color are identity-based communities populated primarily by people that identify as Black or African American, Hispanic or Latino, Indigenous or Native American (see "Indigenous Communities"), Asian, Pacific Islander, and multiracial.[20,68,69] Although race is a social construct and not scientific, social structures often render communities of color more susceptible to the health harms of climate change. The prevalence of systemic disempowerment fuels disproportionate hazardous exposures in communities of color, where it is well established that race is the predominant predictor of the location of toxic facilities, with all races assessed being significantly correlated (African American, Hispanic or Latino, and Asians/Pacific Islanders),[70,71] leaving communities of color with a higher burden of air toxin exposure,[72] as well as a higher threat of toxic exposures during climate events, such as flooding.[20,73] Communities of color generally bear disproportionate exposures to climate hazards and often experience higher burdens of social and health factors that amplify their susceptibility. Climate change exacerbates stressors experienced by communities of color that have been marginalized by pollution, underinvestment, and disproportionate adverse health outcomes.

As discussed in several chapters, redlining was one of many historic racist practices used to segregate communities. Though now illegal, this biased practice of denying certain people access to home loans has had lasting impacts affecting health and wealth in communities of color today.[74] In fact, communities that were formerly redlined continue to experience environmental disparities related to climate change, such as air quality,[75] exposure to heat events,[76] and flooding risk,[77] and have less access to environmental protective features, including tree canopy[78] and green space.[79] Thus, formerly redlined communities have demonstrated disproportionate associations with multiple serious adverse health outcomes, including asthma, diabetes, hypertension, heat-related illness, and preterm birth.[80]

People of color are more likely to live in areas with higher surface urban heat island intensity.[81] Mortality risk associated with rising temperatures is higher among African Americans, Hispanic or Latino Americans, and Native Americans.[69,82] Extreme weather reveals disproportionate flooding risk and recovery resources for communities of color,[69] along with poorer mental health outcomes, including a greater association with PTSD in African Americans following Hurricane Katrina[83,84] and Hurricane Harvey.[85] African Americans also have experienced higher respiratory hospitalization risk associated with wildfire exposure.[69,86]

INDIGENOUS COMMUNITIES

Native American and Indigenous communities have close cultural ties to the land, including engaging in traditional food culture as well as religious traditions. The effects of climate change impede participation in these practices for the current generation and hinder the ability to gather and prepare traditional food and share culturally sacred traditions with future generations. Drought, warming temperatures, melting glaciers, and sea level rise can disrupt ecosystems, impacting native plants and wildlife, thus limiting food access. For example, the Inupiat, a group of Alaska Natives in Nuiqsut, Alaska, face challenges with food storage due to warming temperatures. Historically, these populations have been able to effectively store food during the winter season in traditional underground ice cellars that cut directly into the permafrost.[87] However, the melting permafrost can result in spoilage of the food stored in these cellars, contributing to food insecurity and increasing the risk of infectious diseases due to food-borne illnesses.[87,88]

PEOPLE LIVING WITH DISABILITIES

People living with disabilities can face complex inequities that can intensify the burden of climate events and hinder the ability to adapt to protect their safety and well-being. Factors that further enhance susceptibility among people living with disabilities include female gender, uncoupled status or living alone, low-wealth status, and marginalized racial/ethnic groups. People living with disabilities who are also living with a preexisting illness are more susceptible to climate events. Further, they may have an impaired or constrained ability for extreme weather preparedness actions, have a perceived lack of ability to evacuate, and/or experience reduced recovery capacity.[20,89]

OCCUPATIONAL GROUPS

Multiple climate hazards also facilitate occupational hazards, particularly including poor air quality, extreme heat, extreme weather, and vector-borne disease. By the nature of their work, outdoor workers, including those in agriculture, construction, and utilities, and police officers and firefighters can have increased exposure to unhealthy air quality and extreme heat.[20,90] Health outcomes include heat-related illness and vector-borne diseases, including Lyme disease.[20,90] Links also exist between heat-related acute kidney injury among workers in construction, manufacturing, delivery jobs, and solid waste collection.[91]

RURAL COMMUNITIES

Populations living in rural communities have several factors that render them uniquely susceptible to the health threats of climate change, including older age, lower incomes, more social isolation, reduced access to healthcare, more likely to be underinsured, a lack transportation to essential services,[92] being less well educated and less affluent, higher unemployment, and lower population health status.[93] The vulnerability of emergency response services and physical infrastructure in rural areas can further exacerbate the risk for rural residents.[93]

Rural areas are characterized by having large land areas with low population density. Despite the fact that rural areas have vast land, they often have few transportation routes available for motorists. This lack of transportation options can render rural communities more susceptible to flooding events. Rural water basins can be uniquely susceptible to flooding, relying on low-water crossings as opposed to bridges, which can leave drivers at a higher risk in flooding events.[93]

Agricultural communities and populations with close economic or cultural ties to the land are often located in rural areas.[20] Climate factors, including drought and changing temperatures, are resulting in decreased crop quantity, and warming waters can impair aquatic food safety.[94] These changes are associated with food insecurity and can cause economic uncertainty and hardships in rural communities. Agricultural communities with close ties to the land are also susceptible to mental health burdens linked with the climate-related threat of economic hardship. Crop failures are associated with suicide attempts among farmers. For farmers, changes in crop quantity and quality can increase the expenses of food regionally, cause economic hardship, and lead to displacement and vocation changes. The mental health burdens can be further exacerbated because of reduced access to healthcare facilities in rural areas and warmer temperatures, which are independently associated with an increased suicide risk.[27]

Increased temperatures, deforestation, and land use changes in rural areas can increase exposures to disease-carrying vectors. For example, land-use changes can put humans in closer proximity to tick habitats, raising the risk of Lyme disease.[95] In addition, the drought/flooding cycles in rural areas can facilitate an attractive environment for Culex mosquitoes, the primary vector carrying West Nile virus.[93,96]

PEOPLE IDENTIFYING AS LGBTQIA2S+

The designation *LGBTQIA2S+* includes people who identify as lesbian, gay, bisexual, transgender and/or gender expansive, queer or questioning, intersex, agender or asexual, or two-spirit. People identifying as LGBTQIA2S+ can be uniquely burdened by climate events owing to discrimination, stigma, and violence, each of which is associated with poorer health outcomes and mortality.[97-99] Health impacts include exclusion from shelters after disasters; this population's unique needs being ignored in disaster relief efforts; unequal access to resources following climate events, including access to shelters; harassment at shelters; disrupted access to medical care; failure to meet healthcare needs; and exacerbation of homelessness, displacement, and existing marginalization and vulnerability.[97] Further, the mental health burdens of climate change on LGBTQIA2S+ people may include anxiety, depression, substance use, and suicidality.[97]

PEOPLE EXPERIENCING HOUSING INSECURITY

People experiencing housing insecurity or homelessness may have more exposure to temperature extremes and can be less protected in extreme weather. Further, people who are experiencing housing insecurity or are unhoused may have a number of risk factors that make them more susceptible to climate exposures, including poorly managed chronic illnesses, cigarette smoking, and mental illness.[100]

ENVIRONMENTAL HEALTH INEQUITIES

Thus far we have named, described, and alluded to many ways that health inequities emerge in the context of climate change, many of which relate to underlying conditions. As described in several chapters in this textbook, the Centers for Disease Control and Prevention (CDC) defines social determinants of health (SDOH) as the "conditions in the places where people live, learn, work, play, and worship that affect a wide range of health risks and outcomes."[101] Examples of SDOH linked with climate impacts are described in Table 3.1.

Environmental health disparities are differences and major gaps in health outcomes related to a range of SDOH. Multiple indicators (e.g. community stressors, social processes, physical hazards, and exposures) and measures can contribute to the development of environmental health disparities.[105] Similarly, several factors can contribute to environmental health disparities linked to climate injustice. For example, structural inequalities in housing/land-use policies, disparities in fossil fuel exposure, and the climate gap, which describes the disproportionate impact of climate change on marginalized communities, are major factors that drive health disparities.[106] Likewise, race[107] and socioeconomic status[2] are linked with increased harms associated with climate change. Climate models project that low-wealth countries in tropical areas are particularly susceptible to heat waves and increased temperatures.[2]

Spatial patterns of climate injustice are also observed throughout the United States, as discussed further in Chapter 8. Residential segregation is linked to the race and ethnicity of residents, as well as their proximity to subsequent stressors, resources, structural factors, and pollution exposure.[105] For instance, places with a higher proportion of racially/ethnically diverse residents tend to experience extreme climate disasters more frequently.[107] Although it is not true in all cases, Native American, Black, Hispanic or Latino, Pacific Islander, and Asian communities are often at a higher risk of the impacts of climate change (e.g., hurricanes, flooding, wildfires).[69] Concerns about climate change can prompt distress, anxiety, depressive symptoms, and a range of other mental health challenges that perpetuate climate injustice[108] and health disparities. Research documents major disparities in climate adaptation across U.S. counties, particularly by demographic factors, such as race.[107] Projected changes in climate variability demonstrate inequalities that illustrate concerns in climate injustice.[2] In addition to demographic factors, geographic areas, such as coastal communities, island nations, and cities with high proportions of impervious surfaces, are susceptible to the impacts of climate change.

TABLE 3.1. FACTORS AFFECTING HEALTH EQUITY (SDOH) ACROSS CLIMATE IMPACTS

CLIMATE IMPACT	INCOME AND WEALTH GAPS	SOCIAL AND COMMUNITY CONTEXT	HEALTHCARE ACCESS AND USE	NEIGHBORHOOD AND BUILT ENVIRONMENT	WORKPLACE CONDITIONS
Air Quality	Low-wealth communities have higher exposure to PM.[102] Underresourced populations may lack access to protective features like air filtration devices.[102]	Communities of color experience higher mortality risk associated with PM regardless of wealth.[102] Factors can include closer residential proximity to toxic air emitters, including toxic facilities, major roadways, and bus depots.	People with chronic diseases and those who lack insurance or are underinsured are more susceptible. Underresourced communities have reduced access to medical services.	Homes without air conditioning may use windows for air flow, increasing exposure to toxins that may be in ambient air. Communities with less tree canopy and less access to green space experience higher levels of air pollution.	Outdoor workers, particularly those who engage in strenuous activity, including construction and farming, can face a higher burden of poor air quality.[32]
Extreme Heat	"The difference in the threshold temperature when households begin to use air conditioning," or the energy equity gap, is expanding, resulting in deferred use of air conditioning, and an increasing risk of heat-related illness.[20]	Formerly redlined communities experience a higher burden of heat and have less access to parks, green space, and tree cover. Excess heat-related mortality occurs in communities of color.[32] Energy insecurity, "the inability to meet energy needs," is higher in African American and low-wealth households.[20]	Chronic diseases can be exacerbated by exposure to extreme heat. Access to medical services is not equally distributed across communities, but quick medical attention is essential to treat heat stroke.	Low-wealth and communities of color are more likely to reside in urban heat islands. Factors that contribute to urban heat island effect: lacking green space and tree canopy, pavement that holds heat, and proximity to vehicles and air conditioning units that emit heat. Homes without air conditioning bear greater exposure in heat events.	Outdoor farmworkers have greater exposure to extreme heat and are predominantly Hispanic; occupational heat stress is linked with kidney disease.[32]
Extreme Weather	Displacement may cause economic instability.	Undocumented residents are not eligible for Federal Emergency Management Agency assistance.[32] Low-wealth communities are often underinsured and lack adequate resources for recovery.[32] Emergency information is not always accessible to people living with disabilities.[32]	Displacement can interrupt medical services, including medication and provider access. Disrupted provider and medication access can be uniquely challenging for trans individuals.[97] Undocumented residents and LGBTQIAS2+ individuals may avoid evacuating to shelters to avoid discrimination, thus increasing the risk of injury and death.	Communities with failing protective infrastructure features, like broken levees, are rendered more susceptible in extreme weather events. Infrastructure challenges, like stormwater overflow, can cause exposure to contaminated water, increasing the risk of water-borne diseases.[32]	Destruction to communities can displace workers, contributing to economic insecurity.

(continued)

54

TABLE 3.1. FACTORS AFFECTING HEALTH EQUITY (SDOH) ACROSS CLIMATE IMPACTS *(continued)*

CLIMATE IMPACT	HEALTH EQUITY CONTRIBUTING FACTORS					
	INCOME AND WEALTH GAPS	SOCIAL AND COMMUNITY CONTEXT	HEALTHCARE ACCESS AND USE	NEIGHBORHOOD AND BUILT ENVIRONMENT	WORKPLACE CONDITIONS
Flooding	Communities with close ties to the land may experience income instability.	Formerly redlined communities have a higher flood risk.	Exposure to mold, following flooding, may exacerbate chronic conditions.	Communities lacking robust public transit access can experience impaired evacuation.[32] Flooding can cause drinking water contamination.[32]	Flooding can introduce contaminated water to farmland, affecting economic stability in farmland communities.
Sea Level Rise	Displacement may cause economic instability.	Climate gentrification is occurring, where wealthier communities are able to relocate to higher ground, displacing lower income and historically redlined communities.[32] Indigenous communities that engage in subsistence farming and fishing are susceptible to sea level rise, including its effects on crop production and on fisheries' collapse.[32]	People living with disabilities may have impairments that adversely impact their ability to evacuate to safety.[32] Increased salt water in drinking water heightens the risk of increased blood pressure, kidney disease, and preeclampsia.[32]	Coastal communities have the highest burden of sea level rise.[32] Communities with failing protective infrastructure features like sea walls are rendered more susceptible in sea level rise.[32] Sea level rise can cause drinking water contamination.	Increased salinity in groundwater and well water is resulting in reduced crop yields in agricultural areas, increasing the risk of economic instability among farmworker communities.[32]
Drought	Communities with close ties to the land may experience threats to livelihood and income instability during drought.	African American and Filipino populations are at increased risk of contracting dust-related Valley fever.[32]	Lack of safe drinking water can threaten treatment for kidney disease, including dialysis. Food insecurity can increase the risk of chronic disease.[32] Reduced access to safe drinking water can exacerbate kidney disease.[32]	Rural communities and those reliant on well water can experience water insecurity in drought.[32]	Farmworker communities are more susceptible to economic instability; the majority identify as Hispanic.[32]

(continued)

TABLE 3.1. FACTORS AFFECTING HEALTH EQUITY (SDOH) ACROSS CLIMATE IMPACTS *(continued)*

CLIMATE IMPACT	HEALTH EQUITY CONTRIBUTING FACTORS					
	INCOME AND WEALTH GAPS	SOCIAL AND COMMUNITY CONTEXT	HEALTHCARE ACCESS AND USE	NEIGHBORHOOD AND BUILT ENVIRONMENT	WORKPLACE CONDITIONS
Wildfires	Property destruction and displacement may cause economic instability. Impoverished populations are less likely to have disaster insurance and generally have fewer resources for recovery.[32]	African Americans have an increased sensitivity to wildfire smoke due, in part, to higher rates of cardiovascular disease and asthma.[32] Tribes and Alaska Natives are at increased risk of displacement, smoke exposure, injury, and property loss.[32]	Wildfire smoke can reach well beyond the area burned, harming health in communities long distances from the area affected.[32] Wildfires stress health systems owing to evacuations, increased medical visits, and stress to emergency medical services.[32]	Communities at the wildland–urban interface adjacent to areas of wildland vegetation are at greater risk of wildfires.[32]	Emergency responders have an increased risk of trauma, respiratory and mental health impacts, and death.[32] Outdoor workers, including farmworkers and utility workers, have an increased adverse respiratory risk.[32]
Vector Changes	Impoverished populations and people experiencing homelessness may not be able to access protective resources like window screens and insect repellant.	Gentrification is a social driver that can increase tick-borne disease in communities of color through population displacement or land-use changes.[103]	There are no vaccines or medications to treat West Nile virus, therefore prevention is key.[104]	Neighborhood factors of vector-borne disease include standing water and trash collection services. Impoverished communities may have more standing water, homes without window screens, and less access to trash collection, all of which support vector proliferation.	Outdoor workers bear a higher risk of exposure to vectors.

PM, particulate matter; SDOH, social determinants of health.

WORKING TOWARD ENVIRONMENTAL HEALTH AND JUSTICE

Given its urgency as a societal issue, much work is needed to ensure environmental health in the context of our changing climate as we work toward climate equity and justice. Many related policies are discussed in Chapter 4 that may help to address climate change. According to the U.S. Environmental Protection Agency (EPA), "**Climate equity** is the goal of recognizing and addressing the unequal burdens made worse by climate change, while ensuring that all people share the benefits of climate protection efforts."[109] **Climate justice** "is the principle that the benefits reaped from activities that cause climate change and the burdens of climate change impacts should be distributed fairly."[110] The University of California Center for Climate Justice provides a road map for climate justice solutions through their Six Pillars of Climate Justice to be considered when developing climate solutions[111]:

1. **Just Transition:** Transitioning of fossil-fuel-based economies to renewable-energy-based systems.
2. **Social, Racial, and Environmental Justice:** Connecting the climate crisis to social, racial, and environmental issues.
3. **Indigenous Climate Action:** Partnering collaboratively with Indigenous communities to amplify their voices and promote Indigenous sovereignty.
4. **Community Resilience and Adaptation:** Viewing resilience and adaptation through a social justice and equity lens.
5. **Natural Climate Solutions:** Recognizing forests and agricultural lands as critical climate-action solutions.
6. **Climate Education and Engagement:** Countering denial and misunderstanding with climate education and engagement.

Efforts to advance community resilience in the face of climate change should be approached with deep intention to prevent the worsening of existing inequities. **Climate resilience** describes a community's ability to stay strong or "bounce back" in the face of a changing climate. However, many have noted that this term has been overused and misused. In particular, communities who are affected by environmental injustice may be celebrated for being resilient when they would prefer living in conditions that did not repeatedly require resilience. Climate resilience strategies may be agency or community led. Either way, it is imperative to include not only the best climate-related science, but also the invaluable insights and lived expertise of members directly affected by these issues. Collaborative decision-making is more likely to address concerns related to institutional racism, uneven distribution of resources, and capacity to adapt.[112]

Globally, cities, states, and nations have been working to develop strategies for climate resilience, sometimes in the form of climate action plans that spell out mitigation and adaptation strategies. Climate action plans can range in their goals and length. Often they include information about: (a) current and projected climate impacts locally, (b) data about major sources of greenhouse gas emissions, (c) data that describes populations who are most likely to experience climate-related health impacts, and (d) strategies for local adaptation and mitigation informed by these projections and data.[113]

HEALTH IMPACT ASSESSMENTS TO SUPPORT CLIMATE MITIGATION AND ADAPTATION

Health Impact Assessments (HIAs) are crucial public health tools for informing climate action by assessing projected health impacts from implementing climate policy. As discussed in more detail in Chapter 14, "Healthy Communities for All," an HIA is:

a process which systematically judges the potential, and sometimes unintended, effects of a project, program, plan, policy, or strategy on the health of a population and the distribution of those effects within the population.[114]

(continued)

> In the context of climate change, HIAs can use evidence about relationships between environmental exposures and baseline health to estimate possible climate impacts under different policy scenarios.[115] For instance, in 2012, the Los Angeles County Department of Public Health worked with the County's Sustainability Office to conduct an HIA on the Regional Climate Action Plan (CAP).[116] The team considered the impacts of the plan on air quality, mental health, transportation, physical activity, heat-related illness, and social and economic equity.[116] The HIA showed many health-related cobenefits of the CAP but also noted some potential ways the CAP could worsen health inequities.[116]
>
> We must continue to consider when and how to utilize HIAs to highlight the importance of policies considering climate and health at all stages to maximize benefits.

MITIGATING CLIMATE CHANGE FOR HEALTHIER LIVES

The science is clear: The primary cause of the climate crisis is human-induced greenhouse gas emissions, predominantly from burning fossil fuels. A shift toward renewable energy sources, like wind and solar, not only helps combat climate change, but also yields immediate health benefits by lowering air pollution levels. There is abundant evidence for mitigation actions to prevent catastrophic and irreversible damage from climate change. Effective **climate mitigation** strategies reduce the extraction and burning of fossil fuels or the release of greenhouse gasses and, as such, offer opportunities to protect health and the environment. It is imperative that mitigation strategies be evidence based and community driven.

According to the *Fifth National Climate Assessment*, mitigation strategies that yield substantial health benefits include:

- the reduction of emissions from point sources (e.g., coal-fired power plants) and mobile sources (e.g., trucks, cars);
- promoting active transportation through activities like walking or bicycling; and
- encouraging the shift toward a plant-rich diet high in fruits, vegetables, nuts, and legumes.[117]

Crucially, data show that the economic benefits of mitigation activities outweigh the costs of implementing these interventions, particularly when considering the costs associated with climate-related hospitalizations and premature deaths.[15,118]

With regard to mitigation strategies, the climate and air pollution impacts of electricity production highlight the particularly damaging effects of coal power. By some estimates, a shift away from fossil fuels for electricity generation could save millions of lives globally from lower $PM_{2.5}$ exposure.[119] More information on energy use and production is covered in Chapter 9, "Energy and Health." Relatedly, household energy is also recognized as a contributor to climate change, especially in energy-poor populations relying on wood, charcoal, or other solid fuels for cooking, contributing to highly polluted indoor environments.[120] Health outcomes linked to household air pollution include higher rates of lower respiratory infections, cardiovascular disease, and COPDs.[121] While the ideal transition to cleaner options like electric and induction is optimal for health and climate benefits, it is not universally feasible. Therefore the transition to liquefied petroleum gas (LPG) or gas from the burning of solid fuel presents a realistic alternative in many regions of the globe, offering a net climate benefit.[121] However, the increased identification of gas as a source of indoor air pollution, particularly in poorly ventilated environments, is important to note, particularly its associations with higher rates of childhood asthma.[122]

Urban and regional planning is also a key driver for mitigating climate change and enhancing health outcomes. Redesigning cities to minimize greenhouse gas emissions and maximize health benefits involves policies promoting mixed-use planning, increased active and public transportation, and reduced traffic, yielding health benefits such as reduced traffic fatalities and air pollution, along with increased green space.[123] Planners must also ensure that these actions do not perpetuate green gentrification, however, with increased property values and displacement of existing, often low-wealth, residents. Planners can work with communities to anticipate local climate projections and mitigate their impacts on extreme weather events or sea level rise, for instance. Elected officials, as well as local and state authorities, can also work toward requiring, supporting, or incentivizing local businesses to reduce their emissions through waste management, electrification, shifts to renewable energy, or other sustainable practices.

Our food system accounts for over 25% to 30% of global greenhouse gas emissions,[124] while at the same time unhealthy diets have been identified as a significant contributor to premature mortality linked to close to 11 million deaths annually.[125] For more information on how our food systems impact health, see Chapter 12, "Food Safety, Security, and Sovereignty." Interventions targeting improved diets for health can concurrently mitigate climate impacts, particularly given the detrimental effects of meat-intensive diets on health and the environment. Plant-based diets emerge as the optimal diets for human and planetary health, capable of averting millions of deaths annually and reducing greenhouse gas emissions by gigatons, resulting in trillions in health savings.[126]

ADAPTING TO THE CURRENT REALITY TO PROTECT HEALTH

The decades-long changes to temperature, precipitation, wind patterns, and other weather-related effects from climate change[127,128] are impacting lives in the United States and globally. Action now to mitigate climate change, including reducing greenhouse gas emissions, is urgently required to reduce the risks of the harmful impacts of climate change. In addition to mitigating climate change, adaptation steps are also pertinent for adjusting to the current realities of climate change. **Climate adaptation** is the adjustment in natural or human systems to a new or changing environment that exploits beneficial opportunities or moderates negative effects.[128,129] Adaptation examples can include:

- stormwater management and flood mitigation,
- land-use changes to reduce urban heat islands,
- adjusting forest management in the face of increasing wildfires,
- supporting farmers in managing crops and soil and anticipating extreme weather events, and
- building climate-smart infrastructure.

Workforce development to create economic opportunities, co-governance with communities and agencies, and institutional support are integral components of effective adaptation strategies that are community defined, driven, and led, while also embracing diverse cultures, histories, and knowledge systems to create healthy and equitable climate-resilient communities.[20]

Climate and health adaptation examples are visible throughout the nation. Many state and local health departments nationwide are taking action to adapt to the current reality of climate change to protect health, often in collaboration with other sectors. For instance, local health departments might work with parks and recreation departments to ensure safe, cool spaces during heat events. They may also work with housing and transportation planners to anticipate extreme weather events and ensure that seniors and isolated individuals with underlying health conditions will have access to healthcare and at-home medical services. There can be wide differences in experiences with climate change by region, so it is important that the climate and health adaptation activities are designed with the local community in mind and are specific to the climate exposures faced by that community.[130] These adaptations may be spelled out in climate action plans or sustainability plans and can be similar to emergency preparedness and response measures covered in more detail in Chapter 15, "Preparing for and Recovering From Disasters in Our Changing Climate."

> ### CASE STUDY 3.2: Indigenous Communities and Climate Change Response
>
> Indigenous communities across the United States are disproportionately affected by the impacts of climate change. Coastal Indigenous communities face the added threat of land loss due to rising sea levels, which puts sacred sites and ancestral burial grounds at risk and leads to the displacement of entire communities. Additionally, many Indigenous communities encounter barriers in transitioning to renewable energy, which limits their ability to implement mitigation measures and prevents a just energy transition nationwide.
>
> Despite these challenges, traditional ecological knowledge, passed down through generations, equips many Indigenous communities with valuable insights into local ecosystems and weather patterns, enabling them to anticipate and respond to environmental changes. Many of these communities are implementing innovative strategies, such as restoring traditional land management practices, diversifying and securing food sources, and developing climate-resilient infrastructure.
>
> Collaborative partnerships between Indigenous communities, government agencies, and nonprofit organizations are crucial in developing creative solutions. One example of such a partnership can be seen in southeast Alaska, where harmful algal blooms, which are increasing due to climate change, have long been a problem. These blooms can cause illness, brain damage, and even death when people swim or play in the water, breathe in tiny droplets of water, or consume contaminated shellfish. In 2013, after two cases of paralytic shellfish poisoning in Sitka, regional Tribal communities formed the Southeast Alaska Tribal Toxins partnership, a part of the larger Southeast Alaska Tribal Ocean Research (SEATOR) initiative. SEATOR consists of partnerships between Tribal communities, nonprofit organizations, the University of Alaska, and government agencies like the Alaska Department of Environmental Conservation, the National Oceanic and Atmospheric Administration, and the Environmental Protection Agency (EPA).
>
> The overall goal of SEATOR is to ensure food security. In order to enhance access to traditional foods for Tribal and rural communities, the network focuses on monitoring toxic plankton blooms and ocean chemistry, conducting tests on shellfish to detect harmful toxins, collaborating with the EPA to improve water quality standards, and initiating a heavy metals testing program, among other initiatives. By working together, the partners in SEATOR leverage Tribal knowledge and agency resources to address climate impacts. Furthermore, the comanagement work supports self-determination, whereby Indigenous Peoples can make decisions about how to respond to climate change in ways that reflect community priorities and meet their needs.[131,132]
>
> ### REFLECTION QUESTIONS
>
> *1. How do changes in the oceans due to climate change pose unique challenges to Indigenous communities?*
>
> *2. In what ways does traditional ecological knowledge empower Indigenous communities to adapt to climate change?*
>
> *3. What are the key benefits of collaborative partnerships with Indigenous communities and other agencies in addressing climate impacts?*

Monitoring and surveillance are effective means of understanding climate experiences in a community and can help to shape adaptation efforts.[133] For example, communities can monitor climate events by noting changes in air quality, heat levels, hot or cold weather, flooding, rainfall, drought, sea level, and disease-carrying vectors. In addition, health departments can also track health changes in health outcomes related to climate change, including rates of emergency admissions or deaths from respiratory and cardiovascular conditions, heat-related mortality, cases of gastrointestinal illness, and cases of Lyme disease and West Nile virus. Tracking these conditions may allow for forecasting and projections. Additionally, mapping health outcomes along with other environmental factors can also be useful to identify communities that may be more susceptible to climate and health hazards, providing evidence for these areas to be prioritized for adaptation interventions. Climate and public health scholars Moulton and Schramm note that surveillance systems should capture the expansive scope of climate and health impacts and be adaptive to emergent surveillance needs yet to come.[133]

Adaptation to extreme weather events can look different, and work is needed to support communities with limited resources. Emergency evacuations are a key example of a climate and health adaptation. The sooner and further communities evacuate ahead of extreme weather events, the better the physical and mental health outcomes.[43] Therefore, communicating early about the need for evacuation along with providing a means for evacuation (e.g., providing transportation) will protect communities from experiencing injury and death resulting from direct exposure to extreme weather. Effective evacuations also require cooperation from workplaces, whose employers, when possible, should not penalize employees for evacuating. Also, cooling centers are crucial in providing a lifesaving refuge for local residents during hot weather. These centers can be public spaces, such as air-conditioned libraries, or other public buildings where people can find relief from the heat.[134] They are particularly beneficial for individuals without access to air conditioning in their homes or for people experiencing homelessness. Therefore, cooling centers must be free and easily accessible to the community. This accessibility should cater to individuals with disabilities and ensure proximity to public transportation routes. Importantly, a coordinated strategy should be in place to effectively communicate the location and availability of cooling centers in a variety of media and languages.

With regard to climate-adaptive infrastructure, networks of green spaces (also known as green infrastructure) are particularly important given the increased frequency and intensity of extreme heat and rain events in many communities. Urban green spaces may include different types of vegetated cover, such as parks, greenways, and gardens, and they can mitigate the effects of climate change. For example, canopy cover can buffer the urban heat island effect and decrease the local temperature in urban settings. Also, green infrastructure, including bioswales, some types of trees, and bioretention gardens, can be designed to soak up excess stormwater. However, access to protective green spaces is not equally experienced. A study that used national land cover data[135] observed that residential segregation by racial/ethnic groups was related to increased heat-related risks for Black, Hispanic, and Asian populations. Scholars describe how inequitable access to green spaces can be linked to health disparities in heat-related illnesses, psychological well-being, cardiovascular health, and obesity.[136] In light of their findings, incorporating an environmental justice (EJ) framework as part of greening initiatives is important.[135]

> **IN OTHER WORDS: BIOSWALES**
>
> *Bioswales* are planted areas that are covered in vegetation. They serve the purpose of treating and retaining stormwater as it travels from one location to another. The plants and the structure of the bioswales have the ability to slow down, absorb, and purify stormwater flows. Long, narrow bioswales are especially well suited for placement alongside streets and parking lots.

SUPPORTING CLIMATE ADAPTATION AND MITIGATION THROUGH HEALTHCARE

Many healthcare professionals are advocating for a transformative shift in clinical practice to confront the root causes of both chronic disease and climate change crises, as discussed in Chapters 16 and 17 as well. This advocacy presents an opportunity to prescribe comprehensive interventions, including:

- **Whole-food, plant-rich eating patterns:** Diets low in whole grains, vegetables, fruits, and nuts, and high in red meat, salt, and processed foods result in the annual loss of 11 million lives globally,[125] as discussed in Chapter 12, "Food Safety, Security, and Sovereignty." Meanwhile, the food system also has a profound effect on the Earth's resources; for example, it uses 70% of freshwater and 40% of land, and significantly contributes to biodiversity loss, pollution, and antibiotic resistance.[124,137]

- **Physical activity:** Sedentary lifestyles claim over 3 million lives globally,[138] and only 20% of Americans meet physical activity guidelines, while 25% are classified as physically inactive.[139] Simultaneously, about 29% of greenhouse gas emissions in the United States stem from the transportation sector.[140] Encouraging patients to consider eliminating short car trips (less than 5 miles round trip) can yield air quality and exercise benefits.[141]
- **Strategies to improve sleep, enhance social connection, and manage stress:** For instance, prescribing nature-based treatments that promote the protection of local tree canopies addresses both mental and physical health.[142] Individual and community-level interventions to improve access to green space can reduce exposure to air pollution, lower local temperatures during heat waves, and diminish noise and light pollution, effectively addressing a myriad of health and climate-related issues.[143]

All of these prescriptions can address the specific chronic health concerns relevant to each patient, with the added "side effect" of addressing carbon emissions.[144] Evidence from the *Lancet* Countdown on health and climate change report and other studies reveal that these prescriptions play a crucial role in climate change mitigation and resilience building.[143,145,146]

Although it is necessary that clinicians support climate adaptation, they must be careful not to overlook barriers to "filling a prescription." Not all people have equal access to healthcare, and all of these prescriptions can be greatly affected by one's SDOH. For instance, some neighborhoods may not have access to healthy foods or essential resources to safely and accessibly reach schools, workplaces, or other places by foot or bicycle. Residents of some neighborhoods or individual households face many barriers when working to reduce their exposure to air pollutants, particularly if they are living in a neighborhood overburdened with multiple pollution sources or lack the resources to filter indoor air quality. Thus, programs that move upstream to address these conditions remain essential for promoting health equity.

IN OTHER WORDS: COMMUNICATING ABOUT CLIMATE CHANGE

Despite substantial evidence about the causes and impacts of climate change, communication about climate change and its health implications remains either insufficient or suboptimally effective. Given the urgency for climate action and a closing window of opportunity to stave off the worst impacts of climate change, effective communication about the risks of the climate crisis along with the benefits of climate action is crucial. Effective communication strategies can drive positive individual behavioral change along with public pressure for system-level investments that are necessary to shift from dirty fossil fuels to renewable energy, bolster public health and healthcare infrastructure resilience, and increase support for environmental justice.

Evidence-based resources are available to develop strategies for communicating about climate change. Research by the Yale Program on Climate Change Communication and the George Mason Center for Climate Communication shed light on public opinion; educate the public, the media, and policy makers; and work to build motivation for climate action. Using the evidence and lessons learned from the COVID-19 pandemic, researchers present 11 theory-based strategies for bridging the gap between climate change and health risks in order to build support for climate action.[147] They highlight the role of trusted messengers, including healthcare professionals, in enhancing understanding and prompting actionable responses. The strategies for effective communication on climate change and health risks, as presented by Peters and colleagues, include:

- **Credible sources:** Messages are more impactful when delivered by trusted sources. Healthcare professionals, as credible messengers, can significantly influence the effectiveness of the communication.
- **Social networks:** Social networks greatly influence beliefs and behaviors. Engaging influential individuals within these networks can extend the reach and effectiveness of messages about climate change and health.

(continued)

> **IN OTHER WORDS: COMMUNICATING ABOUT CLIMATE CHANGE** (*continued*)
>
> - **Social norms:** Framing environmentally friendly and health-conscious actions as social norms can encourage adoption of these behaviors by promoting conformity and social approval.
> - **Empowerment and belonging:** Messages that foster a sense of community belonging and empower individuals to make a difference can be highly motivating, promoting positive climate-related behaviors.
> - **Strategic language choices:** The choice of words in communication is crucial. Using language that resonates emotionally with the audience can make messages more compelling.
> - **Emotional appeals:** Messages that evoke emotions like empathy, concern, or hope can be more engaging and motivating.
> - **Visual communication:** Visual elements, such as infographics or images that illustrate the health impacts of climate change, can make communication more effective.
> - **Narrative communication:** Using narrative techniques to connect health outcomes with the broader issue of climate change can make the information more relatable and understandable.
> - **Key statistics:** Clear presentation of data and statistics can help people understand the risks associated with climate change and motivate them to adopt healthier, more climate friendly behaviors.
> - **Overcoming barriers:** Identifying and addressing barriers that hinder health-promoting and environmentally friendly actions can increase the effectiveness of communication.
> - **Message testing:** Testing messages with the target audience fosters their effectiveness, allowing for adjustments based on real-world feedback.
>
> Integrating these strategies into communication efforts may increase the likelihood of effectively conveying the health risks of climate change, encouraging positive behavioral changes, and contributing to a collective response to this global challenge. Improving how we communicate about climate change is essential for mitigating its adverse effects on human health and well-being.

MAIN TAKEAWAYS

In this chapter, we learned that:

- Climate change is real. The science is clear.
- Climate change is happening now.
- Climate change is affecting health today.
- The unequal distribution of climate impacts most distinctly burdens the populations least responsible for the climate crisis.
- There are climate solutions that allow humans to adapt to the climate threats we are currently facing, as well as mitigate climate change to reduce future risk.
- Clear and effective communication is key for minimizing the adverse risks of climate change on health.

SUMMARY

Climate change poses a significant and escalating threat to human health, manifesting through a broad array of direct and indirect pathways that public health and healthcare professionals are still discovering. As discussed in this chapter, human health impacts range from increased disease burdens and deteriorating mental health to amplifying health disparities. Already marginalized and biologically susceptible groups are particularly at risk, for example, people with preexisting health conditions and low-wealth communities who disproportionately suffer the consequences. Beyond the risks to personal health, climate change also puts a strain on healthcare systems and infrastructure. The unequal distribution of climate impacts most distinctly burdens the populations least responsible for the climate crisis, including children, low-wealth communities, and communities of color. Attributing factors include systemic marginalization, socioeconomic disenfranchisement and underinvestment, and environmental injustice. Climate justice requires the fulfillment of EJ to realize healthy communities. This chapter provides examples along with insights to consider when deploying climate adaptation or mitigation to protect health. Although the science of climate change and the solutions to protect health are complex, there are evidence-based approaches that inform effectively conveying the realities of climate change.

END-OF-CHAPTER RESOURCES

DISCUSSION QUESTIONS

1. After reading this chapter, how has your understanding of climate change altered, if at all?
2. Most of us will be affected by climate change, if we aren't already. What are your biggest concerns when it comes to your own community? In what ways do you think your future work will be affected by climate change?
3. In what ways would you like to see your own community work toward climate mitigation? Climate adaptation?
4. As noted in the chapter, "Climate resilience is commonly used to describe a community's ability to stay strong or 'bounce back' in the face of a changing climate. However, many have noted that this term has been overused and misused. In particular, communities who are affected by environmental injustice may be celebrated for being resilient when they would prefer living in conditions that did not repeatedly require it." In your opinion, what should climate resilience look like? Think about your own community.
5. Using the communication strategies recommended in this chapter, how might you craft climate communications about the issues your own community is confronting? Think about different audiences, data you would include, and your overall framing needed to be most effective.

LEARNING ACTIVITIES
THE TIME IS NOW

Think about the communities you are part of and examine how they are planning for climate change.

- Does your city, region, or state have a climate action plan? If so, does it address environmental health and justice issues explicitly? How does it plan for mitigation and adaptation? What does implementation look like? What has been accomplished already?
- Does your university or workplace have a climate action plan? If so, does it address environmental health and justice issues explicitly? How does it plan for mitigation and adaptation? What does implementation look like? What has been accomplished already?

After reading this chapter, what would you ask of or recommend to those leading this work? Are there ways you can engage in the work?

IN REAL LIFE

Write and share your climate story.

The organization Climate Generation explains that a climate story is a person's unique description of their experiences with climate change. The exchange of climate stories can help us connect and relate with one another in our communities as we describe our fears, grief, memories, and how we might cope or adapt.[148]

There is no "right" way or "right" length for your story, but start by drafting a brief essay that expresses your connection to climate change. As you develop your story, you might begin by thinking about:

- the community where you live;
- the people and places you (or your family) are connected to;
- your values;
- the climate-related issues that concern you most;
- how you, your loved ones, or your community have already experienced climate change; and
- strategies to strengthen your community in the face of climate change.

Invite others to write and share their climate stories with you. This could be done with friends and loved ones, in a class, or as part of a larger community initiative.

 A robust set of instructor resources designed to supplement this text is located at http://connect.springerpub.com/content/book/978-0-8261-8353-8. Qualifying instructors may request access by emailing textbook@springerpub.com.

REFERENCES

1. Lee H, Calvin K, Dasgupta D, et al. IPCC, 2023: Summary for Policymakers. In: *Core Writing Team*, Lee H, Romero J, eds. *Climate Change 2023: Synthesis Report. Contribution of Working Groups I, II and III to the Sixth Assessment Report of the Intergovernmental Panel on Climate Change.* IPCC; 2023.
2. Gulev SK, Thorne PW, Ahn J, et al. *Changing State of the Climate System.* Cambridge University Press; 2021.
3. Bathiany S, Dakos V, Scheffer M, Lenton TM. Climate models predict increasing temperature variability in poor countries. *Sci Adv.* 2018;4(5):eaar5809. doi:10.1126/sciadv.aar5809
4. Grineski SE, Collins TW, Ford P, et al. Climate change and environmental injustice in a bi-national context. *Appl Geogr.* 2012;33:25–35. doi:10.1016/j.apgeog.2011.05.013
5. Watts N, Amann M, Arnell N, et al. The 2019 report of The *Lancet* Countdown on health and climate change: ensuring that the health of a child born today is not defined by a changing climate. *Lancet.* 2019;394(10211):1836–1878. doi:10.1016/S0140-6736(19)32596-6
6. Luber G, McGeehin M. Climate change and extreme heat events. *Am J Prev Med.* 2008;35(5): 429–435. doi:10.1016/j.amepre.2008.08.021
7. Heat Island Effect. United States Environmental Protection Agency. Updated March 18, 2024. https://www.epa.gov/heatislands
8. Vicedo-Cabrera AM, Scovronick N, Sera F, et al. The burden of heat-related mortality attributable to recent human-induced climate change. *Nat Clim Chang.* 2021;11(6):492–500. doi:10.1038/s41558-021-01058-x
9. Howard G, Calow R, Macdonald A, Bartram J. Climate change and water and sanitation: likely impacts and emerging trends for action. *Annu Rev Environ Resour.* 2016;41(1):253–276. doi:10.1146/annurev-environ-110615-085856
10. Hsiang S, Greenhill S, Martinich J, et al. Economics. In: Crimmins AR, Avery CW, Easterling DR, Kunkel KE, Stewart BC, Maycock TK, eds. *Fifth National Climate Assessment.* U.S. Global Change Research Program; 2023.
11. Hsiang S, Kopp R, Jina A, et al. Estimating economic damage from climate change in the United States. *Science.* 2017;356(6345):1362–1369. doi:10.1126/science.aal4369
12. Nelson GC, Valin H, Sands RD, et al. Climate change effects on agriculture: economic responses to biophysical shocks. *Proc Nat Acad Sci.* 2014;111(9):3274–3279. doi:10.1073/pnas.1222465110
13. Darwin RF, Tol RSJ. Estimates of the economic effects of sea level rise. *Environ Resour Econ.* 2001;19(2):113–129. doi:10.1023/A:1011136417375

14. Climate action plan: revitalizing efforts to bolster adaptation & increase resilience. United States Department of Transportation. In: Transportation OotSo, ed. 2021. https://www.transportation.gov/sites/dot.gov/files/2022-04/Climate_Action_Plan.pdf
15. Hayden MH, Schramm PJ, Beard CB, et al. Human health. In: Crimmins AR, Avery CW, Easterling DR, Kunkel KE, Stewart BC, Maycock TK, eds. *Fifth National Climate Assessment.* U.S. Global Change Research Program; 2023.
16. Reid CE, Brauer M, Johnston FH, Jerrett M, Balmes JR, Elliott CT. Critical review of health impacts of wildfire smoke exposure. *Environ Health Perspect.* 2016;124(9):1334–1343. doi:10.1289/ehp.1409277
17. Ziska L, Knowlton K, Rogers C, et al. Recent warming by latitude associated with increased length of ragweed pollen season in central North America. *Proc Nat Acad Sci.* 2011;108(10):4248–4251. doi:10.1073/pnas.1014107108
18. D'Amato G, Chong-Neto HJ, Monge Ortega OP, et al. The effects of climate change on respiratory allergy and asthma induced by pollen and mold allergens. *Allergy.* 2020;75(9):2219–2228. doi:10.1111/all.14476
19. Keswani A, Akselrod H, Anenberg SC. Health and clinical impacts of air pollution and linkages with climate change. *NEJM Evid.* 2022;1(7):EVIDra2200068. doi:10.1056/evidra2200068
20. Beyeler N, DeJarnett N, Lester P, Hess J, Salas R. *Lancet* Countdown on health and climate change: Policy brief for the United States of America. *Lancet.* October 2022. https://www.lancetcountdownus.org/2022-lancet-countdown-u-s-brief/#:~:text=The%202022%20Brief%20focuses%20on,infectious%20disease%2C%20and%20mental%20health
21. Climate change indicators: heat-related deaths. United States Environmental Protection Agency. Updated November 1, 2023. https://www.epa.gov/climate-indicators/climate-change-indicators-heat-related-deaths
22. Semenza JC, Rubin CH, Falter KH, et al. Heat-related deaths during the July 1995 heat wave in Chicago. *N Engl J Med.* 1996;335(2):84–90. doi:10.1056/nejm199607113350203
23. Klinenberg E. Denaturalizing disaster: a social autopsy of the 1995 Chicago heat wave. *Theory Soc.* 1999;28(2):239–295. doi:10.1023/A:1006995507723
24. O'Neill MS, Jackman DK, Wyman M, et al. US local action on heat and health: are we prepared for climate change? *Int J Public Health.* 2010;55(2):105–112. doi:10.1007/s00038-009-0071-5
25. How many people die from extreme heat in the US? USAFacts. Updated August 22, 2023. https://usafacts.org/articles/how-many-people-die-from-extreme-heat-in-the-us/
26. Health impacts of extreme weather: climate change and human health. National Institute of Environmental Health Sciences. Updated August 30, 2022. https://www.niehs.nih.gov/research/programs/climatechange/health_impacts/weather_related_morbidity
27. Padhy SK, Sarkar S, Panigrahi M, Paul S. Mental health effects of climate change. *Indian J Occup and Environ Med.* 2015;19(1):3–7. doi:10.4103/0019-5278.156997
28. Weather related fatality and injury statistics. National Weather Service. 2023. Accessed January 26, 2024. https://www.weather.gov/hazstat/
29. Erdman J. America's top weather killer is not tornadoes, flooding, lightning or hurricanes—it's heat. In: *Heat Safety & Prep.* Vol 2024. The Weather Channel; 2023. https://weather.com/safety/heat/news/2021-06-03-heat-america-fatalities
30. Precipitation extremes. Climate and Health website. Centers for Disease Control and Prevention. Updated December 21, 2020. https://www.cdc.gov/climateandhealth/effects/precipitation_extremes.htm
31. American Public Health Association. *Extreme Rainfall and Drought.* American Public Health Association; 2016.
32. Rudolph L, Harrison C, Buckley L, North S. Climate change, health, and equity: a guide for local health departments. *Public Health Inst and Am Public Health Assoc.* 2018;369.
33. Wade T, ClimAtlantic. Health risks associated with sea level rise. National Collaborating Centre for Environmental Health (NCCEH). November 2022. https://ncceh.ca/sites/default/files/Final%20Draft%20-%20Health%20impacts%20of%20SLR_EN%20Dec%207_1.pdf
34. Hayes K, Blashki G, Wiseman J, Burke S, Reifels L. Climate change and mental health: risks, impacts and priority actions. *Int J Ment Health Syst.* 2018;12(1):28. doi:10.1186/s13033-018-0210-6
35. Clayton S, Manning C, Krygsman K, Speiser M. *Mental Health and Our Changing Climate: Impacts, Implications, and Guidance.* American Psychological Association and ecoAmerica; 2017.
36. Albrecht G. Chronic environmental change: emerging 'psychoterratic' syndromes. In: Weissbecker I, ed. *Climate Change and Human Well-Being: Global Challenges and Opportunities.* Springer; 2011:43–56.

37. Albrecht G, Sartore G-M, Connor L, et al. Solastalgia: the distress caused by environmental change. *Australas Psychiatry.* 2007;15(suppl 1):S95–S98. doi:10.1080/10398560701701288
38. Palinkas LA, Wong M. Global climate change and mental health. *Curr Opin Psychol.* 2020;32:12–16. doi:10.1016/j.copsyc.2019.06.023
39. Scheelbeek PFD, Chowdhury MAH, Haines A, et al. Drinking water salinity and raised blood pressure: evidence from a cohort study in coastal Bangladesh. *Environ Health Perspect.* 2017;125(5):057007. doi:10.1289/ehp659
40. Naser AM, Rahman M, Unicomb L, et al. Drinking water salinity and kidney health in southwest coastal Bangladesh: baseline findings of a community-based stepped-wedge randomised trial. *Lancet.* 2017;389:S15. doi:10.1016/S0140-6736(17)31127-3
41. Khan AE, Scheelbeek PFD, Shilpi AB, et al. Salinity in drinking water and the risk of (pre) eclampsia and gestational hypertension in coastal Bangladesh: a case-control study. *PLoS One.* 2014;9(9):e108715. doi:10.1371/journal.pone.0108715
42. Bell JE, Herring SC, Jantarasami L, et al. Impacts of extreme events on human health. In: *The Impacts of Climate Change on Human Health in the United States: A Scientific Assessment.* U.S. Global Change Research Program; 2016:99–128.
43. American Public Health Association, American Psychological Association. Climate for Hhealth, ecoAmerica. *Making the Connection: Climate Changes Mental Health.* American Public Health Association; 2017. https://apha.org/-/media/Files/PDF/topics/climate/Climate_Changes_Mental_Health.pdf
44. Vose JM, Peterson DL, Domke GM, et al. Forests. In: *Impacts, Risks, and Adaptation in the United States: Fourth National Climate Assessment*; 2018;2:232–267.
45. Jolly WM, Cochrane MA, Freeborn PH, et al. Climate-induced variations in global wildfire danger from 1979 to 2013. *Nat Commun.* 2015;6(1):7537. doi:10.1038/ncomms8537
46. Zheng B, Ciais P, Chevallier F, et al. Record-high CO_2 emissions from boreal fires in 2021. *Science.* 2023;379(6635):912–917. doi:10.1126/science.ade0805
47. Shrestha B, Brotzge JA, Wang J. Observations and impacts of long-range transported wildfire smoke on air quality across New York state during july 2021. *Geophys Res Lett.* 2022;49(19):e2022GL100216. doi:10.1029/2022GL100216
48. Wang Z, Wang Z, Zou Z, et al. Severe global environmental issues caused by Canada's record-breaking wildfires in 2023. *Adv Atmos Sci.* 2024;41:565–571. doi:10.1007/s00376-023-3241-0
49. Ceamanos X, Coopman Q, George M, Riedi J, Parrington M, Clerbaux C. Remote sensing and model analysis of biomass burning smoke transported across the Atlantic during the 2020 Western US wildfire season. *Sci Rep.* 2023;13(1):16014. doi:10.1038/s41598-023-39312-1
50. Liu JC, Pereira G, Uhl SA, Bravo MA, Bell ML. A systematic review of the physical health impacts from non-occupational exposure to wildfire smoke. *Environ Res.* 2015;136:120–132. doi:10.1016/j.envres.2014.10.015
51. Duwell M. Notes from the field: locally acquired mosquito-transmitted (autochthonous) plasmodium falciparum malaria—national capital region, Maryland, August 2023. *MMWR Morb Mortal Wkly Rep.* 2023;72(41):1123–1125. doi:10.15585/mmwr.mm7241a3
52. Carlson CJ, Albery GF, Merow C, et al. Climate change increases cross-species viral transmission risk. *Nature.* 2022;607(7919):555–562. doi:10.1038/s41586-022-04788-w
53. Nicholas PK, Breakey S, White BP, et al. Mental health impacts of climate change: perspectives for the ED clinician. *J Emerg Nurs.* 2020;46(5):590–599. doi:10.1016/j.jen.2020.05.014
54. Cianconi P, Betrò S, Janiri L. The impact of climate change on mental health: a systematic descriptive review. *Front Psychiatry.* 2020;11. doi:10.3389/fpsyt.2020.00074
55. Fallon BA, Nields JA. Lyme disease: a neuropsychiatric illness. *Am J Psychiatry.* 1994;151(11):1571–1583. doi:10.1176/ajp.151.11.1571
56. Dewar B-K. Emotional and behavioural difficulties after encephalitis. Encephalitis International; June 2001; 2021.
57. Abdat Y, Butler M, Zandi M, et al. Mental health outcomes of encephalitis: an international web-based study. *Eur J Neurol.* 2024;31(1):e16083. doi:10.1111/ene.16083
58. Hopkins RO, Larson-Lohr V, Weaver LK, Bigler ED. Neuropsychological impairments following hantavirus pulmonary syndrome. *J Int Neuropsychol Soc.* 1998;4(2):190–196. doi:10.1017/s1355617798001908
59. Paixão ES, Rodrigues LC, Costa MdCN, et al. Chikungunya chronic disease: a systematic review and meta-analysis. *Trans R Soc Trop Med Hyg.* 2018;112(7):301–316. doi:10.1093/trstmh/try063

60. Zhang Y, Bi P, Hiller JE. Climate change and disability-adjusted life years. *J Environ Health.* 2007;70(3):32-38.
61. Hoffman JL. Heat-related illness in children. *Clin Pediatr Emerg Med.* 2001;2(3):203-210. doi:10.1016/S1522-8401(01)90006-0
62. Pacheco SE. Catastrophic effects of climate change on children's health start before birth. *J Clin Invest.* 2020;130(2):562-564. doi:10.1172/JCI135005
63. Sorensen C, Murray V, Lemery J, Balbus J. Climate change and women's health: impacts and policy directions. *PLoS Med.* 2018;15(7):e1002603. doi:10.1371/journal.pmed.1002603
64. Peters A, Schneider A. Cardiovascular risks of climate change. *Nat Rev Cardiol.* 2021;18(1):1-2. doi:10.1038/s41569-020-00473-5
65. Vallianou NG, Geladari EV, Kounatidis D, et al. Diabetes mellitus in the era of climate change. *Diabetes Metab.* 2021;47(4):101205. doi:10.1016/j.diabet.2020.10.003
66. Westaway K, Frank O, Husband A, et al. Medicines can affect thermoregulation and accentuate the risk of dehydration and heat-related illness during hot weather. *J Clin Pharm Ther.* 2015;40(4):363-367. doi:10.1111/jcpt.12294
67. Ebi KL, Capon A, Berry P, et al. Hot weather and heat extremes: health risks. *Lancet.* 2021;398(10301):698-708. doi:10.1016/s0140-6736(21)01208-3
68. Balajee SS, Cross T, Curry-Stevens A, et al. *Equity and Empowerment Lens (Racial Justice Focus).* Multnomah County; 2012. https://multco-web7-psh-files-usw2.s3-us-west-2.amazonaws.com/s3fs-public/E%26E%20Lens%20Final-090613.pdf
69. Berberian AG, Gonzalez DJX, Cushing LJ. Racial disparities in climate change-related health effects in the United States. *Curr Environ Health Rep.* 2022;9(3):451-464. doi:10.1007/s40572-022-00360-w
70. Bullard RD, Mohai P, Saha R, Wright B. Toxic wastes and race at twenty: why race still matters after all of these years. *Envtl L.* 2008;38(2):371-412.
71. Mascarenhas M, Grattet R, Mege K. Toxic waste and race in twenty-first century America: neighborhood poverty and racial composition in the siting of hazardous waste facilities. *Environ Soc.* 2021;12(1):108-126. doi:10.3167/ares.2021.120107
72. Mikati I, Benson AF, Luben TJ, Sacks JD, Richmond-Bryant J. Disparities in distribution of particulate matter emission sources by race and poverty status. *Am J Public Health.* 2018;108(4):480-485. doi:10.2105/AJPH.2017.304297
73. Marlow T, Elliott JR, Frickel S. Future flooding increases unequal exposure risks to relic industrial pollution. *Environ Res Lett.* 2022;17(7):074021. doi:10.1088/1748-9326/ac78f7
74. Nelson RK, Winling L, et al. Mapping inequality: redlining in new deal America. Digital Scholarship Lab. American Panorama: An Atlas of United States History website 2023. Accessed January 23, 2024. https://dsl.richmond.edu/panorama/redlining
75. Lane HM, Morello-Frosch R, Marshall JD, Apte JS. Historical redlining is associated with present-day air pollution disparities in U.S. cities. *Environ Sci Technol Lett.* 2022;9(4):345-350. doi:10.1021/acs.estlett.1c01012
76. Hoffman JS, Shandas V, Pendleton N. The effects of historical housing policies on resident exposure to intra-urban heat: a study of 108 US urban areas. *Climate.* 2020;8(1):12. doi:10.3390/cli8010012
77. Nogueira L, White KE, Bell B, et al. The role of behavioral medicine in addressing climate change-related health inequities. *Transl Behav Med.* 2022;12(4):526-534. doi:10.1093/tbm/ibac005
78. Locke DH, Hall B, Grove JM, et al. Residential housing segregation and urban tree canopy in 37 US Cities. *npj Urban Sustain.* 2021;1(1):15. doi:10.1038/s42949-021-00022-0
79. Nardone A, Rudolph KE, Morello-Frosch R, Casey JA. Redlines and greenspace: the relationship between historical redlining and 2010 greenspace across the United States. *Environ Health Perspect.* 2021;129(1):017006. doi:10.1289/ehp7495
80. Lee EK, Donley G, Ciesielski TH, et al. Health outcomes in redlined versus non-redlined neighborhoods: a systematic review and meta-analysis. *Soc Sci Med.* 2022;294:114696. doi:10.1016/j.socscimed.2021.114696
81. Hsu A, Sheriff G, Chakraborty T, Manya D. Disproportionate exposure to urban heat island intensity across major US cities. *Nat Commun.* 2021;12(1):2721. doi:10.1038/s41467-021-22799-5
82. Adams RM, Evans CM, Mathews MC, Wolkin A, Peek L. Mortality from forces of nature among older adults by race/ethnicity and gender. *J Appl Gerontol.* 2021;40(11):1517-1526. doi:10.1177/0733464820954676

83. Ali JS, Farrell AS, Alexander AC, Forde DR, Stockton M, Ward KD. Race differences in depression vulnerability following Hurricane Katrina. *Psychol Trauma.* 2017;9(3):317–324. doi:10.1037/tra0000217
84. Alexander AC, Ali J, McDevitt-Murphy ME, et al. Racial differences in posttraumatic stress disorder vulnerability following Hurricane Katrina among a sample of adult cigarette smokers from New Orleans. *J Racial Ethn Health Disparities.* 2017;4(1):94–103. doi:10.1007/s40615-015-0206-8
85. Flores AB, Collins TW, Grineski SE, Chakraborty J. Disparities in health effects and access to health care among Houston area residents after Hurricane Harvey. *Public Health Rep.* 2020;135(4):511–523. doi:10.1177/0033354920930133
86. Liu JC, Wilson A, Mickley LJ, et al. Who among the elderly is most vulnerable to exposure to and health risks of fine particulate matter from wildfire smoke? *Am J Epidemiol.* 2017;186(6):730–735. doi:10.1093/aje/kwx141
87. United States Global Change Research Program. Iñupiat work to preserve food and traditions on Alaska's North slope. U.S. Climate Resilience Toolkit website. 2017. Accessed January 26, 2024. https://toolkit.climate.gov/case-studies/i%C3%B1upiat-work-preserve-food-and-traditions-alaskas-north-slope#:~:text=View%20looking%20down%20the%20entry,the%20permafrost%20to%20store%20food
88. Ford JD. Indigenous health and climate change. *Am J Public Health.* 2012;102(7):1260–1266. doi:10.2105/ajph.2012.300752
89. Gaskin CJ, Taylor D, Kinnear S, Mann J, Hillman W, Moran M. Factors associated with the climate change vulnerability and the adaptive capacity of people with disability: a systematic review. *Weather Clim Soc.* 2017;9(4):801–814. doi:10.1175/WCAS-D-16-0126.1
90. Balbus JM, Malina C. Identifying vulnerable subpopulations for climate change health effects in the United States. *J Occup Environ Med.* 2009;51(1):33–37. doi:10.1097/jom.0b013e318193e12e
91. Shi DS, Weaver VM, Hodgson MJ, Tustin AW. Hospitalised heat-related acute kidney injury in indoor and outdoor workers in the USA. *Occup Environ Med.* 2022;79(3):184–191. doi:10.1136/oemed-2021-107933
92. Kearney GD, Jones K, Bell RA, Swinker M, Allen TR. Climate change and public health through the lens of rural, eastern North Carolina. *N C Med J.* 2018;79(5):270–277. doi:10.18043/ncm.79.5.270
93. Houghton A, Austin J, Beerman A, Horton C. An approach to developing local climate change environmental public health indicators in a rural district. *J Environ Public Health.* 2017;2017:3407325. doi:10.1155/2017/3407325
94. Gutierrez KS, LePrevost CE. Climate justice in rural southeastern United States: a review of climate change impacts and effects on human health. *Int J Environ Res Public Health.* 2016;13(2):189. doi:10.3390/ijerph13020189
95. Elmieh N, National Collaborating Centre for Environmental Health (NCCEH). Review of environments that exacerbate tick related risks. NCCEH. September 2022. https://ncceh.ca/sites/default/files/Elmieh_ticks%20in%20parks_environmental%20risks_Nov18_mp_1.pdf
96. Beard CB, Eisen RJ, Barker CM, et al. Vectorborne diseases. In: *The Impacts of Climate Change on Human Health in the United States: A Scientific Assessment.* U.S. Global Change Research Program; 2016:129–156.
97. Simmonds KE, Jenkins J, White B, Nicholas PK, Bell J. Health impacts of climate change on gender diverse populations: a scoping review. *J Nurs Scholarsh.* 2022;54(1):81–91. doi:10.1111/jnu.12701
98. Bockting W. How far has transgender health come since stonewall? *Am J Public Health.* 2019;109(6):852–853. doi:10.2105/AJPH.2019.305095
99. Reisner SL, Poteat T, Keatley J, et al. Global health burden and needs of transgender populations: a review. *Lancet.* 2016;388(10042):412–436. doi:10.1016/s0140-6736(16)00684-x
100. Ramin B, Svoboda T. Health of the homeless and climate change. *J Urban Health.* 2009;86(4):654–664. doi:10.1007/s11524-009-9354-7
101. What is health equity? Centers for Disease Control and Prevention. Updated July 1, 2022. https://www.cdc.gov/healthequity/whatis/index.html
102. Patel L, Friedman E, Johannes SA, Lee SS, O'Brien HG, Schear SE. Air pollution as a social and structural determinant of health. *J Clim Chang Health.* 2021;3:100035. doi:10.1016/j.joclim.2021.100035
103. Halsey SJ, VanAcker MC, Harris NC, Lewis KR, Perez L, Smith GS. The public health implications of gentrification: tick-borne disease risks for communities of color. *Front Ecol Environ.* 2023;21(4):191–198. doi:10.1002/fee.2549
104. American Public Health Association. Climate change increases the number and geographic range of disease carrying ticks. April 18, 2016. https://apha.org/-/media/Files/PDF/factsheets/climate/Vector_Borne.pdf

105. Payne-Sturges D, Gee GC. National environmental health measures for minority and low-income populations: tracking social disparities in environmental health. *Environ Res.* 2006;102(2):154–171. doi:10.1016/j.envres.2006.05.014
106. Morello-Frosch R, Obasogie OK. The climate gap and the color line—racial health inequities and climate change. *N Engl J Med.* 2023;388(10):943–949. doi:10.1056/nejmsb2213250
107. Liu T, Fan C. Impacts of disaster exposure on climate adaptation injustice across U.S. cities. *Sustain Cities Soc.* 2023;89:104371. doi:10.1016/j.scs.2022.104371
108. Ingle HE, Mikulewicz M. Mental health and climate change: tackling invisible injustice. *Lancet Planet Health.* 2020;4(4):e128–e130. doi:10.1016/s2542-5196(20)30081-4
109. Climate equity. Climate Change Impacts. United States Environmental Protection Agency. Updated January 2, 2024. https://www.epa.gov/climateimpacts/climate-equity#:~:text=Environmental%20justice%20is%20the%20fair,laws%2C%20regulations%2C%20and%20policies
110. Arcaya M, Gribkoff E. Climate justice. Climate portal website. March 14, 2022. https://climate.mit.edu/explainers/climate-justice
111. What is climate justice? University of California Center for Climate Justice. 2022. Accessed January 26, 2024. https://centerclimatejustice.universityofcalifornia.edu/what-is-climate-justice/
112. Krishnaswami J, Sardana J, Daxini A. Community-Engaged Lifestyle Medicine as a framework for health equity: principles for lifestyle medicine in low-resource settings. *Am J Lifestyle Med.* 2019;13(5):443–450. doi:10.1177/1559827619838469
113. Hughes S, Chu EK, Mason SG. *Climate Change in Cities.* Springer; 2017.
114. Winkler M, Viliani F, Knoblauch A, et al. Health impact assessment international best practice principles. International Association for Impact Assessment; 2021.
115. Ammann P, Dietler D, Winkler MS. Health impact assessment and climate change: a scoping review. *J Clim Chang Health.* 2021;3:100045. doi:10.1016/j.joclim.2021.100045
116. Mendez MA. Assessing local climate action plans for public health co-benefits in environmental justice communities. *Local Environ.* 2015;20(6):637–663. doi:10.1080/13549839.2015.1038227
117. United States Global Change Research Program. *Fifth National Climate Assessment.* U.S. Global Change Research Program; 2023.
118. Shindell D, Ru M, Zhang Y, et al. Temporal and spatial distribution of health, labor, and crop benefits of climate change mitigation in the United States. *Proc Natl Acad Sci USA.* 2021;118(46):e2104061118. doi:10.1073/pnas.2104061118
119. Vohra K, Vodonos A, Schwartz J, Marais EA, Sulprizio MP, Mickley LJ. Global mortality from outdoor fine particle pollution generated by fossil fuel combustion: results from GEOS-Chem. *Environ Res.* 2021;195:110754. doi:10.1016/j.envres.2021.110754
120. Bensch G, Jeuland M, Peters J. Efficient biomass cooking in Africa for climate change mitigation and development. *One Earth.* 2021;4(6):879–890. doi:10.1016/j.oneear.2021.05.015
121. World Health Organization. Achieving universal access and net-zero emissions by 2050: a global roadmap for just and inclusive clean cooking transition. November 28, 2023. https://www.who.int/publications/m/item/achieving-universal-access-by-2030-and-net-zero-emissions-by-2050-a-global-roadmap-for-just-and-inclusive-clean-cooking-transition
122. Gruenwald T, Seals BA, Knibbs LD, Hosgood HD. Population attributable fraction of gas stoves and childhood asthma in the United States. *Int J Environ Res Public Health.* 2023;20(1):75. doi:10.3390/ijerph20010075
123. Baobeid A, Koç M, Al-Ghamdi SG. Walkability and its relationships with health, sustainability, and livability: elements of physical environment and evaluation frameworks. *Front Built Environ.* 2021;7. doi:10.3389/fbuil.2021.721218
124. Rosenzweig C, Mbow C, Barioni LG, et al. Climate change responses benefit from a global food system approach. *Nat Food.* 2020;1(2):94–97. doi:10.1038/s43016-020-0031-z
125. Willett W, Rockström J, Loken B, et al. Food in the anthropocene: the EAT-Lancet Commission on healthy diets from sustainable food systems. *Lancet.* 2019;393(10170):447–492. doi:10.1016/s0140-6736(18)31788-4
126. Lucas E, Guo M, Guillén-Gosálbez G. Low-carbon diets can reduce global ecological and health costs. *Nat Food.* 2023;4(5):394–406. doi:10.1038/s43016-023-00749-2
127. Climate Adaptation and EPA's Role. United States Environmental Protection Agency. Updated September 6, 2023. https://www.epa.gov/climate-adaptation/climate-adaptation-and-epas-role

128. Adaptation in action: grantee success stories from CDC's Climate and Health Program. American Public Health Association. 2015. Accessed December 22, 2023. https://www.apha.org/-/media/Files/PDF/topics/environment/Adapt_In_Action.pdf
129. Wasley E, Dahl TA, Simpson CF, et al. Adaptation. In: Crimmins AR, Avery CW, Easterling DR, Kunkel KE, Stewart BC, Maycock TK, eds. *Fifth National Climate Assessment*. U.S. Global Change Research Program; 2023.
130. Owen G. What makes climate change adaptation effective? A systematic review of the literature. *Glob Environ Change*. 2020;62:102071. doi:10.1016/j.gloenvcha.2020.102071
131. Whyte K, Novak R, Laramie MB, et al. Tribes and Indigenous peoples. In: Crimmins AR, Avery CW, Easterling DR, Kunkel KE, Stewart BC, Maycock TK, eds. *Fifth National Climate Assessment*. U.S. Global Change Research Program; 2023.
132. United States Global Change Research Program. Alaskan Tribes join together to assess harmful algal blooms. U.S. Climate Resilience Toolkit website. 2021. Updated April 24, 2024. https://toolkit.climate.gov/case-studies/alaskan-tribes-join-together-assess-harmful-algal-blooms
133. Moulton AD, Schramm PJ. Climate change and public health surveillance: toward a comprehensive strategy. *J Public Health Manag Pract*. 2017;23(6):618–626. doi:10.1097/PHH.0000000000000550
134. Sampson NR, Gronlund CJ, Buxton MA, et al. Staying cool in a changing climate: reaching vulnerable populations during heat events. *Glob Environ Change*. 2013;23(2):475–484. doi:10.1016/j.gloenvcha.2012.12.011
135. Jesdale BM, Morello-Frosch R, Cushing L. The racial/ethnic distribution of heat risk–related land cover in relation to residential segregation. *Environ Health Perspect*. 2013;121(7):811–817. doi:10.1289/ehp.1205919
136. Jennings V, Gaither CJ. Approaching environmental health disparities and green spaces: an ecosystem services perspective. *Int J Environ Res Public Health*. 2015;12(2):1952–1968. doi:10.3390/ijerph120201952
137. Musicus AA, Wang DD, Janiszewski M, et al. Health and environmental impacts of plant-rich dietary patterns: a US prospective cohort study. *Lancet Planet Health*. 2022;6(11):e892–e900. doi:10.1016/s2542-5196(22)00243-1
138. Physical activity. World Health Organization. Accessed June 10, 2024. https://www.who.int/westernpacific/health-topics/physical-activity#:~:text=Conversely%2C%20physical%20inactivity%20has%20been,as%20stroke%2C%20diabetes%20and%20cancer
139. CDC releases updated maps of America's high levels of inactivity. Centers for Disease Control and Prevention. 2022. Accessed July 11, 2024. https://www.cdc.gov/media/releases/2022/p0120-inactivity-map.html
140. Fast facts on transportation greenhouse gas emissions. United States Environmental Protection Agency. Updated May 14, 2024. Accessed June 11, 2024. https://www.epa.gov/greenvehicles/fast-facts-transportation-greenhouse-gas-emissions
141. Grabow ML, Spak SN, Holloway T, Stone B, Mednick AC, Patz JA. Air quality and exercise-related health benefits from reduced car travel in the midwestern United States. *Environ Health Perspect*. 2012;120(1):68–76. doi:10.1289/ehp.1103440
142. Nguyen P-Y, Astell-Burt T, Rahimi-Ardabili H, Feng X. Effect of nature prescriptions on cardiometabolic and mental health, and physical activity: a systematic review. *Lancet Planet Health*. 2023;7(4):e313–e328. doi:10.1016/s2542-5196(23)00025-6
143. Pathak N, McKinney A. Planetary health, climate change, and lifestyle medicine: threats and opportunities. *Am J Lifestyle Med*. 2021;15(5):541–552. doi:10.1177/15598276211008127
144. Pathak N, Pollard KJ. Lifestyle medicine prescriptions for personal and planetary health. *J Clim Chang Health*. 2021;4:100077. doi:10.1016/j.joclim.2021.100077
145. Romanello M, Napoli Cd, Green C, et al. The 2023 report of the *Lancet* Countdown on health and climate change: the imperative for a health-centred response in a world facing irreversible harms. *Lancet*. 2023;402(10419):2346–2394. doi:10.1016/s0140-6736(23)01859-7
146. Hamilton I, Kennard H, McGushin A, et al. The public health implications of the Paris Agreement: a modelling study. *Lancet Planet Health*. 2021;5(2):e74–e83. doi:10.1016/s2542-5196(20)30249-7
147. Peters E, Boyd P, Cameron LD, et al. Evidence-based recommendations for communicating the impacts of climate change on health. *Transl Behav Med*. 2022;12(4):543–553. doi:10.1093/tbm/ibac029
148. What is a climate story. Climate Generation. Accessed June 10, 2024. https://climategen.org/take-action/storytelling/

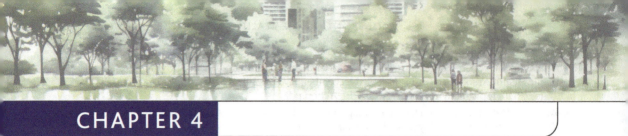

CHAPTER 4

Environmental Health Policies and Protections: Successes and Failures

Adrienne L. Hollis, Vernice Miller-Travis, and Daria E. Neal

LEARNING OBJECTIVES

- Identify laws, statutes, and executive orders that address environmental health and justice in the United States at the federal level.
- Describe the role local governments can play in addressing environmental health and justice.
- Evaluate environmental policies in the United States, understanding how they have been designed to protect public health and how they could be improved to ensure equal protection for all.
- Understand the opportunities and limits of regulatory science, including the role of various types of evidence.
- Learn some key technical and scientific concepts of environmental policies, such as "point" and "nonpoint" sources used when discussing pollution discharges.

KEY TERMS

- advocacy
- amendment
- consent agreement
- environmental policy
- executive orders
- false solutions
- Federal Register
- legislation
- lobbying
- ordinance
- precautionary principle
- presidential memoranda
- public policy
- regulatory science
- rule
- Sustainable Development Goals (SDGs)

OVERVIEW

How is environmental health protected? This question is a complex one given the variety of environmental exposure pathways we face daily. For instance, if there is a high level of air pollution in one's neighborhood, how is it regulated? Is the pollution from diesel trucks whose emissions are regulated by the U.S. Environmental Protection Agency (EPA), which implements laws set by the Congress? Is pollution coming from nearby facilities regulated under the Clean Air Act through their Title V permit, which is overseen by the EPA but likely implemented by your state environmental agency? Is the pollution just in the air ("ambient") and hard to attribute to a single source? If so, it could be regulated under the Clean Air Act's National Ambient Air Quality Standards (NAAQS). Or the pollution could be fugitive dust, and you may not have a local ordinance to address it. It could even be coming from a power plant's activities in another state, which may mean it falls under EPA's Good Neighbor Plan. With this example of possible contributors to neighborhood air pollution, one can quickly see that the system of environmental protections in the United States is hard to navigate for most people.

Throughout the past century, many major environmental regulations were developed, and advances in science, technology, and advocacy generally led to more stringent protections over time. For example, early regulations focused on conservation efforts to support hunting and sport fishing activities and did not focus on environmental health issues. Environmental health-related issues and challenges are much the same today as they were at the start of the modern environmental movement in the 1960s.[1] They are arguably more complex, however, owing to our growing population, the loss of biological diversity, the increasing use of chemicals, and the increasingly threatened climate. Of course, adding to that complexity is an ongoing need to recognize and address environmental injustice.

Communities of color and low-wealth communities are disproportionately burdened by environmental hazards,[2] and the resulting health disparities fall heavily along racial lines.[3,4] For instance, the COVID-19 pandemic most clearly demonstrated in real time how exposure to fine-particle air pollution left Black, Hispanic or Latino, and Indigenous communities particularly susceptible to the severe respiratory virus. Additionally, many communities of color also experience relatively higher rates of asthma and other respiratory conditions, making them especially susceptible to this new deadly virus. Recently, there has been increasing attention to environmental justice (EJ) issues, but a consideration of health equity with respect to all government policies is needed to make real progress.

Beginning in 2021, the Biden–Harris Administration began working with the 117th U.S. Congress to pass several historic bills to advance environmental protections, including establishing the first-ever national *green bank*, which is intended to:

- invest in infrastructure modernization,
- focus on providing expanded access to safe drinking water and wastewater systems,
- expand renewable energy and build a more resilient power grid, and
- support electrification of the transportation system, thereby reducing climate-changing carbon emissions, as well as many other programs.

Many of these bills are aimed at reducing environmental impacts and improving human and ecological health.

With this burst of environmental legislation—together with specific targeted **executive orders,** the Inflation Reduction Act (IRA), and the Bipartisan Infrastructure Law (BIL)—we are poised to see unprecedented efforts to reduce environmental injustice, invest in disadvantaged communities, reduce harmful levels of toxic exposures, and create a record number of jobs in green industries in the United States. This chapter focuses primarily on U.S. federal laws, while noting the role of policy from global to local levels.

GLOBAL ENVIRONMENTAL POLICYMAKING

Globally, there have been many efforts to address environmental issues, particularly climate change, over the past few decades. Global environmental policies, treaties, and charters are often internationally agreed-upon goals, principles, or procedures used to guide environmental decisions and actions. For instance, the United Nations (UN) Environmental Law is a foundation for environmental sustainability,[5] and the UN Environment Programme is a global authority that works toward achieving the **Sustainable Development Goals (SDGs;** Figure 4.1).[6] The SDGs are designed to be achieved by 2030 and serve as a framework for international cooperation to improve the well-being of people and the planet.

Other important global policies are identified in Table 4.1, many which were established through the UN Conference of Parties (COP). The COP is a central component of the UN Framework Convention on Climate Change (UNFCCC), an international treaty aimed at addressing global climate change. The COP meetings are gatherings of representatives from countries that are parties to the UNFCCC, and they play a crucial role in the global efforts to combat climate change. At these meetings, global leaders negotiate on major issues, such as emission reduction targets, climate financing, and strategies for building global capacity and resources for mitigation and adaptation. The Paris Agreement, perhaps the most well known in recent history, was

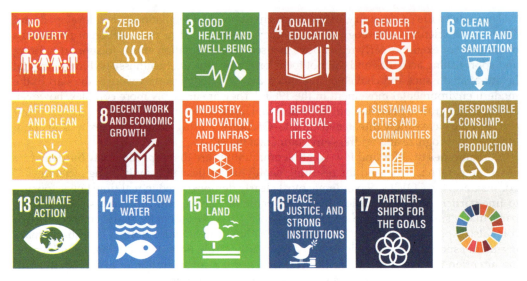

FIGURE 4.1. United Nations 17 Sustainable Development Goals.
Source: The 17 goals. United Nations Department of Economic and Social Affairs: Sustainable Development. 2015. https://sdgs.un.org/goals

TABLE 4.1. MAJOR GLOBAL POLICIES RELATED TO ENVIRONMENTAL HEALTH AND JUSTICE

POLICIES/CHARTER	PURPOSE
UNFCCC: Established in 1992 with near universal membership of 198 parties (or nations).	The Convention is the parent treaty of both the 2015 Paris Agreement and the 1997 Kyoto Protocol.
Kyoto Protocol: Adopted on December 11, 1997, at the UN Climate Change Conference (COP11) in Kyoto, Japan, and entered into force on February 16, 2005.	This international treaty extends the UNFCCC and commits parties to reduce greenhouse gas emissions.
Paris Agreement: Adopted on December 12, 2015, at the UN Climate Change Conference (COP21) in Paris, France, and entered into force on November 4, 2016.[5]	This legally binding international treaty sets an overarching goal to hold "the increase in the global average temperature to well below 2°C above preindustrial levels" and pursue efforts "to limit the temperature increase to 1.5°C above preindustrial levels."[5]
Montreal Protocol: Adopted on September 16, 1987, in Montreal, Canada, and entered into force on January 1, 1989.[1]	This international treaty protects the ozone layer by phasing out the production of numerous substances that are responsible for ozone depletion. It was amended in 2016 with the Kigali Amendment, a legally binding international agreement to gradually reduce the consumption and production of hydrofluorocarbons.[3]
The Basel Convention on the Control of Transboundary Movements of Hazardous Wastes and Their Disposal: Adopted in 1989 in Basel, Switzerland.	The convention establishes a framework for controlling the movement of hazardous waste across international borders. It seeks to prevent the export of hazardous waste from wealthy nations to poorer nations, where inadequate facilities and regulations may lead to environmental injustice.

UN, United Nations; UNFCCC, United Nations Framework Convention on Climate Change.

adopted at the 2015 COP meeting, setting a global goal to limit global warming to well below 2 degrees Celsius above preindustrial levels, with efforts to limit it to 1.5 degrees. Subsequent COP meetings have focused on implementing and strengthening the Paris Agreement.

ENVIRONMENTAL POLICYMAKING IN THE UNITED STATES

The U.S. Constitution does not explicitly address public health in detail. However, it can be interpreted to encompass environmental health concerns. The Preamble to the Constitution states that one of its purposes is to "promote the general Welfare." This clause has been used to justify various federal government interventions in public health matters, such as funding for medical research, public health programs, and healthcare infrastructure. The Commerce Clause (Article I, Section 8) of the Constitution grants Congress the power to regulate commerce among the states. This authority has been used to regulate aspects of public health, including the regulation of food and drugs and the control of infectious diseases. The federal government can use its taxation and spending powers to raise revenue and allocate funds for public health initiatives. It may also act during public health emergencies, for instance, by allocating resources to respond to environmental health emergencies. Although the Constitution provides a broad framework, the specific authority to address environmental health matters often is given to state and local governments.

Specifically, **environmental policy** includes government actions that affect (or attempt to affect) environmental quality or the use of natural resources. Figure 4.2 reminds us of the roles of our three government branches, and Figure 4.3 clarifies a policy versus a program. At the federal level, environmental policy is about the collective decision of society to pursue certain

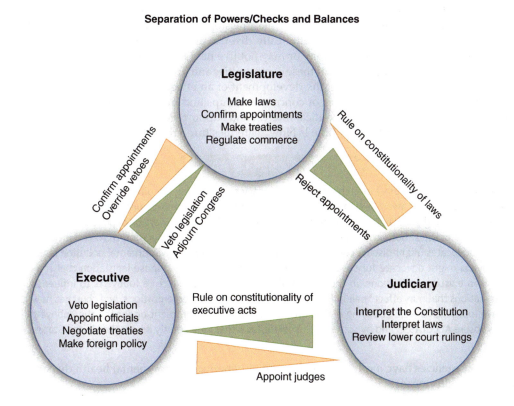

FIGURE 4.2. Back to the basics.

There are three branches of government in the United States: the legislative, executive, and judicial branches. What role do they each play in implementing our environmental protections? They participate in a system of "checks and balances." They can respond to the acts of the other branches and even change those acts through specific processes.

> **A program generally:**
> Addresses a small part of the problem
> Changes individuals or communities
> Meets an immediate need with short-term change

> **A policy may:**
> Address entire process
> Address big picture
> Move toward broader goals
> Change institutions and communities
> Lead to long-term change

FIGURE 4.3. Is that a program or a policy?
Source: Israel BA, Coombe CM, Cheezum RR, Schulz AJ, McGranaghan RJ, Lichtenstein R, Reyes AG, Clement J, Burris A. Community-based participatory research: a capacity-building approach for policy advocacy aimed at eliminating health disparities. *Am J Public Health*. 2010 Nov;100(11):2094–2102. doi:10.2105/AJPH.2009.170506

environmental goals and objectives and to use specific tools to achieve them. These tools may encompass actions like executive orders, presidential memoranda, or **legislation**, which generally includes the introduction of a proposal in one of four principal forms: the bill, the joint resolution, the concurrent resolution, and the simple resolution.

Most environmental policies are developed in response to public mobilization, sometimes entailing decades of advocacy. *Grassroots* and *grasstops* organizations have a role to play in this advocacy work. Historically, grassroots organizations are more often underfunded and composed of people of color, Tribal communities, and those with limited socioeconomic means living on the front lines near hazardous conditions that adversely affect their health and environment. They have much expertise, but they typically have fewer resources or less capacity to achieve protective policies, corrective actions, or funding for environmental amenities when compared to grasstops organizations. Meanwhile, grasstops organizations usually have greater access to wealth, are less racially and ethnically diverse, and have more capacity to impact environmental policymaking. They may or may not live near hazardous conditions, and they may or may not center the priorities of these communities and grassroots organizations in their advocacy efforts. For the most part, the development of an effective environmental health or justice policy depends on the ability of concerned groups and interested community organizations to collaborate and garner political interest and support. For ideas about ways you can engage in advocacy, refer to "The Time Is Now" activities through this book.

IN OTHER WORDS: ADVOCACY VERSUS LOBBYING

Although sometimes used interchangeably, advocacy and lobbying are different. **Advocacy** generally entails raising awareness, mobilizing public support, and educating policymakers on specific issues. **Lobbying** entails attempting to influence policymakers to support or oppose specific legislation or policies. Both could involve meeting with the public and decision makers. However, while advocates might discuss concerns and data related to a local environmental pollution issue, lobbyists might advocate for specific environmental regulations or oppose legislation that may weaken existing protections. In the United States, many companies hire lobbyists to influence regulations that may affect their industry. Universities, nonprofit organizations, and churches may have lobbyists as well. Lobbying is regulated by the federal government under the the Lobbying Disclosure Act of 1995 and by some state-specific laws that vary greatly across the United States.

Federal agencies have a role in reducing and eliminating environmental health disparities through various means:

- grant programs targeting overburdened, marginalized, and disadvantaged communities;
- technical assistance programs that build the capacity of state and local governments and support academic institutions and local nonprofit organizations; and
- collection of critical data that enable the development of new tools, programs, and strategies to remedy existing harms.

Much of this work is determined by appropriations, which is the process of setting aside money for specific projects. In the federal government, appropriations determine how much money is allocated through the federal budget. The president submits a budget to Congress for the federal government every fiscal year (October 1 through September 30). Congress must then pass appropriations bills to provide money to carry out government programs for that year.[7] It is worth noting that the president's budget proposal is really just a request and has no binding authority in Congress. The budget proposal is best understood as a detailed statement by the administration of its fiscal goals and policy preferences.[8]

Further, guided by legislation, agency staff conduct and rely on regulatory science for setting rules and regulations to implement legislation. For instance, agency staff use regulatory science in the process of characterizing the risks associated with drinking water or air pollutants and informing new standards. According to the EPA, **regulatory science** is the use of scientific information from models, assessments, peer-reviewed literature, and other sources that act as a foundation for regulatory decisions. This foundation may include research conducted by academic scholars or scholars at other research institutions.

IN OTHER WORDS: PUBLIC COMMENTS

What are public comments?

Whenever a federal, state, or local government agency proposes a major environmental action, the agency is required to document the action in writing. The actions can have significant impacts on individuals, communities, economies, and the environment, so they are usually accompanied by an open-comment period. The process of allowing for a written commentary allows individuals, organizations, agencies, and businesses to provide feedback on proposed decisions and make their voices heard.

Where can opportunities to comment be found?

The **Federal Register** is a daily publication by the United States government that contains various proposed rules, final rules, notices, and executive orders issued by federal agencies. It serves as a public resource for information about the government's activities and allows the public to participate in the rule-making process by providing comments on proposed rules or policies. Local and state governments may have various systems for communicating their open-comment opportunities. Following trusted organizations via email, newsletters, or social media may also provide notices about comment opportunities related to certain environmental health issues of interest.

Tips for writing effective comments:

In *The Art of Commenting*, Elizabeth Mullin[9] suggests that you do one of the following:

- **Pound the law:** Comment on clear legal omissions or violations if you understand the legalities of the issue under consideration.
- **Pound the facts:** Comment on notably inaccurate or omitted information, or facts that deserve more consideration and elaboration.
- **Pound the table:** If you cannot comment on legal or scientific matters, you may want to critique the process or conclusions.

MAJOR FEDERAL ENVIRONMENTAL HEALTH PROTECTIONS

This section provides an overview of major U.S. environmental policies, starting with what is most likely the oldest legislation "focused directly on environmental issues" not law—the National Environmental Policy Act (NEPA). Many of these policies began to take shape in the mid-1900s alongside the mainstream U.S. environmental movement and formally took shape alongside the birth of the EPA in 1970 under President Nixon. In recent years, attention has focused on increasing either the protections or the enforcement activities provided by several of these existing policies, many of which have been in existence for more than 50 years.

THE NATIONAL ENVIRONMENTAL POLICY ACT

The first piece of official environmental health legislation in the United States was National Environmental Policy Act (NEPA), signed into law on January 1, 1970. NEPA requires federal agencies to assess the environmental effects of proposed major federal actions before making decisions.[10] These actions may include permitting the filling of wetlands, approving highway expansions, or constructing new pipelines to transport fossil fuels. Countries and nongovernmental organizations all over the globe have created their own environmental impact assessment programs, modeled upon NEPA, making NEPA an international catalyst in the field of environmental protection.[11]

Section 102 of NEPA establishes procedural requirements that are applied to proposals for major federal actions that would (or will) significantly affect the quality of the human environment. It does this by requiring federal agencies to prepare a detailed statement on:

- the environmental impact of the proposed action,
- any adverse effects that cannot be avoided,
- alternatives to the proposed action,
- the relationship between local short-term uses of human environments and the maintenance and enhancement of long-term productivity, and
- any irreversible and irretrievable commitments of resources that would be involved in the proposed action.[11]

As one might imagine, these are situations in which community concerns abound and in which communities demand that NEPA be strictly enforced given the extent to which their health, as well their immediate environment, could be at risk.

Many advocates would agree that NEPA falls short in achieving EJ. Although NEPA was designed to ensure that "agencies consider the significant environmental consequences of their proposed actions and inform the public about their decision-making,"[11(para3)] many argue that the process and outcomes are too broad and overlook underlying inequities. For example, in communities where health is already disproportionately impacted by multiple pollution sources, related concerns are not really considered during decision-making. If those concerns were indeed prioritized (or even just considered), then many environmental decisions would err on the side of protecting communities. However, this prioritization and resulting protection often do not occur.

The development of an international border crossing between southwest Detroit, Michigan, USA, and Windsor, Ontario, Canada, illustrates NEPA's failure to consider EJ. Here, the new Gordie Howe International Bridge crossing's environmental impact statement (EIS), prepared by the U.S. Department of Transportation and the Michigan Department of Transportation, concluded from their analysis that air quality would improve *regionally*.[12] However, the prevailing conclusion among residents, community leaders, scientists, and health professionals was that the *neighborhood* air quality could not possibly improve, given the increase of more than 10,000 new trucks a day on the crossing, which would inevitably bring more air pollution to a community already impacted by exposures from more than 40 polluting facilities.[13] The Southwest Detroit Community Benefits Coalition has worked for over 20 years to secure environmental protections, despite this NEPA outcome.

THE CLEAN WATER ACT

About 50 years ago, some U.S. rivers were so polluted with oil and grease that they caught fire.[14] Other rivers were so filled with industrial pollution, untreated sewage, or smelly algal blooms that they were declared "functionally dead," and it was said that they "oozed" instead of flowed. In 1972, Republicans and Democrats, in a bipartisan effort, decided to address this public health crisis by passing the Clean Water Act (CWA), with the specific intention of protecting lakes, rivers, streams, wetlands, and bays from pollution and destruction. The vote in favor was unanimous in the Senate and very nearly so in the House.

The CWA has the enormous task of overseeing the nation's water quality and controlling point-source pollution discharge into surface waters. The EPA defines a *point source* as "any discernible, confined, and discrete conveyance,"[15(para5)] such as a pipe, well, ditch, channel, tunnel, conduit, concentrated animal feeding operation, discrete fissure, rolling stock, or container. It also includes vessels or other floating crafts from which pollutants are or may be discharged. Conversely, nonpoint sources are those that are not discharged at a single outlet or pipe. They may include runoff of pesticides or animal waste from commercial farms into waterways, for instance, or from everyday activities such as lawn fertilization or construction."[15] A nonpoint source is not easily identifiable, which makes enforcement activities harder to carry out.

The CWA gives the EPA the authority to implement pollution-control programs, like setting wastewater standards for industry and establishing water quality standards for all contaminants in surface waters.[16] Under the CWA, specific conditions and permitting for discharges of pollutants into the waters of the United States are defined and described under the National Pollution Discharge Elimination System (NPDES).[17] This system makes it unlawful for any person to discharge any pollutant from a point source into U.S. waters, unless a NPDES permit is first obtained.[16] NPDES permits include limits on what can be discharged, and they contain monitoring and reporting requirements. The CWA has additional provisions that help ensure that any discharge does not negatively affect people's health or water quality generally.

Since it was first established, the CWA has been extremely effective for many but not all waterways. It has kept about 700 billion pounds of pollutants out of our waters each year, slowed the rate of wetland loss, doubled the number of places that meet clean water goals, and, as a result, lowered the cost to treat drinking water. However, while the CWA has been successful for the most part, it has not been as protective as hoped, especially for communities of color. Cities like Jackson, Mississippi,[18] which is nearly 83% Black, with more than 150,000 residents, have had to deal with the shortcomings of race-based unequal CWA enforcement.

In August 2022, after the Pearl River flooded because of severe storms, more than 170,000 residents in Jackson experienced an extreme public health crisis. As a result, they lost access to potable water to drink, wash, or flush their toilets. This crisis was the latest in a series of water-related problems plaguing Jackson, the biggest city in Mississippi. The problems have included frequent line breaks, shut-offs, boil-water notices, and an ongoing exposure to toxic lead and harmful bacteria.[19] Since 2018, the city of Jackson has also consistently violated drinking water standards, and it has been under a federal order to repair the water system since 2020. During the week of January 17, 2023, Jackson had four boil-water notices for areas across the city, and notices had just ended in four other areas the week prior. The Jackson water crisis and accompanying environmental health effects continue as of this writing.[20] Passed in 2021, the BIL was designed to repair failing infrastructure, the main issue in Jackson. The concern for most environmental advocates revolves around the need for appropriate oversight to ensure that this federal money (now in the billions of dollars) is used for places like Jackson, where the population majority is Black.

THE SAFE DRINKING WATER ACT

Originally passed in 1974, the purpose of the Safe Drinking Water Act (SDWA) is to provide public health protection through the nation's drinking water. The EPA does this by developing primary and secondary drinking water standards, which are implemented primarily by state agencies. These standards were created to protect drinking water from more than 90 contaminants. These standards specify the maximum allowable levels of various substances in drinking water, including microbiological contaminants (e.g., bacteria, viruses), chemical contaminants (e.g., lead, arsenic), and radiological contaminants. The SDWA mandates that water suppliers provide the households they service with an annual water quality report (called a Consumer Confidence Report) that outlines the source of their water, any contaminants detected, and whether the water meets federal standards.

Although the EPA reports on its website that over 92% of the population supplied by community water systems receive drinking water that meets all health-based standards, compliance with the standards has not always been the case.[21] For example, in 2014 the city of Flint, Michigan, made the flawed decision to change their municipal water supply source from Lake Huron to the Flint River without any corrosion controls. Because of that decision, residents were exposed to drinking water contaminated with extremely high levels of lead and other contaminants from the resulting corroding water supply pipes. Inadequate and inaccurate water testing and treatment led to serious illnesses from *Legionella* bacteria and lead poisoning, particularly among children. The numerous reports of bad-smelling water, sickness, skin irritation, hair loss, and other health effects were largely ignored by authorities. For almost 2 years, residents were exposed to contaminated water, in flagrant violation of the SDWA.

THE CLEAN AIR ACT

The Clean Air Act (CAA) is the federal law that regulates air emissions from stationary and mobile sources.[22] Stationary sources include factories, refineries, and power plants. Mobile sources include cars, trucks, buses, and marine vessels. Alongside the NEPA and the CWA, the CAA was among the first groundbreaking environmental policies in the United States. It was first enacted in 1963 and has undergone several amendments and updates, with the most significant revisions in 1970 and 1990. Key provisions of the CAA are listed in Table 4.2 and discussed in more detail in Chapter 10, "The Air We Breathe." This law authorizes the EPA to establish NAAQS to protect public health and public welfare and to regulate the emissions of hazardous air pollutants. There are six major pollutants regulated by the NAAQS: ozone (O_3), particulate matter (PM), carbon monoxide (CO), sulfur dioxide (SO_2), nitrogen dioxide (NO_2), and lead (Pb).

In the 50 years during which the EPA has overseen state implementation of the CAA, air quality has dramatically improved in many ways. In the United States, common pollutants such as sulfur dioxide and nitrogen oxide have been controlled, and restrictions have been placed on dangerous air toxics. Between 1990 and 2018, the levels of CO fell by 74%, ground level ozone declined by 21%, and lead levels in ambient air decreased by 82%. The EPA estimates that amendments made to the CAA over time are responsible for preventing over 230,000 early deaths by 2020, and significantly reducing the frequency of respiratory diseases, including chronic bronchitis and asthma exacerbation.[23]

TABLE 4.2. KEY PROVISIONS OF THE CLEAN AIR ACT

CLEAN AIR ACT TITLE	PROGRAMS AND ACTIVITIES COVERED
TITLE I	NAAQS, HAPS, state implementation plans, regulations for smokestack heights, new source review, plans for nonattainment
TITLE II	Emission standards for mobile sources, motor vehicle emissions, aircrafts, "clean" fuel alternatives
TITLE III	General provisions, HAPS continued, risk assessment and technology-based emissions standards (i.e., MACT)
TITLE IV	Noise pollution and acid deposition control, reduction of SO_2 at power plants
TITLE V	Operating permits for polluting facilities issued by state and local agencies to track and report emissions; sets technical standards for facilities, RACT for existing sources, BACT for new sources, and LAER when in nonattainment area
TITLE VI	Stratospheric ozone protection, phased out ozone-depleting HFCs

CAA, Clean Air Act; HAPS, hazardous air pollutants; HFCs, hydrochlorofluorocarbons; LAER, lowest achievable emissions rate; MACT, maximum achievable control technology; NAAQS, National Ambient Air Quality Standards; RACT, reasonably available control technology

The CAA includes a Good Neighbor provision that requires states that are upwind to ensure that the air pollution that they create does not affect downwind states' ability to meet the NAAQS. The Good Neighbor provision helps downwind states protect the environmental health of their residents. In 2023, the EPA announced the final Good Neighbor Plan, which will significantly cut smog-forming nitrogen oxide pollution from power plants and other industrial facilities in 23 states. This rule is expected to save lives, reduce hospitalizations and sick days, and reduce the number and severity of asthma attacks.[24]

> **NATIONAL AMBIENT AIR QUALITY STANDARDS FOR PARTICULATE MATTER: THE "SOOT RULE"**
>
> In January 2023, the Environmental Protection Agency (EPA) introduced a rule designed to strengthen the National Ambient Air Quality Standards (NAAQS) for fine particulate matter (black soot or particulate matter 2.5 [$PM_{2.5}$]). $PM_{2.5}$ designates particulate matter not visible to the human eye at around 2.5 microns in size. The rule was designed to protect communities, particularly those that are disproportionately exposed to pollution.
>
> Soot can penetrate deep into the lungs, resulting in numerous adverse health effects, like asthma, cardiovascular disease, and even death. Special populations that are most susceptible to this type of pollution include children, older people, and those with preexisting respiratory or heart conditions. Pollution exposure is relatively much higher for communities of color and people experiencing poverty.
>
> In March 2023, over 80 House and Senate Democrats pushed for the EPA to aggressively pursue strong national soot standards. In February 2024, the EPA issued the final rule, which significantly lowered the allowable limit for annual $PM_{2.5}$ levels from 12 micrograms per cubic meter to 9. States have several years to reach this new standard, which is expected to save thousands of lives each year once established. As of this writing, many Republican-led states have initiated lawsuits to challenge the rule.

Much like other major environmental protections, however, the CAA has not been a success story for all communities. Even though CAA policies have been effective overall, there has been an increase in dangerous air pollution levels in some communities, accompanied by demands for stronger air quality regulations to mitigate health risks, combat the climate crisis, and support economic growth. Some communities have not met the NAAQS for decades even with plans in place to help them achieve attainment. As seen in the example in Figure 4.4 for the 8-hour ozone standard, several parts of the country do not meet this standard, which is referred to as "nonattainment."

TOXIC SUBSTANCES CONTROL ACT OF 1976

The Toxic Substances Control Act (TSCA) gives the EPA the authority to require manufacturers, distributors, importers, laboratories, and other frequent and heavy chemical users to engage in specific regulated activities like reporting, record-keeping, and testing. TSCA is important for communities, particularly those in proximity to chemical facilities, because it focuses on the production, importation, use, and disposal of specific chemicals including polychlorinated biphenyls (PCBs), asbestos, radon, and lead-based paint, among many others. TSCA includes restrictions related to the use of chemical substances and mixtures. However, TSCA does not include, among other things, food, drugs, cosmetics, and pesticides.[25] Instead, food, food additives, drugs, and cosmetics are regulated by the United States Food and Drug Administration (FDA), and pesticides are regulated by the Federal Insecticide, Fungicide, and Rodenticide Act (FIFRA). In addition, tobacco and tobacco products are regulated by the Bureau of Alcohol, Tobacco, Firearms and Explosives (ATF), and radioactive materials are regulated by the Nuclear Regulatory Commission (NRC).

There are many critiques of TSCA and, after 40 years, it was significantly amended for the first time in 2016. Renamed the Frank R. Lautenberg Chemical Safety for the 21st Century Act,[26]

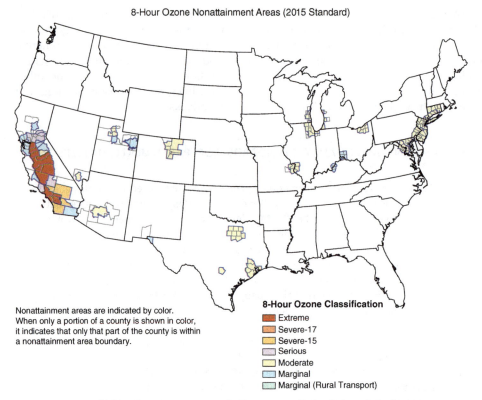

FIGURE 4.4. A snapshot from U.S. Environmental Protection Agency's Green Book, which tracks nonattainment for the National Ambient Air Quality Standards.

Source: Green Book: 8-hour ozone nonattainment areas (2015 standard). United States Environmental Protection Agency. Updated March 31, 2024. https://www3.epa.gov/airquality/greenbook/map8hr_2015.html

the amendments revised the process and the requirements for evaluating and determining whether regulatory control is warranted for manufacturing, distribution, processing, using, and disposing of chemicals. The Act also revised a number of the TSCA provisions, including revisions to chemical testing, the review and regulation of new chemicals, new uses for existing chemicals, information reporting, preemption of state regulations, and fees.[26] In addition, the Act revised TSCA requirements on testing chemicals and authorized the EPA to develop new information for evaluating unreasonable risks to human health and the environment, prioritizing the risk evaluations, and implementing risk-management control actions. The Act also allows the EPA to require the development of information through a **consent agreement,** or an order, which is very important, since prior to the amendments, the EPA was limited to requiring the development of information through a rule.

CASE STUDY 4.1: United States Versus European Union Regulations

The United States' Toxic Substances Control Act (TSCA) and the European Union's Registration, Evaluation, Authorization, and Restriction of Chemicals (REACH) regulation are two significant frameworks that address chemical management. Comparisons can be made between the frameworks to illustrate some of the failures of TSCA and the successes of the REACH regulation.

(continued)

> **CASE STUDY 4.1:** United States Versus European Union Regulations (*continued*)
>
> TSCA was enacted nearly 30 years prior to the implementation of the REACH regulation. Unlike REACH, TSCA did not require comprehensive testing before a chemical was introduced into the market. REACH embraced the **precautionary principle**, which advocates taking preventative action in the face of scientific uncertainty. In other words, it adopts a "better-safe-than-sorry" approach, while TSCA has more of a "wait-and-see" approach. TSCA's lack of a precautionary approach has resulted in little to no information on thousands of chemicals. When TSCA was implemented, over 60,000 chemicals were allowed to remain on the market without careful scrutiny. Furthermore, the burden of proof for demonstrating the safety of these chemicals largely falls on regulatory authorities. Consequently, there has been an extremely slow pace for the review of chemicals and a burdensome process that has prohibited the removal of substances with known hazardous properties. While the 2016 amendments to TSCA were a significant update, the Environmental Protection Agency was left to regulate chemicals and determine the best available science, leaving room for political influence, underestimation of exposures, and lack of protection for highly susceptible populations, like children, and already overburdened environmental justice communities.[27]
>
> In contrast, REACH, which was implemented in 2007, requires manufacturers to provide comprehensive data on chemicals, enabling informed decision-making. The shift of responsibility to manufacturers promotes the development of safer alternatives, encourages sustainable and healthy practices, and reduces the regulatory burden on authorities compared to TSCA. Importantly for the sake of health, many chemicals that are permitted for use in the United States are banned in Europe under REACH. Examples include potentially cancer-causing substances like titanium dioxide and potassium bromate, which are allowed in a number of foods in the United States but not in Europe.

"EVERY SECTOR IS A HEALTH SECTOR": OTHER FEDERAL ENVIRONMENTAL HEALTH PROTECTIONS

As social epidemiologist Sir Michael Marmot has famously stated, "every sector is a health sector."[28] Thus we should also think about the ways in which planning, housing, transportation, education, and other sector's policies shape our communities and are related to environmental health. To this end, although the EPA oversees the majority of environmental protections in the United States, other agencies are certainly implicated. For instance, the United States Department of Agriculture (USDA), which oversees the commercial supply of meat, poultry, and eggs, implements the Farm Bill. The Farm Bill is a package of legislation passed every five years or so to shape how food is grown and accessed in the United States. Many key policies and other legislation are provided in Table 4.3, and even more legislation and policies are referenced throughout this text. This list is by no means exhaustive.

EXECUTIVE ORDERS CALLING FOR ENVIRONMENTAL HEALTH AND JUSTICE

Executive Orders 12898, 13985, 14008, and 14096 represent the Executive Branch's efforts to establish support for environmental health and justice. Executive Order 12898, *Federal Actions to Address Environmental Justice in Minority Populations and Low-Income Populations*, issued in 1994 by President Bill Clinton, directed federal agencies to make achieving EJ part of their mission by identifying and addressing disproportionately high and adverse human health or environmental effects of its programs, policies, and activities on minority populations and low-income populations.[35] In his first two years in office, President Joe Biden published over 100 executive orders, alongside agency regulatory and policy actions that authorize agencies to take affirmative steps to address health disparities.

TABLE 4.3. OTHER LEGISLATION RELATED TO ENVIRONMENTAL HEALTH

OTHER LEGISLATION	DESCRIPTION	AGENCY LEAD
The Methane Rule[29]	Requires the monitoring of emissions from oil and gas wells nationwide, instead of just focusing on new wells.	EPA
The Mercury Air Toxics Standards (MATS)[30]	Limits the emissions of toxic air pollutants like mercury, arsenic, and metals and other toxic substances from fossil fuel power plants.	EPA
Comprehensive Environmental Response, Compensation, and Liability Act (CERCLA)[31]	Provides a federal Superfund to clean up uncontrolled or abandoned hazardous waste sites as well as accidents, spills, and other emergency releases of pollutants and contaminants into the environment; gives the EPA authority to seek out responsible parties responsible for any release and cleanup.	EPA
Resource Conservation and Recovery Act (RCRA)[32]	Manages hazardous and nonhazardous solid waste.	EPA
The Farm Bill[33]	Addresses agricultural and food issues by providing assistance for farms and food; updated every five years; and the current Farm Bill is called the Agriculture Improvement Act of 2018.	USDA
The Food Quality Protection Act of 1996 (FQPA)[34]	Requires safety standards and collection of pesticide residue data on commodities most frequently consumed by infants and children; considers aggregate and cumulative risk assessment.	EPA

EPA, United States Environmental Protection Agency; USDA, United States Department of Agriculture

Twenty-seven years after Executive Order 12898, Executive Order 13985, *Advancing Racial Equity and Support for Underserved Communities Through the Federal Government*, issued in 2021, recognized that the United States was facing "converging economic, health, and climate crises that have exposed and exacerbated inequities, while a historic movement for justice has highlighted the unbearable human costs of systemic racism" and directed agencies to "assess whether, and to what extent, its programs and policies perpetuate systemic barriers to opportunities and benefits for people of color and other underserved groups."[36]

Executive Order 14008, *Tackling the Climate Crisis at Home and Abroad*, is one of the most far-reaching directives that takes a government-wide approach to the climate crises by prioritizing climate in foreign policy and national security as well as securing "environmental justice and . . . economic opportunity for disadvantaged communities that have been historically marginalized and overburdened by pollution and underinvestment in housing, transportation, water and wastewater infrastructure, and health care."[37] It also introduced the Justice40 Initiative (J40). Most notably, J40 establishes a goal that 40% of the overall benefits of certain federal investments must flow to disadvantaged communities that are marginalized, underserved, and overburdened by pollution.[38]

Executive Order 14096, *Revitalizing our Nation's Commitment to Environmental Justice for All*, recognizes that restoring and protecting a healthy environment "is a matter of justice and a fundamental duty that the Federal Government must uphold on behalf of all people."[34] The order acknowledges that "communities with environmental justice concerns face entrenched disparities that are often the legacy of racial discrimination and segregation, redlining, exclusionary zoning, and other discriminatory land use decisions or patterns." To address the persistence of discrimination, EO 14096 did something the first EJ executive order, EO 12898, did not: It specifically directed agencies to act "in accordance with Title VI of the Civil

TABLE 4.4. EXECUTIVE ORDERS RELATED TO ENVIRONMENTAL HEALTH

EXECUTIVE ORDER	RELEVANT LANGUAGE
13990: Protecting Public Health and the Environment and Restoring Science to Tackle the Climate Crisis	Mandates a review of the actions and policies of the Trump administration to ensure compliance with the administration's environmental policies; addresses climate change, and prioritizes environmental justice; issued in 2021.
13995: Ensuring an Equitable Pandemic Response and Recovery	Addresses COVID-19's disproportionate impacts on people of color and other underserved populations and allocates equitable resources; issued in 2021.
14007: President's Council of Advisors on Science and Technology (PCAST)	Established PCAST to advise the president on matters related to informing public policy on the economy, worker empowerment, education, energy, the environment, public health, and other topics; issued in 2021.
13045: Executive Order on the Protection of Children from Environmental Health Risks and Safety Risks	Requires federal agencies to identify disproportionate risks to children that result from environmental health risks or safety risks; issued in 1997.

Rights Act of 1964, 42 U.S.C. 2000d, and agency regulations, [to] ensure that all programs or activities receiving Federal financial assistance that potentially affect human health or the environment do not directly, or through contractual or other arrangements, use criteria, policies, practices, or methods of administration that discriminate on the basis of race, color, or national origin."[34]

These four executive orders mark an intentional effort by the federal government to address the intersection of environmental, health, and racial discrimination. A partial list of other executive orders that include language related to environmental health is provided in Table 4.4.

MAJOR INFRASTRUCTURE AND ECONOMIC LEGISLATION AS ENVIRONMENTAL POLICY

Though many previous administrations have discussed the need to improve the nation's infrastructure, none since the Eisenhower Administration successfully passed significant funding into federal law. As a result of insufficient maintenance and modernization, drinking water systems are failing and sewer systems are collapsing, leading to the discharge of raw sewage and wastewater directly into rivers, streams, and oceans. Additionally, bridges, roadways, and railways are deteriorating, mass transit systems are in decline, and flooding is becoming more frequent across the nation. As discussed in Chapter 15, "Preparing for and Recovering From Disasters in Our Changing Climate," climate-related disasters are also occurring more regularly, impacting fisheries, farmland, forests, and the energy grid. Already overburdened EJ communities are the most impacted and are being called upon again and again to be resilient in the face of repeated infrastructure and social safety net failures.[39]

Without significant investment to maintain, improve, and modernize our infrastructure, these issues have led to major public health failures, including asthma; chronic respiratory, lung, and heart disease; and lead poisoning, among many other issues. These health issues are due to several factors, including air pollution and wildfire smoke, unsafe drinking water contaminated by old lead service lines, chemical spills into water sources, and contaminated sites that are still backlogged and awaiting clean-up. Extensive investments, such as the IRA and the BIL, have long been needed to address these infrastructure challenges and the associated harms, *and* to ensure amenities like green spaces, parks, and other health-promoting environments for everyone.

THE INFLATION REDUCTION ACT

The IRA was signed into law on August 16, 2022. It has been summarized as an Act that will "make a historic down payment on deficit reduction to fight inflation, invest in domestic energy production and manufacturing, and reduce carbon emissions by roughly 40 percent by 2030."[40] It called for comprehensive permitting reform legislation to be passed before the end of fiscal year 2023. This type of reform is described as "essential to unlocking domestic energy and transmission projects."[40] The IRA includes historic investments in EJ, including establishing several new EJ grant programs. The law is intended to significantly improve public health, reduce pollution, and revitalize communities that are marginalized, underserved, and overburdened by pollution while increasing access to affordable and accessible clean energy.[41]

The IRA earmarked $3 billion in Environmental and Climate Justice Block Grants for community-led projects that address EJ concerns. The block grants are described as being "community-led," perhaps a nod to the model of community input used in the design of the Environmental Justice for All Act (EJ4AA). See Case Study 4.2 for more information about the EJ4AA, which was developed over several years but has not made it into law. When it comes to addressing environmental health, the IRA text lists eligible projects including:

- community-led air and other pollution-monitoring, -prevention, and -remediation projects,
- mitigation efforts relating to extreme weather,
- climate resilience and adaptation,
- reduction of indoor air pollution, and
- facilitating engagement of communities w/EJ concerns in federal advisory groups, workshops, rule makings, and other public processes.

It also provides needed funding through Neighborhood Access and Equity Grant programs that will fund programs for:

- remediating/improving infrastructure relating to impacts on human and natural environments,
- monitoring and studying emissions,
- reduction of emissions, and
- other public processes.[41]

Even with all these positive aspects of the IRA, the legislation does not do enough for overburdened communities. Community groups and advocates have pointed out that there are several negative results from the IRA, including the likely creation of sacrifice zones. These are areas where mostly people of color, Indigenous Tribes, and poor people live and have high levels of pollution and environmental hazards from nearby toxic or polluting industrial facilities. For instance, along parts of the Gulf of Mexico and Alaska's Cook Inlet, nearby communities and their environment are repeatedly overburdened by oil and gas development and leasing. The term *sacrifice zones* was coined by EJ activists and communities to reflect the fact that some siting decisions do nothing to improve or even address the exposures these communities continue to face but instead increase their potential for harm. For example, advocates point out that the IRA grants approval for the Mountain Valley pipeline, which would carry natural gas from the Marcellus Shale fields in West Virginia across almost 1,000 streams and wetlands to Virginia and the Thomas Jefferson National Forest. The IRA also includes funding for carbon-capture storage projects that capture carbon dioxide and transport it across pipelines through communities. There have already been instances of problems along both types of pipelines, and future accidents are likely, endangering the lives of residents and causing environmental damage. These approvals and incentives are despite the continued opposition and outcry by environmentalists, civil rights activists, lawmakers, and communities who will be sacrificed.

CASE STUDY 4.2: The Environmental Justice for All Act

The Environmental Justice for All Act (EJ4AA), now renamed the Donald McEachin Environmental Justice for All Act after Representative McEachin's untimely death in 2023, is important for a variety of reasons. First, it was developed through a community-led process, after numerous, detailed conversations and comments from environmental justice (EJ) and other communities. It sets a number of EJ requirements, as well as establishing advisory bodies and programs, the purpose of which are to address the disproportionate adverse health or environmental effects of federal laws and programs on communities of color, low-income communities, or Tribal and Indigenous communities. In addition, it prohibits disparate impacts based on race, color, or national origin as discriminatory, and it provides legal recourse to people affected by that discrimination. The proposed Act also:

- requires that agencies prepare community impact reports to assess the impacts of agency action on EJ communities.
- establishes requirements and programs related to chemicals or toxic ingredients in certain products, like cosmetics.

The EJ4AA requires that a list of ingredients or warnings be included in certain packaging, and it also provides grants for research on designing safer alternatives to chemicals in certain consumer, cleaning, toy, or baby products that are inherently toxic or that are associated with chronic adverse health effects. Although the EJ4AA has not become law, it can stand as a model for the correct way to create effective legislation with community input.

The challenges with the EJ4AA stem from the way the act was created: with direct, regular input from EJ communities. The EJ4AA serves as a much-needed model for partnership, which is the best way to address environmental issues. It identifies the issues about which EJ and other disenfranchised communities are concerned and confront on a daily basis. The problem is that this partnership model may not be in line with congressional or political priorities. Instead of listening to those affected most by environmental contamination and climate change—among other challenges—and welcoming and learning from their input, there will always be individuals and groups who believe they know best what communities need.

REFLECTION QUESTIONS
1. What is unique about the way in which the EJ4AA was developed?

BIPARTISAN INFRASTRUCTURE LAW

The Bipartisan Infrastructure Law (BIL), also known as the Infrastructure Investment and Jobs Act (IIJA), is defined as a once-in-a-generation piece of federal legislation that authorized $1.1 trillion in federal funding to address long-standing needs to improve and upgrade the nation's infrastructure.[42] The BIL takes a broad view of infrastructure and recognizes the harm that many large-scale federally funded projects have inflicted on certain communities and populations in the past. Those harms have manifested as adverse health impacts, including elevated levels of chronic health conditions and shortened life expectancy.[43,44] This Act has a particular focus on environmentally related infrastructure, including access to clean drinking water, enhanced wastewater management systems, and the removal of dangerous persistent chemicals from water, flood mitigation, lead service-line replacement, public transit improvements, carbon emissions reduction via clean energy production, and a more resilient electricity transmission grid. The BIL focuses on building out electric vehicle (EV) infrastructure, including electrifying school and public transit buses, expanding the network of EV charging stations, electrifying ports, and modernizing the rail freight system. There is also a focus on cleaning up and redeveloping hazardous sites, as well as reconnecting communities that have been historically erased or gutted by major transportation infrastructure. Review the history of the Federal-Aid Highway Act of 1956 to learn about how it harmed many communities of color in Detroit, New York, Miami, Chicago, Baltimore, and many other cities.

> **BE WARY OF FALSE SOLUTIONS**
>
> Much of environmental policymaking entails a compromise between policy makers, activists, and industry. As has been said, "Anyone who loves the law or sausages should never watch either being made." In the world of policy advocacy, policymaking or policy implementation, there will be opportunities to witness this process. As policy solutions are proposed, think critically and ask: *Do they improve environmental health for all? Or could they likely perpetuate health inequities?*
>
> Many environmental justice (EJ) organizers warn of **false solutions**, or solutions that do not address the root causes of environmental injustice. For instance, there is waste-to-energy incineration, which many consider a false solution to climate change and plastic pollution. Incinerators are discussed in more detail in Chapter 13, "Waste and Sustainability." These facilities burn garbage to produce steam, which is used to power electric generator turbines. However, this approach often does not consider that incinerators are disproportionately located in low-wealth communities and communities of color, and these facilities emit cancer-causing chemicals, endocrine disruptors, and other toxicants.

WORKING TOWARD ENVIRONMENTAL HEALTH AND JUSTICE

Various initiatives across the United States aim to address EJ concerns through state-level legislation. While the full impact of these policies remains uncertain, there are notable examples of states taking proactive steps. For instance, in 2018, California passed a significant bill, AB617. This legislation mandates that communities selected by the California Air Resources Board (CARB) collaborate with regional air districts to create air-monitoring plans and emissions-reduction programs. To facilitate this collaboration, community steering committees composed of local residents, community organizations, local government officials, and businesses, are responsible for developing plans for CARB approval. This approach distinguishes itself from the conventional air quality management practices in the United States by prioritizing the well-being of communities grappling with the most severe air quality issues within the state.

In another instance, New Jersey made substantial progress in 2020 when it passed groundbreaking legislation: S232/A2212. This law mandates that the New Jersey Department of Environmental Protection assess and consider public health and environmental risks associated with projects seeking permits to operate in communities already burdened by pollution. These overburdened communities are defined as low-income, minority, Tribal, or having limited English proficiency, per the bill.[45] Again, its impacts are yet to be measured, but this legislation signifies a significant shift toward addressing environmental equity in the state.

Local governments do not always recognize their role in advancing EJ. However, there are numerous avenues for cities, counties, or regions to implement policy and programmatic solutions. A comprehensive analysis of local EJ policies identified six distinct categories of policies to address EJ (Box 4.1). For example, cities like Chicago, Detroit, and Oakland have instituted bans on the open storage of petroleum coke, a byproduct of fossil fuel production known to pose severe heart and lung health risks when inhaled. San Francisco, as part of its comprehensive EJ policy, enacted a Public Utilities Commission Resolution in 2009. This resolution mandated EJ training for government personnel, expanded job opportunities within affected EJ communities, implemented strategies to mitigate the utility's disproportionate impacts, and enhanced opportunities for public involvement. Additionally, some cities have updated zoning ordinances and plans to better address EJ impacts, while others have established interagency working groups. It is worth noting that certain EJ policies may face legal challenges or opposition from those concerned about potential declines in tax revenue. Nevertheless, looking at these examples reveals how numerous communities have successfully struck a balance between safeguarding their local environment and supporting economic development.

> **BOX 4.1. LOCAL POLICIES TO ADDRESS ENVIRONMENTAL JUSTICE**
>
> - Bans on specific types of polluting facilities typically sited in environmental justice (EJ) communities.
> - Broad EJ policies that incorporate EJ goals and considerations into a range of municipal activities.
> - Environmental review processes applied to new developments.
> - Proactive planning targeted at future development to address EJ via comprehensive plans, overlay zones, or green zones.
> - Targeted land use measures that address existing sources of pollution, like amortization policies.
> - Enhanced public health codes that reach both existing and new sources of pollution that impact public health.
>
> *Source:* Adapted from Baptista AI, Sachs A, Rot C. Local policies for environmental justice: a national scan. The New School Tishman Environment and Design Center. February 2019. https://doi.org/doi:10.7282/t3-pywf-p055

MAIN TAKEAWAYS

In this chapter, we learned that:

- Early federal environmental policies, such as the NEPA, the CAA, and the CWA have been generally effective at protecting our environment, but they have failed to address environmental injustice in the United States. We have seen improvement in the use of these policies, but more enforcement and more actions directed at protecting people are needed.
- Given the increase in executive orders that directly address health and environmental issues faced by impacted communities, as well as recent funding to address infrastructure and economic opportunities, it seems that environmental health is becoming more of a national priority. However, much more work is needed to ensure that these policies lead to equitable outcomes.
- Policy can be less political and more protective of public health if agencies and regulators applied the precautionary principle and centered EJ in making their decisions.
- Be careful of false solutions. Consider who benefits and who suffers. What can be done to ensure that there are no sacrifice communities? The goal is equal protection under the laws—not equal pollution.
- Every sector is a public health sector with the potential to work toward EJ. We need all sectors to address climate change, environmental contamination, and accompanying adverse health effects. Everything is interconnected.

SUMMARY

This chapter illustrates the protection of environmental health in the United States through a complex system of regulations and policies. Environmental challenges persist, becoming more complex due to factors like climate change, development and growth, and chemicals in the environment. EJ issues highlight and amplify existing disparities, with communities of color and low wealth facing higher exposure to hazards. Many EJ issues are specifically addressed in newer legislation, such as the IRA and the BIL, and historic levels of targeted congressional appropriations, combined with presidential executive orders. The unprecedented focus on addressing long-standing environmental health disparities and community disinvestment is long past due, but it may not solve all problems, still leaving some communities to be sacrificed in the name of progress. Some recent state and city policies provide examples of how to center EJ in creating new policies and procedures.

END-OF-CHAPTER RESOURCES

DISCUSSION QUESTIONS

1. Does the IRA apply the precautionary principle? Why or why not?
2. In recent years, we have seen an unprecedented increase in federal infrastructure spending. How could this increased spending improve the health conditions of historically disadvantaged communities? What are some considerations in ensuring that the funding addresses inequities and does not perpetuate them?
3. Executive orders direct federal agencies to review their policies and practices and take steps to address their adverse impacts. Because executive orders do not apply to states or local governments, the policy priorities may not be quickly realized by the average person. What steps could be taken by state governments to address disparate environmental and health burdens?
4. Numerous screening tools have been developed to assist the public in identifying the proximity of polluting facilities and other environmental threats in their community (covered in detail in Chapter 8, "Mapping Environmental Health and Justice Issues"). For instance, EPA's EJSCREEN is an EJ mapping and screening tool that provides the EPA with a national data set and approach for combining environmental and demographic socioeconomic indicators.[46] This mapping tool identifies areas across the nation where communities are faced with one or more of eight categories of burdens: climate change, energy, health, housing, legacy pollution, transportation, water and wastewater, and workforce development.[47] How might these tools be used to inform health policies to remedy existing negative burdens and prevent future ones?
5. The spending for EJ-related initiatives under the IRA and BIL is unprecedented. In your opinion, how can we ensure that these dollars are achieving the goals of Justice40? How can we make progress toward environmental health equity that can be sustained?

LEARNING ACTIVITIES

THE TIME IS NOW

Visit the Federal Register or your state's environmental agency webpage. Do a bit of searching to find an environmental health or justice issue open for public comment. Use the tips presented in this chapter to prepare your own public comments. As Elizabeth Mullin suggests, pound the law, pound the facts, or pound the table. Will you show support for the proposed action? Will you request minor or major changes to the proposed action? Or, will you downright oppose it? Be clear and direct. If you need examples, you can browse through comments submitted on closed items in the Federal Register. You will see a range of examples from industry spokespeople, policy advocates, researchers, legal experts, and the general public. Tell decision makers what you think!

IN REAL LIFE

"Budgets are moral documents," so the saying goes. (The origin of this saying is unknown, but many attribute it to Reverend Martin Luther King Jr.) In other words, city, state, and federal budgets give us pretty clear indicators of our government's priorities. How we appropriate our tax dollars indicates which policies and programs can be implemented and sustained.

Have you ever looked at your city or hometown's annual budget? These are generally publicly available with a quick online search. Once you find it, ask yourself how well it reflects your own values and priorities. What services receive the majority of the funding dollars? What seems to be left off? Directly or indirectly, how do environmental health or justice issues show up in the budget? If you were in charge, would you change how funding was distributed? How so?

A robust set of instructor resources designed to supplement this text is located at http://connect.springerpub.com/content/book/978-0-8261-8353-8. Qualifying instructors may request access by emailing textbook@springerpub.com.

REFERENCES

1. Kamieniecki S, Kraft ME. *The Oxford Handbook of U.S. Environmental Policy*. Oxford University Press; 2016.
2. Tessum CW, Paolella DA, Chambliss SE, Apte JS, Hill JD, Marshall JD. PM$_{2.5}$ polluters disproportionately and systemically affect people of color in the United States. *Sci Adv*. 2021;7(18):eabf4491. doi:10.1126/sciadv.abf4491
3. Mikati I, Benson AF, Luben TJ, Sacks JD, Richmond-Bryant J. Disparities in distribution of particulate matter emission sources by race and poverty status. *Am J Public Health*. 2018;108(4):480–485. doi:10.2105/ajph.2017.304297
4. Bullard R, Mohai P, Saha R, Wright B. *Toxic Wastes and Race at Twenty, 1987–2007: A Report Prepared for the United Church of Christ Justice & Witness Ministries*. United Church of Christ; March 2007. https://www.ucc.org/wp-content/uploads/2021/03/toxic-wastes-and-race-at-twenty-1987-2007.pdf
5. Rashid NM. Environmental law. United Nations and the Rule of Law. Accessed June 17, 2024. https://www.un.org/ruleoflaw/thematic-areas/land-property-environment/environmental-law/
6. The 17 Goals. United Nations; 2015. Accessed June 17, 2024. https://sdgs.un.org/goals
7. Appropriations. U.S. Senate. Accessed June 17, 2024. https://www.senate.gov/legislative/common/generic/bills_acts_laws_appropriations.htm
8. A brief guide to the federal budget and appropriations process. American Council on Education. 2019. Accessed June 17, 2024. https://www.acenet.edu/Policy-Advocacy/Pages/Budget-Appropriations/Brief-Guide-to-Budget-Appropriations.aspx
9. Mullin ED. *The Art of Commenting: How to Influence Environmental Decisionmaking with Effective Comments*. 2nd ed. Environmental Law Institute; 2013.
10. What is the National Environmental Policy Act? United States Environmental Protection Agency. July 31, 2013. Updated October 5, 2023. https://www.epa.gov/nepa/what-national-environmental-policy-act
11. National Environmental Policy Act. Accessed June 17, 2024. https://ceq.doe.gov/#:~:text=Section%20102%20of
12. Detroit River International Crossing Project. Final environmental impact statement. Accessed June 17, 2024. http://www.partnershipborderstudycom/reports_us.asp#feis
13. Sampson N, Sagovac S, Schulz A, et al. Mobilizing for community benefits to assess health and promote environmental justice near the Gordie Howe international bridge. *Int J Environ Res Public Health*. 2020;17(13):4680. doi:10.3390/ijerph17134680
14. The 1969 Cuyahoga River fire. National Park Service. Updated May 3, 2022. https://www.nps.gov/articles/story-of-the-fire.htm
15. Basic information about nonpoint source (NPS) pollution. United States Environmental Protection Agency. Updated December 4, 2023. https://www.epa.gov/nps/basic-information-about-nonpoint-source-nps-pollution
16. Summary of the Clean Water Act, 33 U.S.C. §1251 et seq. (1972). United States Environmental Protection Agency. Updated June 22, 2023. https://www.epa.gov/laws-regulations/summary-clean-water-act#:~:text=%22Clean%20Water%20Act%22%20became%20the,for%20pollutants%20in%20surface%20waters
17. National Pollution Discharge Elimination System (NPDES). United States Environmental Protection Agency. Updated March 22, 2024. https://www.epa.gov/npdes
18. Adams C. Jackson's water crisis persists as national attention and help fade away. *NBC News*. January 17, 2023. https://www.nbcnews.com/news/nbcblk/jackson-mississippi-still-dealing-water-crisis-rcna65563
19. Coz EL, Connolly D, Hitson H, Mealins E, USA Today. Jackson water crisis flows from century of poverty, neglect and racism. *Mississippi Today*. November 7, 2022. https://mississippitoday.org/2022/11/07/jackson-water-crisis-poverty-neglect-racism/

20. Scott R, Stewart B. "Through the cracks": inside the fight to fix Jackson's water crisis. *ABC News*. February 6, 2023. https://abcnews.go.com/US/cracks-inside-fight-fix-jacksons-water-crisis/story?id=96922793
21. Safe Drinking Water Act (SDWA). United States Environmental Protection Agency. February 2, 2018. Updated April 10, 2024. https://www.epa.gov/sdwa
22. Summary of the Clean Air Act, 42 U.S.C. §7401 et seq. (1970). United States Environmental Protection Agency. February 22, 2013. Updated September 6, 2023. https://www.epa.gov/laws-regulations/summary-clean-air-act#:~:text=The%20Clean%20Air%20Act%20(CAA
23. Progress cleaning the air and improving people's health. United States Environmental Protection Agency. March 14, 2019. Updated April 30, 2024. https://www.epa.gov/clean-air-act-overview/progress-cleaning-air-and-improving-peoples-health
24. EPA announces final "Good Neighbor" plan to cut harmful smog, protecting health of millions from power plant, industrial air pollution. United States Environmental Protection Agency. Updated March 15, 2023. https://www.epa.gov/newsreleases/epa-announces-final-good-neighbor-plan-cut-harmful-smog-protecting-health-millions
25. Summary of the Toxic Substances Control Act. United States Environmental Protection Agency. February 22, 2013. Updated September 29, 2023. https://www.epa.gov/laws-regulations/summary-toxic-substances-control-act
26. Shimkus J. H.R.2576—114th Congress (2015–2016): Frank R. Lautenberg Chemical Safety for the 21st Century Act. Congress.gov. June 22, 2016. https://www.congress.gov/bill/114th-congress/house-bill/2576
27. Rayasam SDG, Koman PD, Axelrad DA, Woodruff TJ, Chartres N. Toxic Substances Control Act (TSCA) implementation: how the amended law has failed to protect vulnerable populations from toxic chemicals in the United States. *Environ Sci Technol*. 2022;56(17):11969–11982. doi:10.1021/acs.est.2c02079
28. Marmot M. Social determinants of health inequalities. *Lancet*. 2005;365:1099–1104. doi:10.1016/s0140-6736(05)71146-6
29. U.S. to sharply cut methane pollution that threatens the climate and public health. United States Environmental Protection Agency. November 2, 2021. Updated September 26, 2023. https://www.epa.gov/newsreleases/us-sharply-cut-methane-pollution-threatens-climate-and-public-health
30. Basic information about mercury and air toxics standards. United States Environmental Protection Agency. January 18, 2023. Updated January 8, 2024. https://www.epa.gov/mats/basic-information-about-mercury-and-air-toxics-standards
31. Summary of the Comprehensive Environmental Response, Compensation, and Liability Act (Superfund) 42 U.S.C. §9601 et seq. (1980). United States Environmental Protection Agency. February 22, 2013. Updated September 6, 2023. https://www.epa.gov/laws-regulations/summary-comprehensive-environmental-response-compensation-and-liability-act
32. Resource Conservation and Recovery Act (RCRA) laws and regulations. United States Environmental Protection Agency. February 12, 2019. Updated February 13, 2024. https://www.epa.gov/rcra
33. White C. The farm bill: what will 2023 bring? The Council of State Governments. September 7, 2022. https://www.csg.org/2022/09/07/the-farm-bill-what-will-2023-bring/
34. Biden JR Jr. EO 14096. Revitalizing our nation's commitment to environmental justice for all. The White House. April 21, 2023. https://www.govinfo.gov/content/pkg/DCPD-202300319/pdf/DCPD-202300319.pdf
35. EO 12898. Federal actions to address environmental justice in minority populations and low-income populations. February 11, 1994. https://www.archives.gov/files/federal-register/executive-orders/pdf/12898.pdf
36. EO 13985. Advancing racial equity and support for underserved communities through the federal government. January 20, 2021. https://www.govinfo.gov/content/pkg/FR-2021-01-25/pdf/2021-01753.pdf
37. EO 14008. Tackling the climate crisis at home and abroad. January 27, 2021. https://www.govinfo.gov/content/pkg/FR-2021-02-01/pdf/2021-02177.pdf
38. The White House. Justice40 initiative. 2022. https://www.whitehouse.gov/environmentaljustice/justice40/
39. Centers for Disease Control and Prevention. Flint water crisis. May 28, 2020. https://www.cdc.gov/nceh/casper/pdf-html/flint_water_crisis_pdf.html

40. Summary: the Inflation Reduction Act of 2022. 2022. https://www.democrats.senate.gov/imo/media/doc/inflation_reduction_act_one_page_summary.pdf
41. The White House. Fact sheet: Inflation Reduction Act advances environmental justice. August 17, 2022. https://www.whitehouse.gov/briefing-room/statements-releases/2022/08/17/fact-sheet-inflation-reduction-act-advances-environmental-justice/#:~:text=The%20Inflation%20Reduction%20Act%20includes
42. The White House. Fact sheet: the bipartisan infrastructure deal. November 6, 2021. https://www.whitehouse.gov/briefing-room/statements-releases/2021/11/06/fact-sheet-the-bipartisan-infrastructure-deal/
43. Finkelstein MM, Jerrett M, Sears MR. Traffic air pollution and mortality rate advancement periods. *Am J Epidemiol*. 2004;160(2):173–177. doi:10.1093/aje/kwh181
44. Hoek G, Brunekreef B, Goldbohm S, Fischer P, van den Brandt PA. Association between mortality and indicators of traffic-related air pollution in the Netherlands: a cohort study. *Lancet*. 2002;360(9341):1203–1209. doi:10.1016/s0140-6736(02)11280-3
45. Assembly Committee Substitute for Assembly, No. 2212. State of New Jersey 219th Legislature. 2020. Accessed June 17, 2024. https://pub.njleg.gov/bills/2020/A2500/2212_R1.PDF
46. United States Environmental Protection Agency. EJScreen: environmental justice screening and mapping tool. August 2, 2018. https://www.epa.gov/ejscreen
47. Climate and economic justice screening tool. U.S. Climate Resilience Toolkit. https://toolkit.climate.gov/tool/climate-and-economic-justice-screening-tool
48. United States Environmental Protection Agency. Summary of the Food Quality Protection Act. March 2019. https://www.epa.gov/laws-regulations/summary-food-quality-protection-act

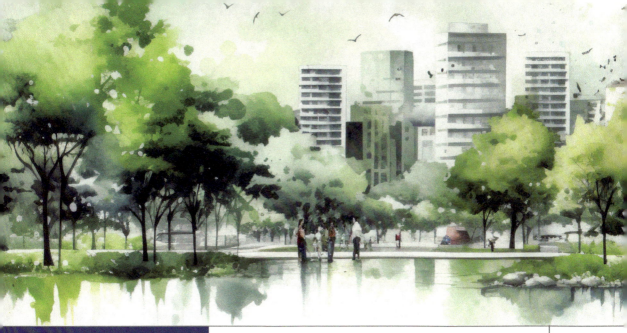

SECTION II

The Environmental Health Science Toolkit

THE SCIENCE OF PFAS DETECTION

Hosts Natalie Conti and Anchal Malh are back for another educational episode on per- and polyfluoroalkyl substances (PFAS). This time, they investigate how PFAS are studied and monitored. In this conversation with Dr. Katherine Manz, Assistant Professor of Environmental Sciences at the University of Michigan School of Public Health, they begin to explore how PFAS contaminates water and soil with implications for environmental health and justice. Tune in to explore how the human body responds to PFAS exposure.

Access the podcast via the QR code or http://connect.springerpub.com/content/book/978-0-8261-8353-8/chapter/ch00

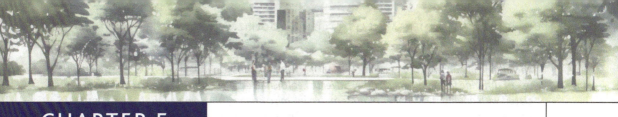

CHAPTER 5

Environmental Health Science for the People

Monica Unseld and Omega Wilson

LEARNING OBJECTIVES

- Describe the history of health-related science and the ways in which it has led to harm and mistrust for many historically marginalized communities.
- Acknowledge society's failure to address harms of racism, which is illustrated by long-standing and intersecting issues such as environmental injustice, police brutality, and many health inequities.
- Explain the concepts of data justice and epistemic justice, which have great relevance when conducting science related to environmental health and justice.
- Identify research principles and practices that may help to achieve structural changes and environmental justice through authentic community–academic partnerships.
- Share tips and resources, particularly for those starting their journey in environmental health and justice-related research, practice, and advocacy.

KEY TERMS

- anti-racist research
- data justice
- data residency
- data sovereignty
- community-based participatory research
- community engagement
- community-owned and -managed research
- environmental justice
- epistemic justice
- implicit bias
- structural violence
- syndemic

AUTHOR'S NOTE

Monica Unseld

Years ago, while working on my doctorate in biology at the University of Louisville, I attended a conference presentation by a "DES Daughter." DES Daughters are the daughters of mothers who took diethylstilbestrol (DES), a drug prescribed to pregnant people to prevent miscarriages between 1938 and 1971 in the United States and until 1978 in Europe. I later read about someone who goes by the name "Domino" who was born in France in 1971. When Domino was 30, she experienced a miscarriage and infertility. She was subsequently diagnosed with a T-shaped uterus and a uterine septate. The septate divided her uterus into two cavities, and the hallmark T-shape of her uterus indicated in utero exposure to DES. Domino's story and the impacts to her health and fertility began decades before she was even born.

In 1947, the U.S. Food and Drug Administration approved DES to prevent miscarriages. During the next decade, controlled academic studies found mixed results that cast doubts on the drug's ability to prevent miscarriages. More disturbingly, pregnant patients participated in the study without their

(continued)

knowledge or consent. Today we know that the children of those patients given DES are at a higher risk of suffering from cancer and other adverse health impacts. Research has shown that DES is associated with double the number of preterm births, miscarriages, and low-weight babies. Many DES children and grandchildren have concerns—not just about the cross-generational health effects of DES—but about the unethical behavior of researchers who studied DES, the healthcare professionals who prescribed it, and the decision makers who failed to ban it sooner.[1]

In my graduate studies, I learned about endocrine disruptors and how long-term, low-dose exposure to chemicals that mimic or inhibit our body's hormones can lead to negative health outcomes. I attended other scholarly conferences where I engaged with countless academic and institutional researchers. At the sessions I attended, researchers made little to no mention of how to effectively engage and share our findings with healthcare providers, communities, study participants, and those most impacted by the study results, like Domino and her family.

Domino was able to have three daughters of her own after much trauma, surgery, and work to educate her doctors and to advocate for the care she needed and deserved as a DES daughter. Domino now openly shares her concerns for her daughters, who are DES granddaughters. When I learned of her story, I realized I shared many of her concerns. I was growing increasingly concerned that science—while vital and amazing in many ways—might also be complicit in creating and perpetuating harm. How and why did science and policy get this so wrong? How can we make sure that environmental health science is designed, carried out, and shared in ways that work to promote environmental justice for all?

Editors' Note: As a leader at Until Justice Data Partners and Coming Clean Inc., Dr. Unseld has brought her expertise to various policy conversations, for instance, by serving on the Environmental Protection Agency's Science Advisory Committee on Chemicals.

OVERVIEW

In this chapter, we critically explore the role of environmental health science in society. To accomplish this task, we need to investigate the ways it has led to harm and created mistrust among historically marginalized communities. We examine the concepts of data justice and epistemic justice, which are key concepts when conducting research that is equitable and solutions oriented. Additionally, we explore various approaches that have the potential to promote equity and address past harms. It is important to understand the roles and responsibilities of environmental health scientists in advancing **environmental justice (EJ)**. Scientific partnerships must be built on sustained community engagement, mutual respect, and trust, and also be grounded in anti-racist principles. Lastly, we consider how to effectively communicate environmental health science with the collective goal of EJ.

We must also recognize the role of environmental health science in our current moment with major pandemics; pressing concerns about climate change; and a renewed focus on intersecting social, environmental, and racial justice issues. In 2020, the global COVID-19 pandemic and demonstrations against racism and police brutality, particularly in the United States, emphasized long-standing patterns of discrimination against Black, Brown, and Indigenous communities. This structural violence has been well documented. Over a 40-year study period (1980–2019), Black Americans were estimated to be 3.5 times more likely to die from police violence than White Americans.[2] In 2020, COVID-19 infection and death rates in Black counties were three-to-six times higher than the rates in predominantly White counties.[3] Meanwhile, communities historically burdened by relatively higher levels of air pollution and environmental injustice saw higher rates of COVID-19. Some activists and scholars dubbed this a **syndemic**, or synergistic epidemic in which two or more ills (e.g., racism, COVID-19, police brutality, climate change) affect each other and worsen impacts.[4]

This chapter explores the role of public and environmental health research in society from past to present. How can we effectively translate scientific knowledge into solutions for communities that need it the most? How can science guide efforts toward corrective action and the creation of thriving environments for all? If not for the greater good, then why do research? These broader questions should be kept in mind while reading and thinking about how science affects the communities where we live, work, and play.

SCIENCE AND SOCIETY

Science plays a crucial but complex role in society. Science has allowed us to explore questions about how the world works—from the cellular level to the universal. It has allowed us to develop interventions that protect and sustain us—from vaccines to lifesaving medical devices. Science has made our lives easier with the development of technologies that transport us and our ideas at rapid speed.

However, science can cause harm in society, too. Science can be biased, exploitative, and practiced in discriminatory ways. In the past, scientific research was conducted in colonized regions of the world without the consent of or benefit to the local populations. These studies often disregarded the knowledge and rights of Indigenous Peoples. Throughout history, scientists have repeatedly exploited communities of color in various ways, including unethical medical experiments, forced sterilizations, and unauthorized collection of biological samples. The COVID-19 pandemic highlighted the level of distrust some communities understandably feel toward science and scientists, as many people were skeptical of the state and federal policy response, as well as the science related to infection and vaccines. For many, trust was broken decades ago and felt across generations.

HISTORICAL EXAMPLES OF UNETHICAL MEDICAL AND PUBLIC HEALTH RESEARCH

Tuskegee Syphilis Study

In 1932, the United States Public Health Services and Centers for Disease Control and Prevention (CDC) began working with the Tuskegee Institute to record the natural history of syphilis, a sexually transmitted disease. The initial study included 600 Black men, 399 of whom had syphilis and 201 of whom did not. No informed consent was collected, and researchers told the participants they were being treated for "bad blood"—a general term used for ailments. The study incentives only included free medical exams, free meals, and burial insurance. By the mid-1940s penicillin became the preferred treatment for syphilis, but the men in the study with syphilis were not told there was treatment and it was purposely withheld. The study continued until 1972 when a press leak resulted in the study's termination. Due to the unethically justified lack of treatment, 28 participants had directly died from syphilis, 100 died from complications related to syphilis, 40 of the participants' wives were infected with syphilis, and 19 children were born with congenital syphilis. This 40-year study is considered one of the most infamous violations of ethical standards of biomedical research in U.S. history and led to the creation of the 1979 Belmont Report, the establishment of the Office for Human Research Protections, and federal regulations requiring institutional review boards for protecting human subjects in studies. Additionally, the Tuskegee Syphilis Study has resulted in the continued mistrust of medical and public health researchers and institutions by some people in the Black community.[5,6]

Gynecological Research on Enslaved Black Women and Immigrants

Dr. J. Marion Sims, referred to as the "Father of Modern Gynecology" and a celebrated physician of his time, holding elected positions within the American Medical Association, was discovered to have used unethical research in surgical techniques. Vesicovaginal fistula was common among American women in the 1800s, and Dr. Sims managed to perfect a surgical technique in 1849 after only a 4-year experimentation period (1845–1849) on Black female slaves and immigrant Irish women who had not given consent, were not seen as autonomous persons, and were denied pain-relieving measures (e.g., anesthesia) during surgical experimentation. In hindsight, Sims's practice has been condemned because progress in medical research was made at the expense of a marginalized population. This research is another example of an unethical study within a community that has led to continued distrust of medical and research institutions, and the hesitancy of particular racial/ethnic groups to participate in medical research.[7,8]

Researchers and clinicians have helped to perpetuate health disparities, sometimes by relying on racist, classist, and other dangerous assumptions. For example, healthcare providers' implicit bias can lead to differences in the diagnosis and treatment of patients of different racial backgrounds, as well as to inaccurate medical research findings. In another example, pulse oximeters operate in a way that may lead to inaccurate findings for those with more melanin (the pigment responsible for skin color). Pulse oximeter devices typically shine a light through the skin to measure the amount of oxygen in the blood. However, these devices do not work as accurately on individuals with darker skin tones because the absorption of light by melanin can affect the accuracy of readings. Biased data have created and sustained inaccurate and false representations of marginalized communities, potentially costing them money on ineffective public health interventions.

IN OTHER WORDS: RACISM, NOT RACE

Let us take a moment to clarify that when we see racial disparities that the issue is racism—not race. Racial health disparities—defined as unequal health outcomes between different population groups—are primarily driven by societal power imbalances and not by biological or genetic differences. Dr. Joia Crear-Perry's model adapted from Hofrichter and Bhatia (Figure 5.1) emphasizes that health disparities stem from root causes like racism, White supremacy, class oppression, gender discrimination, and exploitation, which shape social determinants of health (SDOH).[9] When researchers and clinicians conflate race with biology, they perpetuate racism and fail to address the real causes of health disparities.

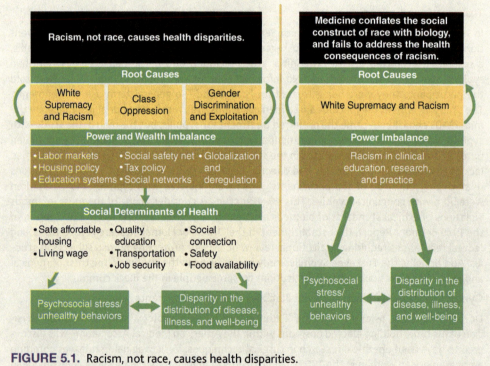

FIGURE 5.1. Racism, not race, causes health disparities.
Source: Courtesy of Dr. Joia Crear-Perry.

Academic researchers sometimes metaphorically "gatekeep" from their "ivory tower," by "parachuting" into communities to collect data. In other words, they conduct disconnected and esoteric research, often targeting marginalized communities with little collaboration. They analyze and publish their findings to advance their careers, while deciding who has access to knowledge. Data collected on the populations they study are often hidden behind the expensive paywalls owned by prestigious publishers. These publications are typically written in technical terms that only those in a specific field can easily understand. Research is presented at expensive conferences organized by academic associations that dismiss the expertise and knowledge of the communities being studied, who are often not invited to present, engage, or attend. Furthermore, those most disproportionately impacted by societal struggles, like COVID-19, environmental racism, and climate change, have long been intentionally excluded from solution-seeking discussions and plans that may be informed by this research.

> **THE ROLE OF INSTITUTIONAL REVIEW BOARDS IN RESEARCH**
>
> In 1972, the National Research Act established the National Commission for the Protection of Human Subjects of Biomedical and Behavioral Research. A few years later in 1979, the Commission released the Belmont Report, which focuses on three core principles: respect for persons, beneficence, and justice. At this time, Institutional Review Boards (IRBs) were first required. Several regulations and guidelines soon followed, marking significant milestones in the history of ethical oversight in research.
>
> *IRBs* are committees that provide ethical oversight of research involving human participants. IRBs are typically established by institutions such as universities, hospitals, and research organizations to ensure that research studies are conducted in a manner that protects the rights, safety, and well-being of research participants. They are composed of a diverse group of individuals, including scientists, ethicists, medical professionals, and community representatives. This diversity helps ensure that a wide range of perspectives is considered when evaluating research proposals.
>
> IRBs have not prevented exploitative research approaches or corrected for past harms that communities have experienced. They have required that researchers communicate with study participants about all of the potential risks and benefits of a study, about how their privacy will be protected, and about how they will be compensated appropriately. All researchers must participate in ethics training and report any major issues that emerge related to the study.
>
> In recent years, Community Institutional Review Boards, often referred to as a Community IRBs or CIRBs, have become more common. Similarly, CIRBs are ethical oversight bodies responsible for reviewing and approving research involving human participants that is conducted within or in collaboration with community-based organizations or communities themselves.

SCIENCE AND ENVIRONMENTAL JUSTICE

Epidemiologist Steve Wing called on the field of public health to challenge its core beliefs about science if we are to achieve EJ.[10] He explained:

> *Epidemiology is the study of health and disease in populations. It serves as one basis for making public policy, including environmental and occupational regulations. Epidemiological knowledge claims a prestige and dominance over knowledge of workers, community members, journalists, and even medical doctors, by using scientific methods of study design, measurement, and quantitative analysis. Science purports to discover truths about how the world works in an objective and value-free manner that does not take sides with any particular groups in society. Scientists are supposed to produce these truths with a scientific method that involves use of theory, principles of logic, and techniques of data collection and analysis, to ensure valid findings. This is believed to result in knowledge with a status and legitimacy that is unattainable through any other approach.*
>
> *The view that science can describe and explain the natural world from a uniquely valid and objective standpoint is widely accepted among scientists and among much of the public as well. However, science is associated with many modern technological developments, including nuclear, chemical, and biological weapons, which are perceived as political projects that threaten humans and the complex web of life on Earth. The neutrality of science is threatened by the fact that these immensely profitable industries support scientific research.*[10]

In his 2005 essay titled "Environmental Justice, Science, and Public Health," Wing examined the relationships between science, industry, and government, which have historically done little to disrupt environmental injustice.[11] The study of complex, interacting, and inequitable exposures is often reduced to a study on a single exposure that does little to inform solutions toward EJ. He puts this "traditional" research approach in opposition to the EJ movement, which has primarily been led by people of color and those identifying as women, who prioritize seeking and creating solutions. (This chapter's first case study takes readers to North Carolina to learn about the work of Wing and community partners Naeema Muhammad and Gary Grant of Concerned Citizens of Tillery. Also in North Carolina, the second case study describes the work of Omega and Brenda Wilson of the West End Revitalization Association [WERA] to implement community-owned and -managed research.)

Furthermore, as Wing emphasizes, the myth of objectivity often paralyzes researchers from listening to frontline communities. He explains that science has long held onto the "naive" perception of objectivity. This perception effectively removes science from historical, political, and social contexts, and it often leads to flawed research questions, experimental designs, data collection, and interpretation.[11]

> **AUTHOR REFLECTIONS: THE INTERSECTION OF SCIENCE AND POLICY**
> *Monica Unseld*
>
> In graduate school, I often heard researchers at conferences discuss their need to refrain from taking a stand on issues, including publicly stating that a chemical or product is dangerous. Researchers were to report the data, but refrain from making broad conclusions, even if the data supported this.
>
> Due to the nature of science and the fact that "facts" can change with new information, a certain level of conservatism in reaching conclusions might be understood. However, what if the evidence was consistent and showed clear trends and predictable findings?
>
> Even today, I meet researchers who believe it is best to remain neutral to protect access and influence decision makers. I'm not convinced that the practice and myth of objective neutrality have helped society or the planet. While many researchers avoided speaking with decision makers, powerful lobbying groups were forming trusted relationships with them, and they were reaching conclusions that would benefit them for decades.
>
> My career has led me to often work at the intersection of science and policy. Unfortunately, I discovered that science as it is taught in the academy is not the science that appears in government spaces. Agencies are often understaffed and underbudgeted. As a result, they will not devote too much time to search through high-cost, pay-walled, peer-reviewed databases to find someone's latest research. While many researchers avoid speaking with policy-makers, powerful industrial lobbying groups work hard to form relationships with them to influence policymaking.
>
> For years, I've heard scientists claim that they must not engage in politics (policy) in order to protect their access to politicians. Unfortunately, too many scientists never took advantage of that access and became almost invisible in comparison to the chemical industry lobbyists who had professional, and sometimes personal, relationships within agencies.
>
> The academy must engage in some urgent and important conversations to determine what role it will play in society that is currently experiencing daily emergencies on a global scale. How will your research help us put out the "fires?" How can scientists, like myself, take your research into policy meetings to assist agencies in relying less on the chemical industry for data and information? We are currently in an "all-hands-on-deck" point in history. You do not have to publicly advocate but you can make your findings accessible to the masses.

TYPES OF JUSTICE

Scientists and policy makers working toward EJ must commit to various types of justice in their work, including:

- **Data justice:** The fair and equitable treatment of individuals and communities in the context of data collection, processing, and usage.
- **Distributive justice:** The fair distribution of resources, benefits, and burdens within a society.

- **Epistemic justice:** The opportunity for all to participate in knowledge production and dissemination.
- **Language justice:** Equitable access to information, services, and opportunities to participate in society for speakers of all languages, regardless of their linguistic background.
- **Procedural justice:** Just processes and procedures used to make decisions.
- **Structural justice:** Just social, economic, and political systems and institutions.

Next we examine data justice and epistemic justice more closely, as they are particularly relevant when conducting environmental health science.

Data Justice

Whether a researcher is collecting data on environmental exposures, a community organization is leading a local monitoring project, or a state agency scientist is reviewing studies to inform rule making, **data justice** should be a key consideration. It entails issues related to data privacy, access, and control, as well as data residency and data sovereignty. Data justice is closely tied to broader discussions about ethics, human rights, and social justice in the digital age. As data-driven technologies, big data, and open data systems continue to grow and shape our society, the concept of data justice may be increasingly important.

> **IN OTHER WORDS: DATA RESIDENCY VERSUS DATA SOVEREIGNTY**
>
> **Data residency** refers to where data are stored and used. **Data sovereignty** refers to who controls the data, which can be affected by laws in the country where the study occurs. For example, data collected and stored in the United States fall under the jurisdiction of its applicable laws, including privacy laws. In some instances, it is useful to consult with legal experts because related laws change as technology evolves. Environmental health researchers must consider both concepts before starting their studies, during their studies, and after completing their studies to ensure that the communities under study remain protected.

In practice, data justice may entail partners having a transparent and agreed-upon data justice statement or plan. These documents are sometimes published in public-facing ways to ensure transparency and accountability by all involved. For instance, the Coalition for Communities of Color website states, "The fundamental premises of data justice are that data should: (a) make visible community-driven needs, challenges, and strengths; (b) be representative of community; and (c) treat data in ways that promote community self-determination."[12] The Minneapolis organization Metropolitan Alliance of Connected Communities[13] lists its own set of data justice principles for human services organizations on its website. These address how data are collected, used, secured, and shared. For instance, principles include that "data that does not serve clients/communities should not be collected," and to "consider the emotional impact that the act of data collection can have on a person, particularly as it relates to sensitive topics."[13(p2)] Such documents may be one way to uphold the right to self-determination for marginalized communities involved in research.

In recent years, Indigenous communities worldwide have begun to establish their own sovereign data policies. In 2018, the National Congress of American Indians (NCAI), the largest Tribal membership organization in the United States, accepted and released a statement titled *Support of U.S. Indigenous Data Sovereignty and Inclusion of Tribes in the Development of Tribal Data Governance Principles*.[14] Through the statement, the NCAI reaffirmed support for Tribal initiatives promoting Indigenous data sovereignty and governance, endorsing advocacy and research in this field, and advocating for Tribal participation in shaping related key principles. Carroll, Rodriquez-Lonebear, and Martinez further explain that Indigenous data governance should lead with Indigenous values, value epistemic justice, use existing Tribal procedures, promote Indigenous scholarship, and be in service to communities.[15]

> **FURTHER READING ON INDIGENOUS SCIENCE AND COMMUNITY-ORIENTED RESEARCH**
> *Fresh Banana Leaves: Healing Indigenous Landscapes Through Indigenous Science* by Jessica Hernandez, PhD. From Penguin Random House: "... holistic land, water, and forest management practices born from millennia of Indigenous knowledge systems have much to teach all of us, Indigenous science has long been ignored, otherized, or perceived as "soft"—the product of a systematic, centuries-long campaign of racism, colonialism, extractive capitalism, and delegitimization."[16]

Epistemic Justice

In the context of environmental health science, *epistemic justice* particularly calls for the valuing of diverse forms and sources of knowledge—including the experiences of those most impacted by environmental issues. It addresses the ways in which knowledge is produced, disseminated, and recognized within society.

Epistemic injustice can occur through various means, including testimonial injustice, where someone's testimony is not believed or taken seriously because of their social identity. For instance, imagine a scenario in which a resident attends a permit hearing for a facility in their community that is seeking to expand its operations. Their testimony speaks to the challenges faced by their neighbors dealing with a variety of health issues, such as high rates of asthma and cancer. However, owing to their lack of higher education and the fact that their testimony is based on their lived experience, it is dismissed.

Another form of epistemic injustice is *hermeneutical injustice*, which arises when a person's experiences cannot be fully understood due to a lack of shared experiences. For example, a community leader may be describing concerns about the high number of cancer cases in their neighborhood. However, an academic or agency researcher may respond that there is not enough statistical power to test the hypothesis that a cancer cluster is present, which is a common jargon-filled response. Rather than discussing shared concerns and ways to document local health issues, a disconnect occurs and the community leader's request is dismissed.

Last, *epistemic exclusion occurs* when certain voices and perspectives are systematically ignored or excluded from knowledge production. It can also occur when individuals or communities are not given proper recognition for their contributions, which has happened often in the history of research. This exclusion not only does a disservice to those left out, but it also limits the diversity of perspectives that can enrich our global and collective understanding of environmental health issues and solutions.

WORKING TOWARD ENVIRONMENTAL HEALTH AND JUSTICE

The United Nations Educational, Scientific and Cultural Organization (UNESCO) describes "science for society" as "the greatest collective endeavor."[17] Science provides countless benefits to society through healthcare and public health and in many other ways, such as how we communicate and engage with each other through sports, music, and entertainment.

Although much more work is needed, there has been great progress in community, academic, and agency settings to conduct science for the benefit of society and to decolonize the practice of research, taking into account epistemic and data justice. Working to decolonize research means recognizing that traditional research methodologies have often:

- perpetuated unequal power relations,
- marginalized Indigenous and underrepresented knowledge systems, and
- failed to adequately address the priorities and perspectives of many communities of color or low-wealth communities.

Academic environments often teach researchers to operate from an expert's mindset that leads them to: (a) act as saviors or heroes, (b) overspeak and miss learning from community partners, and (c) fail to yield power in decision-making. Decolonizing research means challenging and dismantling the historically embedded biases, power dynamics, and colonial legacies that have influenced the way research is conducted, knowledge is produced, and communities are studied. Taking this one step farther, indigenization means working to value Indigenous perspectives in policies and daily practices.

PARTICIPATORY RESEARCH FOR ENVIRONMENTAL HEALTH AND JUSTICE

In the past few decades, many have proposed research approaches that may support overall efforts toward EJ. A review by Davis and Ramírez-Andreotta[18] summarized many of these approaches, as described in Table 5.1. They argued that academic institutions could indeed use these approaches to "leverage their positions of power through collaboration with environmental justice communities in ways that work 'upstream' to structurally address the systems that perpetuate environmental injustice."[18] After their close review of many participatory studies, they noted that EJ can be achieved when it is the primary goal of a research project. They learned that reseach projects are most effective at doing this when:

- formal project leadership includes community members,
- the project includes policy goals and involves decision makers, and
- partnerships are sustained beyond one grant or study.

TABLE 5.1. PARTICIPATORY RESEARCH TERMS AND DEFINITIONS[18]

TERM	DEFINITION
Participatory research (PR)	*Participatory research* is used as an umbrella term for various research methodologies, which all share a philosophy of valuing local people and communities as beneficiaries, contributors, users, and stakeholders of the research. These methodologies may include community-based participatory research, participatory action research, community-engaged research, community-directed research, community-owned and -managed research, citizen science, photovoice, and participatory geographic information systems.[19-21] Participatory research may be initiated and/or led by an academic research institution with community partners (see community–academic partnership) or initiated and/or led by members of the affected community themselves (see community-driven research, community-owned and -managed research).
Community-based participatory research (CBPR)	*Community-based participatory research* emphasizes community involvement in determining the issue addressed through the research, the design and process of research, and action to effect change as a part of the research process.[22,23]
Participatory action research (PAR)	*Participatory action research* involves researchers and participants working together to understand a problematic situation for participants and to act to improve the situation. Methods are context specific and iterative throughout the research process, relying on a cycle of reflection and action. Through this process, participants gain access to power and increased control of their lives.[24,25]
Community-engaged research (CEnR)	*Community-engaged research* involves researchers working collaboratively with and through groups of people affiliated by location, interest, or their position to address relevant issues. It is typically initiated by academic researchers and centered on scientific questions, with publication and dissemination of results often being the final desired outcome. However, community partners may identify new questions or inform the research process in a variety of ways.[26,27] Community engagement may happen at various levels, from community outreach to shared leadership.[28]
Community-driven research (CDR)	*Community-driven research* involves community members affected by a suspected or identified problem initiating the research effort to address the problem.[29,30]

(continued)

TABLE 5.1. PARTICIPATORY RESEARCH TERMS AND DEFINITIONS (*continued*)

TERM	DEFINITION
Community-owned and -managed research (COMR)	The community-owned and -managed research approach builds on the principles of CBPR and CDR, but is defined by community ownership and management at each stage of the research process, including community members or staff at a community-based organization acting in the roles of principal investigator(s) and project manager(s).[31-33]
Citizen science (CS) (Also referred to as *civic science* or *volunteer monitoring*)	Citizen science is scientific research conducted with nonprofessional volunteers, who may contribute to data collection, data analysis, or generation of theory or hypothesis. CS is a term more commonly used in ecological research, although it may be employed in environmental health research.[27,34,35] Similar to CEnR, CS projects may involve varying levels of community participation from "contributory" to "collaborative."[36,37]
Photovoice/videovoice	Photovoice enables community members to document their own reality through providing cameras and uses community photographs or videos to both identify relevant problems and prompt public dialogue. It relies on the immediacy of visual evidence to promote discussion and action.[38,39]
Participatory geographic information systems (PGIS)	PGIS uses geographic information technologies with the aim of creating community-centered spatial information gathering, awareness, and decision-making. PGIS attempts to reverse the trend of inequitable access to GIS technologies through using more inexpensive and accessible 3D mapping and modeling tools.[40-42]
Community–academic partnership (Also referred to as *community–university partnership* or *community–academic collaboration*)	Any partnership between an academic institution and a community-based organization or group may be defined as a community–academic partnership. These partnerships are typically centered on a shared goal, may share a funding source to pursue that goal, and may formalize their working relationship through an interorganizational agreement and/or committee with representatives from all partnering organizations.[43,44]

Source: Davis LF, Ramírez-Andreotta MD. Participatory research for environmental justice: a critical interpretive synthesis. *Environ Health Perspec.* 2021;129(2):026001. doi:10.1289/ehp6274.

As also described in Chapter 7, "Understanding the Environment and How It Relates to Health Using Toxicology and Epidemiology Research Methods," the practice of **community-based participatory research (CBPR)** is a vital tool that fills data gaps and creates effective interventions. The beginnings of CBPR can be traced to German American psychologist Kurt Lewin, who developed this approach in the 1940s as a tool for social change to go further than data collection or discovery. Orlando Fals Borda, a Colombian researcher and sociologist, and Paolo Friere, a Brazilian educator and philosopher who led the popular education movement in Latin America, are also credited with the origins of CBPR.[45]

Today, the Detroit Community-Academic Urban Research Center defines CBPR as "a partnership approach to research that equitably involves, for example, community members, organizational representatives, and researchers in all aspects of the research process and in which all partners contribute expertise and share decision-making and ownership."[46] Key CBPR principles include:

- promoting collaborative and equitable partnerships in all research phases,
- building on strengths and resources within the community,
- facilitating colearning and capacity building among all partners,
- balancing research and action for the mutual benefit of all partners,
- disseminating findings and knowledge gained to the broader community and involving all partners in the dissemination process, and
- promoting a long-term process and commitment to sustainability.

CASE STUDY 5.1: Community Health Effects of Industrial Livestock Operations

In the early 2000s, the Community Health Effects of Industrial Hog Operations (CHEIHO) study began measuring health issues related to livestock-related air pollution. The community–academic team was able to show that increased air pollution was linked to eye, nose, and throat irritation, respiratory symptoms, higher blood pressure, and reduced quality of life.

CHEIHO grew out of a collaboration between academic researchers and the Concerned Citizens of Tillery (CCT). Established in 1978, CCT initially focused on preserving a community school, preventing the loss of land owned by Black residents, and improving economic prospects and healthcare access. In the early 1990s, CCT extended its involvement to address environmental concerns when Tillery, a rural and predominantly Black community in eastern North Carolina, was chosen as the site for multiple industrial hog operations.

These hog operations are considered concentrated animal feeding operations (also known as CAFOs), meaning that they hold thousands of hogs in close confinement. At CAFOs in North Carolina, billions of gallons of animal waste are dumped into nearby lagoons each year. Often located in flood plains, these lagoons are a constant threat to nearby watersheds.

Meanwhile, in the early 1990s, Steve Wing, an epidemiologist at the University of North Carolina began attending CCT meetings. Wing connected with Gary Grant of the CCT, Naeema Muhammad, and Nan Freehand, among others, to establish the North Carolina Environmental Justice Network (NCEJN). Together they developed a community-based participatory research (CBPR) "doorstep epidemiology" approach to identify and address the following research questions through interviews, participant diaries, surveys, saliva collection, and air monitoring:

- What was the frequency, magnitude, and duration of swine odors experienced by the operations' neighbors?
- What were the levels of particulate matter less than 10 μm in aerodynamic diameter, hydrogen sulfide, and endotoxin in communities near industrial hog operations, and were these pollutants associated with residents' reports of odor?
- How were pollution levels and malodors related to the lung function, blood pressure, symptoms, mood, and quality of life of neighbors?
- How were odors related to stress reported by residents?
- How were odors or reported stress related to levels of salivary immunoglobulin A (IgA)?
- How were the cultural and social contexts of rural life related to experiences of environmental exposures and quality of life?[47(p1391)]

As a CBPR study, the team was comprehensive in attempting to understand the many threats to quality of life. Also, the study sought to inform efforts toward environmental justice. For instance, after years of research, the NCEJN has filed several civil rights complaints to the U.S. Environmental Protection Agency with the data in hand.[47–49]

CASE STUDY 5.2: Learning From West End Revitalization Association's Community-Owned and -Managed Research

In 1994, Omega and Brenda Wilson, Marilyn Holt-Snipes, and several neighbors founded the West End Revitalization Association (WERA) to address systemic environmental racism and ensure the right to basic public health amenities for all in Mebane, North Carolina.

Environmental justice (EJ) requires understanding historical context, as is the case for WERA's work that is rooted in Alamance County, North Carolina. In 1870, the first Black appointed official in the county, Wyatt Outlaw, was lynched by the Ku Klux Klan. This murder and other lynchings motivated the "The Kirk–Holden War," which spread across into nearby counties and resulted in the impeachment of Governor William Holden, a critic of the Confederacy. Today, in Alamance County, a Confederate monument remains on the courthouse steps. This is a mere snapshot of the racist systems that have persisted across centuries and harmed Mebane's residents.

(continued)

CASE STUDY 5.2: Learning From West End Revitalization Association's Community-Owned and -Managed Research (continued)

Omega Wilson grew up in the segregated Mebane area, attended segregated schools, and eventually returned with Brenda after college. At this time, Omega worked as an insurance broker. WERA's mission began to take shape, as many neighbors began approaching the Wilsons with concerns: *My yard is under water from a recent rainstorm, and now there's sewage backing up on my lawn from a failed septic tank. My road has never been paved. We have dust and stormwater problems with no ditches. Can you help to get our roads paved? We've been living with these problems for way too long. The city doesn't listen to us.*

For over 30 years, WERA has made an impact on environmental health and justice through research, advocacy, legal action, and outreach, as well as through advising agency leaders and elected officials. These impacts have included:

- saving homes, churches, and a cemetery from demolition as a result of a planned highway project, preserving the heritage of Black and Indigenous communities;
- influencing street design to improve emergency response in historically disinvested communities;
- informing EJ mapping tools in North Carolina's Alamance and Orange counties;
- collaborating with public health and legal experts to develop policy statements on key issues related to waste and EJ; and
- assisting over a hundred homeowners in getting sewer lines and paved streets through federally funded development grants, among many other accomplishments.

In 2023, Governor Roy Cooper's Health and Human Services staff recognized WERA's model for addressing health disparities with an EJ lens and began extending this approach to all counties in North Carolina.

WERA has offered a new model for conducting research on EJ issues, known as community-owned and -managed research (COMR). As Omega Wilson, Chris Heaney, and Sacoby Wilson explain:

The COMR model evolved from the lived experience of WERA members and neighborhood residents to address EJ and community planning and development inequities at the local level. The COMR model goes beyond traditional UMRMs [university-managed research models], including CBPR . . ., by emphasizing the credibility and capacity of the community to develop, manage, and sustain a research agenda and establishes that universities and other research institutions are not the sole purveyors of valid scientific research.[31]

COMR looks different from most other scholarly research in that:

- The lead community-based organizations have authority to select the university experts whom they identify as appropriate to collaborate with to address prioritized EJ or health issues.
- There is community management of the research collaboration process to prioritize, maximize, and leverage available funding.
- There is community ownership of data to ensure implementation of solutions for evolving community issues and corrective actions (after initial research and data generation activities are completed).

WERA's research approach, which includes many examples from their own work in Mebane, has been shared with the National Institute of Environmental Health and countless academic institutions.

As cofounders of WERA, the Wilsons have been recognized with several awards for their dedicated work. They continue to fight against structural racism, striving for equitable access to basic public health amenities for communities of color in Mebane and beyond. Learn more about WERA at https://weranc.org.[31–33,50]

ANTI-RACIST RESEARCH AND ENGAGEMENT FOR ENVIRONMENTAL HEALTH AND JUSTICE

Engaging communities in research, on its own, is not anti-racist. Anti-racism entails a commitment to actively question, analyze, and challenge racist policies and practices.[51] The Environmental Justice Principles (described several times throughout this textbook) and the Jemez Principles for Democratic Organizing both provide a strong foundation for authentic anti-racist engagement. In 1996, the Jemez Principles were created by Black, Brown, and Indigenous EJ advocates who were frustrated with being the subjects of various research projects without respect or collaboration. The document has six principles, including the belief that communities can and must speak for themselves, and that partnerships can be created and sustained when mutually beneficial and based on trust, respect, and power sharing. Many nonprofits across the United States have adopted the principles as they try to improve their efforts in working with communities, ensuring benefits without causing harm.

Since many of society's EJ issues are rooted in racism, anti-racist research and engagement practices are likely needed to address them. Wilkins and Schulz explain how researchers and funders, including the National Institutes of Health and foundations, must move beyond the performative and commit to this work with concrete actions.[52] Adapted from their article "Anti-racist Research and Practice for Environmental Health: Implications for Community Engagement," Table 5.2 provides examples of anti-racist approaches to environmental health research and practice. Like CBPR and the Environmental Justice and Jemez Principles, these approaches call for shared power, shared decision-making, and accountability structures.

In pursuing anti-racist science, community–academic teams should also decide together who will fund the research they seek to conduct. For some teams, working with and receiving funding from foundations, private industries, or agencies that do not share the same values may be problematic. While many funders claim to be community servants, many uphold the

TABLE 5.2. ENVIRONMENTAL RACISM AND CHARACTERISTICS OF ANTI-RACIST APPROACHES TO ENVIRONMENTAL HEALTH RESEARCH AND PRACTICE

FORMS OF RACIAL DISCRIMINATION IDENTIFIED BY CHAVIS THAT DEFINE ENVIRONMENTAL RACISM	ANTI-RACIST APPROACHES
Environmental policymaking	Identify, document, and work to address policies and practices that create and maintain inequities between racial groups.
Enforcement of regulations and laws	Identify, document, and work to address differential enforcement of regulations and laws across racialized communities.
Targeting of communities of color for toxic waste disposal and the siting of polluting industries	Identify, document, and work to address the targeting of communities of color for siting toxic waste disposal facilities and polluting industries.
Official sanctioning of life-threatening presence of toxicants and pollutants in communities of color	Identify, document, and work to address the presence of toxicants and pollutants in communities of color.
Exclusion of people of color from mainstream environmental groups, decision-making boards, commissions, and regulatory bodies	Actively work to promote the inclusion of people of color in decision-making and regulatory bodies, including involvement in funding and research priority setting at the institutional level.

Source: Chavis Rev BF Jr. Preface. In: Bullard RD, ed. *Unequal Protection: Environmental Justice and Communities of Color.* Sierra Club Books; 1994; Wilkins D, Schulz AJ. Antiracist research and practice for environmental health: implications for community engagement. *Environ Health Perspect.* 2023;131(5). doi:10.1289/ehp11384.

very oppressions they claim to oppose. In many instances, their wealth was made possible through exploitative economic practices, from enslavement to harmful labor practices. They may continue to protect this wealth through complicated grant application processes or backing certain policies and political candidates. Again, community–academic teams must determine how they will work to identify and choose the funding opportunities they will pursue.

SHARING AND USING ENVIRONMENTAL HEALTH SCIENCE FOR GOOD

The COVID-19 pandemic highlighted that public health experts often struggle to communicate science in ways that promote trust and understanding. While we were learning about disease transmission, potential prevention strategies, and vaccine trials in real time in those first few years of the pandemic, officials often failed to effectively communicate the rapidly evolving science. There were challenges in combating disinformation, which has been referred to as an infodemic, or a rapid and confusing spread of both accurate and inaccurate information. In addition to the ongoing COVID-19 pandemic, our society has been grappling with the impacts of climate change, racial and social justice reckonings, high costs of living, unemployment, housing shortages, and threats to democracy. Therefore, it comes as no surprise that many people have lost (or have further lost) trust or hope in our governmental systems, including public health, in recent years.

Communicating Uncertainty and Building Trust

As seen with the COVID-19 pandemic, and in the context of environmental health and justice issues, scientific uncertainty is particularly difficult to communicate and accept. Scientists are generally hesitant to suggest there is a causal relationship between a specific environmental exposure and health outcome without first having lots of evidence collected over multiple studies. In the case of environmental exposures, understanding and communicating the impact of cumulative exposures has proven difficult because of shortcomings in traditional study designs. Additionally, there is a long latency period in many cases in which environmentally related health issues may not be seen until years after exposure. For instance, one cannot prove with certainty that an exposure in utero caused cancer later in life. (These complex issues are discussed at length in Chapter 7, "Understanding the Environment and How It Relates to Health Using Toxicology and Epidemiology Research Methods.")

Yet, according to Dan Noyes of the European Molecular Biology Laboratory (EMBL), "scientists should be more honest about the nature of the research and the uncertainties involved, even at risk of sowing confusion."[53] When scientists or agencies communicate honestly about uncertainties through more common outlets like community meetings, multimedia, and brief reports, they can foster trust and maintain partnerships for EJ. Failure to communicate beyond traditional academic means, such as research journals and professional association conferences, can also perpetuate mistrust and cause harm by restricting access to information that could improve quality of life or even save lives.

Making Environmental Health Science Accessible and Actionable

Environmental health researchers and practitioners have a responsibility to effectively communicate scientific information so that it is accessible and actionable. Effective communication does not necessarily mean oversimplifying the content, but rather using language that can be understood by your audience—whether they are scientists, the general public, or decision makers who may not have a background in environmental health science. It is important to consider the primary languages spoken among your audience and to ensure that study findings are translated appropriately in written documents and media content and at public meetings. For example, when informing residents about a public hearing regarding a potentially polluting facility in their community, the notice should clearly convey the environmental health issues and provide information on how residents can participate in the decision-making process. Often, these written documents have technical or legal terminology that may be difficult for individuals without a background in industrial engineering or law to understand. Additionally, when conducting a study in a community, it is crucial to share the findings in ways that will reach and resonate with those who participated and are affected by the issues. Engaging the most relevant forums and voices can help to ensure that these messages reach the right people.

Environmental health researchers and practitioners should continue to track opportunities to communicate science better—whether communicating general information or study findings. To begin with, the federal government's *plainlanguage.gov* has many basic tips for how to use "plain language," including suggestions for how to use headers and active voice and how to organize text to prioritize the reader's needs. With regard to study findings, approaches such as CBPR emphasize shared dissemination to all partners from the outset. Although national and international agencies strongly recommend that researchers share findings with participants, this practice is often inadequate or nonexistent.[54] Report backs can and should include information about how individuals and communities can protect themselves, while also spelling out necessary policy changes to underlying environmental health and justice issues.

Public health practitioners should also consider structural factors, or SDOH, in their messaging. For instance, during the early days of the COVID-19 pandemic, public health messages reminded everyone to wash their hands thoroughly. However, some communities only had access to contaminated water supplies or faced water shut-offs due to high water bills. Similarly, it may be illogical to solely promote healthy eating without also addressing racist planning policies that lead to food apartheid—a system of institutional segregation that separates those who have access to abundant, healthy, and culturally appropriate food options from those who do not.

Using Media to Share Environmental Health Science

Effective science communication requires the strategic use of media as well. Of course, social media is also a powerful tool—good and bad—for communicating science. We live in a society where millions of people can go on social media outlets, say anything, and have what they say go viral. More concerning, their followers will listen to what they say, regardless of its accuracy, and take action. Environmental health scientists and researchers have the power to use these outlets as well, but often do not.

The mainstream media still plays a vital role in science communication, and environmental health scientists can benefit from learning to write press releases, op-eds, and brief talking points, as well as from media training. Journalists, and specifically science reporters, have a key role to play in our democracy by holding scientists accountable. Science journalist Peter Aldhous explains, "journalists should serve the public rather than science . . . part of my job as a science journalist is to report on wrongdoing by scientists, triggering a number of retractions and corrections in the scientific literature."[53]

Finally, it is crucial for environmental health researchers and practitioners to always remember whose stories they are conveying through their data. Many universities and research institutions have specific offices or staff members dedicated to disseminating new discoveries to the press. While these offices can provide an opportunity to share vital information with the public, they also serve as a means for public relations officials to portray the institutions in a positive manner. It is important to acknowledge that journalism and public relations have different agendas with respect to communication in the scientific field. On the other hand, EJ advocates actively strive to establish and maintain relationships with journalists in order to establish their presence and influence in the media. These relationships are essential for exercising some control over the narrative.

MAIN TAKEAWAYS

In this chapter, we learned that:

- Science is central to public health. However, science—even the most ethical, community-centered, and anti-racist science—is not enough to ensure environmental health and justice.

- EJ issues are rooted in racism. Predominantly Black, Brown, and Indigenous communities, as well as low-wealth communities, do not deserve the negative impacts of discriminatory policies.
- There is a need for both individual and systemic approaches to address and find solutions for environmental health exposures. While individual behaviors are important, they cannot undo structural inequalities. Without a consideration of historical, political, and social factors, public health professionals may fall into patterns of victim blaming.
- Scientific objectivity is a myth. To achieve EJ, science must be community centered or led and solutions oriented.
- The public health community cannot develop prolonged community relationships based on trust and respect without doing deep reflective work at the individual, organizational, and institutional levels. By first establishing a strong anti-racist foundation, environmental health practitioners can focus on systemic change.

SUMMARY

Science in service to EJ requires working collaboratively to create change. Now perhaps more than ever in recent times, the world needs solutions. Community-led and community-serving research can lead to new research questions, new data sets, and new, more effective interventions. The same communities historically marginalized and dehumanized by society often already have solutions. It is essential for scientists, community leaders, agency staff, and officials to work without ego in service of the greater good in order for equitable research to take place. Researchers, whether they are university scholars, community scientists, or agency staff, can fulfill various roles. They can partner with communities to develop research programs that address the needs of all and ensure epistemic and data justice. To facilitate collaboration, experts can also become involved in government and media sectors. They can write op-eds and letters to the editor, provide courtroom testimony, serve as trusted media sources to discuss findings, and assist in community-led investigations. Ultimately, this chapter emphasizes the importance of using one's knowledge, privilege, and courage to commit to environmental health science that is equitable, anti-racist, and solutions driven.

> **ENVIRONMENTAL HEALTH IN PRACTICE**
>
> Communicating Environmental Health Science in Society: Five Questions Scientists Should Ask
>
> 1. *What formats should you use to communicate science?* Ask communities the best way to communicate with them. Do they watch specific news channels, or are they more likely to find information on social media? Remember that all communication does not have to be given in the form of a paper or presentation. Consider other forms of media that are convenient, accessible, and culturally welcoming. Your materials may include multimedia, infographics, and other visual images. Why would we want to lock our work behind a paywall or conference fee if it has the power to transform the world. Share it.
>
> 2. *Whether written or oral, is your scientific information accessible?* Using plain language is *not* about "dumbing down" content. It is meant to ensure that intended readers, viewers, or listeners can easily find, understand, and use the information they are provided. There are many resources to help you with formatting, word choice, and understanding the literacy levels of your content. To this end, practice explaining technical research work to friends who are not familiar with the work or the field and ask for feedback.
>
> 3. *What languages should you present your findings in?* Remember that everyone does not speak English or one of the major European languages. Language justice is real. Everyone has a right to this scientific information. Plan accordingly from the beginning of your study
>
> *(continued)*

to ensure that you have resources for translation. Also, using plain language typically makes translation easier.

4. *Have you recognized the weight of your findings for those most affected?* If your research might create fear or a sense of overwhelming powerlessness among the general public, consider how you phrase the findings and be cognizant that people may respond with emotion. When giving a public presentation, for instance, it is okay to pause and even skip slides. Take time to talk about how the data make everyone feel. If you continue to plow through charts and tables without recognizing the weight of the information, it may come off as uncaring and rude, thus furthering public mistrust.

5. *How can your science be used for good to improve environmental health and justice?* For instance, always end a talk with actions people can take. Think about how you can inspire partnerships and support others working on these issues. Will you commit to being a resource? Do not overpromise. The goal is to meet your audience where they are at. Then, in the future, you might have stronger relationships that allow for even better pathways of communication, making it easier to convey the complexity of science in a trustworthy and actionable way.

For more, check out: Olson R. *Don't Be Such a Scientist: Talking Substance in an Age of Style.* Island Press; 2018.[55]

END-OF-CHAPTER RESOURCES

DISCUSSION QUESTIONS

1. Review the Jemez Principles for Democratic Organizing. Reflect on this document. Why do you think it is relevant to environmental health and justice? Why do you think its relevant to environmental health and justice-related research?

2. Dan Noyes of the EMBL states, ". . . scientists should be more honest about the nature of the research and the uncertainties involved, even at risk of sowing confusion."[53(p1515)] Do you agree or disagree? Can you share an example of what this approach could look like in the context of environmental health science?

3. The following is a quotation featured on the Coalition for Communities of Color webpage: "Research Justice is a strategic framework that seeks to achieve self-determination for marginalized communities. It centralizes community voices and leadership in an effort to facilitate genuine, lasting social change."[56(p1)] In your opinion, what would efforts to support self-determination in environmental health science look like?

4. Refer back to the case studies in this chapter:
   A. Steve Wing stated: "By joining movements for human rights and social justice, health scientists can identify research questions that are relevant to public health, develop methods that are appropriate to answering those questions, and contribute to efforts to reduce health inequalities."[57(p103)] What do you think is the most effective way to identify research questions?
   B. Discuss "doorstep epidemiology" and its importance in supporting communities.
   C. Discuss the myth of objectivity in science. What are the implications of this myth?

LEARNING ACTIVITIES

THE TIME IS NOW

If you are reading this chapter as a student, reflect on your own college major or areas of study. Look at syllabi across your courses. Are different ways of knowing valued? What principles, norms, values, and worldviews about science are conveyed? Whose voices are present in the readings, podcasts, or videos you are assigned? Whose voices are missing? *If you feel comfortable doing so,* discuss your reflections with other students, faculty, or leaders on campus.

IN REAL LIFE

Are there communities or organizations near you that conduct CBPR or COMR? Do some online searching to see where you might engage in environmental health science with communities. Find inspiration in these examples:

- Engage with grassroots efforts: River Valley Organizing (RVO; www.rivervalleyorganizing.org).
    - Explore the key tenets of RVO.
    - Why are these tenets important?
    - What was RVO's role in the wider discussion in EJ around the East Palestine, Ohio, train derailment?
- Engage with grassroots efforts: WERA (original website: www.wera-nc.org).
    - Explore the mission statement of WERA.
    - Discuss environmental protection and the importance of community-based expertise.
    - How has WERA engaged in or led research that is solutions-oriented towards EJ?

A robust set of instructor resources designed to supplement this text is located at http://connect.springerpub.com/content/book/978-0-8261-8353-8. Qualifying instructors may request access by emailing textbook@springerpub.com.

REFERENCES

1. DES Daughter. DES tested on pregnant women without consent: ethical violations. Diethylstilbestrol DES. February 6, 2016. https://diethylstilbestrol.co.uk/des-tested-on-pregnant-women-without-consent/
2. GBD 2019 Police Violence US Subnational Collaborators. Fatal police violence by race and state in the USA, 1980–2019: a network meta-regression. *Lancet*. 2021;398(10307):1239–1255. doi:10.1016/S0140-6736(21)01609-3
3. Yancy CW. COVID-19 and African Americans. *JAMA*. 2020;323(19):1891–1892. doi:10.1001/jama.2020.6548
4. Lee, C. Confronting disproportionate impacts and systemic racism in environmental policy. *Environ Law Rep*. 2021;51:10207.
5. Shavers VL, Lynch CF, Burmeister LF. Knowledge of the Tuskegee study and its impact on the willingness to participate in medical research studies. *J Natl Med Assoc*. 2000;92(12):563–572.
6. Brandon DT, Isaac LA, LaVeist TA. The legacy of Tuskegee and trust in medical care: is Tuskegee responsible for race differences in mistrust of medical care? *J Natl Med Assoc*. 2005;97(7):951–956.
7. Ojanuga D. The medical ethics of the 'father of gynaecology', Dr J Marion Sims. *J Med Ethics*. 1993;19(1):28–31. doi:10.1136/jme.19.1.28
8. Wall LL. The medical ethics of Dr J Marion Sims: a fresh look at the historical record. *J Med Ethics*. 2006;32(6):346–350. doi:10.1136/jme.2005.012559
9. Hofrichter R, Bhatia R, National Association of County & City Health Officials. *U.S. Tackling Health Inequities Through Public Health Practice: Theory to Action*. Oxford University Press; 2010.
10. Wing S. Whose epidemiology, whose health? *Int J Health Serv*. 1998;28(2):241—252. doi:10.2190/Y3GE-NQCK-0LNR-T126
11. Wing S. Environmental justice, science, and public health. *Environ Health Perspect*. Published online 2005. doi:10.1289/ehp.7900
12. Research & data justice. Coalition for Communities of Color. Accessed June 20, 2024. https://www.coalitioncommunitiescolor.org/-why-research-data-justice
13. Data justice. Metropolitan Alliance of Connected Communities. 2023. Accessed June 20, 2024. https://macc-mn.org/WhatsNew/DataJustice.aspx#:~:text=Data%20justice%20is%20the%20collection
14. Resolution. National Congress of American Indians. 2018. Accessed June 20, 2024. https://www.ncai.org/resources/resolutions/support-of-us-indigenous-data-sovereignty-and-inclusion-of-tribes-in-the-development-of-tribal-data

15. Carroll SR, Rodriguez-Lonebear D, Martinez A. Indigenous data governance: strategies from United States native nations. *Data Sci J*. 2019;18:31. doi:10.5334/dsj-2019-031
16. Hernandez J. *Fresh Banana Leaves*. North Atlantic Books; 2022.
17. Science for society. UNESCO. June 6, 2013. https://en.unesco.org/themes/science-society#:~:text=Science%20generates%20solutions%20for%20everyday
18. Davis LF, Ramírez-Andreotta MD. Participatory research for environmental justice: a critical interpretive synthesis. *Environ Health Perspect*. 2021;129(2):26001. doi:10.1289/EHP6274
19. Cargo M, Mercer SL. The value and challenges of participatory research: strengthening its practice. *Annu Rev Public Health*. 2008;29:325–350. doi:10.1146/annurev.publhealth.29.091307.083824
20. English PB, Richardson MJ, Garzón-Galvis C. From crowdsourcing to extreme citizen science: participatory research for environmental health. *Annu Rev Public Health*. 2018;39:335–350. doi:10.1146/annurev-publhealth-040617-013702
21. Macaulay AC, Jagosh J, Seller R, et al. Assessing the benefits of participatory research: a rationale for a realist review. *Glob Health Promot*. 2011;18(2):45–48. doi:10.1177/1757975910383936
22. Israel BA, Eng E, Schulz AJ, Parker EA. *Methods for Community-Based Participatory Research for Health*. 2nd ed. John Wiley & Sons; 2012.
23. Wallerstein N, Duran B, Oetzel JG, Minkler M. *Community-Based Participatory Research for Health: Advancing Social and Health Equity*. John Wiley & Sons; 2017.
24. Baum F, MacDougall C, Smith D. Participatory action research. *J Epidemiol Community Health*. 2006;60(10):854–857. doi:10.1136/jech.2004.028662
25. Friere P. *Pedagogy of the Oppressed*. Seabury; 1970.
26. Michener L, Cook J, Ahmed SM, Yonas MA, Coyne-Beasley T, Aguilar-Gaxiola S. Aligning the goals of community-engaged research: why and how academic health centers can successfully engage with communities to improve health. *Acad Med*. 2012;87(3):285–291. doi:10.1097/ACM.0b013e3182441680
27. O'Fallon L, Finn S. Citizen science and community-engaged research in environmental public health. *Lab Matters*. 2015;4:5.
28. McCloskey DJ, Akintobi TH, Bonham A, Cook J, Coyne-Beasley T. *Principles of Community Engagement*. 2nd ed. National Institutes of Health; 2011.
29. Eisinger A, Senturia K. Doing community-driven research: a description of Seattle partners for healthy communities. *J Urban Health*. 2001;78(3):519–534. doi:10.1093/jurban/78.3.519
30. Wing S. Social responsibility and research ethics in community-driven studies of industrialized hog production. *Environ Health Perspect*. 2002;110(5):437–444. doi:10.1289/ehp.02110437
31. Heaney CD, Wilson SM, Wilson OR. The West End Revitalization Association's community-owned and -managed research model: development, implementation, and action. *Prog Community Health Partnersh*. 2007;1(4):339–349. doi:10.1353/cpr.2007.0037
32. Heaney C, Wilson S, Wilson O, Cooper J, Bumpass N, Snipes M. Use of community-owned and -managed research to assess the vulnerability of water and sewer services in marginalized and underserved environmental justice communities. *J Environ Health*. 2011;74(1):8–17.
33. Wilson OR, Bumpass NG, Wilson OM, Snipes MH. The West End Revitalization Association (WERA)'s right to basic amenities movement: voice and language of ownership and management of public health solutions in Mebane, North Carolina. *Prog Community Health Partnersh*. 2008;2(3):237–243. doi:10.1353/cpr.0.0027
34. Bonney R, Shirk JL, Phillips TB, et al. Citizen science. Next steps for citizen science. *Science*. 2014;343(6178):1436–1437. doi:10.1126/science.1251554
35. Ramirez-Andreotta MD, Brusseau ML, Artiola JF, Maier RM, Gandolfi AJ, Caron RM. Building a co-created citizen science program with gardeners neighboring a Superfund site: the Gardenroots case study. *Int Public Health J*. 2015;7(1):13.
36. Haklay M. Citizen science and volunteered geographic information: overview and typology of participation. In: Sui D, Elwood S, Goodchild M, eds. *Crowdsourcing Geographic Knowledge: Volunteered Geographic Information (VGI) in Theory and Practice*. Springer; 2013:105–122.
37. Shirk JL, Ballard HL, Wilderman CC, et al. Public participation in scientific research: a framework for deliberate design. *Ecol Soc*. 2012;7(2). doi:10.5751/ES-04705-170229
38. Catalani C, Minkler M. Photovoice: a review of the literature in health and public health. *Health Educ Behav*. 2009;37(3):424–451. doi:10.1177/1090198109342084

39. Wang C, Burris MA. Photovoice: concept, methodology, and use for participatory needs assessment. *Health Educ* Behav. 1997;24(3):369–387. doi:10.1177/109019819702400309
40. Corbett JM, Keller CP. An analytical framework to examine empowerment associated with participatory geographic information systems (PGIS). *Cartographica*. 2005;40(4):91–102. doi:10.3138/J590-6354-P38V-4269
41. Jiao Y, Bower JK, Im W, et al. Application of citizen science risk communication tools in a vulnerable urban community. *Int J Environ Res Public Health*. 2015;13(1):11. doi:10.3390/ijerph13010011
42. Radil SM, Anderson MB. Rethinking PGIS: participatory or (post)political GIS? *Prog Human Geog*. 2018;43(2):195–213. doi:10.1177/0309132517750774
43. Brush BL, Mentz G, Jensen M, et al. Success in long-standing community-based participatory research (CBPR) partnerships: a scoping literature review. *Health Educ Behav*. 2019;47(4):556–568. doi:10.1177/1090198119882989
44. Coombe CM, Schulz AJ, Guluma L, et al. Enhancing capacity of community–academic partnerships to achieve health equity: results from the CBPR Partnership Academy. *Health Promot Pract*. 2020;21(4):552–563. doi:10.1177/1524839918818830
45. Gray MN. *Arbitrary Lines: How Zoning Broke the American City and How to Fix It*. Island Press; 2022.
46. What is CBPR? The Detroit Community-Academic Urban Research Center University of Michigan School of Public Health (U-M SPH) January 20, 2011. https://detroiturc.org/about-cbpr/what-is-cbpr
47. Wing S, Horton RA, Muhammad N, Grant GR, Tajik M, Thu K. Integrating epidemiology, education, and organizing for environmental justice: community health effects of industrial hog operations. *Am J Public Health*. 2008;98(8):1390–1397. doi:10.2105/AJPH.2007.110486
48. Alvarez R. Study confirms waste from industrial hog farms creates life-threatening hazards for nearby residents. *The Washington Spectator*. September 17, 2021. https://washingtonspectator.org/industrial-hog-farm-alvarez
49. Guidry VT. In memoriam: Steve Wing. *Environ Health Perspect*. 2017;125(1):A1–A2. doi:10.1289/EHP1406
50. Wilson O, Wilson B. Our right to basic public health amenities. Harvard Medical School Primary Care Review. Published online December 16, 2022:1–9. https://info.primarycare.hms.harvard.edu/review/our-right-to-basic-public-health-amenities
51. Kendi IX. *How to Be an Antiracist*. One World; 2019.
52. Wilkins D, Schulz AJ. Antiracist research and practice for environmental health: implications for community engagement. *Environ Health Perspect*. 2023;131(5). doi:10.1289/ehp11384
53. Hunter P. The communications gap between scientists and public. *EMBO Rep*. 2016;17(11):1513–1515. doi:10.15252/embr.201643379
54. Lebow-Skelley E, Yelton S, Janssen B, Erdei E, Pearson MA. Identifying issues and priorities in reporting back environmental health data. *Int J Environ Res Public Health*. 2020;17(18):6742. doi:10.3390/ijerph17186742
55. Olson R. *Don't Be Such a Scientist: Talking Substance in an Age of Style*. Island Press; 2018.
56. DataCenter. An introduction to research justice. DataCenter: Research for Justice. 2015. https://www.powershift.org/sites/default/files/resources/files/Intro_Research_Justice_Toolkit_FINAL1.pdf
57. Wing S. Science for reducing health inequalities emerges from social justice movements. *New Solut*. 2016 May;6(1):103–114. doi:10.1177/1048291116634098

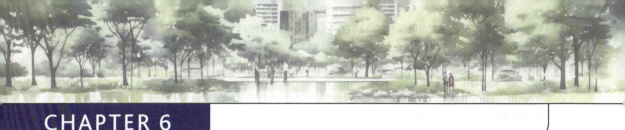

CHAPTER 6

Understanding (Unequal and Cumulative) Risks in Our Daily Environment

Cielo A. Sharkus, Tatiana C. Height, April M. Ballard, Ami Zota, Wilma Subra, and Lariah Edwards

LEARNING OBJECTIVES

- Understand how environmental exposures can accumulate over the course of one's life, starting from prenatal and early childhood experiences, and how these exposures can contribute to adult health burdens.
- Recognize the ways in which multiple intersecting factors, such as race, class, and cultural contexts, shape an individual's exposure and the impacts of environmental health risks.
- Recognize the ways that racism, classism, sexism, and other forms of discrimination contribute to environmental health disparities and inequities.
- Explain the basic science and goals of traditional risk assessment, including an overview of exposure assessment.
- Understand the current approaches used for risk assessment as part of regulatory science, including the ways these approaches have both protected health and contributed to health inequities.
- Explain why the public health and healthcare workforce needs to consider social determinants of health (SDOH) to address unequal risks and health inequities.

KEY TERMS

- allostatic load
- cumulative risk
- exposure assessment
- intersectionality
- life-course exposure
- prenatal and early-life exposures
- risk
- risk assessment
- stressors
- unequal risk

OVERVIEW

As emphasized throughout this textbook, our daily environment is full of potential hazards or **stressors** that can affect our health and well-being. These hazards or stressors in the environment pose risks to health daily—when we take a deep breath, grab a glass of water, eat a meal, and use personal products to care for ourselves. **Risks** include the myriad of harmful effects to human health or ecological systems that can result from exposure to hazards or stressors. A life-course approach to assess exposures and health outcomes offers a framework for understanding how the risks that we encounter in our environment over time cumulatively impact health. It considers the fact that we are exposed to environmental hazards from the moment we are conceived, and exposures continue throughout the rest of our lives. Some of these risks are inconsequential and incalculable, while others are more serious and may cause immediate and long-lasting impacts. Some of these risks are within our control, though sometimes limited, and many are beyond our control. Regardless of severity, the risks that we encounter accumulate over our lifetime (i.e., **cumulative risk**). However, we do not all share the burden in the same way (i.e., some of us have an unequal risk).

Further, in recent years, a growing body of scientific research has shed light on the ways in which intersecting social determinants of health (SDOH; as described in earlier chapters and later in this chapter) shape exposure to environmental hazards and health outcomes. This research shows that unequal and cumulative exposures to environmental risks have significant impacts on health, particularly in communities of color and low-wealth communities. Psychosocial stressors such as family turmoil, violence, poverty, and household food insecurity can have a significant impact on fetal development and allostatic load, which can increase the risk of chronic health conditions, such as cardiovascular disease and obesity, and cumulative health over time. These stressors can also impact the development of the hypothalamic-pituitary-adrenal (HPA) axis, which is responsible for regulating the body's response to stress, leading to an increased risk of chronic health conditions later in life.

This chapter introduces the concepts of cumulative and unequal risk. **Unequal risk** describes how historically marginalized populations, such as Black, Brown, and Indigenous communities or lower wealth communities, are more likely to be exposed to multiple and higher levels of environmental risks over time. Some of these risks compound on intersecting issues, leaving a larger impact. Although we all face cumulative health burdens from environmental chemicals and harms, unequal risk arises from systemic factors, such as environmental racism. Understanding cumulative and unequal risks is essential for addressing the root causes of environmental health inequities and promoting health and well-being for all.

WHAT ARE ENVIRONMENTAL HEALTH RISKS?

In this chapter, **risk** is defined as the probability, or chance, of harmful effects to human health or ecological systems resulting from exposure to an environmental stressor or hazard. Risks can be related to various chemical or nonchemical hazards. Chemical stressors include heavy metals, pesticides, substances found in consumer products, and contaminants in the air. Nonchemical stressors can be natural threats, such as extreme temperatures, weather events, and biological agents (e.g., bacteria, viruses, parasites). Nonchemical stressors can also be other factors or SDOH—conditions in an environment where people are born or spend their lives that affect a wide range of health outcomes, as well as overall quality of life.

Examples of environmental risks that people may encounter on a typical day include common chemical (per- and polyfluoroalkyl substances [PFAS]) and nonchemical (norovirus) hazards.

- **Chemical hazard:** *PFAS* are widely used chemicals that persist in the environment and may lead to harmful health outcomes such as an increased risk of high blood pressure and preeclampsia in pregnant people. PFAS are in consumer, commercial, and industrial products, and are found in air, water, and soil throughout the United States and the world. Because of the widespread use of PFAS chemicals and their ability to persist in the environment, human exposure is universal, and most people will encounter them on a typical day. An exposure to PFAS may occur when someone washes their hair with shampoo at home, wears a stain-resistant shirt or waterproof coat, or eats dinner where a nonstick pan was used to prepare their meal.[1]
- **Nonchemical hazard:** Norovirus is the most common food- and waterborne illness in the United States. Norovirus can be transmitted from person to person, but environmental contamination from, for example, sewage overflows can contaminate food,

water, and the environment. An exposure to norovirus may occur while eating food at a restaurant where a worker is infected, when touching a fomite (a doorknob or surface that an infected person has left virus on), or when drinking water with contaminated ice or from a local water treatment plant that has not properly treated the water, for instance.[2]

As environmental health scientists work hard to characterize and reduce environmental risks, we must emphasize that the concept of risk is *socially constructed* in practice. Risk is a product of human definition and interpretation, and it is determined by societal, cultural, and historical contexts. As a result, each person may define and navigate risks in their daily life differently. For example, while one person may opt to grow a garden organically because they consider the use of pesticides to be a substantial risk to health, another person may deem it unnecessary and think eating conventionally grown produce poses a minimal risk.

Personal, societal, and cultural beliefs and values can also influence which hazards or stressors are considered risks from a regulatory standpoint. For example, in an effort to protect industry interests, particularly those of an industry deemed economically vital to society, decision makers may influence who is consulted and who is excluded from the process of risk assessment. If a decision maker or risk assessor does not determine that a risk is present, there will be no regulatory action enacted to manage the risks. Identifying, assessing, and mitigating environmental health risks, therefore, is not always straightforward, may be political, and may be limited in many ways.

RACISM THAT UNDERLIES ENVIRONMENTAL RISK

When discussing environmental risk in the United States, we must discuss racism. Racial disparities in environmental health stem from systemic factors like institutional racism, denying marginalized groups fair access to resources like healthcare, education, and stable living environments. Historical government-backed segregation and unequal distribution of assets during the Jim Crow era sustained racial inequalities. Despite civil rights acts, racial health disparities persist due to largely unchanged social structures.[3-6]

The root causes of environmental health inequities, including structural racism, persist today. Social determinants of health (SDOH)—economic stability, education, social context, healthcare access, and neighborhood environments—significantly shape exposure and health outcomes for communities of color and low-wealth communities.[7-9] Structural racism impacts housing, education, employment, and public health. Redlining following the Great Depression led to enduring effects: increased pollution exposure and health disparities in marginalized and excluded communities.[10]

Interpersonal, intrapersonal, and institutional racism further perpetuate discrimination. SDOH, intersecting with race and class, magnifies environmental exposure impacts. For instance, economic instability limits healthcare access.[11,12] Quality education positively impacts well-being but remains unequal across demographics. Social contexts affect mental health; systemic racism's chronic stressors contribute to allostatic load, impacting long-term health.

Healthcare disparities, exacerbated by socioeconomic conditions, hinder access to care and the quality of care that communities of color receive. Neighborhood environments, influenced by systemic racism, lack resources, perpetuating inequality.[13] Cumulative stress from poverty, discrimination, and inadequate resources contributes to allostatic load (described later in this chapter), leading to severe health conditions like cardiovascular diseases and mental disorders. Structural inequalities and racism continue to perpetuate health disparities today (Figure 6.1).

(continued)

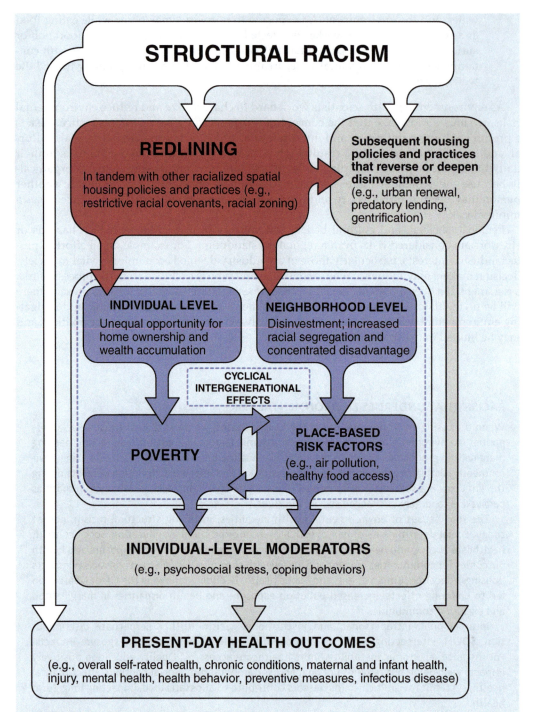

FIGURE 6.1. Structural racism is embedded in our society and continues to affect our lives presently. This figure outlines the cyclical intergenerational impacts of structural racism and how they impact present-day health outcomes.

Source: Swope CB, Hernández D, Cushing LJ. The relationship of historical redlining with present-day neighborhood environmental and health outcomes: a scoping review and conceptual model. *J Urban Health*. 2022;99(6):959–983. doi:10.1007/s11524-022-00665-z.

TRADITIONAL ASSESSMENT OF ENVIRONMENTAL HEALTH RISKS

The assessment of the human health risks associated with hazards or stressors is critical to environmental health research and practice. Environmental health uses an interdisciplinary approach—including toxicology, epidemiology, exposure science, and risk assessment—to reduce exposure to hazards or stressors to promote and protect human health. Chapter 7, "Understanding the Environment and How It Relates to Health Using Toxicology and Epidemiology Research Methods," discusses how toxicology is used to understand if and how an exposure could cause a specific outcome. The same chapter also covers how environmental epidemiology can be used to assess the relationship between exposures and health outcomes. Exposure science examines the types and nature of human exposure, and risk assessment determines whether exposure is a significant risk to human health.

Historically, toxicology, epidemiology, and exposure science studies have been used to characterize environmental health risks through a process called risk assessment. **Risk assessment** is "the use of the factual base to define the health effects of exposure of individuals or populations to hazardous materials and situations."[14] To identify potential ways that humans are exposed to hazards and determine if they pose a danger to health, risk assessment specifically examines existing evidence about a particular chemical or nonchemical hazard or stressor and narrates its flow through the environment. A **stressor** is any physical, chemical, radiological, or biological entity that can induce an adverse effect in humans or ecosystems. The U.S. Environmental Protection Agency (EPA) environmental assessments typically fall into two types: human health risk or ecological risk assessments, as stressors may adversely affect specific natural resources or entire ecosystems, including flora and fauna and their environment.

The human health risk-assessment process was formalized in the 1980s by the National Academies of Sciences, Engineering, and Medicine in their report called "Risk Assessment in the Federal Government: Managing the Process," also known as the Red Book.[14] The process has largely remained unchanged since that time.[15] However, the type, number, and complexity of environmental health risks, as well as the scientific knowledge about these risks, have increased dramatically.

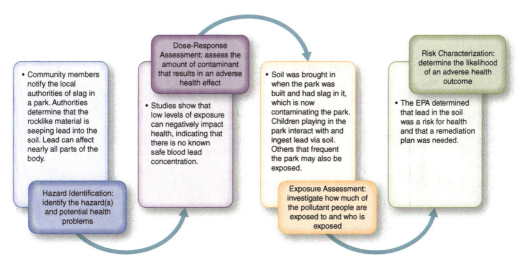

FIGURE 6.2. Risk assessment, which is the science of quantifying risk, is a four-step process. This example illustrates how it is used to make sense of an emerging environmental concern in a community.
EPA, U.S. Environmental Protection Agency.

Briefly, there are four steps involved in risk assessment; they are also shown in Figure 6.2, using an example:

1. **Hazard identification:** Identify the hazard or stressor.
2. **Dose-response assessment:** Determine the amount of the stressor that negatively impacts human health, investigate how we are exposed to it, and combine all the information to decide on the likelihood of adverse human effects.
3. **Exposure assessment:** Estimates or measures the magnitude, frequency, and duration of exposure to a hazard.
   - *Magnitude* is the amount of a hazard that is available. This is dependent on the timeframe and the route of exposure.
   - *Routes of exposure* can include breathing (inhalation), eating (ingestion), through our skin (dermal exposure), and via the bloodstream (by injection).
4. **Risk characterization:** Determines the likelihood that exposure will lead to harm (e.g., a 1-in-5 cancer risk).

DOSE-RESPONSE ASSESSMENT

A *dose-response assessment* looks at what can happen if we are exposed to a hazard or stressor and how much it takes to cause harm or make us sick. Each pollutant can cause different types of harm at the cellular to organ to system level, and each of us may respond differently (Figure 6.3).

THE BASICS OF EXPOSURE ASSESSMENT

As part of risk assessment, environmental health scientists typically get extensive training in exposure assessment. It allows us to ask: *How much of a pollutant is present in the environment? Are we exposed? If so, how and how much are we exposed to?*

Exposure assessment involves looking at how much of a pollutant is present in the environment and how someone might be exposed. This information is then used to calculate and estimate the exposure. The pollutant has to be in the same place and time as the person or population.

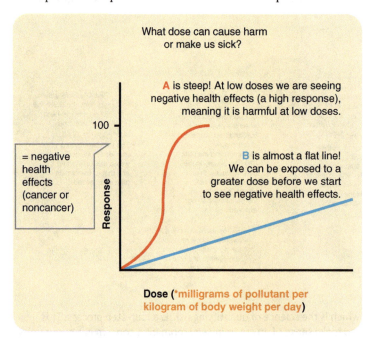

FIGURE 6.3. What dose can cause harm or make us sick?

Source: Kaufmann D, Ramirez-Andreotta MD. Communicating the environmental health risk assessment process: formative evaluation and increasing comprehension through visual design. *J Risk Res.* 2020;23(9):1177-1194. doi:10.1080/13669877.2019.1628098.

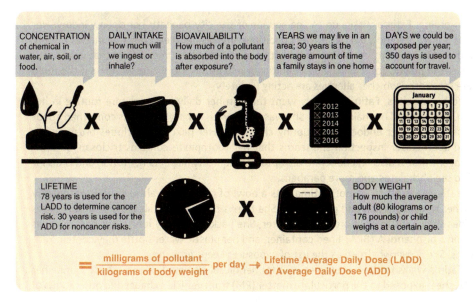

FIGURE 6.4. The basics of exposure assessment.
Source: Ramirez-Andreotta MD, Kaufmann D. Understanding environmental health risk assessment. The University of Arizona Superfund Research Program. 2016. https://superfund.arizona.edu/sites/superfund.cals.arizona.edu/files/8.5x14v9final.pdf

We need to be extra careful with sensitive populations such as children, older people, people who are already sick, and pregnant people because they may be harmed more than an average, healthy adult.

An exposure assessment calculation includes two types of numbers: the *lifetime average daily dose* (LADD; when we know that the pollutant can cause cancer) and the *average daily dose* (ADD; when the pollutant has not been proven to cause cancer). Figure 6.4 shows what goes into an exposure assessment. The numbers used are based on average human activities.

ASSESSING CUMULATIVE AND UNEQUAL RISKS

Although traditional risk assessment is extremely important to understanding environmental health, it is often focused on a single exposure and a single outcome rather than the messy reality of daily life. People encounter countless environmental stressors each day that could lead to infectious and chronic diseases.[16] Whether or not a person encounters many or few environmental contaminants or stressors is influenced by individual, interpersonal, institutional, community, and policy factors—meaning that risk and exposure are not the result of one, but many, factors. As illustrated by the following story of Fatima, multiple exposures occur at the same time and over the life course (i.e., **cumulative risks**). Additionally, the type, number, and magnitude of risks differ across populations because different factors drive these differences (i.e., **unequal risks**). Effectively reducing environmental health risks in today's world therefore necessitates assessment beyond that of a single hazard's flow through the environment.[17]

> **THE STORY OF FATIMA AND HER DAILY EXPOSURES**
>
> Fatima is a young woman who lives in the bustling city of Philadelphia, Pennsylvania. She recently took a class on environmental health and started to look more critically at potential exposure pathways throughout her day. Like most people, before this class, she did not always think about how her daily activities could impact her exposure to harmful chemicals.

(continued)

Every morning, Fatima wakes up to the sounds of the city beneath her open window. Her apartment is always so hot, but her old air conditioner makes her feel drowsy whenever it is on. She wonders if it is leaking coolant or maybe it needs a new filter. She notices that water condenses over the plastic cover on the air conditioner and grows mold. She wonders if the mold spores are the reason why her allergies are acting up lately.

Inspired by her class, Fatima recently went through her daily personal care routine in her bathroom. She just had her hair relaxed. She was happy with her style but was concerned about the parabens and other endocrine-disrupting chemicals. Her next step includes brushing her teeth, and upon closer inspection she learns that her toothpaste contains triclosan, an antibacterial agent that is also an endocrine disruptor. She quickly inspects her lotion and is disappointed to see phthalates and more parabens.

Before she heads off to school, Fatima eats a bowl of cereal with almond milk, potentially exposing her to carrageenan and glyphosate. She thinks these chemicals are safe in low doses but decides she needs to do more research later. She packs a healthy lunch, but her soup was packaged in a bisphenol A (BPA)-lined container, and her plastic water bottle may contain xenoestrogens. She is overwhelmed as the list of exposures keeps growing.

Next Fatima walks to the bus stop to wait for her diesel-powered ride to school. During her commute, she is exposed to the particulate matter (PM) from vehicle exhaust and other forms of outdoor air pollution. Once she arrives at school, she looks at the old painted walls and wonders if there is lead-based paint on the walls of the old building. She sighs as she fills up her water bottle in the sink, thinking about whether lead exposure was possible from the drinking water here.

After school, Fatima changes into her work clothes. She wears a button-down shirt and matching skirt she recently purchased from an online fashion company. Looking in the mirror, she vows to stop buying from fast fashion companies that have questionable labor and environmental practices, even though they fit her budget and style needed for her job. This company allegedly had been using lead, per- and polyfluoroalkyl substances (PFAS), and other chemicals in their clothing.

Fatima works at a jewelry shop, which means she likely has occupational exposures to beryllium and nickel that have been linked to cancer. Fatima also loves keeping the shop smelling lovely for her customers. She always keeps a scented candle lit, but often does not think about the PM or volatile organic compounds that it releases into the air. At the end of the day, Fatima wipes the counters and cleans her work area. However, she was not aware that her likely exposure to disinfectants, aldehydes, and fragrances in the cleaning products that are irritants might be contributing to her adult-onset asthma.

Later in the day, Fatima is tired but stops in the grocery store to pick up some ingredients to make dinner: salmon pinwheels stuffed with crab and a side salad. She is worried that some of the food she purchases may contain heavy metals, such as lead and mercury that had accumulated in the food chain. The crab, which came packaged in a BPA-lined can, also contains chromium, copper, and cadmium. She has been craving this meal and decides she will stay away from seafood for the rest of the week.

Fatima turns on the burner of her gas stove. She just recently read a news article that said gas stoves release indoor air pollutants like nitrogen dioxide and $PM_{2.5}$ indoor air pollutants, which is another chemical linked to asthma. She rents her apartment and does not see getting a new electric or induction stove any time soon.

Finally, Fatima sits down to relax and eat her dinner. She thinks about how environmental health risks are everywhere! As she reflects on her daily routine, Fatima knows she was exposed to a variety of environmental pollutants through different pathways. From the products she uses to the air she breathes, every aspect of her life is impacted by the environment around her. Fatima recognizes that cumulative exposure to these environmental stressors could have long-term consequences for her health and well-being. She vows to make more informed choices in the future where she can, but she also realizes how much of this feels out of her control.

Over the past few decades, environmental health experts have begun to change their belief that *one* exposure stressor causes *one* health outcome in isolation. This change is largely in response to modern scientific advances, the increasingly complex world we live in, and the realization that historic approaches have many limitations,[16] as well as ongoing mobilization of overburdened communities that call on leaders to better address cumulative impacts and environmental injustice. New frameworks and approaches that identify and investigate the impacts of cumulative and unequal risks may allow us to better predict, prevent, and reduce environmental health risks. In *Exposure Science in the 21st Century: A Vision and a Strategy*, the National Research Council highlighted that environmental health and risk assessment must account for the complexity among the various human and nonhuman components of the world to enhance responses to risks.[17] Researchers and practitioners have also emphasized the need for methodological approaches that place people in the context where exposure, biological responses, and ultimately health outcomes occur to improve the identification of the causes of risks and of the strategies to mitigate them.[16-18] As such, we next examine three key frameworks that may help us to contextualize and humanize risks: (1) a life-course perspective, (2) intersectionality, and (3) the social-ecological model.

ENVIRONMENTAL HEALTH ACROSS THE LIFE COURSE

Exposure to environmental chemicals begins before birth. The placenta and blood–brain barrier do not fully protect the fetus from exposure to all environmental chemicals. As a result, developing fetuses often experience all the same chemical exposures as the mother. After birth, children are both more vulnerable and susceptible to the health risks posed by environmental chemical stressors.[19] Children are often more heavily exposed to chemical stressors in their environments because of differences in physiology and behavior. See Chapter 17, "Ensuring Children's Environmental Health and Justice," for more discussion of childhood exposures.

Scientists are particularly concerned about environmental chemical stressors that can affect children's rapidly developing bodies because they are especially susceptible. Heavy metals such as cadmium, arsenic, mercury, and lead are of particular concern because they can affect children's developing nervous systems.[20] These naturally occurring metals are found in food, water, and household dust. In addition, industrial chemicals such as phthalates have been linked to impaired child brain development and increased risks for learning, attention, and behavioral disorders.[21] Phthalates are widely used in various consumer products, including food production and packaging materials, medical supplies, flooring and other home materials, and personal care products.[22]

Imagine now that the same child, who was exposed to phthalates during their younger years, is living in Springfield, Massachusetts, for example, where roadway traffic is substantial and is assumed to be the greatest source of air pollution for city residents. Springfield residents are exposed to high levels of air pollution throughout their lifetime simply from breathing. As discussed in Chapter 10, "The Air We Breathe," exposure to air pollution can cause respiratory problems (e.g., asthma, decreased lung function) and other negative health effects (e.g., cardiovascular disease, cognitive impacts, and breast cancer). In fact, Springfield has an elevated prevalence of pediatric asthma (19%) compared to the state average (11%), leading to a range of health issues, including a disproportionately higher burden of illness and death. Such a pattern is not unique to Springfield. The cumulative burden of early childhood exposures combined with air pollution and other life stressors is a global concern that is largely a consequence of our industrial development.

Exposure to environmental risks and pollutants throughout life can have long-lasting impacts on health and well-being. Addressing these risks requires a comprehensive and integrated approach that considers the unique experiences and needs of different populations and communities. **Life-course exposure** to environmental hazards can greatly influence adult disease risk. Exposure to toxic substances and pollutants throughout life can accumulate in the body and increase the risk of developing chronic conditions such as heart disease, respiratory problems, cancers, and other diseases. Understanding the role of life-course exposure in shaping lifelong disease risk is essential for addressing the root causes of cumulative and unequal risks in environmental health and promoting health and well-being for all.

IN OTHER WORDS: ACCUMULATING PSYCHOLOGICAL STRESSORS ACROSS THE LIFE COURSE: THE CONCEPT OF ALLOSTATIC LOAD

Over the course of life, social determinants of health (SDOH) intertwine, intersecting to impact various life aspects. For instance, discrimination and poverty can hinder education, affecting academic performance. These factors, along with others, contribute to **allostatic load**, or cumulative stress on the body.[23]

Allostatic overload occurs when challenges surpass coping abilities, causing chronic stress-related health issues like cardiovascular disease, diabetes, and mental disorders.[23-25] This wear and tear from sustained stress negatively affects overall health, akin to a car's engine that is under constant pressure. Research demonstrates how structural inequalities and racism disproportionately affect marginalized groups and groups with poor socioeconomic status, leading to health disparities.[26]

INTEGRATING INTERSECTIONALITY INTO ENVIRONMENTAL HEALTH SCIENCE

Intersectionality is a theoretical framework that emphasizes the influence of intersecting systems of oppression that many people experience. First coined by Kimberlé Crenshaw to address the synergistic experiences of Black women who endure multiple forms of oppression as being both Black and female,[27] *intersectionality* is a critical, theoretical framework that has been expanded to examine how multiple social identities, such as race, gender, sexual orientation, (dis)ability, and socioeconomic status, intersect at the micro level of individual experience to reflect interlocking systems of privilege and oppression (i.e. racism, sexism, heterosexism, classism) at the macro social-structural level.[28]

Although applications of intersectionality have increased in public health, this framework has been underutilized in environmental health. Environmental health has increasingly acknowledged the exposome, a paradigm that considers the totality of an individual's environmental exposures across the life course (described in Chapter 1, "Fundamentals of Environmental Health and Justice"). Despite advancements in the biological complexity of exposome models, these models continue to fall short in addressing health inequities. Therefore, we highlight the need for integrating intersectionality into the exposome. The integration of intersectionality into the environmental health paradigm has the potential to enrich the field through:

- greater attention to causal processes that produce health inequities,
- identification of overlooked populations, and
- the development of more effective interventions and public policy.

Next we introduce some key concepts and tools for environmental health scientists who are interested in operationalizing intersectionality in their studies, and discuss examples of this innovative approach from our work on addressing racial inequities in environmental exposures arising from consumer and personal care products.

IN OTHER WORDS: INTERSECTIONALITY

Intersectionality is recognizing that each person is a unique mix of different identities, such as race, gender, class, sexuality, and more. Our intersecting identities can bring unique challenges or advantages. Ultimately, intersectionality is about understanding that there is a connection between these different social identities, and that they work together in complex ways to shape our experiences and well-being.

CASE STUDY 6.1: Applying Intersectionality to Understand Environmental Injustice of Beauty

Although environmental chemicals in cosmetics and other consumer products are commonly included in the exposome, the social context of these exposures is rarely considered. Zota and Shamasunder explain that elevated exposures to beauty product chemicals in women of color are, in part, attributable to the "Environmental Injustice of Beauty"—a framework that links intersectional systems of oppression (i.e., racism, sexism, classism) to racialized beauty practices, which in turn, leads to unequal environmental exposures and poor health.[29] Due to historical and ongoing racial discrimination and cultural imperialism, there is a hierarchy of global beauty norms that prioritizes Whiteness and White femininity. For example, racism, sexism, and classism intersect in Black hair discrimination, which penalizes Black people, especially Black women, for wearing their hair in natural styles. Black hair discrimination often operates in the workplace; some employers discourage, or even prohibit, natural hairstyles worn by Black women. This form of intersectional discrimination can negatively impact professional opportunities for Black women and consequently their long-term wealth. To comply with racialized beauty norms, Black women may feel pressure to straighten their hair using beauty products that contain harmful endocrine-disrupting chemicals, such as phthalates and parabens, which can impact reproductive health. Indeed, hair relaxer use is associated with an increased risk of fibroids, uterine cancer, and breast cancer.[30]

Products sold and used to lighten skin are another example of the environmental injustice of beauty. *Colorism* is prejudice or discrimination toward individuals with darker skin, with benefits accruing to people with lighter or whiter skin. Due to the enduring power of colorism, there is an extensive global market for skin-lightening products.[31] Skin lighteners can contain chemicals that are known human hazards, including hydroquinone, corticosteroids, and mercury.[32] In the United States, these products are disproportionately used by communities of color and immigrant populations.

Several community-based research collaboratives are working to reduce risks from unregulated chemicals in consumer products among Black, Hispanic or Latino, and Asian women and femme-identifying individuals. For example, the Beauty Inside Out Campaign recently published a community-based study of personal care product use among a diverse group in Northern Manhattan and the South Bronx.[33] Their study found that compared to non-Asian respondents and respondents born in the United States, Asian respondents and respondents born in other countries, respectively, had over threefold higher odds of ever using skin lighteners. Respondents' perceptions that others believe straight hair or lighter skin confer benefits such as beauty, professionalism, or youth were associated with a greater use of chemical straighteners and skin lighteners. These data further reinforce the fact that structural determinants, such as racialized beauty norms, influence personal decisions around personal care product use. WE ACT for Environmental Justice, the grassroots organization that leads the Beauty Inside Out Campaign, recently leveraged the skin-lightening use data to help advocate for more health-protective state regulations. As a result, New York became the third state to ban the sale of mercury-containing beauty products in 2022.

WANT TO ADDRESS THE ENVIRONMENTAL INJUSTICE OF BEAUTY?

- Research and choose brands that have sustainable practices and do not disproportionately harm communities of color.
- Follow @VeladyaOrganica on Instagram and YouTube to learn more about holistic and herbal health.
- Critically examine advertisements for implicit messaging about beauty standards based upon identity groups. Visit the Media Literacy Clearinghouse for more information on deconstructing television advertisements (www.frankwbaker.com/mlc/advertising-deconstructing-commercial).
- Engage with community-based organizations that are advocating for Beauty Inside Out, such as WE ACT for Environmental Justice in New York.

APPLYING THE SOCIAL-ECOLOGICAL MODEL TO ENVIRONMENTAL HEALTH

Another model that helps environmental health to contextualize cumulative and unequal risks is the social-ecological model. The *social-ecological model* describes how intersecting personal and environmental factors are related to, interact with, and influence each other. Ecological, or ecology, refers to relationships between living organisms and their physical environment. Social ecology expands this focus to include humans as living organisms and forms the sociocultural environment. The environment, from a social-ecological perspective, therefore, consists of physical, social, and cultural elements.[34]

The application of the social-ecological model to environmental health is appropriate given that, by design, the discipline is concerned with health risks and outcomes that result from peoples' relationships and interactions with all aspects of their environment. Viewing environmental health issues through a social-ecological lens can allow scientists to understand the range of factors that put people at risk and cause adverse health outcomes. It can also permit scientists to examine how factors are experienced and impact people and populations differently to show if, how, and why risks are unequal and cumulative.[34,35]

Figure 6.5 depicts how the social-ecological model applies to environmental health—delineating the interplay between risk and exposure and specific factors at multiple levels.

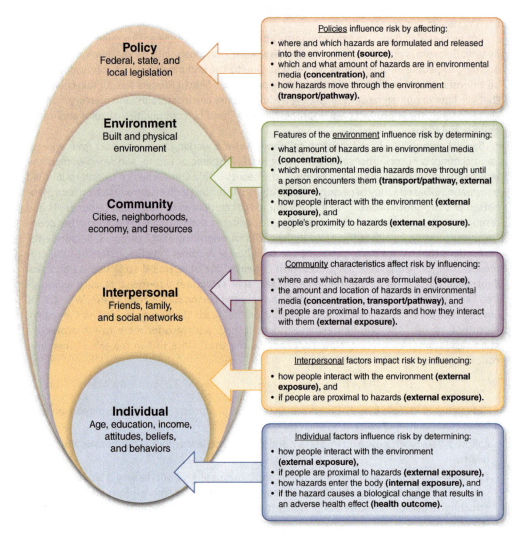

FIGURE 6.5. A social-ecological approach to environmental health that assesses the interplay between risk and exposure and specific factors at multiple levels.

Specifically, the model considers how individual, interpersonal, community, environment, and policy factors influence environmental risks and exposures:

- Individual-level factors include biological and personal characteristics (e.g., age, occupation, and behaviors) that influence exposure to hazards and health risks. Individual determinants impact the specific dose that someone is exposed to, and if that dose results in an adverse health effect biologically.
- Interpersonal factors are factors related to other people in an individual's life (e.g., who they interact with and social norms and practices). Interpersonal determinants, for example, can influence how people interact with their environment, which may be contaminated with hazards or stressors.
- Community characteristics include development patterns and the availability of resources, among others, and can impact where and which hazard stressors are produced and contaminate the environment, as well as if people are proximal to them. The environment includes both built (e.g., infrastructure) and physical (e.g., rivers) characteristics.
- Environmental characteristics impact the flow of hazards or stressors and how people may interact with them.
- Policy, the outermost layer, includes federal, state, and local legislation. Historical and current policy (e.g., redlining, zoning regulations) determine which hazards are produced and where, and what environmental media hazards can be legal and at what concentrations.

Case Study 6.2 applies the concepts presented in Figure 6.5. It provides an example of how the social-ecological framework can be used to understand cumulative and unequal risks, specifically applied to exposure to sewage pollution in the city of Atlanta, Georgia, in the United States.

CASE STUDY 6.2: Pollution in Atlanta's Watershed

In the city of Atlanta, Georgia, sewage pollution in the Proctor Creek and South River watersheds is an ongoing issue that disproportionately impacts Black and low-wealth communities (Figure 6.6).[36,37] Combined sewer systems (CSSs) are present in the communities surrounding Proctor Creek and South River, even though their construction is no longer permitted in the United States. As described in Chapter 11, "Clean Water for All," CSSs collect sewage, rainwater drainage, and other wastewater in the same pipes that flow to a plant for treatment. Spillage of sewage into the watersheds from CSSs occurs during heavy rainfall when the volume of water flowing through pipes exceeds the wastewater plant's capacity.[36]

The city of Atlanta has made drastic improvements to its sewage system since the 1990s.[36] However, pollution in Black and low-wealth communities in west and south Atlanta remains unaddressed, largely due to discriminatory policies and unequal enforcement of sewage waste policies.[38] In addition to sewage pollution, many other environmental hazards are found in the Proctor Creek and South River watersheds because of illegal dumping, industrial pollution, and the proximity of toxic waste sites. Residents may therefore be exposed to environmental hazards daily. New development resulting from gentrification in the area has increased the vulnerability to flooding and CSS overflow events owing to expanded areas of nonporous concrete and asphalt.[39]

As an example of using the social-ecological framework to understand unequal and cumulative environmental risks—Black and low-wealth communities surrounding the Proctor Creek and South River waterways in Atlanta, Georgia, are disproportionately impacted by unequal and cumulative risks. Specific factors impacting exposures include:

- individual: age, income, occupation, behaviors, biological susceptibility;
- interpersonal: social norms, social capital;
- community: development patterns, gentrification, crowding, distribution of resources;

(continued)

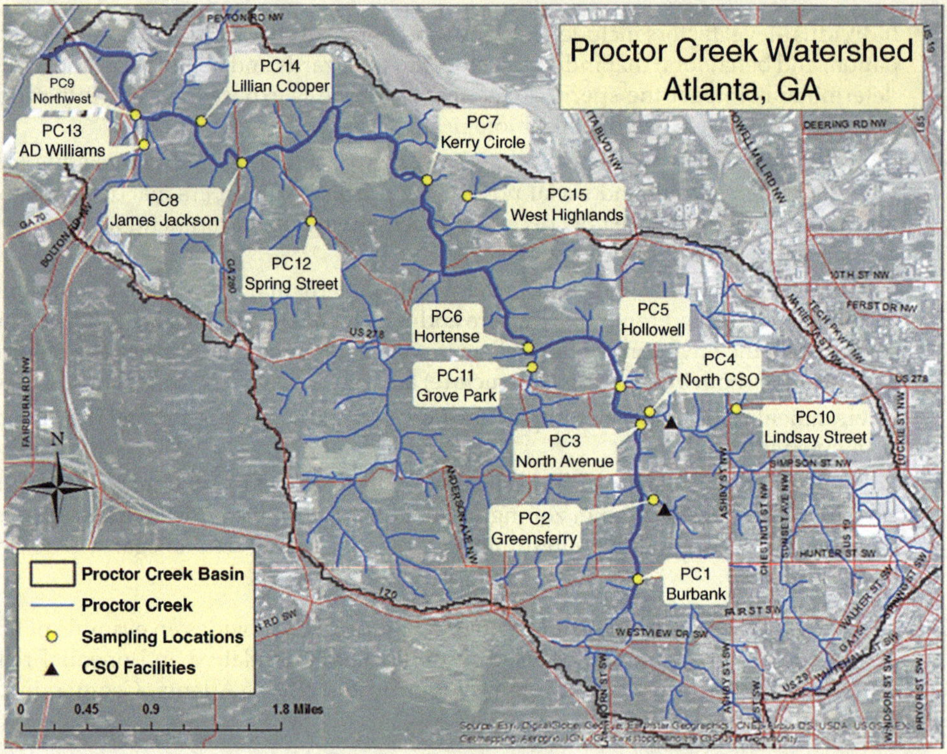

FIGURE 6.6. Proctor Creek Watershed, Atlanta, Georgia.
CSO, Combined Sewer Overflow; PC, Proctor Creek.
Source: Proctor Creek water monitoring activity. U.S. Environmental Protection Agency: Urban Waters Partnership. Updated June 6, 2023. https://www.epa.gov/urbanwaterspartners/proctor-creek-water-monitoring-activity

- environment: infrastructure, general environmental (air, water, etc.) quality, natural elements (e.g., trees, water), parks, walkability, proximity to hazards; and
- policy: sewage and dumping policies and regulations, legacy of structural and institutional racism, and current and historical zoning regulations in predominantly Black communities (e.g., redlining, location of hazardous industry).

Community members have forged partnerships to raise awareness and build support for clean, safe water. This effort has led to several community-led projects to address various environmental risks with leaders from the West Atlanta Watershed Alliance and many other grassroots groups. Much work remains to ensure healthy waterways and environmental justice in the region.[37,40]

REFLECTION QUESTION

1. How can community-led initiatives in Atlanta effectively address the challenges of sewage pollution and environmental hazards in Black and low-wealth communities?

ENVIRONMENTAL HEALTH POLICY: PROTECTING SOME BUT NOT ALL FROM RISKS AND IMPACTS

The unequal protection of marginalized groups under the current regulatory space has caused many scientists, community leaders, and advocates to criticize the risk-assessment process. They raise valid concerns about the process and its utility. Often, the process of evaluating a chemical stressor through the traditional risk assessment approach is lengthy and can take years to complete. If regulatory action is dependent upon this risk judgment, communities can be left suffering until this process is completed and can produce a value that can inform regulations. Also, lack of data on a specific chemical or class of chemicals does not necessarily mean there is no risk, and this situation is common given the thousands of chemicals on the market today.

The process of risk assessment described in Figure 6.2 is used across federal and state agencies to evaluate environmental health concerns. This four-step risk-assessment process is used in whole or in part by different agencies to understand the risk that various environmental stressors pose to public health (Table 6.1). Some agencies may include additional steps, but these four steps are traditionally seen as the basis of risk assessment. Throughout the risk-assessment process, agencies make important decisions and assumptions that are reflected in the final risk judgment. Once the risk has been quantified, regulatory agencies evaluate and select the appropriate policy and regulatory actions to manage the environmental stressor in a way that protects health. This risk-management step combines the risk decision with other factors, such as political, social, economic, and engineering information.

For example, a risk assessment can determine whether phthalates, a group of chemicals commonly used in plastic products, present a risk to the health of children in their toys and child-care items. In 2014, the CPSC concluded that certain phthalates could cause adverse health effects on the male reproductive system and recommended a ban on several phthalates, which was enacted in 2017. The CPSC's risk-management decisions were directly informed by recommendations made by the expert panel responsible for conducting the risk assessment.[41] The phthalates and CPSC example not only showcases effective risk assessment and management, but also serves as a rare example of an agency implementing a cumulative risk approach. The expert panel convened by the CPSC evaluated how multiple phthalates negatively affect male reproductive health, which is important because it reflects real-world experience.

Again, however, traditional risk assessment, and thus the resulting regulatory actions, has not historically considered the cumulative and unequal risks or the needs of specific populations, such as pregnant people.[42] As a result, some individuals, neighborhoods, and communities will experience greater exposures to environmental stressors, more health risks, and unequal impacts. Too often and for too long, it is people of color who are left unprotected, a situation that has caused environmental scientists, advocates, and communities to question

TABLE 6.1. FEDERAL AGENCIES AND RISK ASSESSMENT RESPONSIBILITIES

AGENCY	RESPONSIBILITIES
Environmental Protection Agency (EPA)	Evaluates chemicals in commerce, pesticides, water, and air and hazardous waste sites
Food and Drug Administration (FDA)	Focuses on the safety of food, drugs, and cosmetics
Agency for Toxic Substances and Disease Registry (ATSDR)	Focuses on hazardous waste sites
Occupational Safety and Health Administration (OSHA)	Evaluates the risk of workplace exposures
Consumer Product Safety Commission (CPSC)	Determines the safety of consumer products
National Institute for Occupational Safety and Health (NIOSH)	Informs occupational safety and health standards
National Institutes of Health (NIH)/ National Institute of Environmental Health Sciences (NIEHS)	Communicates information on human health concerns

regulatory actions. For instance, many assessments of chemical stressors solely focus on the chemical of interest that is undergoing assessment. This overly narrow scope does not reflect any population's lived experiences. An analysis of the first 10 chemical risk assessments conducted by the EPA under the Toxic Substances Control Act, the main U.S. chemical safety law, after it was amended in 2016 revealed that none of the assessments were considered coexposures to other relevant chemical stressors. Additionally, none of these assessments accounted for nonchemical stressors.[43] The resulting risk-management actions taken by the EPA will not benefit populations who are at the greatest risk.

Also, as discussed throughout this text, current environmental regulations have allowed cumulative impacts from the unequal placement of toxic chemical facilities in communities of color. The disproportionate placement of industrial facilities, hazardous waste landfills, and other undesirable polluting sources in marginalized communities was one of the founding issues of the environmental justice (EJ) movement. However, new hazardous chemical facilities continue to be built, and existing facilities continue to expand in communities where predominantly people of color live, play, pray, and work.[44] For example, in 2018, in Houston, Texas, 75% of the city's population lived within three miles of a facility—a 92% increase above the national average. Latinos make up 39% of the city's population but represent 56% of the residents living in low-income and low-food access zones within three miles of a facility.[44] The purposeful nature of these facility placements clearly shows that regulations by federal, state, and local governments have historically failed people of color, and the effects can still be seen today.

WORKING TOWARD ENVIRONMENTAL HEALTH AND JUSTICE

THE PRECAUTIONARY PRINCIPLE

Critics question the overall framework of the risk-assessment process, which inherently asks, "How much risk can we tolerate?" or put another way "How many excess cancer cases will we tolerate as a result of exposure to this chemical?" A different approach to consider is the precautionary principle, which was proposed at the turn of the century and remains relevant in theory. The *precautionary principle* broadly shifts the focus to "What can we do to prevent risk altogether?" As an approach to environmental regulation, it has four components:

1. taking preventative action even if we are uncertain about risks,
2. exploring a wide variety of alternatives to potentially harmful actions,
3. requiring the proponents of the activity to be in charge of burdening the proof, and
4. increasing public participation in the decision-making process.[45]

With this approach, risk assessors might consider a chemical to be toxic to human health on the basis of a few scientific studies, even if there are some uncertainties in the scientific evidence base. A company would be required to prove that the chemical they want to use in their products is not toxic to people before the use of said chemical is approved by a regulatory agency. Additionally, the company would be required to explore available safer alternatives for this chemical. Although, the industry may find alternatives that are harmful as well if regulators are not fully engaged. For instance, the United States, Canada, and the European Union have banned bisphenol A (BPA) in baby bottles, yet many companies have continued to use BPA analogues (BPS, BPF) that also behave like endocrine disruptors in their effects on the body.[46]

The precautionary approach also echoes what many advocates and communities have long been calling for: meaningful engagement and communication between researchers and communities. Community members are often the first to become aware of environmental stressors, yet they are frequently excluded from the research process. Instead of the traditional "investigator-initiated" approach, increasingly, there has been a stronger emphasis on centering community leadership and voices in research projects, as discussed in Chapter 5.[47]

ADDITIONAL INTERDISCIPLINARY APPROACHES TO ASSESSING CUMULATIVE RISK AND IMPACTS

Multiple authoritative scientific bodies, including the EPA and the National Academy of Sciences, have provided guidance and recommendations for advancing cumulative risk assessment of chemicals.[48,49] One issue impeding progress is the logistical challenge of incorporating nonchemical stressors into the risk-assessment process. A risk assessment that adequately reflects the complexity of the modern environment is inherently more complicated to conduct. Although scientific evidence suggests that nonchemical stressors amplify health outcomes caused by chemicals, there is a lack of consensus on how to include these stressors in the risk-assessment process, especially in assessing risk quantitatively. For example, risk assessors would have to determine how to account for exposure to stress, experienced either on the individual or community level, in risk-assessment models.

Although several conceptual models that support cumulative risk assessment have been proposed, and to some extent utilized, regulatory agencies have yet to consistently conduct this type of assessment. Some potential tools include[50]:

- **Biomonitoring:** "Body burden" studies allow us to efficiently measure multiple chemicals in humans using biomarkers in urine, baby teeth, blood, or hair, for instance. They may help us to understand the combined exposures experienced by individuals or a population. However, they often lack the ability to pinpoint sources of these exposures.
- **Mapping:** As described in Chapter 8, "Mapping Environmental Health and Justice Issues," recent mapping approaches use geographic information science (GISc) to assess cumulative impacts by integrating various stressors and demographic factors. These tools can help to identify areas for EJ concerns, allocate funds for environmental programs, and improve land use planning by providing a comprehensive and visual representation of cumulative impacts based on health, environmental, and social vulnerability indicators at the census-tract level.
- **Health Impact Assessments (HIAs):** HIAs evaluate the human health consequences of decisions or projects stemming from environmental impact assessment practices as part of the National Environmental Policy Act (see Chapter 4, "Environmental Health Policies and Protections: Successes and Failures"). Developed in the 1990s, HIAs examine the potential effects of policies or projects on population health using diverse data sources and community input. Unlike health risk assessments, HIAs can include qualitative outcomes that consider environmental, social, economic, and psychological factors and emphasize public participation and equity in impact distribution.
- **Quantitative Structure-Activity Relationship (QSAR) modeling:** QSAR modeling is a predictive tool used in environmental risk assessment to estimate the potential effects of chemicals on the environment. Although QSAR modeling itself does not directly assess cumulative environmental impacts, it can contribute to understanding the potential cumulative effects by providing crucial information about individual chemicals. By analyzing the structural characteristics of chemicals and their known effects, QSAR models can identify chemicals with similar structures and potentially similar impacts. QSAR models can reduce the need for extensive testing by predicting the behavior of chemicals, thereby minimizing costs, and reducing the number of experiments required to evaluate multiple substances.

Furthermore, reimagining risk assessment requires expertise and collaboration with frontline community members and with people across sectors and disciplines. There is a need to develop innovative concepts for solutions that combine several viewpoints and disciplines to deal with urgent concerns relating to human and environmental health.[51] There is evidence that systems-based transdisciplinary learning may facilitate a deeper understanding of complex factors across many contexts. Facing 21st-century environmental health challenges will require environmental health scientists, policy makers, practitioners, and advocates to be knowledgeable about the social, cultural, economic, political, and historical context from which environmental health burdens arise and grow. The ability to leverage multiple knowledge systems will promote a more holistic way of assessing risk and contribute to positive changes for those most impacted by these environmental health challenges.

MAIN TAKEAWAYS

In this chapter we learned that:

- Environmental risks and exposures can accumulate over the course of one's life, starting from prenatal and early childhood experiences, and these exposures can contribute to adverse health outcomes that last for a lifetime.
- Risk is a social construct, and those living in communities frontline to cumulative impacts should be heard when naming environmental health risks.
- Multiple intersecting factors, such as race, class, and cultural contexts, shape an individual's experience with and impact from environmental stressors.
- Countless examples exist to highlight the ways that structural racism has led to the unequal distribution of environmental risks and thus health disparities, from the purposeful siting of toxic waste facilities in communities of color to glorification of Eurocentric beauty standards by the beauty industry.
- Much work is being done to rethink risk assessment, including considering SDOH and introducing cumulative approaches, and overall, we would benefit from application of the precautionary principle in policy and practice.
- Current regulatory approaches that assess and manage environmental health risks largely have not kept up with the more recent scientific evidence that suggests that cumulative exposures and risks need to be considered because doing so is the only way to truly estimate public health impact.

SUMMARY

The environmental risks and exposures present in our daily environment are not equally distributed. Historically excluded groups, such as Black, Brown, Indigenous, and low-wealth communities, are often the ones who are disproportionately exposed to multiple higher levels of environmental stressors. This exposure increases the chance of adverse health outcomes that can be long lasting and are often disproportionately experienced by these same communities.

Cumulative risk is the combination of different environmental stressors and exposures that can increase the likelihood of negative health outcomes. It describes what frontline communities and activists have been voicing for years—it is not just one chemical or nonchemical stressor that impacts our health. Rather, there are multiple stressors and SDOH that influence our risk. Furthermore, intersecting factors, such as race, class, and cultural contexts, shape an individual's experience with environmental stressors and their perception of risk. Years of structural racism that are so deeply embedded in our society have created health disparities that burden historically excluded communities.

Models such as the social-ecological model or intersectionality are helpful tools to use when trying to understand an individual's risk for environmental stressors in the context of their entire lived experience. The traditional four-step risk-assessment process that is used to quantify risk to environmental stressors fails to account for cumulative risk and impacts. By incorporating cumulative approaches, risk assessors have a greater chance of adequately assessing the risks for all, particularly for communities who are experiencing health and exposure disparities. These changes could lead to regulatory actions that will manage environmental risks in a way that is protective of public health for everyone.

END-OF-CHAPTER RESOURCES

DISCUSSION QUESTIONS

1. Going back to the vignette in this chapter, describe the environmental risks Fatima faces. For instance, she encountered sources of air pollution, both inside her apartment and outdoors. What were some of the specific sources? How can her risks and any health impacts be reduced?
2. Imagine there is a large storm that has caused severe flooding in a community where you serve as an environmental health scientist. Many households have likely been exposed to sewage. What might your team learn by conducting a traditional risk assessment? What might be missed if this assessment is not approached with attention to the social-ecological model?
3. Explain how SDOH relate to allostatic load. Explain how allostatic load contributes to the distribution of environmental health risks and impacts. Use examples.
4. In practice, how could environmental health practitioners reimagine risk assessment in ways that improve EJ? What could this look like in a local or state health department, for instance?

LEARNING ACTIVITIES

THE TIME IS NOW

Consider the nearest facility that releases toxic chemicals into the air and water near where you live, study, work, or play. Using resources like the EPA's Toxic Release Inventory (TRI), look up what toxic chemicals are released.

According to the EPA, "There are currently [over 790] individually listed chemicals and 33 chemical categories covered by the TRI Program. Facilities that manufacture, process, or otherwise use these chemicals in amounts above established levels must submit annual reporting forms for each chemical. Note that the TRI chemical list doesn't include all toxic chemicals used in the [United States]."[52 (para4)]

Ask yourself:

- What are the acute and chronic health impacts associated with each of the chemicals being released?
- Are there standards for what is deemed "safe" and allowable for release into the air or water? Do you think these standards are protective?
- What can you do to reduce your exposure to the toxic chemicals being released in your area?
- What can you do to educate community members like your family and neighbors, other students, and coworkers about their risks?

If you are concerned about the related risks, contact the EPA or your state's environmental agency's staff scientists to ask how regulatory science was used to set these standards. Ask them if there is a timeline for when new evidence will be assessed to reevaluate these standards or for the public to comment.

IN REAL LIFE

While reading this textbook, you have undoubtedly had moments like Fatima, whose story you read earlier in the chapter. Take a day (or even a few hours) and document your environmental exposures. Think about your built environment, food, personal care products, occupational hazards, transportation, clothing, and more. When you are done, ask yourself:

1. Which of these exposures can I reduce easily?
2. Which would present many challenges when trying to reduce?
3. Which requires community or policy changes?

A robust set of instructor resources designed to supplement this text is located at http://connect.springerpub.com/content/book/978-0-8261-8353-8. Qualifying instructors may request access by emailing textbook@springerpub.com.

REFERENCES

1. Preston EV, Hivert MF, Fleisch AF, et al. Early-pregnancy plasma per- and polyfluoroalkyl substance (PFAS) concentrations and hypertensive disorders of pregnancy in the Project Viva cohort. *Environ Int*. 2022;165:107335. doi:10.1016/j.envint.2022.107335
2. Norovirus. Centers for Disease Control and Prevention. 2022. Updated January 18, 2024. https://www.cdc.gov/norovirus/index.html
3. Yearby R. Racial disparities in health status and access to healthcare: the continuation of inequality in the United States due to structural racism. *Am J Econ Sociol*. 2018;77(3–4):1113–1152. doi:10.1111/ajes.12230
4. Katie R. The new Jim Crow is the old Jim Crow. *Yale Law J*. 2019;128(4):76.
5. Bullard R. Addressing environmental racism. *J Int Aff*. 2019;73(1):237–242.
6. Bullard RD. Environmental racism and invisibe communities. *West VA Law Rev*. 1993;96:1037.
7. Lane HM, Morello-Frosch R, Marshall JD, Apte JS. Historical redlining is associated with present-day air pollution disparities in U.S. cities. *Environ Sci Technol Lett*. 2022;9(4):345–350. doi:10.1021/acs.estlett.1c01012
8. Nardone A, Rudolph KE, Morello-Frosch R, Casey JA. Redlines and greenspace: the relationship between historical redlining and 2010 greenspace across the United States. *Environ Health Perspect*. 2021;129(1):17006. doi:10.1289/EHP7495
9. Lee EK, Donley G, Ciesielski TH, et al. Health outcomes in redlined versus non-redlined neighborhoods: a systematic review and meta-analysis. *Soc Sci Med*. 2022;294:114696. doi:10.1016/j.socscimed.2021.114696
10. Swope CB, Hernández D, Cushing LJ. The relationship of historical redlining with present-day neighborhood environmental and health outcomes: a scoping review and conceptual model. *J Urban Health*. 2022;99(6):959–983. doi:10.1007/s11524-022-00665-z
11. Rethorn ZD, Cook C, Reneker JC. Social determinants of health: if you aren't measuring them, you aren't seeing the big picture. *J Orthop & Sports Phys Ther*. 2019;49(12):872–874. doi:10.2519/jospt.2019.0613
12. Singh R, Javed Z, Yahya T, et al. Community and social context: an important social determinant of cardiovascular disease. *Methodist DeBakey Cardiovasc J*. 2021;17(4):15–27. doi:10.14797/mdcvj.846
13. Morello-Frosch R, Zuk M, Jerrett M, Shamasunder B, Kyle AD. Understanding the cumulative impacts of inequalities in environmental health: implications for policy. *Health Aff*. 2011;30(5):879–887. doi:10.1377/hlthaff.2011.0153
14. National Research Council (US) Committee on the Institutional Means for Assessment of Risks to Public Health. *Risk Assessment in the Federal Government: Managing the Process*. National Academies Press; 1983.
15. Shaffer RM. Environmental health risk assessment in the federal government: a visual overview and a renewed call for coordination. *Environ Sci Technol*. 2021;55(16):10923–10927. doi:10.1021/acs.est.1c01955
16. Wild CP. The exposome: from concept to utility. *Int J Epidemiol*. 2012;41(1):24–32. doi:10.1093/ije/dyr236
17. Committee on Human and Environmental Exposure Science in the 21st Century, Board on Environmental Studies and Toxicology, Division on Earth and Life Studies, National Research Council. *Exposure Science in the 21st Century: A Vision and a Strategy*. National Academies Press; 2012.
18. Balazs CL, Morello-Frosch R. The three R's: how community-based participatory research strengthens the rigor, relevance, and reach of science. *Environ Justice*. 2013;6(1):9–16. doi:10.1089/env.2012.0017

19. Hauptman M, Woolf AD. Childhood ingestions of environmental toxins: what are the risks? *Pediatr Ann*. 2017;46(12):e466–e471. doi:10.3928/19382359-20171116-01
20. Bellinger DC. An overview of environmental chemical exposures and neurodevelopment impairments in children. *Pediatr Med*. 2018;1:1–9. doi:10.21037/pm.2018.11.03
21. Engel SM, Patisaul HB, Brody C, et al. Neurotoxicity of ortho-phthalates: recommendations for critical policy reforms to protect brain development in children. *Am J Public Health*. 2021;111(4): 687–695. doi:10.2105/AJPH.2020.306014
22. Chronic Hazard Advisory Panel on Phthalates and Phthalate Alternatives. US Consumer Product Safety Commision. 2014. Accessed June 21, 2024. https://www.cpsc.gov/chap
23. Guidi J, Lucente M, Sonino N, Fava GA. Allostatic load and its impact on health: a systematic review. *Psychother Psychosom*. 2021;90(1):11–27. doi:10.1159/000510696
24. Parker HW, Abreu AM, Sullivan MC, Vadiveloo MK. Allostatic load and mortality: a systematic review and meta-analysis. *Am J Prev Med*. 2022;63(1):131–140. doi:10.1016/j.amepre.2022.02.003
25. Finlay S, Roth C, Zimsen T, Bridson TL, Sarnyai Z, McDermott B. Adverse childhood experiences and allostatic load: a systematic review. *Neurosci Biobehav Rev*. 2022;136:104605. doi:10.1016/j.neubiorev.2022.104605
26. Smith GS, Anjum E, Francis C, Deanes L, Acey C. Climate change, environmental disasters, and health inequities: the underlying role of structural inequalities. *Curr Environl Health Rep*. 2022;9(1):80–89. doi:10.1007/s40572-022-00336-w
27. Crenshaw K. Mapping the margins—intersectionality, identity politics, and violence against women of color. *Stanford Law Rev*. 1991;43(6):1241–1299. doi:10.2307/1229039
28. Bowleg L. The problem with the phrase women and minorities: intersectionality—an important theoretical framework for public health. *Am J Public Health*. 2012;102(7):1267–1273. doi:10.2105/ajph.2012.300750
29. Zota AR, Shamasunder B. The environmental injustice of beauty: framing chemical exposures from beauty products as a health disparities concern. *Am J Obstet Gynecol*. 2017;217(4):418.e1–418.e6. doi:10.1016/j.ajog.2017.07.020
30. Zota AR, VanNoy BN. Integrating intersectionality into the exposome paradigm: a novel approach to racial inequities in uterine fibroids. *Am J Public Health*. 2021;111(1):104–109. doi:10.2105/AJPH.2020.305979
31. Pollock S, Taylor S, Oyerinde O, et al. The dark side of skin lightening: an international collaboration and review of a public health issue affecting dermatology. *Int J Women's Dermatol*. 2021;7(2):158–164. doi:10.1016/j.ijwd.2020.09.006
32. Masub N, Khachemoune A. Cosmetic skin lightening use and side effects. *J Dermatolog Treat*. 2022;33(3):1287–1292. doi:10.1080/09546634.2020.1845597
33. Edwards L, Ahmed L, Martinez L, et al. Beauty inside out: examining beauty product use among diverse women and femme-identifying individuals in northern Manhattan and South Bronx through an environmental justice framework. *Environ Justice*. 2023;16(6):449–460. doi:10.1089/env.2022.0053
34. Kilanowski JF. Breadth of the socio-ecological model. *J Agromedicine*. 2017;22(4):295–297. doi:10.1080/1059924x.2017.1358971
35. Golden SD, McLeroy KR, Green LW, Earp JAL, Lieberman LD. Upending the social ecological model to guide health promotion efforts toward policy and environmental change. *Health Educ Behav*. 2015;42(suppl 1):8S–14S. doi:10.1177/1090198115575098
36. Miller AG, Ebelt S, Levy K. Combined sewer overflows and gastrointestinal illness in Atlanta, 2002–2013: evaluating the impact of infrastructure improvements. *Environ Health Perspect*. 2022;130(5):57009. doi:10.1289/EHP10399
37. Milligan R, McCreary T, Jelks NTO. Improvising against the racial state in Atlanta: reimagining agency in environmental justice. *Environ Plann C: Politics Space*. 2021;39(7):1586–1605. doi:10.1177/23996544211038944
38. Jelks N, Hawthorne T, Dai D, Fuller C, Stauber C. Mapping the hidden hazards: community-led spatial data collection of street-level environmental stressors in a degraded, urban watershed. *Int J Environ Res Public Health*. 2018;15(4):825. doi:10.3390/ijerph15040825
39. Jelks NO, Jennings V, Rigolon A. Green gentrification and health: a scoping review. *Int J Environ Res Public Health*. 2021;18(3):907. doi:10.3390/ijerph18030907

40. Urban waters and the proctor Creek Watershed/Atlanta (Georgia), urban waters partnership. United States Environmental Protection Agency. Updated July 26, 2021. https://www.epa.gov/urbanwaterspartners/urban-waters-and-proctor-creek-watershedatlanta-georgia
41. Consumer Products Safety Commission. Prohibition of children's toys and child care articles containing specified phthalates. *Fed Regist*. 2017;82:49938–49982. https://www.federalregister.gov/documents/2017/10/27/2017-23267/prohibition-of-childrens-toys-and-child-care-articles-containing-specified-phthalates
42. Koman PD, Hogan KA, Sampson N, et al. Examining joint effects of air pollution exposure and social determinants of health in defining "at-risk" populations under the Clean Air Act: susceptibility of pregnant women to hypertensive disorders of pregnancy. *World Med Health Policy*. 2018;10(1):7–54. doi:10.1002/wmh3.257
43. McPartland J, Shaffer RM, Fox MA, Nachman KE, Burke TA, Denison RA. Charting a path forward: assessing the science of chemical risk evaluations under the Toxic Substances Control Act in the context of recent national academies recommendations. *Environ Health Perspect*. 2022;130(2):25003. doi:10.1289/EHP9649
44. Life at the fenceline: understanding cumulative health hazards in environmental justice communities. Environmental Justice Health Alliance for Chemical Policy Reform Coming Clean. Campaign for Healthier Solutions. 2018. Accessed June 21, 2024. https://ej4all.org/life-at-the-fenceline
45. Kriebel D, Tickner J, Epstein P, et al. The precautionary principle in environmental science. *Environ Health Perspect*. 2001;109(9):871–876. doi:10.1289/ehp.01109871
46. Siddique S, Zhang G, Coleman K, Kubwabo C. Investigation of the migration of bisphenols from baby bottles and sippy cups. *Curr Res Food Sci*. 2021;4:619–626. doi:10.1016/j.crfs.2021.08.006
47. Van Horne YO, Alcala CS, Peltier RE, et al. An applied environmental justice framework for exposure science. *J Expo Sci Environ Epidemiol*. 2023;33(1):1–11. doi:10.1038/s41370-022-00422-z
48. U.S. EPA. Framework for Cumulative Risk Assessment. U.S. Environmental Protection Agency, Office of Research and Development, Center for Public Health and Environmental Assessment (CPHEA), formerly known as the National Center for Environmental Assessment (NCEA), Washington Office, Washington, DC, EPA/600/P-02/001F. May 2003. Accessed June 21, 2024. https://www.epa.gov/risk/framework-cumulative-risk-assessment
49. National Research Council (US) Committee on Improving Risk Analysis Approaches Used by the U.S. EPA. *Science and Decisions: Advancing Risk Assessment*. National Academies Press (US); 2009. doi:10.17226/12209
50. Solomon GM, Morello-Frosch R, Zeise L, Faust JB. Cumulative environmental impacts: science and policy to protect communities. *Annu Rev Public Health*. 2016;37:83–96. doi:10.1146/annurev-publhealth-032315-021807
51. Capetola T, Noy S, Patrick R. Planetary health pedagogy: preparing health promoters for 21st-century environmental challenges. *Health Promot J Austr*. 2022;33(suppl 1):17–21. doi:10.1002/hpja.641
52. What is the Toxics Release Inventory? U.S. Environmental Protection Agency. Updated April 4, 2024. https://www.epa.gov/toxics-release-inventory-tri-program/what-toxics-release-inventory

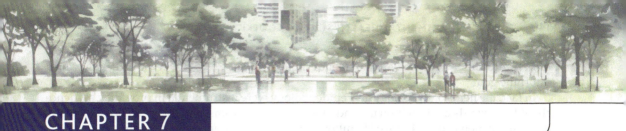

CHAPTER 7

Understanding the Environment and How It Relates to Health Using Toxicology and Epidemiology Research Methods

Chanese A. Forté, Aurora B. Le, Dana C. Dolinoy, and Jaclyn M. Goodrich

LEARNING OBJECTIVES

- Understand the general concepts of toxicology and epidemiology and how these scientific fields are used to identify health hazards in our environment.
- Identify the major types of epidemiologic studies, their applications to environmental health, and their limitations.
- Describe and apply the absorption, distribution, metabolism, and elimination process for toxicological exposures.
- Understand why in utero development and early life are susceptible time periods for environmental exposures.
- Understand the value of community-based participatory research and similar research approaches when identifying environmental hazards.
- Describe and begin to evaluate how toxicology and epidemiology are used in environmental policymaking.
- Examine the key principles and practices for conducting justice-informed research focused on environmental hazards.

KEY TERMS

- absorption, distribution, metabolism, and elimination (ADME)
- cohort study
- community-based participatory research (CBPR)
- developmental origins of health and disease (DOHaD)
- environmental justice
- epidemiology
- epigenetics
- exposome
- exposure
- toxicant
- toxicology
- toxin

OVERVIEW

Human civilizations have used the metal lead (Pb) for at least 5,000 years, and there is evidence that its hazardous qualities were known for most of this time. In the Roman Empire, Pb had many uses, including as a food and wine additive and a major material component of pipes.[1] Because acute Pb poisoning caused "madness," enslaved people, rather than the wealthy aristocracy, were forced to work in the Pb mines. Chronic subtle exposure to Pb through water and food was not considered hazardous. However, many aristocrats experienced gout (a painful form of arthritis).[2] Epidemiologic evidence in 1876 linked Pb to a type of gout now called saturnine gout.[3]

In fact, the fields of toxicology and epidemiology were instrumental in providing evidence about the hazards of Pb in humans and other living organisms, and this evidence eventually drove regulations. In 1914, Alice Hamilton, considered the founder of occupational medicine, profiled Pb poisoning symptoms in industrial workers (see Chapter 16, "Ensuring Occupational Health").[4] In the last half of the 20th century, an explosion of experimental toxicology (e.g., animal studies, cell studies) and epidemiology (e.g., human-cohort, case-control) studies provided evidence that Pb is toxic to nearly every system in the body, conveys no health benefit, and is likely toxic at any dose. This knowledge shaped the regulatory landscape of Pb around the world. In the United States, Pb was first restricted or banned from paint, then gasoline, followed by toys, plumbing, and industrial emissions. Declines in blood Pb levels among the general population track directly with major regulations, giving hope to environmental health professionals that science *can* drive policy and protect public health.

For legacy pollutants such as Pb with known toxicity, toxicology and epidemiology remain important in pushing the scientific, medical, and regulatory fields in taking steps to protect all individuals. In the case of Pb, environmental injustice has led to communities with disproportionate exposure burdens due to historic sources or industrial uses.[5,6] For example, childhood Pb exposure from contaminated water or housing with historic leaded paint and plumbing can still result in toxic Pb levels and sometimes Pb poisoning. In the United States, this exposure is more common in neighborhoods with economic stress and high proportions of people of color, such as was the case with the Flint Water Crisis (see Chapter 11, "Clean Water for All"). Thus, modern toxicologists and environmental epidemiologists continue work that provides evidence of the damage that chronic low-dose Pb exposure causes to children and evidence to support potential protective measures (e.g., certain diets, educational enrichment programs) that can support communities continuing to face an unacceptable burden of Pb exposure.

For emerging exposures about which less is known, toxicology and epidemiology are essential for providing the evidence that environmental health professionals rely upon to inform regulations and intervention strategies, as well as medical care for people who have been exposed. For instance, in the late 20th century, per- and polyfluoroalkyl substances (PFAS) in the human bloodstream were observed by researchers in occupational health studies and eventually in studies of the general population. *PFAS are a large group of thousands of human-made, synthetic chemicals that help make products water resistant.* They have been used in many industries for decades, including in the aerospace, semiconductor, healthcare, automotive, construction, and electronic industries. PFAS are commonly found in consumer products, including carpets, clothing, furniture, outdoor equipment, food packaging, and firefighting foam. Often called "forever chemicals," the United States is currently grappling with how best to regulate PFAS and address the harms they have already caused.

This chapter provides a high-level overview of toxicology and epidemiology, including the key concepts for characterizing the toxicity of an agent (toxicology) and common study designs (epidemiology). The reader is oriented around applications of toxicology and epidemiology in identifying hazardous environmental agents and in determining how exposure occurs. Several specific types of studies that are especially important to environmental health and justice are covered; they include studies that examine population health and the origins of health and disease and provide an introduction to epigenetics. The importance of solutions-oriented science—which may entail applying a community-based participatory research approach—is emphasized. The chapter also covers the important role that evidence from toxicology and epidemiology can play in shaping protective policies and reversing environmental injustices.

USING TOXICOLOGY AND EPIDEMIOLOGY TO UNDERSTAND ENVIRONMENTAL HAZARDS

Environmental health science is all around us, and how we study and understand this science is often through the use of toxicology and epidemiology research methods.

Toxicology is the study of poisons. More specifically, environmental toxicologists study the poisons people may encounter within their environment. Here environment means anywhere people exist, which can be either indoors (e.g., workplace, apartment, or school) or outdoors (e.g., city streets, a farm, or even a hiking trail). As discussed in other chapters, these environments can include one's natural, built, or social environments.

The poisons we study in toxicology are often referred to as toxicants. As opposed to a natural **toxin**, such as snake venom, a **toxicant** is any poison placed in the environment, usually by industry or otherhuman actions, that has the potential to harm living beings. In public health, researchers have numerous ways to study these toxicants. This chapter focuses on environmental **epidemiology**, which in the context of environmental toxicology is more narrowly defined as the study of environmental hazards across a human population.

The many subfields that make up toxicology, and related fields, such as environmental epidemiology, regulatory science, and pharmacology, are referenced throughout this chapter. It is important to understand that regulatory science is defined by environmental toxicology or epidemiology findings that are used as the evidence base for developing policies or laws (i.e., from local or national governments). See Chapter 4, "Environmental Health Policies and Protections: Successes and Failures," for more information on regulatory science. All of these subfields approach environmental toxicology in different ways, and all may be relevant to the work of environmental health researchers, practitioners, or advocates.

TYPES OF ENVIRONMENTAL HAZARDS

Hazards are anything harmful in the environment that may potentially come into contact with people. Environmental exposures typically fall into five categories of hazards:

- biological,
- physical,
- chemical,
- psychosocial, and
- radiological.

Biological hazards are naturally occurring biological toxins that can harm the health of humans, such as a virus, bacteria, or other microbes. Microbes are living organisms that cannot be seen by the naked eye and can be found in water, soil, and air and on the surfaces we touch every day. Microbes can be good, bad, or unaffecting to human health. Biological hazards also include poisons or venom of bacterial, plant, or animal origin.

Chemical hazards include chemical toxicants placed into the environment, such as pesticides or plastics (e.g., phthalates, polychlorinated biphenyls [PCBs]), but they can also include naturally occurring elements like arsenic, mercury, Pb, or radon. Many chemical hazards are found in consumer products (e.g., bisphenol A [BPA]) and may be released from products during usage or over time. It is important to note that of the 85,000 and counting chemicals sold on the global market, we only have human health data on less than 1% of these chemicals.

Physical hazards are anything in the environment that can cause harm to the human body, such as noise like the siren from an ambulance, the shaking from an earthquake, or physical stressors in the workplace due to repetitive motion. Additional physical hazards include extreme temperatures, electricity, and fire.

Psychosocial harm is increasingly recognized as another important hazard category that can impact health. It accounts for the mental health effects of social exclusion, marginalization, or discrimination. Although it is an important aspect of public health, it is not a focus of this chapter.

Radiological or radioactive hazards are defined as any toxic material that emits radiation. Radiation can include the emission of radioactive particles or waves such as alpha and beta particles and gamma waves released during reaction or decay. Radioisotopes or radionuclides are compounds prone to radioactive decay and differ from their elemental form by the number of protons in the nucleus and by weight. Radioisotopes include uranium, plutonium, strontium-90, iodine-131, tritium (a form of hydrogen), and various decay products. However, nuclear fission reactions are not the only sources for environmental exposure; other sources include cosmic rays in airplanes, x-rays, or medical treatments, and even substances like radon or uranium that occur naturally in sediment or rock (Case Study 7.1).

CASE STUDY 7.1: Understanding Radiation Hazards—Indigenous Health and Uranium Mining in the United States

The *nuclear weapons complex* refers to all processes related to nuclear weapons, such as the mining, production, storage, and disposal of nuclear weapons. The governments of the nuclear-weapons states (NWS) like the United States have often targeted Indigenous communities for nuclear weapons waste and exposure—such as uranium mining in the Navajo Nation, nuclear weapons testing on Shoshone land, and intercontinental ballistic missile silos on Tribal land in the Great Plains.

In 1948, after years of dependence on foreign uranium sources, the U.S. Atomic Energy Commission declared it would create a guaranteed price and purchase for all uranium mined in the United States. From 1948 until 1971, uranium mines sprung up across Arizona, Utah, and New Mexico. Today, the U.S. government is still working to clean up some 27,000 square miles of contaminated sites, which are home to roughly 250,000 people.

Overall, four million tons of uranium ore were removed from Navajo land from 1944 to 1986. The exposure to uranium is so severe and long lasting that new U.S. Centers for Disease Control and Prevention (CDC) research finds that Navajo babies have evidence of uranium exposure at birth that is 3.7 times higher than the general population.[7] Even after the mines were closed, decades of spills, accidents, and legacy exposures would continue to plague the Navajo Nation. To this day, the Navajo Nation has increased rates of kidney failure, thyroid disease, and cancers.

Many Indigenous community members and leaders—many of whom continue to reside in contaminated land—have fought long and hard for the rights of miners and surrounding communities. The Radiation Exposure Compensation Act (RECA) was passed in 1990, and the mines were defined as Superfund sites. Since the United States was the sole purchaser of uranium from 1948 to 1971, this action was upheld by the U.S. Supreme Court ruling. Today, residents continue to fight for recognition under and expansion of RECA.

To date, cleanup of the mines remains incomplete, and aging methods of storing waste are still releasing nuclear materials into the environment. Specifically, uranium mill tailings when they are not properly capped can release radioactive uranium and other decay products into the nearby environment. Many community leaders and organizers are still pushing to expand and develop both current and new laws, cleanup site delegation, and treaties.[8]

Hazards related to nuclear weapons or nuclear energy are often only studied by nuclear engineers, radiation health scientists, or health physicists. Yet, as toxicologists increasingly engage in related research, there is so much to learn about nuclear radioactive hazards, such as how low-dose radiation impacts human health. Nuclear toxicology is the study of nuclear materials put in the environment by humans (anthropogenic origins) and their effect(s) on the human body. Nuclear toxicologists are engaged on topics related to fission and fusion reactions and the resultant materials, such as those created in nuclear reactors and nuclear weapons.

Across the United States and many other former and current locations of NWS, nuclear-weapons exposure affects all races, ethnicities, economic groups, and regions. However, cumulative exposures and disparities, like exposure to other industry chemicals, or access to food, shelter, or healthcare, can exacerbate the burden on some communities.

(continued)

> **CASE STUDY 7.1: Understanding Radiation Hazards—Indigenous Health and Uranium Mining in the United States** (*continued*)
>
> **REFLECTION QUESTIONS**
> 1. Who is most affected by the "nuclear-weapons complex" for the sake of national security?
> 2. How did the Navajo Nation get exposed to uranium?
> 3. What are some types of health outcomes related to uranium mining exposure?

THE EXPOSOME AND TOTALITY OF EXPOSURES

Remember that a hazard is a toxin or toxicant that can cause harm upon contact. An **exposure** occurs whenever a person comes into contact with a hazardous substance. People are simultaneously exposed to more than one hazard, and this complex reality brings about the concept of the exposome. The **exposome** refers to the totality of all exposures to which an individual person may be exposed over their life span, including through daily activities (e.g., diet, personal care), school, and work and in their various social or physical environments.

The exposome remains something of a far-off dream for toxicologists to fully measure and quantify using current scientific methods. The exposome interacts at multiple biological levels. These levels include impacts on the genome and epigenome (described in "In Other Words: What Is Epigenetics?"), as well as impacts on various organ systems, such as the reproductive, cardiovascular, nervous, or respiratory systems. Disease risk is largely determined by interacting environmental factors. An understanding of the environment's contribution will continue to grow as better methods are developed to evaluate the exposome and our many daily exposures over the life course.

FROM EXPOSURE TO DISEASE

Core to toxicology is the use of a wide range of toxicological concepts and methods to understand how exposure leads to disease. How a toxin or toxicant exposure harms the human body is often determined by:

- the type of hazard,
- the route or pathway of the exposure,
- the site of the exposure (or how it is absorbed),
- the duration of the exposure, and
- the frequency of the exposure.

The pathway from exposure to disease is represented in Figure 7.1. Individual and society-level factors influence each point along the continuum, contributing to differences in how disease manifests. Factors that shape how a dose of exposure may lead to disease include:

- **individual susceptibility factors:** Can include one's unique combination of exposures (chemical and nonchemical), preexisting diseases, age, and sex, as well as genetic factors.
- **societal factors:** Can include neighborhoods and the built environment, access to healthcare and to education and resources, policies governing environmental hazards, and racism.
- **subclinical biological effects:** Can include a range of outcomes in the body, such as molecular changes, metabolic changes, disruption of enzyme function, and subtle organ damage, among others.

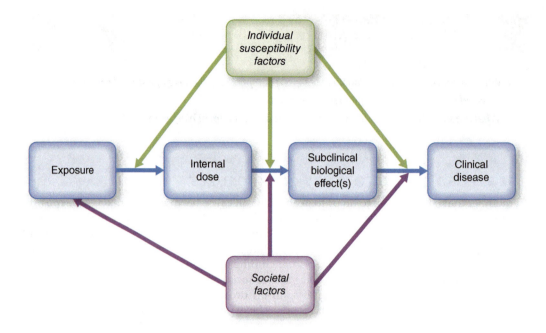

FIGURE 7.1. The exposure to disease continuum.
This is a simplistic representation of how an exposure can result in human disease. How much of a chemical exposure gets into the body (internal dose) is influenced by the amount (dose, duration, frequency) and the route of original exposure.

ABSORPTION, DISTRIBUTION, METABOLISM, AND ELIMINATION

How a toxin, toxicant, or other exposure harms the human body is often dependent on the **absorption, distribution, metabolism, and elimination** (**ADME**) of the poison. In other words, it matters how people are exposed to something and how the body circulates, recognizes, and removes poisons from the body (Figure 7.2).

Absorption is how a toxin or toxicant enters the human body. The routes an exposure can take are often referred to as the absorption pathways. These pathways are usually categorized as inhalation (lungs), dermal contact (skin), ingestion (gastrointestinal tract—esophagus, stomach, small intestine), and injection (muscle). Some exposures can also enter the body through exposed mucus membranes (e.g., eye, vagina, open wound).

Distribution is how a toxicant moves throughout the body. In which organs is it most likely to be stored (e.g., Pb in bone)? How does it circulate and at what amount (e.g., alcohol in blood, pesticides in brain or blood)?

Metabolism refers to how the body recognizes and uses a chemical once it has entered the human body. This process can occur through biotransformation, which is the alteration of toxins and toxicants into different compounds. Sometimes these compounds are more easily excreted, occasionally making them biologically active and harmful. For example, vinyl chloride (an industrially produced colorless gas) can transform into vinyl chloride epoxide and bind to DNA and RNA, which can contribute to cancer.

Elimination is the process by which the toxin or toxicant is removed from the body such as through urine, feces, or other waste matter. Elimination can also refer to the removal of toxins or toxicants from circulation into specific organs, tissues, or fat cells. Some toxicants are eliminated slowly or not at all, such as Pb in bone or organophosphates in fat cells. Others, such as phthalate chemicals (often found in plastics), are rapidly excreted. Even so, phthalates are added to many consumer products and can be harmful given one's likelihood of frequent exposures.

DOSE-RESPONSE CURVES AND TOXICOLOGY

An understanding of ADME helps inform the dose-response curve for target organs—the organs that hazards most actively affect and accumulate in. A dose-response curve represents the quantifiable toxicological response a body, cell, or animal may have with increasing dosage. The typical dose-response curve has no or very low response at low doses, followed by a rapidly increasing response with an increased dosage. A plateau is then often seen for all higher doses, sometimes owing to cellular or tissue death. A simple example is given in Figure 7.3.

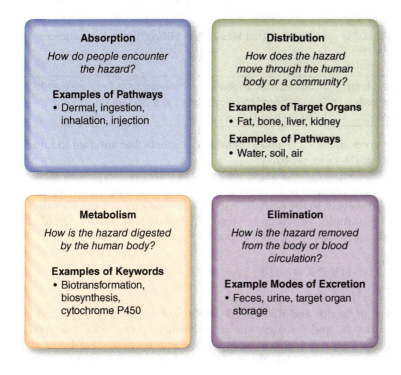

FIGURE 7.2. Absorption, distribution, metabolism, and elimination: How exposures get in and out of the body.

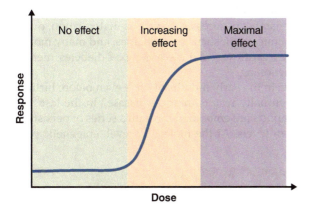

FIGURE 7.3. An example of a dose-response curve.

This image is a general representation of a dose-response curve, where dose is presented on the x-axis and measured on a logarithmic scale. Lower doses are toward the left of the axis, and the higher doses are toward the right. Response is presented on the y-axis, with higher responses representing an adverse biological effect toward the top. Not all dose-response curves look like this one, but this example is considered the typical shape of the dose-response curve for an exposure that has no effect at certain low doses and a maximal effect that tapers off at high doses (usually due to cell death or organ failure).

TABLE 7.1. KEY TERMS IN DOSE-RESPONSE CURVES

TERM	DEFINITION
Limit of detection (LOD)	The minimal measurement the method quantifying the substance can measure with accuracy and precision.
No observed-effect limit (NOEL)	The highest dose at which a response is not observed.
Lowest-observed-effect limit (LOEL)	The lowest dose at which a measured response is observed.
Lethal dose (LD) or lethal concentration (LC)	The concentration at which death begins to occur.
Median lethal dose of 25% (LD25) and median lethal dose of 50% (LD50)	The dose that kills 25% or 50% of the test population.
No observed-adverse-effect limit (NOAEL) and lowest-observed-adverse-effect limit (LOAEL)	Sometimes responses are referred to as "adverse events" as opposed to effects, and the terms are then called NOAEL and LOAEL instead.

Related to dose-response curves, Table 7.1 details several key concepts that are used to understand the toxicology of the substance or exposure.

Dose-response curves can help to characterize all types of hazards. Responses include health outcomes like molecular changes (e.g., cellular changes to DNA, RNA, or proteins), phenotypic changes (e.g., differences in the body or organ), and many more (e.g., prevalence or incidence of disease). For example, we can understand or estimate how much noise (dose) leads to an increase in heart rate (outcome) within a specific population.

DEVELOPMENTAL ORIGINS OF HEALTH AND DISEASE AND EPIGENETICS

The **developmental origins of health and disease (DOHaD)** was a theory first posited by David Barker through a series of epidemiologic studies published in the 1980s that linked poor gestational or infant growth and nutrition to heart disease and mortality decades later.[9,10] Accumulating evidence solidified the DOHaD theory. Fetal undernutrition leads to systemic changes during development that result in long-term metabolic adaptations in the offspring. These adaptations increase the risk for developing adult diseases such as diabetes and cardiovascular disease.

Critically for environmental health, we now know that the nutritional *and* the chemical environments during gestation and early postnatal life can cause physiological changes that lead to chronic disease of adulthood.[11,12] Prenatal exposures as diverse as malnutrition, overnutrition, chemicals (e.g., metals, organic chemicals, plasticizers, pesticides, and many more), and stress have been linked to later life obesity, cardiovascular disease, type 2 diabetes, mental health outcomes, and poor neurological functioning.

So how does an exposure or circumstance in the early months of life—even before birth—leave a lasting impact on the body that eventually results in adult disease? In the last few decades, we have learned that exposures' impacts are embodied through a series of persistent changes at the molecular, cellular, and organ levels. At the molecular level, epigenetic programming is particularly important.

IN OTHER WORDS: WHAT IS EPIGENETICS?

Epigenetics is the study of modifications that impact gene expression without altering the underlying genetic sequence. These modifications change how the DNA is packaged within a cell and influence whether a gene will be turned on or "expressed."

Importantly, epigenetic modifications are heritable when a cell divides into a new cell. However, epigenetic marks can be changed by environmental exposures, and disruptions can lead to

(continued)

> ### IN OTHER WORDS: WHAT IS EPIGENETICS? (continued)
>
> disease. Many disease states are characterized by wildly varied epigenetic profiles.[13] For example, tumors have epigenomes that are drastically different from the healthy tissues from which they originated.
>
> Epigenetics are similar to the software that programs the hardware of a computer. Software is necessary for the computer to perform various functions and tasks. The epigenome is like the software of a computer, while the genome is the hardware. The epigenome controls how the genome is used to carry out biological functions.

Epigenetic modifications influence how genes are expressed or "turned on and off." The epigenome controls cellular processes, such as gene expression, independent of the genetic (DNA) sequence itself. Most important, the epigenome is modified by environmental factors. Unlike some other biological processes that undergo rapid or short-lived changes following exposures, the epigenome can hold onto changes. Each cell and tissue type in the body carries the same DNA sequence but can have widely different functions. The epigenome differs across the approximatey 200 human cell types. It plays a major role in ensuring that the right genes are turned on or off at the right time to perform a needed function.

Environmental exposures can disrupt epigenetic programming, leading to changes in biological function and eventually disease.[14] Early gestation is a particularly vulnerable period for epigenetic changes due to environmental exposures because epigenetic profiles in the early embryo set up the instructions for how the body should work. These instructions are the building parts for different tissues throughout the body. Even small changes at this early stage can result in genes with the "wrong" regulatory structure. Later in life when those genes need to be expressed or repressed, problems can occur, resulting in dysfunction and illness.

> ### AGOUTI MICE
>
> In toxicology research, scientists use a special type of mouse, called the yellow agouti mouse, to show how exposures during pregnancy can influence the long-term health of offspring. This mouse is helpful for studying how early-life exposures result in epigenetic changes (Figure 7.4). These mice have a particular gene that can be turned on or off, affecting phenotype, including coat color, body size, and the risk for developing tumors in adulthood. It is important to note that the epigenetic regulation of this gene is set very early in pregnancy and remains stable through adulthood.
>
>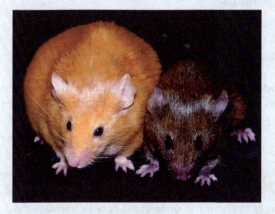
>
> **FIGURE 7.4.** Agouti mouse sisters: epigenetic differences lead to biological differences.
> One-year-old female, genetically identical, viable yellow agouti mice. Maternal dietary supplementation with methyl donors, such as folic acid, choline, and betaine or the phytoestrogen, genistein, shifts the coat color of the offspring from yellow to brown and reduces the incidence of obesity, diabetes, and cancer.[15–17]
> *Source:* Image courtesy of Dana Dolinoy and Randy Jirtle.

(continued)

Researchers have conducted studies with agouti mice in which they exposed pregnant mice to bisphenol A (BPA). BPA was a common chemical found in many products until it was restricted in some countries. The result was that the offspring that were exposed had a gene that was always expressed, resulting in problems like obesity throughout their lives. Interestingly, when the mice were exposed to nutrients rich in methyl (found in some foods like eggs) or genistein (found in soy and soy products) at the same time as BPA, this exposure canceled out the bad effects.[15]

In humans, there is evidence that prenatal exposures to cigarette smoking, other toxicants, stress, trauma, and more can impact the epigenome for both the baby and their future offspring.[18] While we have not found a single exposure–gene combination in humans that has such a large impact on health as in the mice, the mouse experiments demonstrate how early life exposures can affect health for a lifetime.

Epigenetics is one mechanism through which the environment can work to impact health. It is a tool that helps researchers understand what exposures harm human health, how they do so, and at which life stages. With this information, environmental researchers, practitioners, advocates, and policy makers can better monitor and regulate harmful exposures. In particular, if society can prevent exposure to chemicals or other harmful exposures prenatally or early in life, the population burden of many chronic diseases could be greatly reduced. The next sections discuss the methods and study designs that environmental health researchers use to elucidate the human health impact of the environment.

ENVIRONMENTAL EPIDEMIOLOGY AND POPULATION HEALTH

Epidemiology seeks to understand health outcomes or disease across a population, and environmental epidemiology often focuses on understanding associations between environmental exposures and health outcomes. Overall, the study of health outcomes are often defined as:

- **incidence:** The quantification of *new* disease,
- **prevalence:** The quantification of *existing* disease,
- **mortality:** The quantification of *death* due to disease, and
- **morbidity:** The quantification of *illness* due to disease.

Additionally, epidemiology seeks to address factors contributing to health disparities by analyzing social demographics like race and ethnicity, economic status, education attainment, access to healthcare, and many more factors.[19,20]

IN OTHER WORDS: TRANSLATING PUBLIC HEALTH DATA

When translating public health data, it is very important to understand how to translate the outcomes. There are many ways to present measurements of disease occurrence and the association between exposures and outcomes, and understanding how to translate these terms that are usually present in case-control or cohort studies is important. The outcomes of interest for these types of studies often include a disease, but outcomes can also include treatments, behaviors, and much more.

(continued)

IN OTHER WORDS: TRANSLATING PUBLIC HEALTH DATA (*continued*)

COMMON ENVIRONMENTAL EPIDEMIOLOGY VALUES AND HOW TO TRANSLATE THE OUTCOMES

OUTCOME VALUE	WHAT DOES THIS VALUE MEASURE?	HOW DO YOU TRANSLATE THIS VALUE?
Measuring Disease Occurrence		
Incidence	Quantification of a newly diagnosed disease across a population over time.	Over a period of time, X number of people will develop the outcome of interest.
Prevalence	Quantification of a currently diagnosed disease across a population over time.	Over a period of time, X number of people are living with the outcome of interest.
Point prevalence	Quantification of a currently diagnosed disease across a population at one time point.	At a specific time point, X number of people are living with the outcome of interest.
Odds	Ratio of the probability of an event of interest to that of a nonevent.	The odds of developing a disorder is X times higher after exposure.
Associations Between Exposures and Outcomes		
Point prevalence rate ratio	Estimation of relative risk for a point in time (e.g., cross-sectional studies).	At a specific time point, among participants who are exposed, X number of people are living with the outcome of interest.
Relative risk ratio	Risk of developing the disease of interest.	Those who are exposed are X times at risk of having the outcome of interest compared to people who are not exposed.
Odds ratio	Ratio of the odds of developing the outcome of interest in exposed participants to the odds of developing the same outcome in unexposed participants.	The odds of a disorder after being exposed is X times greater than the odds of the disorder if a participant was never exposed.
Attributable risk or odds ratio	Absolute excess risk or odds of an outcome associated with a particular exposure.	Among participants who are exposed, X number of additional people will develop the disease due to that exposure.

TYPES OF ENVIRONMENTAL TOXICOLOGY AND EPIDEMIOLOGY STUDIES

Epidemiologic research can be descriptive or analytical. *Descriptive epidemiology* quantifies trends in time, place, or a population, and it can be used to create hypotheses. An example of descriptive epidemiology includes single-variable (univariate) counts, such as the number and percentage of women with a specific disease, and cross-tabulations (bivariate counts), such as the number and percentage of women across different racial or ethnic groups with that disease. *Analytical epidemiology*, on the other hand, is used to test hypotheses, usually with the use of a comparison group. It is either (1) observational, a study of what is occurring; or (2) experimental, a study of outcomes related to the manipulation of what is occurring, for instance, when a research team assigns exposure and nonexposure.

This chapter predominantly outlines the *primary research* methods used in toxicology and epidemiology. Primary research is any research that produces original data or results. Primary research adds to the overall published body of literature on a topic. Academic and industry researchers often conduct primary research studies with new research ideas and outcomes. Additionally, *secondary research* usually involves a summarization or analysis of primary research that results in new outcomes. Many regulatory scientists at federal agencies conduct secondary research by summarizing existing studies to develop science-informed policies that affect people locally and nationally.

CORRELATION VERSUS CAUSATION

As a society, we strive to understand the etiology (or causes) of health and disease. Many people think that epidemiology is a magic black box. Researchers put exposure information into the box. They use fancy statistical methods. Out pops information about how exposures and health outcomes are related. However, within epidemiology, we know there is much uncertainty, and we need to understand that biases and limitations underlie all research. No single study is perfect, but we design studies as best we can to investigate possible correlations.

It is also imperative to understand that association is not causation. For example, if you did a study on the relationship between getting fresh air and getting a skin tan, you may think that getting fresh air *causes* the skin to tan. However, this is not true. We know that sunshine causes the skin to tan; although when you get fresh air, you are more likely to be outside (in the sun). This example may not seem life or death, but say you are studying more nuanced things like the effects of systemic racism or the effectiveness of planting new forests to uptake toxins? Even with something so closely associated like cigarettes and lung cancer, still there are multiple requirements that must be met for causation to be determined.[21]

Correlation: X and Y are related (statistically, there is an "association").

Causation: X caused Y to happen.

Many studies must be done before scientists declare a causal relationship between X and Y. Throughout history, researchers have generated some criteria that can help us to determine when a causal relationship exists. Perhaps the most well-known criteria are the Bradford Hill criteria proposed in 1965:

- **Temporality:** Does the cause precede the effect?
- **Plausibility:** Is the association consistent with existing knowledge?
- **Consistency:** What is the strength of association between the cause and effect?
- **Dose-response:** Does increased exposure = increased effect?
- **Reversibility:** Does removal of a cause decrease the risk of the effect?
- **Study design:** Is the evidence based on a robust study design?
- **Evidence:** How many lines of evidence lead to the conclusion?

For example, it took decades of observational and experimental studies before the scientific community and the general public accepted the fact that smoking *causes* lung cancer. After noticing a potential relationship, researchers showed that it was biologically plausible. They studied which chemicals within cigarettes were most likely to cause lung cancer. They found that many of the additives are carcinogenic, that the particulates and burnt carbon that lodge in the lungs are carcinogenic, and that in large quantities, nicotine worsens these effects and can also be carcinogenic. Across these studies, researchers accounted for additional factors, including comorbidities like lung disease, confounders like a family history of cancer, and factors like personal enzymatic makeup. There was consistent and strong evidence across many study types that smoking increased the risk of lung cancer.

All studies have bias, but it is important to understand, anticipate, and prevent (when possible) the various types of bias in a research plan, methods, and analysis. Bias creates a lack of validity in study results and is defined not by the results of the study, but as the

TABLE 7.2. TYPES OF BIAS IN ENVIRONMENTAL EPIDEMIOLOGY RESEARCH

TYPE OF BIAS	DEFINITION	EXAMPLE
Selection bias	Participants have different probabilities of being included based on study characteristics.	Healthy workers are the workers who are at work, so studying them produces a selection bias known as the healthy-worker effect, in which the study population may be healthier than the overall population.
Information bias	Imperfect definitions of variables or flawed data-collection methods.	Recall bias, interviewer bias, and exposure misclassification.
Combined selection–information bias	Some studies can have both types of bias, more often in medical surveillance and cross-sectional studies or in screening program evaluations.	Medical surveillance or detection bias, in which participants with a specific condition may be selected for a study and may be monitored differently due to their medical history.

systematic error in the design or procedures of a study.[22] Bias can lead to inaccurate or misleading results. It is imperative to make sure that biases are minimized and acknowledged when reporting results. Some common biases are introduced in Table 7.2.[22] Researchers planning to conduct or interpret epidemiologic studies should learn about these and other types of biases, such as researcher bias or type I and type II errors. For example, to help avoid exposure misclassification—a type of information bias in which exposures for each individual in a study are not accurately measured—more accurate and precise methods for measuring exposures can be used.

Furthermore, the validity, sensitivity, specificity, and reliability of a study can be affected by these underlying study biases. Study *validity* is the ability to correctly determine who has the exposure or outcome of interest and involves sensitivity and specificity. *Sensitivity* is the ability to correctly identify people with a disease or an exposure of interest, and *specificity* is the way to correctly determine when people do not have a disease or an exposure of interest. Finally, *reliability* refers to an experiment that, when repeated, provides the same results again and again.

EXPERIMENTAL STUDIES

Trials make up the majority of experimental studies. Experimental trials are often used in environmental toxicology to understand the dosage of various hazards and their resulting harms. In the field of environmental toxicology, the terms *wet lab* (referring to in vivo or in vitro experiments) and *dry lab* (pertaining to *in silico* experiments) are used to describe the methods used. Experimental trials can occur in vivo (in living organisms), in vitro (in cells or tissue), *in silico* (estimates or modeling using data), or across populations (epidemiology). The main experimental studies outlined in this chapter include experimental trials, such as clinical trials, community trials, and randomized controlled trials (RCTs).

Clinical trials are most often used to understand how a drug or medical device (also referred to as therapeutics) directly affects the human body and at what dose. Clinical trials are also used to understand how new food items, products used on food, and cosmetics may affect the human body. Clinical trials occur in distinct phases that build on each other. They typically begin with preclinical animal or cell studies, and then generally include a larger group of people in each subsequent phase. One consideration of these preclinical studies is that animal and cell models are not perfect predictors of the effect of these therapeutics on humans and are a source of uncertainty in determining the health effects in human populations.

> **CLINICAL TRIALS FOR COSMETICS**
>
> Safety tests for products usually focus on active ingredients only since these ingredients are thought to be the most biologically active (also known as bioactive) in the human body. However, inactive ingredients, even if they have known effects in other products or on their own, are rarely tested for human health effects within a specific product.
>
> In cosmetics, many inactive ingredients are not studied or regulated. For instance, the ingredient known for adding sun protection or plumping skin is labeled as the active ingredient. However, all of the ingredients used in the mixture may still have effects on the human body. Certain shades of red lipstick include the highly toxic substance lead (Pb). Many over-the-counter moisturizers contain parabens, which are carcinogenic compounds, and many fragrances contain phthalates and volatile organic compounds (VOCs) as well as parabens. Surprisingly, these harmful ingredients are not closely regulated or tested like the active ingredients in these products.

Community trials are used to assess an intervention or mitigation strategy that will minimize the effects a hazard may have on a community. *Community trials* typically involve creating an intervention in one geographic area and comparing it to a similar region without the intervention to understand the effects on the community. Researchers must find two regions that are similar in their environment, population, and other factors to make the comparison meaningful. These community trials are also helpful when trying to understand how an environmental intervention (e.g., amenities such as a park) or the lack of that intervention affects a community.

Owing to ethical concerns, RCTs are rarely used in environmental toxicology to test the impact of exposures like Pb unless they are being used to test protective interventions (e.g., access to tree canopy). One cautionary tale of an unethical study that studied Pb exposures in children was the Baltimore Lead Paint Study conducted by the Kennedy Kreiger Institute at Johns Hopkins University during the 1990s. In the study, young children and their families, the majority of whom were Black children from lower income households, were recruited to live in homes with varying levels of partial Pb abatement. Court cases brought against the researchers found alarming ethical concerns about the way that they had conducted the research, drawing parallels to past infamous instances of research abuse, such as the Tuskegee Syphilis Study and exposure of Navajo miners to radiation.[23]

When conducted ethically, RCTs are the only epidemiologic studies that can actually test for causation; all other types of studies in epidemiology test for correlation between exposures and outcomes. In an RCT, researchers can fully manipulate the exposure randomly to create cases and controls, and, thus, they have enough certainty built into their design to assert causation. RCTs create experimental groups of people or "cells" to be randomly assigned to an exposure or therapeutic category. Like most experimental studies, RCTs are dependent on a good comparison group such as a placebo.

RCTs occur in seven steps: (1) eligibility requirements must be met by participants; (2) and (3) participants are randomly assigned to an intervention; (4) participants are observed for a baseline assessment; (5) the intervention (e.g. medicine, exercise) is prescribed and given to those in the intervention group; (6) the participants are observed to determine if outcomes are differed across all groups; and finally (7) analyses are completed for the outcomes of interest, such as dose-response curves, biological activity and pathways, and more (Figure 7.5).

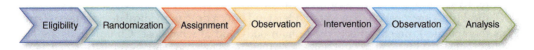

FIGURE 7.5. The process for RCT selection and completion.
This graphic is a quick-and-easy reference to the steps of RCTs. Following this order and the process of randomized intervention assignment are what give RCTs the ability to test causality.
RCT, randomized controlled trial.

TABLE 7.3. BRIEF SUMMARY OF STUDY TYPES COVERED IN THIS CHAPTER

STUDY TYPE	STUDY DESCRIPTION	WHAT CAN WE LEARN?
Experimental Studies		
Clinical trial	Trials that are completed in individuals to understand dose-response in animals, humans, or cells	Dose-response associations, therapeutics
Community trial	Trials that are completed in communities to understand exposures and outcomes on the community	Intervention effect, program evaluation
Randomized controlled trials	Trials that involve randomly assigning an intervention or exposure and measuring the resulting health outcome in animals, humans, or cells	Causality, dose-response associations
Observational Studies		
Cohort study	Follows a sample of people to understand exposure or outcome over time	May result in generalizable outcomes
Case study	Follows a single case or case sample to understand exposure or outcome	Specific exposure and outcomes
Case series	Reports a series of cases to understand exposure and outcome.	A pattern of specific exposures and outcomes
Case-control study	Investigates groups of people who do and do not have a health outcome to understand exposure	Understanding odds and odds ratios
Cross-sectional study	Measures exposure and health outcomes at a certain time point across sample groups.	Understanding point prevalence and exposure events
Epidemiologic triangulation	Uses big data and other publicly available sources to understand exposure and resulting health outcomes across a specific population that is not possible with one of the data sets alone.	Often specific outcomes for a specific population

OBSERVATIONAL STUDIES

Observational studies are often categorized by the group that researchers are observing: cohort, case, case-control, or cross-sectional samples. These studies are used when we want to understand exposure–disease associations, and each of the study types differ by study features and by what can be studied (see Table 7.3).

Table 7.3 presents a brief summary of the basic types of toxicology and epidemiology studies used to understand human health and the environment. (Other study types and substudy types that exist are not presented in this chapter or table.) Additionally, there are more detailed attributes and outcomes that can be studied as you learn more about environmental toxicology and epidemiology.

Cohort Study

A **cohort study** involves following a sample of the population (both exposed and unexposed) over time to observe the health outcomes of the population. This sample is referred to as a cohort and is usually a sample of healthy individuals, or people who do not have the outcome of interest at enrollment in the study. For instance, if you are studying heart disease, you would not enroll people who already have heart disease or related conditions. Cohort studies observe events during a follow-up time period.

Cohort studies are often distinguished as:

- **Retrospective:** Looking back in time to investigate past exposures' associations with current outcomes.
- **Prospective:** Following a group over time to research the associations between current exposures and future outcomes.

Retrospective cohorts can be limited by bias. Recall bias refers to an event or exposure that is either harder or easier to remember, depending on the current diagnosis. For instance, a person who suffers with a complex or traumatic health issue may try recalling every food, drink, or medicine they have recently had, whereas someone without health issues may not recall everything they ate or drank in such detail. Recall bias can often lead to reporting a larger association between exposure and outcome than is actually present. Similarly, a strong assumption is made that those lost to follow-up are similar to those who remain in the study. In fact, there may be similarities among people who decide to leave the study or remain in the study, and the study results can become severely biased.

Case Study

Case studies, case series, and case-control studies are particularly useful when dealing with new environmental exposures to assess their effects on human health before a substantial body of evidence is available. Cases are essential components of case studies, case series, and case-control studies. A case refers to an individual who exhibits the exposure or outcome of interest at the beginning of a study. A *case study* aims to understand how an exposure or disease presents in an individual or population. A *case series study* is a collection of case studies with similarities, used collectively to understand an exposure's effect on the human body. A *case-control study* compares the health outcomes between cases (individuals with the outcome at the start of the study) and controls (individuals without the outcome at the start). Researchers investigate the two groups to try to understand their related exposures.

Cross-Sectional Studies

Cross-sectional studies are often used in occupational health and for exploration of new or uncommon hazards or illnesses. Often referred to as a "snapshot," they include sampling from a population at one time point for an exposure or health outcome of interest. This single time point can represent various scenarios, such as the total exposure during a work shift, exposure levels on a specific day, or the health of a particular group of people.

Epidemiologic Triangulation

Epidemiologic triangulation is loosely defined as the use of data from multiple data sources and studies to more holistically quantify exposure and outcomes across populations. Epidemiologic triangulation strongly depends on publicly available (or open source) big data (any data set with more than 200 data lines). By combining data from different reliable and valid sources, the synthesis may help to counter each data set or study's biases and limitations. Although epidemiologic triangulation is far from ready to use in regulatory science, researchers interested in mapping the human exposome and its effects believe that triangulation will be necessary to do so. For instance, the National Academies of Sciences, Engineering, and Medicine recently convened a workshop to understand and explore triangulation opportunities to enhance the Environmental Protection Agency's (EPA) risk-assessment processes.

Ecological Studies

Ecological studies observe geographic regions or similarly defined geographic risk factors and assess their association with disease outcomes. Ecological studies use measures that fall into three categories:

- **aggregate:** measures summarized across a region, such as prevalence or incidence;
- **environmental:** physical aspects of the region, such as mountains, lakes, hospitals, and so forth; and
- **global:** measures with regional perspectives of the community that stretch beyond boundaries, such as political parties or laws affecting the region.

Researchers must be careful not to make assumptions about individuals based on aggregated data or assume that patterns of aggregate data represent individuals.

COMMUNITY-BASED PARTICIPATORY RESEARCH

Even though environmental health scientists frequently use animal models or large data sets to address research questions, we cannot forget that this work is about real people and environments. As described in Chapter 5, "Environmental Health Science for the People," there are many community-centered ways to approach research with communities and people who are most affected by environmental exposures. Participatory research methods are commonly used in the social sciences, education, organizational science, nursing, and public health. Other terms for this approach include but are not limited to: action research, participatory research, participatory action research, community-based research, community-engaged research, action science, action inquiry, and cooperative inquiry.[24]

Many researchers have metaphorically helicoptered into communities—sometimes without the community's knowledge, acceptance, or full consent—and collected data, published the findings to their own benefit, and had little to no follow-up with the community. This type of research approach is not only unethical, but also undermines trust with these communities, potentially increasing skepticism toward research and government institutions. For example, if researchers confirm that there is a toxic chemical in the community's drinking water but fail to warn the community or bring the issue to the right decision makers to address it, their behavior constitutes unethical conduct and poor research practice.

One approach that environmental health researchers should know about and consider, especially when conducting interventions, is **community-based participatory research (CBPR)**. See Chapter 5, "Environmental Health Science for the People," for an explanation of CBPR principles. *CBPR* is a collaborative research approach that aims to enhance knowledge and understanding of an issue, phenomena, or research question(s) by translating findings to develop an intervention that leads to positive health outcomes, social or political changes, or fewer health disparities that benefit community members, through the equitable involvement of all partners in the research process, and that recognizes the unique strengths each brings.[25]

Again, a CBPR approach works *with* communities rather than *on* communities. In CBPR, it is critical to equitably involve representatives from the research population, community members, organizational representatives, and other key players in all aspects of the research process (e.g., study design, protocol development, disseminating findings). For instance, if researchers are studying the health effects of urban flooding due to the impacts of climate change, have they connected with residents and local organizational leaders to understand their experiences, concerns, and priorities? When all partners contribute and share their expertise, research is more likely lead to equitable decision-making, ownership of the findings, and effective use of findings for social change.[26]

Case Study 7.2 gives an example of successful CBPR in action. In this example, CBPR was used to identify an important issue using epidemiologic data. This case is relevant to environmental health since most cases of cancer are exacerbated by environmental exposures.

CASE STUDY 7.2: Increasing Cervical Cancer Screening Among Vietnamese American Women

Vietnamese American women have some of the highest rates of cervical cancer among all ethnic groups and, at the same time, some of the lowest rates of Pap testing in the United States. This low rate of cancer screening has been attributed to:

- sociodemographic characteristics,
- beliefs around female chastity,
- access, and
- physician characteristics.

(continued)

> **CASE STUDY 7.2: Increasing Cervical Cancer Screening Among Vietnamese American Women** (*continued*)
>
> Previous attempts to increase screening among Vietnamese American women through media messages and lay health-worker interventions have been effective but have not fully addressed access barriers.[27]
>
> In response, a community-based participatory research (CBPR) partnership evolved in Santa Clara County (SCC), California, which at the time of the 2006 study was one of the largest Vietnamese communities in the United States. This community has many social support services, such as churches, temples, stores, restaurants, ethnically representative healthcare providers, and community-based organizations.
>
> This CBPR study involved many partners who formed a coalition to address cervical cancer among Vietnamese women in the county. The coalition included the Vietnamese Community Health Promotion Project, University of California San Francisco, and nine SCC organizations (e.g., Blue Cross of California, Immigrant Resettlement & Cultural Center, Inc., Department of Public Health, Vietnamese Physician Association of Northern California).
>
> The coalition established a Community Action Plan with detailed plans for their interventions and evaluation. Community forums were held to obtain feedback, share results, and obtain input and approval during the study process and planning. The intervention had multiple components:
>
> - media campaigns,
> - lay health worker outreach,
> - continuing medical education for Vietnamese physicians,
> - the restoration of a Breast and Cervical Cancer Control Program,
> - the creation of a Vietnamese Pap clinic and patient navigator, and
> - a Pap test registry and reminder system.
>
> To measure impacts, this CBPR study used a quasi-experimental, controlled trial designed by the coalition. This included:
>
> - **Process measures:** Pre- and postintervention, community-wide cross-sectional telephone surveys in the intervention and control community to document Pap test receipts and the number of registrants for the Pap registry and reminder system.
> - Outcome measures: Pap test recognition, receipts, how recent, and plans for continued testing.
>
> Ultimately, Pap testing increased in SCC when compared with a nearby county. Through continued funding for the program, availability of media products, and provision of long-term screening to the community, the work was sustained. The coalition also obtained funding to address other issues in the community, such as breast cancer screening and hepatitis B prevention.
>
> **REFLECTION QUESTIONS**
>
> 1. Why do you think previous attempts to increase Pap testing among Vietnamese American women in SCC were unsuccessful?

THE ROLE OF ENVIRONMENTAL HEALTH SCIENCE IN POLICYMAKING

As introduced briefly in Chapter 4, "Environmental Health Policies and Protections: Successes and Failures," regulatory science determines the type and amount of toxicants allowed in the general public's air, water, homes, parks, schools, and more. Regulatory scientists, who often staff federal agencies, seek to inform environmental policies through environmental health sciences, toxicology, and epidemiology research. This work is done for many major environmental policies, such as the Clean Air Act, Toxic Substances Control Act, Radiation Exposure Compensation Act, among many others, as well as for some Supreme Court rulings (e.g., on policies to reduce greenhouse gas emissions). For instance, regulatory science is used to inform the way that food and drugs are approved for the market. In another example, every five or so years, each of our National Ambient Air Quality Standards undergoes a scientific review to understand if the standards for air pollutants, including sulfur dioxide, particulate matter, and ozone, should change.

Regulatory scientists often have limited data, research, and funding, and still must implement generalizable effective public health and environmental policy decisions. Methods differ by government, scientist, agency, and fields of research. (We encourage you to learn more about meta-analyses, systematic review, sensitivity analysis, and publication bias if you are interested in the methods and considerations used in regulatory science.) Regulatory scientists often teeter between what is scientifically novel and what are tried-and-true methods (or a gold standard). While a gold standard can be great for comparing differences across regions and time, it can also often mean excluding innovative, community-led, or non-Western research methods that also provide vital information for our environmental regulations. The regulatory science gold standard has historically relied on study samples of healthy White males for understanding exposure and population health outcomes—also known as the "reference man" standard. Regulatory science based on the reference man standard may perpetuate inequities without giving due consideration to diverse populations or variability across a general population.

In particular, it is important to center the experiences of those most marginalized when relying on science for policymaking by learning from theories and frameworks such as *Black Feminist Thought* (e.g., tent theory, which is a framework that analyzes how each of our identities impacts the way we view, understand, and interact with the world).[28] Many modern environmental justice (EJ) organizations are pushing for more inclusive reference models as well. The Tewa Women United organization offers *Nava To'l Jiya* (Tewa word meaning *Land Worker Mother*) as the universal standard for environmental protections. The Land Worker Mother model focuses on the exposures and health outcomes of a pregnant Indigenous woman who works the land. Many organizations, particularly those led by people of color, encourage rethinking regulatory science in ways that could more meaningfully address environmental racism.

WORKING TOWARD ENVIRONMENTAL HEALTH AND JUSTICE

In this chapter, we focus on toxicology and epidemiology as tools for understanding environmental hazards. There is more to protecting public health than naming and characterizing patterns of these toxic exposures; thus, toxicological and epidemiologic methods need to be better harnessed to evaluate health inequities tied to exposures. All of the example environmental chemicals and occupational hazards discussed in this chapter—including Pb, BPA, pesticides, and uranium—are known to be toxic; yet groups of people within the United States and in nearly every country around the world are still exposed to these substances at hazardous levels. It is known that environmental exposures are not evenly distributed across populations owing to geographic, socioeconomic, and other demographic factors, including environmental injustice.[29,30] Many low-wealth communities are often frontline and face environmental health inequities, such as greater exposure to air pollution and other toxicants from industry and less access to preventive methods or healthcare, which result in health disparities driven by environmental exposures. Also, as discussed throughout this textbook, we must recognize interdependent systems of discrimination or disadvantage that act across social categories of race, ethnicity, gender, and others to shape these patterns.

It must be clearly stated: Racism is an insidious concept and strongly influences these environmental exposures, resulting in injustice within disenfranchised racial and ethnic groups. Environmental racism generates health-related inequities, including toxic exposures, unsafe workplaces, food and energy insecurities, and increased risks from global climate change hazards. Also, many people of color and those who are from low-wealth communities have experienced various forms of exclusion and marginalization that affect their environmental health. These injustices may include historical practices like redlining, political gerrymandering, or forced migration of ethnic groups, as well as modern forced displacement due to xenophobic deportation practices or neocolonialist trends like gentrification.

We must strive for inclusive research. For example, there are researchers who do not know how to statistically consider all possible genders because they have not taken the time to learn how to do so. They may believe it must be impossible; it is not. It is also a very common mistake in environmental toxicology to confuse sex and gender. *Sex* is the biological concept defined by chromosomal makeup for genotypic expression and phenotypic presentation often assigned to humans at birth (e.g., male, female, intersex, assigned female at birth). *Gender* is a social construct describing how someone socially and physically expresses a balance or negation of feminine and masculine traits (e.g., man, woman, transgender, nonbinary).[29,30] By understanding and using the language and phrases that people feel the safest hearing, environmental health experts can honor their history, culture, and humanity.

In environmental health and toxicology, we now take into account the impact that environmental exposures have on health or disease varies among individuals and across populations and time, as well as across life stages.[31,32] Specific life stages, such as during embryo and fetal development, early postnatal life, or late adulthood, have been proposed as sensitive time periods.[32] This knowledge needs to be considered when seeking our ultimate goal: protecting the health of *all* people. Achieving EJ will require new knowledge, computational approaches and technologies, and policies to protect individuals and populations. All of these initiatives will be needed to evolve our understanding of the relationships between environmental exposures and health and translate that understanding into effective and precise real-life applications.

MAIN TAKEAWAYS

In this chapter, we learned that:

- Environmental toxicology is the study of poisons in the environment, and epidemiology is the study of disease across a population.
- The major types of hazards include biological, chemical, physical, psychosocial, and radiological hazards.
- Toxicology principles including ADME refer to the basic toxicological concepts of how a substance enters and moves through the body.
- Early life, including gestation, is a susceptible life period when environmental exposures can modify the epigenome and other physiological processes, leading to increased risk for adult diseases later in life.
- Major types of epidemiologic studies that can be used to identify environmental hazards are clinical trials, community trials, RCTs, cohort studies, case studies, case series, case-control studies, and cross-sectional studies.
- Ultimately, findings from toxicology and epidemiology studies on hazardous exposures should be used to inform policies that protect the most disenfranchised people across a population. In doing so, we protect the mainstream population better than by using only the average person's experience. Not everyone is an activist, but there are still ways we can all contribute to uplifting ethical research and understand how public health policies are created.
- It is essential that we conduct environmental health research to address policy-relevant questions. In many instances, CBPR approaches are imperative because they foster equitable research partnerships that inform policy changes needed to achieve environmental health and justice.
- Environmental racism has both historical and current implications for many people of the global majority. Many environmental injustices can also be traced back to environmental racism and monetary gains. Environmental health researchers and practitioners should

strive to use their knowledge to protect all populations from hazardous exposures—with particular attention to populations facing an undue burden of multiple hazards.

SUMMARY

Combining key concepts used in characterizing the toxicity of an agent (toxicology) with common study designs (epidemiology)—including those focused on the DOHaD as well as population health studies—is especially important for environmental health and justice. Evidence from toxicology and epidemiology is critical for shaping protective policies and reversing environmental injustices. Success in reducing the impacts of toxin and toxicant exposures will depend not only on scientific and technological advances, but also on society's capacity to incorporate advances in toxicology and epidemiology into public health strategies that prioritize EJ.

ENVIRONMENTAL HEALTH IN PRACTICE

A few more suggestions for current or future environmental health scientists include:

- Recognize your limitations as a researcher and the privileges of your position. This may require personal work to determine your biases and knowledge gaps.
- Do not forget that data are representations of peoples. You may be telling parts of someone's story with your study findings. Be respectful and careful not to speak for them.
- When working with communities, recognize stories of strength and joy and community-identified solutions to environmental health issues. Researchers regularly pile on negative study findings about environmental health risks and impacts into presentation slides. Do not start and end conversations there.
- It is also important to note that *you will likely make mistakes*, especially when just starting out. Learn from those mistakes. Always be willing to listen and hold yourself accountable in a way that is serving collaborators and research participants. Together with your team members, discuss what should be done when a misstep has occurred. Apologizing and changing unacceptable behavior are pivotal in addressing injustice. Never be afraid to do and be better.

END-OF-CHAPTER RESOURCES

DISCUSSION QUESTIONS

1. Imagine that you want to study the relationship between air pollution and asthma. What would an experimental study look like? What would a cohort or case-control study look like? Which would be most appropriate and why?
2. Practice reading and explaining takeaways from peer-reviewed research studies. For instance, how would you describe this research project to the general public? Forté CA, Millar JA, Colacino JA. Integrating NHANES and toxicity forecaster data to compare pesticide exposure and bioactivity by farmwork history and US citizenship. *J Expo Sci Environ Epidemiol*. 2023. doi:10.1038/s41370-023-00583-5. You might review this guidance first: www.science.org/content/article/how-read-scientific-paper.
3. Why do you think that previous attempts to increase Pap testing among Vietnamese American women in SCC were unsuccessful?
4. Who is the reference man, and how does he inform regulatory science in the past and today? Are there other approaches to understanding human health that may be of interest?

LEARNING ACTIVITIES
THE TIME IS NOW FOR NUCLEAR WEAPONS ABOLITION AND COMPENSATION

Learn more about nuclear weapons abolition and compensation. Read how nuclear weapons affect communities and human health in journals like the *Bulletin of the Atomic Scientists* or novels such as:

- *Plutopia* by Kate Brown,
- *Yellow Dirt* by Judy Pasternak,
- *African Americans Against the Bomb* by Vincent J. Intondi, and
- *Hiroshima* by John Hersey.

Listen to communities living near nuclear waste sites, and speak to legislators on issues such as:

- a timeline for cleanup of nuclear waste sites—even when done expeditiously it can take up to 50 years;
- standards for cleanup that account for those nearby who are most vulnerable; and
- adequate compensation for residents under the Radiation Exposure Compensation Act, the Energy Employees Occupational Illness Compensation Program Act, and the Formerly Utilized Sites Remedial Action Program.

IN REAL LIFE

What environmental health research studies have been done in your community or nearby? Using Google Scholar or databases at your campus or local library, do a search, and report to your family, friends, or classmates what you learn.

For instance, if you live in or near Detroit, Michigan, you might look closely at one of these studies:

1. Franzblau A, Demond AH, Sayler SK, D'Arcy H, Neitzel RL. Asbestos-containing materials in abandoned residential dwellings in Detroit. *Sci Total Environ*. 2020;714: 136580.
2. Orta OR, Wesselink AK, Bethea TN, et al. Correlates of plasma concentrations of brominated flame retardants in a cohort of U.S. Black women residing in the Detroit, Michigan, metropolitan area. *Sci Total Environ*. 2020;714:136777.
3. Schulz AJ, Omari A, Ward M, et al. Independent and joint contributions of economic, social and physical environmental characteristics to mortality in the Detroit Metropolitan area: a study of cumulative effects. *Health Place*. 2020;65:102391.

After reading one chapter, you may not feel like you are an environmental epidemiologist or toxicologist just yet. Do your best! In simple terms, discuss:

- the goals of the study and the environmental health or justice issues under study,
- the type of study (e.g., observational, experimental),
- practices used to ensure the study methods were ethical,
- key findings, and
- implications of the study (i.e., "so what" can we do with this information).

Finally, considering that this study is about your city, region, or state, does it reflect your reality? If you are reading about a nearby community, do you think it respectfully presents the people affected by the issue?

A robust set of instructor resources designed to supplement this text is located at http://connect.springerpub.com/content/book/978-0-8261-8353-8. Qualifying instructors may request access by emailing textbook@springerpub.com.

REFERENCES

1. Lewis J. Lead poisoning: a historical perspective. *EPA J.* 1985;11:15.
2. Nriagu JO. Saturnine gout among Roman aristocrats. Did lead poisoning contribute to the fall of the Empire? *N Engl J Med.* 1983;308(11):660–663. doi:10.1056/nejm198303173081123
3. Garrod AB. *A Treatise on Gout and Rheumatic Gout (Rheumatoid Arthritis).* 3rd ed. Green & Co.; 1876.
4. Baron SL, Brown TM. Alice Hamilton (1869–1970): mother of US occupational medicine. *Am J Public Health.* 2009;99(suppl 3):S548. doi:10.2105%2FAJPH.2009.177394
5. Whitehead LS, Buchanan SD. Childhood lead poisoning: a perpetual environmental justice issue? *J Public Health Manag Pract.* 2019;25(suppl 1):S115–S120. doi:10.1097/PHH.0000000000000891
6. McClure LF, Niles JK, Kaufman HW. Blood lead levels in young children: US, 2009–2015. *J Pediatr.* 2016;175:173–181. doi:10.1016/j.jpeds.2016.05.005
7. Erdei E, Qeadan F, Miller CP, et al. Environmental uranium exposures and cytokine profiles among mother-newborn baby pairs from the Navajo Birth Cohort Study. *Toxicol Appl Pharmacol.* 2022;456:116292. doi:10.1016/j.taap.2022.116292
8. Brugge D, Goble R. The history of uranium mining and the Navajo people. *Am J Public Health.* 2002;92(9):1410–1419. doi:10.2105/ajph.92.9.1410
9. Barker DJ, Osmond C. Infant mortality, childhood nutrition, and ischaemic heart disease in England and Wales. *Lancet.* 1986;1(8489):1077–1081. doi:10.1016/s0140-6736(86)91340-1
10. Barker DJ, Winter PD, Osmond C, Margetts B, Simmonds SJ. Weight in infancy and death from ischaemic heart disease. *Lancet.* 1989;2(8663):577–580. doi:10.1016/s0140-6736(89)90710-1
11. Haugen AC, Schug TT, Collman G, Heindel JJ. Evolution of DOHaD: the impact of environmental health sciences. *J Dev Orig Health Dis.* 2015;6(2):55–64. doi:10.1017/s2040174414000580
12. Roseboom T, de Rooij S, Painter R. The Dutch famine and its long-term consequences for adult health. *Early Hum Dev.* 2006;82(8):485–491. doi:10.1016/j.earlhumdev.2006.07.001
13. Feinberg AP. The key role of epigenetics in human disease prevention and mitigation. *N Engl J Med.* 2018;378(14):1323–1334. doi:10.1056/nejmra1402513
14. Walker CL, Ho S-m. Developmental reprogramming of cancer susceptibility. *Nat Rev Cancer.* 2012;12(7):479–486. doi:10.1038/nrc3220
15. Dolinoy DC, Huang D, Jirtle RL. Maternal nutrient supplementation counteracts bisphenol A-induced DNA hypomethylation in early development. *Proc Natl Acad Sci USA.* 2007;104(32): 13056–13061. doi:10.1073/pnas.0703739104
16. Dolinoy DC, Weidman JR, Waterland RA, Jirtle RL. Maternal genistein alters coat color and protects Avy mouse offspring from obesity by modifying the fetal epigenome. *Environ Health Perspect.* 2006;114(4):567–572. doi:10.1289/ehp.8700
17. Waterland RA, Jirtle RL. Transposable elements: targets for early nutritional effects on epigenetic gene regulation. *Mol Cell Biol.* 2003;23(15):5293–5300. doi:10.1128/mcb.23.15.5293-5300.2003
18. Breton CV, Landon R, Kahn LG, et al. Exploring the evidence for epigenetic regulation of environmental influences on child health across generations. *Commun Biol.* 2021;4(1):769. doi:10.1038/s42003-021-02316-6
19. Payne-Sturges DC, Gee GC, Cory-Slechta DA. Confronting racism in environmental health sciences: moving the science forward for eliminating racial inequities. *Environ Health Perspect.* 2021;129(5):55002. doi:10.1289/ehp8186
20. Zota AR, Shamasunder B. The environmental injustice of beauty: framing chemical exposures from beauty products as a health disparities concern. *Am J Obstet Gynecol.* 2017;217(4):418.e1–418. e6. doi:10.1016/j.ajog.2017.07.020
21. Chambliss DF, Schutt RK. Sampling and generalizability. In: Chambliss DF, Schutt RK, eds. *Causation and Experimental Design. Making Sense of the Social World: Methods of Investigation.* SAGE Publications, Inc; 2018:106–135.

22. Skzlo M, Nieto FJ. *Epidemiology: Beyond the Basics*. Jones & Bartlett Publishers; 2019.
23. Rosner D, Markowitz G. With the best intentions: lead research and the challenge to public health. *Am J Public Health*. 2012;102(11):e19–e33. https://www.ncbi.nlm.nih.gov/pmc/articles/PMC3477943/
24. Holkup PA, Tripp-Reimer T, Salois EM, Weinert C. Community-based participatory research: an approach to intervention research with a Native American community. *ANS Adv Nurs Sci*. 2004;27(3):162–175. doi:10.1097/00012272-200407000-00002
25. Collins SE, Clifasefi SL, Stanton J, et al. Community-based participatory research (CBPR): towards equitable involvement of community in psychology research. *Am Psychol*. 2018;73(7):884–898. doi:10.1037/amp0000167
26. Wallerstein NB, Duran B. Using community-based participatory research to address health disparities. *Health Promot Pract*. 2006;7(3):312–323. doi:10.1177/1524839906289376
27. Nguyen TT, McPhee SJ, Bui-Tong N, et al. Community-based participatory research increases cervical cancer screening among Vietnamese-Americans. *J Health Care Poor Underserved*. 2006;17(suppl 2):31–54. doi:10.1353/hpu.2006.0091
28. hooks b. *Feminist Theory: From Margin to Center*. South End Press; 1984.
29. Goldsmith L, Bell ML. Queering environmental justice: unequal environmental health burden on the LGBTQ+ community. *Am J Public Health*. 2022;112(1):79–87. doi:10.2105/ajph.2021.306406
30. Masri S, LeBron AMW, Logue MD, et al. Risk assessment of soil heavy metal contamination at the census tract level in the city of Santa Ana, CA: implications for health and environmental justice. *Environ Sci Process Impacts*. 2021;23(6):812–830. doi:10.1039/d1em00007a
31. Hsu A, Sheriff G, Chakraborty T, Manya D. Disproportionate exposure to urban heat island intensity across major US cities. *Nat Commun*. 2021;12(1):2721. doi:10.1038/s41467-021-22799-5
32. Wright RO. Environment, susceptibility windows, development, and child health. *Curr Opin Pediatr*. 2017;29(2):211–217. doi:10.1097/mop.0000000000000465

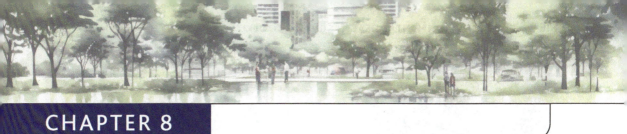

CHAPTER 8

Mapping Environmental Health and Justice Issues

Juliana Maantay and Mozhgon Rajaee

LEARNING OBJECTIVES

- Understand how geographic information science (GISc) can be used to understand, analyze, and visualize public health issues.
- Examine the role of spatial analysis in the history of the environmental justice (EJ) movement, as well its potential for advancing environmental health and justice today.
- Explain the concept and application of participatory geographic information systems (PGIS).
- Understand the basics of geospatial analysis in order to critically interpret spatially based environmental health research.
- Examine and propose ways to integrate geospatial analysis and GISc applications in an interdisciplinary manner for solving real world problems by incorporating information from fields like public health, demography, epidemiology, environmental science, sociology, and urban planning.

KEY TERMS

- climate gentrification
- data aggregation
- geographic information science (GISc)
- participatory geographic information systems (PGIS)
- reference maps
- thematic maps
- vulnerability index

OVERVIEW

The art and science of disease mapping has a long history, dating back at least to the 17th century.[1] Historic examples include the health-related mapping of:

- the 1690 outbreak of the Plague and the consequent quarantine boundaries in Bari, a city near Naples, Italy;
- the 1793 Yellow Fever epidemic in New York City, which killed nearly 5,000 people and led to the city's first Board of Health Department;
- the 1840 spatial study of the incidence of hernia in France, by Dr. Malgaigne, a military surgeon, in which the maps were used to test hypotheses of causes based on regional differences;[2] and
- the well-known spatial analysis of cholera deaths and public water sources in Soho, London, in 1854 by Dr. John Snow, which helped demonstrate that cholera was a waterborne illness, and not due to atmospheric "miasmas."

Several other mapping efforts in the mid-19th century in the United Kingdom also showed the connections between disease and environmental and social conditions, such as Edwin Chadwick's 1842 map of the relationship of mortality to both social class and sanitary conditions; a similar study of Dublin, Ireland, in 1841, linking mortality to living conditions and class; and Robert Perry's 1843 map of a typhus outbreak in Glasgow, Scotland, and its correspondence to residential overcrowding and other environmental conditions (Figure 8.1).

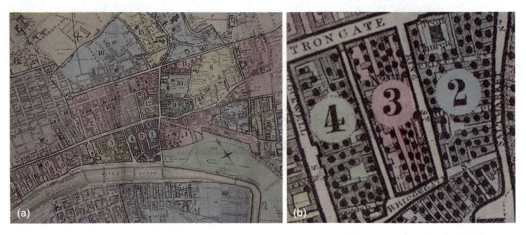

FIGURE 8.1. Mapping neighborhood conditions and fever epidemic in 1844 Glasgow, Scotland, with detail.

This study, *Facts and Observations on the Sanitary State of Glasgow*, published in 1844, relates to the fever epidemic that struck the city in the previous year. Written by Dr. Robert Perry (President of the Faculty of Physicians and Surgeons and Senior Physician to the Glasgow Royal Infirmary), it uses local medical reports, statistical tables, and a color-coded map of the city to highlight the link between poor sanitation, poverty, and poor health. It is an excellent example of early thematic mapping, and predates both Charles Booth's Poverty Maps of London (1886–1903) and John Snow's cholera maps of Soho, London (1854). Dr. Perry's map, with different neighborhood areas colored to designate the severity of the epidemic (a), made it obvious that the effects of the epidemic were not distributed evenly throughout the city, but disproportionately affected the poorest, most densely settled areas, where as many as 20% of the population had succumbed to the disease. The detail of the map shows three of the districts most affected by the epidemic (b).

Source: Hepworth S. Facts and observations on the sanitary state of Glasgow. Glasgow University Library Special Collections Department. February 2006. http://special.lib.gla.ac.uk/exhibns/month/feb2006.html

WHAT IS GEOGRAPHIC INFORMATION SCIENCE?

These historical instances of disease mapping and spatial analyses of health were done the old-fashioned way with pen and paper, but the resultant maps use remarkably similar methods to those now used in **geographic information science (GISc)**. The discipline of *GISc* is a broad field that includes a number of technologies, analytical approaches, and research methods. It encompasses *geographic information systems* (GIS), which are remotely sensed images from satellites, global positioning systems (GPS), photogrammetry, geostatistics, cartography, artificial intelligence, data management, geospatial analysis, spatial modeling, and many varieties of mapping and data visualization.

WE ARE ALL ON NATIVE LAND

Native Land Digital is a Canadian nonprofit organization that works to highlight the history of colonialism, Indigenous ways of knowing, and settler–Indigenous relations. They provide one of many mapping tools that have been developed to show the past and present of the land upon which we live.

Native Land Digital explains on its website that "Land is something sacred to all of us, whether we consciously appreciate it or not…"[3(para2)] Maps are simplified depictions of the places to which we are connected and where we experience our daily lives. As such, Native Land Digital explains that we must honor and treasure land rather than claim and exploit it.

In the United States, there are 574 federally recognized American Indian Tribes and Alaska Native villages. Mapping this land is not just a matter of recognizing history, but also of recognizing the colonization that continues today. See Native Land Digital's mapping tool (https://native-land.ca) to learn more.

Spatial analyses and visualizations have become increasingly common in environmental health research and practice in which it is vital to have an appreciation of GISc capabilities, along with some of its limitations. This chapter covers:

- how GISc is used to analyze environmental health and justice,
- the major concepts of GISc,
- important considerations in GISc research design,
- policymaking with GISc (including community participatory GISc), and
- the limitations and ethical concerns related to GISc.

This chapter mainly focuses on GISc in terms of GIS mapping and analysis, and how these methods can be used in addressing environmental health issues with a focus on environmental justice (EJ) and health equity.

BACKGROUND OF GEOGRAPHIC INFORMATION SCIENCE IN ENVIRONMENTAL HEALTH AND JUSTICE

GISc has played a pivotal role in the advancement of the EJ movement. The EJ movement started in the United States alongside the civil rights and environmental movements. It reached prominence largely as a result of the groundbreaking reports by the United Church of Christ (UCC) Commission on Racial Justice and the U.S. General Accounting Office (GAO), as described in several chapters throughout this text. Both reports revealed the extent of the disproportionate environmental burdens borne by communities of color.[4,5] "Three out of every five Black and Hispanic Americans lived in communities with uncontrolled toxic waste sites."[5] This finding was just one of the shocking outcomes of the UCC report. These studies and the ones that followed coincided with the advent of early forms of basic computerized mapping.

In the decades immediately after publication of the UCC's *Toxic Wastes and Race in the United States* report, many similar studies were conducted, some at the national level and many more at the state or city levels. Virtually every one of these studies pointed to the existence of environmental racism. Race (above and beyond income or other variables) consistently emerged as a key predictor for unequal exposure to environmental contamination and hazards of all sorts, including air and water pollution, soil contamination, flooding, and other environmental issues. In addition to the studies finding disproportionate proximity to adverse environmental conditions, other studies found disproportionately less access to environmental "goods" or amenities by historically marginalized populations. These disparities encompass essential factors that are crucial for healthy living and overall well-being, such as access to nutritious food options, green spaces for recreational activities, and healthcare providers.

Today, the spatial evidence is overwhelming: People of color and people who have less access to wealth live in much less health-supportive places. They live in places that are more polluted, with less access to beneficial features that could improve lives and health. Early EJ studies generally focused on describing the subpopulations in closest proximity to environmental hazards, for instance, by race, ethnicity, income, and education. In time, researchers began trying to parse out the actual exposures and health impacts resulting from the contaminated environments, rather than merely documenting proximity to the hazards (or *potential* exposure). Demonstrating adverse health effects from environmental conditions proves to be challenging. Researchers can establish strong spatial relationships, but definitively proving causality remains harder, as discussed in Chapter 7, "Understanding the Environment and How It Relates to Health Using Toxicology and Epidemiology Research Methods."[6]

The EJ movement coincided with the availability of more accessible user-friendly desktop mapping software, which enabled GIS studies to proliferate. GIS makes it possible to visualize spatial relationships between adverse environmental conditions and human health, making complex data more accessible and understandable to a broader audience in a way that would not have been possible without mapping the data. GIS has made it possible to quantify EJ impacts in a measurable way, taking EJ research beyond anecdotal evidence that is too often dismissed by researchers and policy makers. (See Chapter 5, "Environmental Health Science for the People.") It has also made EJ-related research more apt to be incorporated into policymaking processes that influence government decisions, environmental analyses, urban planning, and public health strategies.[7] GIS serves as a powerful tool for visually illustrating the magnitude of a problem to both the public and policy makers.

GISc is frequently used today in many types of public health research studies. It works best at answering questions about connections between environmental conditions and health outcomes in specific places. For example, it can:

- show how locations of low-wealth communities, pollution sources, and health outcomes (e.g., asthma hospitalizations) are related,
- create visual depictions of human–environment relationships or conduct more quantitative examinations using geostatistical tests and other spatial techniques, and
- identify populations potentially exposed to or impacted by a hazard event or environmental condition, as well as analyzing the spatial (i.e., across spaces) and temporal (i.e., over time) patterns of how diseases and health outcome clusters illustrate change over time. For instance, what percentage of the population is exposed to air pollution concentrations above the U.S. Environmental Protection Agency (EPA) standard now, as compared with 10 years ago? How have the land use, traffic volumes, and other environmental conditions changed in the study area in those 10 years?

These types of analyses can assist policy makers, health experts, and public officials in improving health outcomes, reducing inequity, and mitigating vulnerability.

HOW GEOGRAPHIC INFORMATION SYSTEMS WORK

GIS is a system that integrates various types of information about the real world. This information is abstracted or simplified into a digital database of spatial features (e.g., distance to a healthcare facility) and nonspatial features (e.g., age). With specialized software and computer hardware, coupled with the expert judgment of the GIS user or analyst, we can investigate a variety of environmental issues that may be related to place.

Nonspatial data is commonly referred to as *attribute data,* which are data that would commonly be seen in a spreadsheet. These data can be classified as quantitative (data represented with numbers) or qualitative (data represented by a specific quality). Qualitative attributes can be nominal (e.g., names of places or types of land uses) or ordinal (ranked, e.g., low, medium, or high). *Spatial data* refers to the geographic location of interest. Depending on the format of this spatial data, attributes can be connected to it by a point, line, or polygon or by a cell or pixel.

The main organizing framework of GIS is a layers format, whereby information is separated by thematic content into its constituent parts and then recombined by overlaying one layer on top of the other (Figure 8.2). In this way, the data are merged, leading to the generation of new information that was not available before and the ability to visualize relationships that were not obvious when looking at each layer individually.

WORKING WITH MAPS AND DATA

Mapping data for spatial analyses serves three main functions:

1. **Data visualization and exploratory spatial data analysis (ESDA).** The maps are used for hypothesis development and for generating appropriate research questions. ESDA uses what are generally considered to be "working maps" that are typically not intended for publication or presentation. This ESDA research phase also entails a

8 MAPPING ENVIRONMENTAL HEALTH AND JUSTICE ISSUES ■ 167

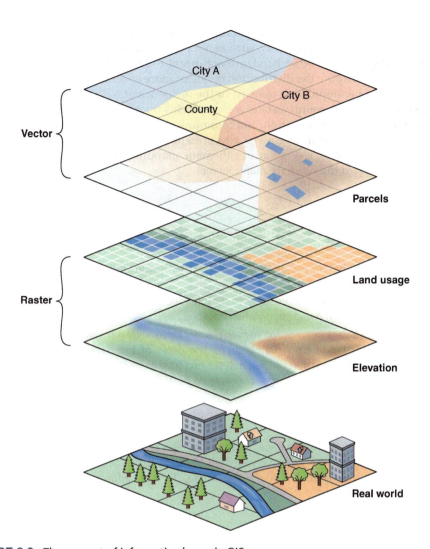

FIGURE 8.2. The concept of information layers in GIS.

Information about the real world is disaggregated into its constituent layers, each of which represents a different set of geographic information. Individual layers can then be recombined in GIS, so that relationships between different aspects of geographic reality become clear. This figure also shows the difference between the vector and raster data formats.

GIS, geographic information systems.

rigorous evaluation of the data to ensure its fitness for the study design and to assess any data deficiencies or incompleteness.

2. **Spatial analysis in research.** In this phase, the data are mapped and analyzed on the basis of the information provided by the ESDA phase and provide a further refinement of the ESDA findings.

3. **Presentation and communication of data and spatial analyses.** The maps used for this phase of a research project need to be designed with the intended audience in mind, whether that be the public or experts. The maps must be designed ethically and honestly with no misleading aspects about how the data are presented, and they must also be culturally appropriate for the audience, clear and understandable, and impart the information in an unbiased and straightforward way. The maps also must be designed in such a way that ensures that they are easily understandable and can assist decision makers and policy makers in effectively integrating a study's results into their decisions.

There are two main categories of maps: reference maps and thematic maps. **Reference maps** are those we use to find our way, such as a road map, or a navigational map for air or sea. **Thematic maps**, on the other hand, are not meant to locate anything with high precision, but are used to display the distribution of one or more specific variables, such as average household income, population density, or the incidence of a disease, as aggregated by a geographic unit, such as country, state, county, census tract, or ZIP code. Maps for ESDA, detailed spatial analyses, presentation, and communication are typically created as thematic maps. Thematic maps offer different ways to present data, each with its own advantages and drawbacks (Figure 8.3). Using various thematic mapping techniques can be beneficial for both the analyst and the ultimate map viewer.

IN OTHER WORDS: HOW TO MAKE ACCESSIBLE MAPS

- *Do you need a map?* Before you develop or share a map, decide if it is a helpful way to share information.
- *Who is your audience?* Maps should speak to the intended audience—policy makers, the public, or a specific community. Avoid jargon when possible.
- *Do you provide relevant information so map viewers can decide if the map is valid and trustworthy?* The map should have data sources, the dates of the data collection and map creation, a simple explanation of the analyses undertaken, a clear legend of the symbols used, the scale and unit of analysis, and caveats outlining any limitations of the data or analyses.
- *Is the map accessible?* For instance, use color-blind-friendly color schemes, as well as contrasts so that labels and text are easy to read.
- *Whose story are you telling?* Remember that the map represents real people and real places. Be respectful and intentional in how maps are designed and shared. (See the lessons from Chapter 5, "Environmental Health Science for the People," for more information about partnering with communities.)

SPATIAL METHODS FOR ASSESSING RISK, EXPOSURE, AND ACCESS

Risk and vulnerability assessments play a large role in many environmental health and justice analyses, as discussed in Chapter 6, "Understanding (Unequal and Cumulative) Risks in Our Daily Environment." These studies evaluate the geographic extent of risk, identify who is at risk, and determine who is exposed to the hazard or condition.

These *prospective studies* often use the technique of spatial coexistence. In other words, where do these criteria or phenomena overlap in space? Source pathway models, often referred to as "fate and transport" models, are instrumental in mapping out the actual extent of the hazard or contaminant. These models simulate the movement of the hazard from its source and illustrate whether the hazard is diffused into the atmosphere, into surface waters, through the soil, or over land. This comprehensive approach aids researchers in predicting the places and populations that are at the greatest risk.

In contrast, *retrospective studies* of risk rely on existing information about a health outcome, such as the actual location of patients with that particular health issue. These studies then conduct analyses, like cluster detection, to explore the spatial patterns and distribution of the health outcome. The ultimate goal is to utilize this information in shaping policies and interventions aimed at enhancing future outcomes.

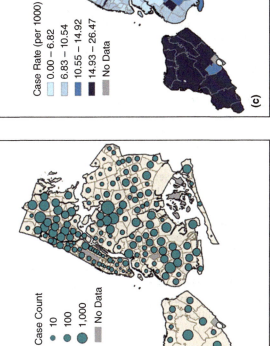

Positive SARS-CoV-2 Cases in New York City

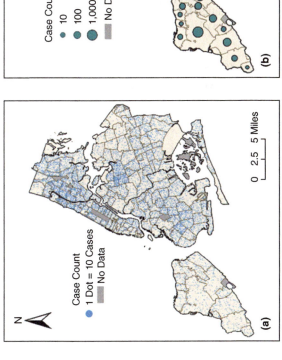

FIGURE 8.3. Types of thematic maps.

These three maps use the same data set but show different aspects of the data: one shows rates (the choropleth map "b") and the other two show the absolute numbers of cases (the dot density map "a" and the proportional symbol map "b"). It is helpful to see both absolute numbers and rates since they can serve different purposes for policymaking and decision-making. Together they provide a more complete picture of the SARS epidemic in New York City.

SARS-CoV-2 (also known as COVID-19) is a communicable disease that was first identified in late 2019. Communicable diseases are often associated with environmental conditions such as population density, as well as various social determinants of health including race/ethnicity and poverty. The maps above depict COVID-19 case counts and cumulative case rates per ZIP Code Tabulation Area (ZCTA), as of April 13, 2020. The case rate is calculated per 1,000 residents.

Data sources: SARS-CoV-2 data from Incident Command System for COVID-19 Response as of 4/13/20. Population Data from American Community Survey 2018, 5-year estimates.
Credit: Jocelyn Rajabelley (2023), Research Assistant, CUNY Institute for Health Equity; and the Urban GISc Lab, Lehman College, CUNY.

IN OTHER WORDS: A NOTE ABOUT VULNERABILITY

Although it is quite common in public health to use the term *vulnerable communities*, be sure to think about what you mean when you say or use this term. *What makes a community or population vulnerable?*

It may not be your intent, but this framing can imply that the people in the community or who are part of a population are the problem. More likely, the problem results from other structural factors that led to unequal risk or impacts, such as historic marginalization, disinvestment in communities of color, or discriminatory policies.

The term *vulnerable* may be appropriate but be sure to explain who you are talking about, their specific risks, and the root causes of these risks whenever possible.

CASE STUDY 8.1: Access to Healthy Foods in New York City

In addition to proximity to environmentally harmful facilities and land uses, access to environmentally beneficial locations, such as healthy food options, is also a way to quantify environmental justice (EJ). The issue of access to healthy foods has implications for health outcomes such as diabetes and cardiovascular disease. Many urban areas have been described as experiencing *food apartheid*, a system of segregation separating residents from supermarkets or other healthy fresh food options that are convenient for everyday shopping, while fast food restaurants or small shops with poor choices in terms of healthy food options are often the only readily available food sources.

Network analysis can help to investigate food access in cities, such as New York. Network analysis measures distances along an existing pedestrian street network. This approach avoids the oversimplification and inaccuracies of other types of analyses that might measure distance "as the crow flies," without regard for the reality of how people are able to walk in cities to access different amenities. Network analysis can also be used to look at vehicular access, although, in the case of New York, walkability to supermarkets is a better indicator of access.[8]

Areas without walkable access to a supermarket may be experiencing food apartheid. Although there may be a vibrant network of food growers that are unaccounted for, findings suggest that underserved populations are likely at risk for diet-related adverse health outcomes, especially those areas with a high percentage of households below the poverty line. It is important to keep in mind that there are several types of "access," all of which may play a part in hindering the availability of health-promoting facilities or services. In addition to geographic access, we must also consider economic and cultural access, any combination of which can block true access.

REFLECTION QUESTIONS

1. What factors influence true access to healthy and affordable foods?
2. What are different ways you might use spatial analyses to explore or communicate these issues in this case or your own community?

GEOGRAPHIC INFORMATION SCIENCE RESEARCH DESIGN

In designing spatial analysis for a research project or public health intervention, several important decisions must be made. These decisions can greatly affect the reliability and accuracy of the analysis. Some of these considerations will be predetermined, meaning that analysts must work with certain limitations. These limitations can stem from the available data, the already established general location of the study area, and the overarching goals of the analysis. Mapmakers must decide on:

- **Geographic extent:** This is the total area under investigation. This area can be the whole country, a state, a county, a neighborhood, or a specific case-study area.
- **Resolution:** The fineness or coarseness of the data and spatial unit.
- **Unit of analysis:** The geographic size used to organize attribute data and perform numerical analysis. These are smaller units within the geographic area; for example, a

state could be the unit of analysis if it is a country-wide analysis or an analysis of census tracts within a neighborhood. Generally, it is accepted that smaller units of analysis provide more detailed results because there is less averaging of quantitative data.

Deciding upon the right spatial unit of analysis is a critical decision because it will affect both the accuracy and the statistical significance of the results. In general, opting for a smaller spatial unit will yield more accurate results, whereas larger units can strengthen the statistical relationships between environmental hazards and sociodemographic factors.[9] However, when using population data aggregated at higher levels like counties or metropolitan areas, it will be harder to detect if specific population groups are disproportionately affected by environmental hazards. This difficulty arises because the values get averaged out within these larger units, making it difficult to detect variations within them.

Data aggregation is an important concept to understand in GISc, whereby the data of interest about the study extent have been aggregated into larger units. Typically, this aggregation is based on established geographic boundaries, like census tracts for population data or health districts for health outcomes (Figure 8.4). In environmental impact assessments, data may be aggregated based on natural boundaries, reflecting the underlying geography of the observed phenomena, such as watersheds, flood plains, or wetlands, rather than arbitrary political or other artificial divisions. Many research projects work with multiple data sets with differing units of analysis or resolutions. Differing units of analysis are problematic when performing statistical tests on the data because the spatial units do not align. For instance, if population data are reported by census tract, but health-outcomes data are reported by health districts, the boundaries of these units will not match. Special analytical techniques are needed to harmonize these data sets for meaningful analysis.

ISSUES UNIQUE TO SPATIAL STATISTICS

There are many types of spatial analytical tools that can be used, and determining the most appropriate ones for a specific study must be considered early in the research design process. Generally, it is better to use more than one analytical method because more meaningful results will often be produced when examining data from multiple perspectives. Spatial statistics have certain pitfalls that do not occur with regular statistics, such as spatial autocorrelation, nonuniformity of space, and the modifiable areal unit problem (MAUP).

Spatial data do not follow the typical randomness assumed by traditional statistical methods because of a concept called *spatial autocorrelation.* This principle states that data from locations close to each other in space tend to be more similar than data in locations that are farther apart.[10] Since geographic data naturally exhibit this pattern, applying traditional statistical tests is challenging. In other words, traditional statistical methods may not work as effectively when dealing with spatial data due to spatial autocorrelation.

Spatial statistics introduce another challenge that is distinct from conventional statistics: *non uniformity of space.* This concept means that space is not uniform, and any distribution of points, such as disease cases or other phenomena, often simply reflects the underlying geography of population distribution rather than indicating relevant relationships or trends. In other words, there should not be an expectation to see the same number of disease cases in an unpopulated area like an industrial district as there would be in a densely settled residential area. Disease cases tend to cluster in areas where people are clustered. Therefore, when examining the distribution of cases, it is essential to take into account the underlying population distribution.

The *MAUP* refers to the fact that the way boundaries are drawn can significantly impact the results of the analysis, as shown in Figure 8.5. Depending on the unit of analysis chosen, results can vary widely. Therefore, selecting the correct unit of analysis becomes very important. MAUP is closely related to a more general statistical problem, known as the *ecological fallacy.* This fallacy assumes that a relationship between variables observed at one level of aggregation holds true for those variables at more detailed levels. An ecological fallacy involves making an inference about individuals based on aggregated data for a group. For instance, there may be a significant relationship between a poor health outcome and poverty

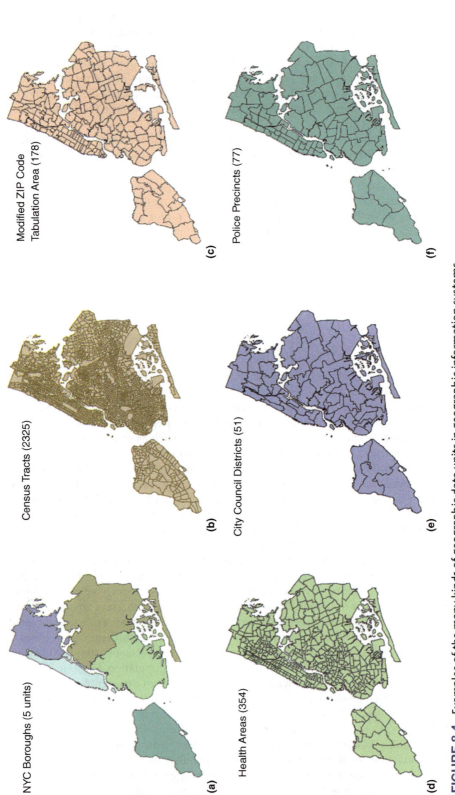

FIGURE 8.4. Examples of the many kinds of geographic data units in geographic information systems.

Data are often reported by different agencies and organizations for specific objectives. Each data set can be accessed based on the unit of aggregation in which it was compiled, which can include county, census tract, ZIP code, health district, and political jurisdictions, as well as natural boundaries with environmental impacts (e.g., watersheds, urban forests, flood zones, and air pollution plumes). The challenge arises when conducting spatial analysis using multiple units of aggregation because the data need to be "harmonized" to a standard unit of aggregation.

Data sources: Bytes of the Big Apple, NYC Dept. of City Planning, https://www.nyc.gov/site/planning/data-maps/open-data.page. *Credit*: Jocelyn Rajabelley (2023), Research Assistant, CUNY Institute for Health Equity; and the Urban GISc Lab, Lehman College, CUNY.

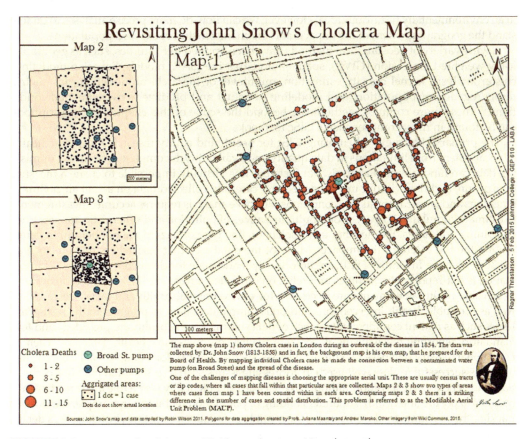

FIGURE 8.5. An example of the modifiable areal unit problem (MAUP).

In 1854, an area in London suffered an outbreak of cholera that killed hundreds of people. Map 1 contains data collected by Dr. Snow, which locates each death by the victim's residential location. By mapping cholera deaths, he connected the disease to a specific water pump. When we aggregate the same death location data using two different units of aggregation with differently drawn boundaries, we can explore the ramifications of the MAUP. Map 2 shows a diffuse pattern of deaths based on how the space has been divided into units, whereas Map 3 shows a clear cluster around the Broad Street Pump. Keep in mind that although Map 1 shows the actual location of the cholera deaths, Maps 2 and 3 are dot-density maps, with the dots representing the correct number of deaths for each unit, but the placement of the dots is random within each unit of aggregation.

Source: Ragnar Thrastarson (2015), MS-GISc graduate student at Lehman College, CUNY, as part of the course "Spatial Analysis of Urban Health."

at the county level. However, it would be incorrect to assume that this relationship holds true at the census-tract level or for an individual. In other words, just because some relationship is observed at one geographic level does not mean it applies to all individuals within that geographic area.

LIMITATIONS OF GEOGRAPHIC INFORMATION SCIENCE

Although many environmental health practitioners and advocates may not directly use GISc for their research, GISc has become a common tool in health policy and research. Having a solid grasp of fundamental geographic analysis concepts is essential to make informed decisions. It is also crucial to appreciate what is possible with GISc analyses, along with some of the typical limitations.

The most common types of analysis in environmental health and justice research and practice are estimates of exposure, risk, and vulnerability. Actual exposure is much less straightforward to measure and prove than simple proximity to a hazard. There are also many confounding variables and limitations in trying to show correlation between adverse health outcomes and living in an environmentally hazardous area. However, we can now do more precise analyses to understand the geographic extent of the impacts and the characteristics of exposed populations.

A wide variety of geostatistical methods have been applied to EJ studies, such as geographically weighted regression (GWR), spatial autoregressive (SAR) models, Bayesian modeling, cluster analysis, kernel density estimation, multilevel or hierarchical modeling, dasymetric disaggregation of population, and modeling of actual and predicted environmental conditions.[11] These more complex methods are beyond the scope of this chapter, but descriptions can be found in most comprehensive GISc textbooks.

The primary challenges when using GISc for health and equity research and public health advocacy stem from limitations in data quality and availability. Incomplete, inaccurate, or missing data can hinder spatial analysis. For instance, it is virtually impossible to create a measure of exposure and risk without more detailed and carefully collected data on actual air pollution emissions and ambient air quality conditions. Effective analysis requires accurate measurements to estimate cumulative impacts from multiple sources of pollution and synergistic impacts from combining pollutants. Studies that focus solely on one type of hazard are not helpful in determining the full extent of the impacts. Many of the databases that researchers rely on, such as the Toxic Release Inventory (TRI), are notoriously inadequate for detailed modeling. TRI information is self-reported by facilities and relies on estimated emissions, not measured quantities.

Reliable health assessments are necessary for environmental health and justice research, as well as for public health interventions and policy implementation to progress to the next level. Issues such as patient confidentiality, a lack of data sharing among healthcare providers, and few mandatory reporting mechanisms all conspire against comprehensive health databases. There is no national registry database for chronic diseases such as asthma, for example. GISc analysis has been less successful (or less well used) in addressing issues such as population mobility, occupation, and genetic predisposition, although these issues all potentially play a role in the relationship between exposure and health. An understanding of population mobility, for example, is crucial to tracking the environmental exposures of susceptible populations over time, but databases detailing population movement have not been widely developed. An index of residential neighborhood stability could be created for community-comparison purposes, but this index would be of limited value in monitoring spatial correspondence of specific hazards and health outcomes. Some of the same data deficiency problems exist for attempts to spatially link occupation and health hazards and to monitor specific populations by residence location.[12] Because many hazardous facilities are not tracked at a national, statewide, or municipal level, community-led inventories and monitoring of local conditions are essential in assessing environmental loads.

Since the use of GISc, mapping, and spatial analyses has become ubiquitous in environmental health research, policymaking, and public health interventions, it is crucial for people working in this field to have some familiarity with how GISc can contribute to furthering the goals of environmental health and justice. GISc has been democratized to the extent that nearly anyone can now make simple maps and think about their work in a spatial context. This brief overview of GISc provides the basis for understanding the current uses of the techniques and methods and aims to direct those interested in expanding on and applying the information in this section to their research, policymaking, or implementation efforts to be able to do so.

ENVIRONMENTAL HEALTH POLICIES WITH SPATIAL CONSIDERATIONS

Local ordinances are often created to reduce exposures to dangers or contaminants. For example, a municipality may limit the number of bars with liquor licenses to curb alcohol issues. Zoning laws regulate land use and typically categorize land for residential, industrial, commercial, agricultural, or recreational purposes. In environmental health, special attention is paid to facility *siting*, or where a facility is located, as well as to the *expansion* of facilities or increases in their air pollution emissions or water pollution discharges. As described in Chapter 4, "Environmental Health Policies and Protections: Successes and Failures," local ordinances and state, federal, and Tribal policies may all regulate the siting of hazardous facilities to ensure that people are not exposed to harmful levels of pollution. Without appropriate, enforced regulations, communities can become overburdened with pollution.

The mapping of environmental health and justice issues has been integrated into some important federal guidelines. The Emergency Planning and Community Right-to-Know Act (EPCRA) of 1986 requires that pollution data that meet certain designations under the TRI must be made publicly available, along with plans for managing and responding to environmental crises. Data from the EPCRA provided some of the first interactive U.S. government data portals and maps on environmental hazards. The TRI data has fueled foundational EJ research and is accessible through EPA tools like the TRI Explorer, the Risk Screening Environmental Indicators (RSEI), the National Air Toxics Assessment (NATA), and EJScreen.

In response to Executive Order 12898 in 1994, which required federal agencies to promote EJ, 18 states (California, Washington, Colorado, New Mexico, Minnesota, Missouri, Illinois, Indiana, Michigan, Pennsylvania, New York, Massachusetts, Connecticut, New Jersey, Delaware, Maryland, Virginia, and North Carolina) produced and shared information and maps of environmental hazards.[13] The specific format and dissemination depended on the use of the data for: (a) government permitting, (b) financial resource allocation, or (c) community engagement. Many government-run, state-level EJ mapping tools provide opportunities for communities to engage in the development of the tool, such as through workshops, partnerships, and EJ advisory councils.[13]

In the absence of enforceable regulations, the U.S. EPA has issued documents that offer guidance on some issues, like school-siting guidelines.[14] The school-siting guidelines encourage school districts to account for exposure to hazardous substances, transportation modes, energy efficiency, and potential emergency shelter uses when siting a new school or determining the closure of existing schools.[14]

Besides federal and state regulations, some municipalities have taken steps to address and prevent disproportionate environmental burdens and to promote environmental health and justice. For example, in 1991, New York City introduced "The Criteria for the Locations of City Facilities (The Fair Share Criteria)," to ensure that neighborhoods, especially those already having a high concentration of environmentally burdensome facilities and land uses, did not continue to be the default host of such facilities when future needs arose, and the city would make siting decisions. The routine practice of saturating specific communities with noxious land uses, resulting in increased exposure, risk, and adverse health impacts to the people in those areas, was not factored into the siting decision-making process before these criteria were issued. The criteria are not perfect, as they are mainly advisory, but they do allow for a process of public involvement and engagement and require a higher level of justification by the city for siting decisions. Importantly, they have brought siting decisions of public facilities into the public eye with increased transparency and options for mitigation.

MAPPING PATTERNS OF ENVIRONMENTAL HEALTH INEQUITIES

HISTORY

The EJ movement established itself after seminal EJ studies were published on the spatial distribution of pollution. In 1983, the U.S. GAO completed a review of four hazardous waste landfills in EPA Region 4 in the Southeastern United States and found that three were located in communities that were majority Black and all had at least one-fourth of the population living below the poverty level.[4] A few years later, in 1987, the UCC released its first *Toxic Wastes and Race in the United States* report, which examined the sociodemographics near treatment, storage, and disposal facilities (TSDFs).[5] The UCC's finding that race was the strongest predictor of whether a community was a "host" to a TSDF, not poverty, galvanized the movement. Following the UCC report, Dr. Robert D. Bullard published *Dumping in Dixie: Race, Class, and Environmental Quality* examining the connections between civil rights, social justice, and environmental contamination in five predominantly Black southern communities. The UCC report and Dr. Bullard's work laid the foundation for the larger EJ movement and the fourth wave of the environmental movement.

After the movement was established, research continued to examine the relationship between hazardous siting patterns and low-wealth and Black, Indigenous, and People of Color (BIPOC) communities to better understand "who came first" (the hazardous facility or the people living there).[15] Two decades after their groundbreaking first analysis, the UCC released the *Toxic Wastes and Race at Twenty: 1987–2007* report, which observed more pronounced siting disparities by race.[16] Questions of whether the disparities were driven by disproportionate siting or move-in by people of color were dispelled, as researchers confirmed that disproportionate siting and siting in areas with recent demographic changes were to blame, not people of color moving to areas with TSDFs.[17,18] While some studies have observed the greatest relationship by race and other studies by income, the inextricable links between the two factors make it difficult to parse out.

Policies and practices promoting racial segregation, such as racially restrictive zoning, redlining, and racially restrictive covenants, were the precursors to hazardous siting disparities. Despite the Civil Rights Act of 1866, which granted "full and equal benefit of all laws and proceedings for security of person and property" to all people born in the United States, except American Indians (14 Stat. 27–30),[19] some municipalities enacted *racially restrictive zoning* policies to prohibit property ownership by people of color. These policies and practices began in the late 1800s but ramped up as the Great Migration brought more people of color to northern communities.[20] The first such ordinance, the Bingham Ordinance of 1890 in San Francisco, only permitted Chinese residents to live and work in one designated area of the city. Similar ordinances that designated neighborhood blocks for "White" and "Black" or other racial and ethnic groups were passed in other cities and towns, such as the Baltimore Ordinance of 1910 that prohibited Black Americans from moving into a neighborhood block with a majority of White residents, and vice versa. Real estate boards and neighborhood associations also utilized *racially restrictive covenants*, a legal contract, which required a property to be sold to only specific racial groups. In 1933, the Home Owners' Loan Corporation (HOLC) took racist zoning a step further by developing and releasing "residential security maps" for over 200 cities across the United States. These maps formed the basis of *redlining*, wherein areas designated as "hazardous" for mortgages were the least likely to receive financial backing and reinvestment. Many of the communities that were redlined decades ago are still segregated today in alignment with the HOLC patterns.[21] The legacy of redlining is also associated with a number of social determinants of health, including elevated heat risks,[22] reduced tree cover and green space,[23,24] and air pollution.[25]

Despite the fact that these practices and policies have been banned, residential segregation has persisted in the United States. This is due in part to the ineffective enforcement of laws, inadequate penalties for infractions, and the difficulties of changing long-entrenched circumstances and behaviors. These siting disparities put marginalized communities at risk of experiencing economic disinvestment, disproportionate pollution exposure burdens, and poor health outcomes.

IMPACTS OF DISPARATE SITING AND EXPOSURES

Researchers have utilized GISc software to reveal spatial pollution patterns to better understand its implications on health outcomes and disparities. Living near hazardous sites increases the risk of experiencing asthma, respiratory diseases, cardiovascular disease, end-stage renal disease, childhood cancers, and certain adverse reproductive outcomes.[6] Approximately 24 million people in the United States live within a 1-mile radius of a *Superfund site*, or sites with significant contamination of hazardous materials designated under the Comprehensive Environmental Response, Compensation, and Liability Act.[26] Comprising 7% of the U.S. population, these residents are disproportionately linguistically isolated, have low-education levels, live below the poverty level, and are communities of color.[26] People living near Superfund sites and/or mining areas are at a greater risk of exposure to environmental hazards, particularly metals such as manganese, copper, zinc, cadmium, arsenic, and lead.[27–29] Exposure to lead, cadmium, chromium, copper, manganese, and phthalates is associated with preterm birth and other outcomes.[30,31] A noteworthy study by Tessum et al. went beyond traditional mapping techniques to examine mortality from particulate matter 2.5 ($PM_{2.5}$) emission sources and exposures by race and ethnicity, while adjusting for consumption factors.[32] The researchers utilized maps and data visualizations to showcase $PM_{2.5}$-attributable premature deaths and pollution inequity. PM$_{2.5}$ burdens were 63% higher for Hispanic or Latino Americans, 56% higher for Black Americans, and 17% lower for non-Hispanic White Americans given their consumption.[32] This use of visualizations paired with maps has proliferated in recent years to enhance the storytelling of environmental health and justice issues.

Some low-wealth communities have experienced *gentrification*, a process in which higher wealth residents displace lower wealth residents as they are priced out of a neighborhood undergoing new business development and improved housing. Gentrification also occurs in relation to environmental amenities such as new green spaces, parks, and clean-up of contaminated sites. One phenomenon that is increasingly observed as the world grapples with the "symptoms" of climate change is *climate gentrification*, whereby low-wealth people and communities of color are displaced from neighborhoods with parks, green infrastructure, or minimal flood risks.[33] This displacement has been documented in the Little Haiti neighborhood of Miami, Florida, where property values are rising because it sits at twice the elevation of Miami Beach.[34] Similar green gentrification occurs in areas that experience urban "renewal" through additional greenways or parks,[35] which attracts wealthier residents and triggers rental-cost increases that are out of reach for many existing residents. Displaced residents may be forced to relocate to environmentally hazardous or precarious areas, thus putting their health at risk. Mapping initiatives have helped to bring this information to the public. The *Toxic Tides* program, for example, maps areas in California that are at risk from hazardous facility contamination after flooding due to rising sea levels (Figure 8.6).[36]

More recently, researchers have explored not just the physical health impacts of environmental hazards, but also the psychological impact and stigma of living near contamination or a hazardous facility. The stigma of living near contaminated sites causes people to experience embarrassment or fear of rejection.[37] Chronic environmental contamination exposure has been associated with moderate increases in symptoms of anxiety, stress, depression, and posttraumatic stress disorder.[38,39] Communities whose concerns are delegitimized or

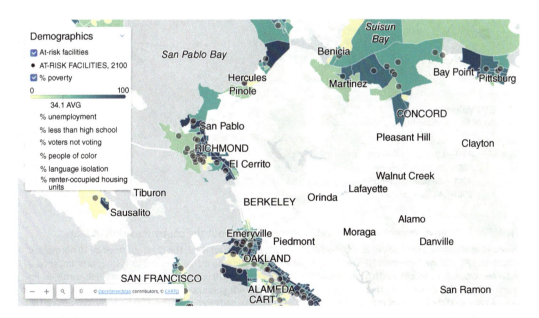

FIGURE 8.6. Flood risks near hazardous facilities and social vulnerability in the Bay Area of California.
The Toxic Tides Project showcases flood risks at hazardous facilities within California through interactive maps of high greenhouse gas emission scenarios for 2050 and 2100. This map shows the Census block groups with at least one at-risk facility within 1 km by the year 2100 by poverty prevalence. Data by Census block groups are taken from the 2017 American Community Survey 5-year estimates and the California Statewide Database, with no change in population growth by 2100. The interactive tool allows for selecting other demographic factors, such as the percentage of eligible voters who do not vote, language isolation, and people of color.

Source: Flood risk & demographics: demographics of census block groups with at least one at-risk facility within 1 km by the year 2100. Toxic Tides. 2022. https://sites.google.com/berkeley.edu/toxictides/flood-risk-demographics

who perceive severe physical health impacts from the environmental contamination are at a greater likelihood of experiencing adverse psychological effects.[38,40]

VULNERABILITY INDICES

Highly representative maps and EJ research can encompass and visualize numerous factors that affect a person's health and well-being. **Vulnerability indices** provide this opportunity by analyzing more than one sociodemographic factor at a time. *Social vulnerability* is defined as the potential negative impacts from external social, economic, and natural stressors on communities.[41] *Social vulnerability indices* (SVIs) therefore, categorize neighborhoods or census tracks based on U.S. Census data about poverty, housing crowding, transportation access, language, race, ethnicity, and education. The CDC's Agency for Toxic Substances and Disease Registry (ATSDR) SVI is used to allocate resources and plan for emergency responses to disasters and hazardous spills.[41] The U.S. EPA's EJScreen similarly combines environmental pollution and socioeconomic factors with vulnerability into one score that ranks vulnerability to environmental pollution.[42] The CDC's ATSDR released the *Environmental Justice Index* (EJI) in 2022, which created an overall EJ score that takes into account social vulnerability, environmental pollution burden, and health vulnerability (Figure 8.7).[43] The EJI is the first EJ index to factor in population-level health

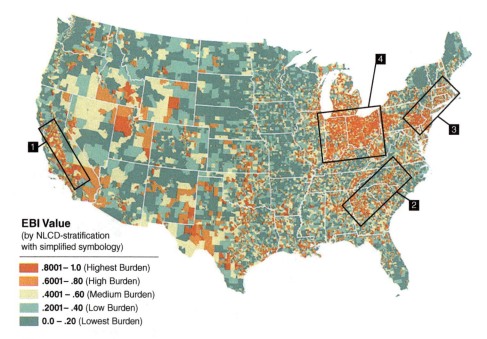

FIGURE 8.7. Environmental burden index ratings throughout the contiguous United States.

Owusu et al. developed methods to assess the EBI at the U.S. census-tract level. The EBI is informed by 10 normalized indicators: $PM_{2.5}$, ozone, Superfund NPL sites, TRI facilities, recreational parks, railways, highways, airports, impaired water sources, and TSD facilities. This map shows the NLCD-stratified EBI scores. Higher EBI scores indicate higher environmental burdens relative to other peer census-tract groups. The highest burden tracts are located in (1) California's Central Valley; (2) the Piedmont regions of Georgia, South Carolina, and North Carolina; (3) the areas surrounding the Northeast Megalopolis (from Philadelphia to Boston); and (4) the easternmost portion of the Midwest between the Ohio River Valley and the Great Lakes, primarily in Indiana, Ohio, and Michigan. This map communicates EBI effectively through a simplified legend and dichromatic color selections. Dichromatic colors (i.e., two distinct color families) help communicate differences more effectively than monochromatic colors.

EBI, environmental burden index; EJI, Environmental Justice Index; NLCD, National Land Cover Database; NPL, National Priority List; PM, particulate matter; TRI, Toxic Release Inventory; TSD, treatment, storage, and disposal.

Source: Owusu C, Flanagan B, Lavery AM, et al. Developing a granular scale environmental burden index (EBI) for diverse land cover types across the contiguous United States. *Sci Total Environ.* 2022;838. doi:10.1016/j.scitotenv.2022.155908.

conditions, including asthma, mental health, diabetes, cancer, and high blood pressure. In addition to factoring in health vulnerability, the EJI factors in lack of health insurance, lack of broadband internet access, housing type (e.g., mobile home), recreational parks, and walkability.[44]

Many of these indices or scores attempt to combine multiple vulnerabilities or risks to showcase cumulative risk or vulnerability (that is, risks to the multitude of hazards people are exposed to in their daily lives). *Cumulative risk assessments* account for multiple exposures in an additive matter. However, the cumulative risk does not account for synergistic interactions of certain hazards or social conditions, which can amplify outcomes beyond a simple additive approach. For example, the risk for lung cancer is 10 times higher if you are exposed to high levels of radon in your home *and* you smoke cigarettes.[45] Currently, there are a wide range of methodologies for cumulative assessments of environmental and social risks, as explored in Chapter 6.

CASE STUDY 8.2: Occupational and Residential Environmental Justice

The study "Occupational Groups and Environmental Justice: A Case Study in the Bronx, New York City,"[12] used spatial analysis to examine the exposure of people in vulnerable occupational groups to two environmental pollutants, particulate matter 2.5 ($PM_{2.5}$) and black carbon, both implicated in serious respiratory and cardiovascular diseases. This ecological study questioned whether people in occupational groups with potentially higher-than-average exposures to pollutants in the workplace could be overexposed to environmental pollutants based on their residential locations in the Bronx. Correlations revealed that areas with high environmental exposures also had high proportions of people working in service industries and manufacturing and high proportions of socioeconomically susceptible populations. This combination of vulnerabilities may be cumulative, suggesting that residents could have both high occupational and residential exposures, in addition to sociodemographic-related inequity.

Environmental exposures were developed and mapped from 300-meter resolution land-use regression model outputs. *Land-use regression* is a statistical model that estimates ambient pollutant concentrations as a function of land use (e.g., vehicle traffic, building emissions, population density). The data were obtained from the city's 60-to-100 air-quality monitors—the exact number of monitors with usable data varied by year. The data were used to estimate pollutant concentrations around the city where no measurements were available (areas not close to one of the air quality monitors).

These maps depict some of the typical variables used in environmental justice (EJ) studies, such as poverty and race, along with less typical variables like occupation, all juxtaposed against concentrations of black carbon and $PM_{2.5}$ (Figure 8.8). Including variables related to occupation is more unusual in EJ studies because exposures are typically considered to be based on residential locations (i.e., nighttime, rather than workplace or daytime, exposures). This study is important because it includes both residential and workplace exposures, capturing more of a comprehensive picture of total exposure.

Health outcomes are also influenced by other social and structural factors often not captured in vulnerability indices, such as health insurance coverage, proximity to hospitals or healthcare centers, bias in treatment recommendations, and immigration status. Structural factors are the drivers of social vulnerabilities, so their absence in these indices can make it easy to overlook them in efforts to address the environmental health or justice issue. *Structural vulnerabilities* occur through a population's interactions with socioeconomic, political, cultural, and normative hierarchies (e.g., heteronormativity, structural racism), which can overlap and reinforce power systems.[46] These additional vulnerabilities can result in a continuation of environmental health and justice issues and health disparities. It is in many ways a perpetration and perpetuation of environmental injustices.

(continued)

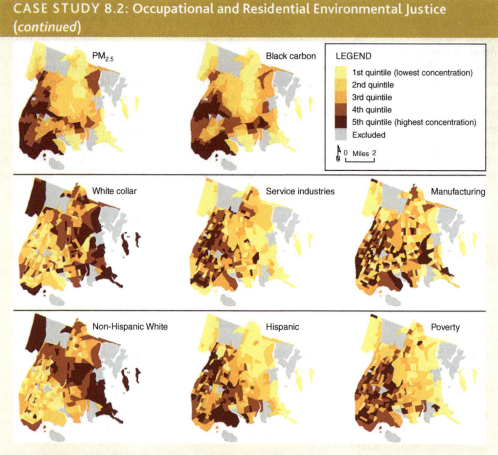

FIGURE 8.8. Case study of occupational environmental justice.

Data sources: American Community Survey 2011–2015 ACS 5-Year Estimates via the National Historic Geographic Information System (5), New York City Community Air Survey 2011–2015 (10).

PM, particulate matter.

Source: Maroko AR, Pavilonis BT. Occupational groups and environmental justice: a case study in the Bronx, New York. *Prev Chronic Dis.* 2018;15:180344. doi:10.5888/pcd15.180344.

REFLECTION QUESTIONS

1. Many mapping studies only account for home (nighttime) exposures. How does this limitation affect our understanding of people's true exposures?

WORKING TOWARD ENVIRONMENTAL HEALTH AND JUSTICE

MAPS AS SIMPLE DATA VISUALIZATIONS

Spatial representations afford unique opportunities to visualize and communicate data. Many people are familiar with *choropleth maps*, which use colors or shading to represent different data. These maps are frequently used in elections to designate winning candidates and therefore can quickly and easily communicate information. Maps can be particularly useful for conveying multiple sets of data and identifying hot spots of environmental burdens. Community groups can use these resources for advocacy, education, and accountability.

PUBLIC AND COMMUNITY-DRIVEN MAPPING

Government agencies at all levels, researchers, private companies, and community-led organizations all utilize and disseminate information through mapping projects. National, state, and local governments implement interactive mapping resources and downloadable data that can be utilized by planners, researchers, and the public (e.g., EJScreen and ECHO, Michigan's MiEJScreen). State and local environmental-quality government agencies (e.g., county, large cities) play an important role here, as they may have greater interfaces with residents and a more granular understanding of each situation. Of the 18 state-level EJ mapping tools available in the United States in 2021, 3 were operated by nongovernmental organizations in Colorado, Illinois, and Indiana.[13]

> **JUSTICE40 INITIATIVE**
>
> Under President Biden, the Justice40 Initiative pledged 40% of federal infrastructure benefits to disadvantaged communities. To identify these communities, the White House began developing the Climate and Economic Justice Screening Tool (CEJST) in 2021. The spatial mapping tool is intended for federal agencies to identify priority communities for investment—the first screening tool designed for these purposes at the federal level. The tool has faced some controversy, however, for not explicitly considering race, despite long-standing patterns of environmental racism in the United States. Refinement continues as the advocates, scientists, and policy makers decide which data to include and which data to leave out, as well as how to consider cumulative impacts.

Common Mapping Tools

In recent years, organizations, government agencies, and researchers have used "StoryMaps" to tell digital stories of environmental injustice through a mixture of interactive maps, photos, and text. In 2021, the U.S. EPA and the Louisiana Department of Environmental Quality used a StoryMap to share federal and state responses to Hurricane Ida.[47] This map, and others like it, allow the public to see event-specific data on air monitoring and chemical releases from industrial facilities.[47,48] This combination of pictures, maps, historical context, health, environment, social, and economic concerns can provide accessible information on issues that are not easily communicated in a single fact sheet or map. One example here demonstrates the impact of the HOLC's 1933 "residential security maps" on current tree cover and land surface temperatures in the Greater Boston area, by explaining the historical context of this disparity (Figure 8.9).[49]

Grassroots, community-based organizations have applied mapping to visualize pollution hot spots, inform communities of contamination risks, and galvanize action to hold polluters accountable. *Public participation GIS* (PPGIS), or **participatory GIS (PGIS),** provides opportunities to incorporate local knowledge, offer contextual information to spatial data, and allows for users to interact with or use data for grassroots, community-led initiatives to leverage requests for changes.[50] PPGIS grew out of critiques that GIS practitioners failed to ground their work in social and political contexts. PPGIS, therefore, is used to enhance public involvement in policymaking and planning and enrich the work of grassroots and nongovernmental organizations.[50] However, PPGIS is not inherently able to affect decision-making. PPGIS that only adds spatial data to an undemocratic process cannot effectively incorporate public opinion into the decision-making process.[51]

Volunteered geographic information (VGI) has grown out of the proliferation of "citizen science" and web technology platforms (e.g., geotagging, sharing Google maps), not academia or government decision-making, as a GIS approach for gathering local residents' spatial knowledge.[52] VGI provides opportunities for the general public to create, collect, analyze, and share spatial data, often referred to as "crowdsourcing" data. The Louisiana Bucket Brigade, for example, allows community members to report and crowdsource pollution data through their iWitness Pollution map.[53] Private companies have also provided similar opportunities, wherein consumers can

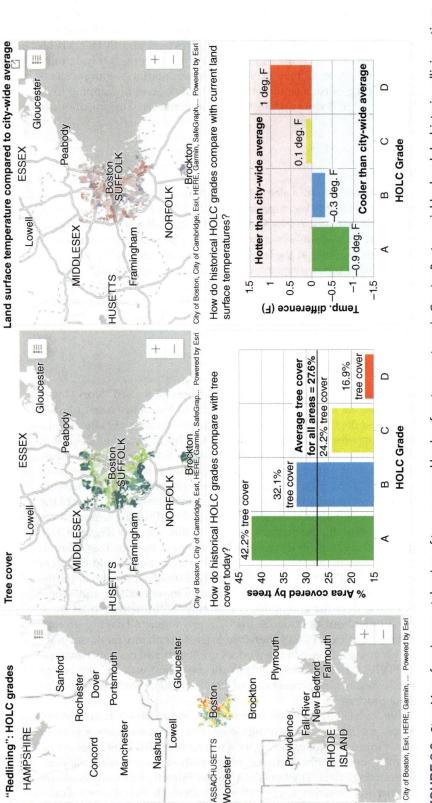

FIGURE 8.9. StoryMap of environmental racism of tree cover and land surface temperatures in Greater Boston neighborhoods by historic redlining ratings.

The Harvard Chan-NIEHS Center for Environmental Health published a StoryMap series on Environmental Racism in Greater Boston, with Part 2 focused on environmental racism at the neighborhood level. The StoryMap combines redlining HOLC maps of the Boston area with more recent data about tree coverage and land surface temperatures. Each map and graph are interactive for the user. Their StoryMap shows how areas rated well by the HOLC (i.e., not redlined or given an "A" grade) have more tree coverage and are, on average, 0.9 degrees cooler than the citywide average temperature. Areas rated with a "D" grade by the HOLC have less tree cover and are, on average, 1 degree warmer than the citywide average temperature. Other maps showcase race and ethnicity in these same areas, noting that areas with low HOLC grades have larger numbers of people of color and low-income people. These temperature differences increase the risk of death for susceptible populations, especially during heat waves.

HOLC, Home Owners' Loan Corporation; NIEHS, National Institute of Environmental Health Science.

Source: HOLC map—University of Richmond; Tree cover & land surface temperature—National Land Cover Database; *see also* Hoffman JS, Shandas V, Pendleton N. The effects of historical housing policies on resident exposure to intra-urban heat: a study of 108 US urban areas. *Climate.* 2020;8:12. doi:10.3390/cli8010012. Created as part of the Environmental Racism in Greater Boston Story-Map; Lisa Frueh, Marissa Chan, Jahred Liddie, Tamarra James-Todd, Gary Adamkiewicz. https://www.hsph.harvard.edu/niehs/environmental-racism-project

participate in crowdsourced data, such as air-quality data maps with Purple Air, Inc.[54] Researchers also collaborate with community-based organizations to develop and disseminate mapping tools for risks that have been understudied or are not captured in government tools.

> ### CASE STUDY 8.3: Participatory Environmental Justice Radar in Charleston, South Carolina
>
> After environmental health and justice concerns were raised in the Charleston area of South Carolina, about the proposed expansion of the Port of Charleston, a partnership was formed between impacted residents at the Low Country Alliance for Model Communities, the South Carolina Department of Health and Environmental Control, and university academics at the Community Engagement, Environmental Justice, and Health Center of the University of Maryland-College Park School of Public Health; and the University of South Carolina's Institute for Partnerships to Eliminate Health Disparities.[55,56] This collaborative group, known as the Charleston Area Pollution Prevention Partnership (CAPs), led a conference to discuss collaboration and mitigation strategies through the Charleston Community Research to Action Board. CAPs also developed a tool for residents, Environmental Justice Radar (EJ Radar), which is a public participation geographic information systems (PPGIS) project and website that allows South Carolina residents to discover and share information about their experiences of environmental and social hazards and health outcomes. The project aimed to increase the capability of and empower residents to be more engaged in environmental decision-making through mapping environmental health data.
>
> EJ Radar allows users to display specific pollution sources and sociodemographic information; interact with the data by visualizing facility density within a designated buffer; and include point, line, and area pollution data with photos via the website. The CAPs evaluated the first version of EJ Radar and recommended: (a) including other disamenities within the map, such as liquor stores and fast-food restaurants; (b) the development and dissemination of a training manual and an online training video; (c) clear pollution categories and color coding; and (d) the ability to include queries and spatial statistics with the data. Despite these limitations in the first iteration, residents appreciated the ability to add qualitative data, which is uncommon for most government-run EJ or environmental health spatial visualization tools. The EJ Radar website is, unfortunately, no longer active. Data for web mapping projects must be hosted somewhere and need to be updated periodically, so sustainability plans for financial and technological resources are required to maintain and continue these types of projects.
>
> As technology and social media platforms change how we interact with each other and share information, platforms and software have started to adapt to the public's uses and demands. Esri's ArcGIS has been the dominant software for mapping in recent decades, but open-sourced, free platforms like QGIS have gained popularity due to their economic accessibility. Although ArcGIS and QGIS have more extensive user expertise requirements, tools like Google Maps can be used by the public much more easily to create and share maps. Tools like StoryMapping have proliferated to tell stories in addition to what can be conveyed in a map and its layers. Despite the advantages and disadvantages of these platforms, their popularity has helped to create easier communication of complex information.
>
> #### REFLECTION QUESTIONS
> 1. What are challenges you may face with participatory geographic information systems (PGIS) initiatives?
> 2. How should "sustainability" be accounted for when planning PGIS programs, such as EJ Radar?

ETHICAL CONSIDERATIONS OF MAPPING

Maps depicting a "snapshot" of environmental and human factors should be developed, used, and interpreted with caution. No one set of data or map layer can comprehensively or cumulatively represent social and economic vulnerability or pollution burdens. Without longitudinal data, maps of specific time points may misrepresent a person or population's risk. While a map may indicate an area as low vulnerability, it may rely on inadequate measures. For instance,

Middle Eastern Americans have been categorized as "White" in many data sets, such as the U.S. Census, but in the United States they are often marginalized. Additionally, we often have insufficient measures of local pollution burdens, which can minimize or inflate the actual risk.

Maps can also perpetuate and exacerbate negative stereotypes and stigmatize those who the spatial depiction represents. Communities may be characterized in ways that do not align with their perception of the community. These characterizations may contribute to harmful stigmas of the area and residents. Just as redlining maps influenced mortgaging and disinvestment practices, developers, realtors, insurance companies, and individuals may inadvertently or intentionally use these maps to further disinvestment.[13] Careful consideration should be used when selecting colors for maps, so that map colors do not perpetuate racial biases. Maps of pollution burden and/or vulnerability may also lack information on power and historical context for contemporary problems.

Given the technological and access barriers inherent in using GISc and GIS for EJ, it is important to create "honest" and culturally appropriate maps. Use a thoughtful and critical approach when examining, using, or designing maps. Maps can tell stories in compelling ways, so proficiency with maps and GISc will help advocate for environmental health and justice.

MAIN TAKEAWAYS

In this chapter, we learned that:

- GISc allows for visualizations of the spatial relationships between features in the environment and people.
- GISc and maps are frequently used in public health and environmental health and justice research projects, including in foundational EJ research.
- Familiarity with the spatial research process is helpful for all environmental health and justice advocates, scholars and practitioners, and even for non-GISc professionals. There are many ways to display spatial data, and understanding the different methods can help you understand a map's limitations and interpret its results.
- Although there are no national policies guiding mapping or the spatial representation of environmental health and justice data, some policies and guidelines have helped to make more spatial data publicly available. Despite this availability, spatial health and equity research is limited by data availability.
- The EJI rates census tracts based on their social vulnerability, environmental pollution burden, and health vulnerabilities. The EJI and other similar indices have recently been developed to assess cumulative impacts. Although these indices are useful for advocacy and policymaking, they may miss structural vulnerabilities.
- Maps are widely used by government agencies, researchers, private companies, and grassroots organizations to share information and promote collaborations.
- Maps need to be culturally appropriate. Mapmakers must consider the ethical implications of the maps they create and ensure that they include adequate context to reduce stigmatization and stereotypes.

SUMMARY

Spatial analyses and GISc are useful for visualizing the spatial relationship between environmental conditions and people. They help us to estimate risks and communicate about environmental exposures and impacts, as well as gaps in resources. Understanding the basic concepts of geographic analysis provides a foundation for understanding the limits and possibilities of maps and GISc. As part of the history of the EJ movement and GIS, maps and spatial analyses are used by many different groups to organize, share information, and influence policies. It is therefore important that maps be more accessible, representative, and ethical to further EJ. Finally, if you are doing this work, also do the work to understand the past and present of the land you are mapping.

ENVIRONMENTAL HEALTH IN PRACTICE

Common mapping tools and resources are summarized in Table 8.1.

TABLE 8.1. COMMON MAPPING TOOLS AND RESOURCES

	RESOURCE NAME	DESCRIPTION
Mapping software and programs	Esri ArcGIS	Common mapping software; license required
	QGIS	Mapping software; open source
	Google Maps	Common mapping web tool; account required
Key national governmental mapping tools	*Toxic Release Inventory (TRI) Explorer* (EPA)	Data portal on TRI facilities' chemical releases, transfers, and managed waste, including facility, waste transfer, and waste quantity reports
	Enforcement and Compliance History Online (ECHO) (EPA)	Data and maps on facilities' compliance with environmental regulations within the most recent three years
	Risk-Screening Environmental Indicators (RSEI) Model (EPA)	Map of modeled, scored data on toxic releases from TRI facilities
	National Air Toxics Assessment (NATA) (EPA)	Interactive mapping tool that showcases cancer risks from exposure to air pollution
	AirToxScreen (EPA)	Mapping tool that combines ambient air emissions and cancer risks
	Environmental Justice Index (CDC ATSDR)	Interactive mapping tool of census-tract-level risks based on environmental, social, and health factors
	EJScreen (EPA)	Interactive mapping and screening tool of environmental justice vulnerability scores
	Smart Location Mapping (EPA)	Suite of interactive maps and data on the built environment, including the *Smart Location Database* of location efficiency indicators; the *Access to Jobs and Workers via Transit*, which assesses accessibility to destinations by public transit; and the *National Walkability Index* of walk scores by Census block groups
	Heat.gov (National Integrated Heat Health Information System)	Interactive data portal on extreme heat risks, vulnerabilities, and heat forecasts
	U.S. Disaster and Risk Mapping (NOAA)	Interactive mapping and data tools to visualize and map the frequency, cost, and vulnerability to billion-dollar weather and climate events

(continued)

	RESOURCE NAME	DESCRIPTION
Key national governmental mapping tools (*cont.*)	*Climate and Economic Justice Screening Tool* (U.S. Office of the President)	Interactive map and screening tool of climate-related burdens and vulnerabilities
	Food Access Research Atlas (USDA)	Interactive map of food indicators by census tracts, including data about supermarket accessibility and food access
	National Priority List (NPL) Sites (EPA)	NPL Superfund sites across the United States and by state
Nongovernmental mapping tools	*EJ Atlas: A Global Atlas of Environmental Justice*	Summarizes cases of environmental injustice around the world and allows users to explore data based on characteristics of the issue, the issue's impacts, and resistance efforts
	Walk Score	Promotes walkable neighborhoods by creating a walkability score by address, neighborhood, or city
U.S. Census Bureau demographic data	*TIGER (topologically integrated geographic encoding and referencing) geodatabases*	Census data, including sociodemographic and housing data
	American Community Survey	Annual Census survey data, including sociodemographic and housing data

CDC ATSDR, Centers for Disease Control and Prevention Agency for Toxic Substances and Disease Registry; EPA, U.S. Environmental Protection Agency; NOAA, National Oceanic and Atmospheric Administration; USDA, United States Department of Agriculture.

ACKNOWLEDGMENTS

Special thanks to Jocelyn Rajabelley (research assistant at the CUNY Institute for Health Equity and the Urban GISc Lab, Lehman College, CUNY) and Ragnar Thrastarson (MS-GISc graduate student at Lehman College, CUNY, as part of the course "Spatial Analysis of Urban Health") for their development of included maps.

END-OF-CHAPTER RESOURCES

DISCUSSION QUESTIONS

1. What are a few research questions you might pursue about your own community using GIS? What types of data would you need to understand the issues that concern you (e.g., health data, U.S. Census data, environmental exposure data)? Think about the different ways you can use GIS, such as to identify hot spots, distances to hazards or amenities, and so forth.
2. In GISc, sometimes we reduce communities to a single demographic variable. Throughout this textbook, we discuss the concept of intersectionality. How can we apply the concept of intersectionality when using GISc?

LEARNING ACTIVITIES

THE TIME IS NOW

Select a mapping tool from the examples provided in Table 8.1 and explore the data available through the map. Are there any data gaps? Can users provide input about qualitative data? Are some of the data hard to understand or interpret? If you see any gaps or issues, contact the map developers or program leads to advocate for more holistic approaches to sharing and communicating about environmental health and justice.

If your state does not have an existing mapping tool, contact your environmental quality and/or health department to encourage them to produce and share environmental health and justice measures through interactive maps.

IN REAL LIFE

There are many GIS environmental health and justice data sources at the national, state, local, Tribal, or other regional levels. The following are commonly used tools for mapping environmental hazards and vulnerability indices, as well as data sources for conducting GISc. These tools are increasingly available and accessible to the public and researchers.

Explore the pollution risks and environmental vulnerabilities near your home or hometown. Look for patterns and areas with the greatest risks and/or vulnerabilities. Note that some mapping tools may not include vulnerability data, so it may help to look at a few different mapping tools. The following are suggestions for the different types of maps:

1. **EJ, EJScreen, or CEJST:** Identifies areas of high risk in your community or region and note any patterns.
2. **NATA or AirToxScreen:** Explores areas with high air pollution burdens and related health and cancer risks.
3. **EJAtlas or National Priority List (NPL):** Explores the different characteristics of EJ issues and NPL sites.
4. **TRI:** Identifies the type of polluting industry, the chemicals emitted (on site), and associated health concerns.
5. **ECHO:** Examines the compliance history for major environmental statutes (e.g., the Clean Air Act, the Resource Conservation and Recovery Act, the Clean Water Act) for qualifying facilities near your home.
6. **Smart Location Mapping or Walk Score:** Examines areas with low walkability and those lacking access to destinations via public transit.
7. **Heat.gov, Disaster and Risk Mapping, or CEJST:** Explores states with the highest heat or disaster burdens (by cost and number of incidents), and type of disaster. Which areas are most vulnerable to climate and weather hazards?
8. **Food Access Research Atlas:** Identifies low-income areas with low access to affordable food through supermarkets.

 A robust set of instructor resources designed to supplement this text is located at http://connect.springerpub.com/content/book/978-0-8261-8353-8. Qualifying instructors may request access by emailing textbook@springerpub.com.

REFERENCES

1. Koch T. *Cartography of Disease: Maps, Mapping, and Medicine.* 2nd ed. Environmental Systems Research Institute (ESRI) Press; 2017.
2. Malgaigne JF. Recherche sur la fréquence des hernies, selon les sexes, les âges, et relativement à la population. *Ann Hygiène Publique Médecine Légale.* 1840;24:5–54.

3. Why it matters. Native Land Digital. Accessed May 23, 2024. https://native-land.ca/about/why-it-matters/
4. US GAO. Siting of hazardous waste landfills and their correlation with racial and economic status of surrounding communities. June 1, 1983. https://www.gao.gov/products/rced-83-168
5. Chavis BF Jr, Lee C. *Toxic Wastes and Race in the United States: A National Report on the Racial and Socio-Economic Characteristics of Communities with Hazardous Waste Sites.* United Church of Christ Commission for Racial Justice; 1987. https://www.ucc.org/wp-content/uploads/2020/12/ToxicWastesRace.pdf
6. Brender JD, Maantay JA, Chakraborty J. Residential proximity to environmental hazards and adverse health outcomes. *Am J Public Health.* 2011;101(suppl 1):S37–S52. doi:10.2105/AJPH.2011.300183
7. Maantay JA. Environmental justice and fairness. In: *Routledge Companion to Environmental Planning.* Routledge; 2019.
8. Maantay JA, Winner A, Maroko AR. Geospatial analysis of the urban health environment. In: Faruque F, ed. *Geospatial Technology for Human Well-Being and Health.* Springer-Verlag; 2022:151–183.
9. Maantay J. Asthma and air pollution in the Bronx: methodological and data considerations in using GIS for environmental justice and health research. *Health Place.* 2007;13(1):32–56. doi:10.1016/j.healthplace.2005.09.009
10. Tobler WR. Cellular geography. In: Gale S, Olsson G, eds. *Philosophyin Geography.* Reidel Publishing Company; 1979:379–386.
11. Chakraborty J, Maantay JA, Brender JD. Disproportionate proximity to environmental health hazards: methods, models, and measurement. *Am J Public Health.* 2011;101(suppl 1):S27–S36. doi:10.2105/AJPH.2010.300109
12. Maroko AR, Pavilonis BT. Occupational groups and environmental justice: a case study in the Bronx, New York. *Prev Chronic Dis.* 2018;15:180344. doi:10.5888/pcd15.180344
13. Konisky D, Gonzalez D, Leatherman K. *Mapping for Environmental Justice: An Analysis of State Level Tools.* Indiana University Environmental Resilience Institute; 2021. https://eri.iu.edu/research/projects/environmental-justice-mapping-tools.html
14. U.S. Environmental Protection Agency. School siting guidelines. 2015. https://www.epa.gov/sites/default/files/2015-06/documents/school_siting_guidelines-2.pdf
15. Maantay J. Mapping environmental injustices: pitfalls and potential of geographic information systems in assessing environmental health and equity. *Environ Health Perspect.* 2002;110(suppl 2):161–171. doi:10.1289/ehp.02110s2161
16. Bullard RD, Mohai P, Saha R, Wright B. *Toxic Wastes and Race at Twenty, 1987–2007: A Report Prepared for the United Church of Christ Justice & Witness Ministries.* United Church of Christ; March 2007. https://www.ucc.org/wp-content/uploads/2021/03/toxic-wastes-and-race-at-twenty-1987-2007.pdf
17. Pastor M, Sadd J, Hipp J. Which came first? Toxic facilities, minority move-in, and environmental justice. *J Urban Aff.* 2001;23(1):1–21. doi:10.1111/0735-2166.00072
18. Mohai P, Saha R. Which came first, people or pollution? Assessing the disparate siting and post-siting demographic change hypotheses of environmental injustice. *Environ Res Lett.* 2015;10(11):115008. doi:10.1088/1748-9326/10/11/115008
19. US House of Representatives: History, Art & Archives. US House of Representatives Office of the Historian. Accessed June 17, 2024. https://history.house.gov/
20. Rothstein R. *The Color of Law: A Forgotten History of How Our Government Segregated America.* Liveright; 2017.
21. Mitchell B, Franco J. HOLC "redlining" maps: the persistent structure of segregation and economic inequality. NCRC. 2018. Accessed June 17, 2024. https://ncrc.org/holc/
22. Hoffman JS, Shandas V, Pendleton N. The effects of historical housing policies on residential exposure to intra-urban heat: a study of 108 US urban areas. *Climate.* 2020;8(12). doi:10.3390/cli8010012
23. Nowak DJ, Ellis A, Greenfield EJ. The disparity in tree cover and ecosystem service values among redlining classes in the United States. *Landsc Urban Plan.* 2022;221(3):104370. doi:10.1016/j.landurbplan.2022.104370
24. Nardone A, Rudolph KE, Morello-Frosch R, Casey JA. Redlines and greenspace: the relationship between historical redlining and 2010 greenspace across the United States. *Environ Health Perspect.* 2021;129(1):17006. doi:10.1289/EHP7495

25. Lane HM, Morello-Frosch R, Marshall JD, Apte JS. Historical redlining is associated with present-day air pollution in U.S. cities. *Environ Sci Technol Lett*. 2022;9:345–350. doi:10.1021/acs.estlett.1c01012
26. Population surrounding 1,877 Superfund sites. U.S. Environmental Protection Agency. 2022. Updated October 30, 2023. https://www.epa.gov/superfund/population-surrounding-1877-superfund-sites
27. Little BB, Reilly R, Walsh B, Vu GT. Cadmium is associated with type 2 diabetes in a Superfund site lead smelter community in Dallas, Texas. *Int J Environ Res Public Health*. 2020;17(12):4558. doi:10.3390/ijerph17124558
28. McDermott S, Hailer MK, Lead JR. Meconium identifies high levels of metals in newborns from a mining community in the U.S. *Sci Total Environ*. 2020;707:135528. doi:10.1016/j.scitotenv.2019.135528
29. Zota AR, Schaider LA, Ettinger AS, Wright RO, Shine JP, Spengler JD. Metal sources and exposures in the homes of young children living near a mining-impacted Superfund site. *J Expo Sci Environ Epidemiol*. 2011;21:495–505. doi:10.1038/jes.2011.21
30. Wu Y, Wang J, Wei Y, et al. Maternal exposure to endocrine disrupting chemicals (EDCs) and preterm birth: a systematic review, meta-analysis, and meta-regression analysis. *Environ Pollut*. 2022;292:118264. doi:10.1016/j.envpol.2021.118264
31. Okorie CN, Thomas MD, Méndez RM, Di Giuseppe EC, Roberts NS, Márquez-Magaña L. Geospatial distributions of lead levels found in human hair and preterm birth in San Francisco neighborhoods. *Int J Environ Res Public Health*. 2021;19(1):86. doi:10.3390/ijerph19010086
32. Tessum CW, Apte JS, Goodkind AL, et al. Inequity in consumption of goods and services adds to racial–ethnic disparities in air pollution exposure. *Proc Natl Acad Sci U S A*. 2019;116(13):6001–6006. doi:10.1073/pnas.1818859116
33. Anguelovski I, Connolly JJT, Pearsall H, et al. Why green "climate gentrification" threatens poor and vulnerable populations. *Proc Natl Acad Sci U S A*. 2019;116(52):26139–26143. doi:10.1073/pnas.1920490117
34. Keenan JM, Hill TS, Gumber A. Climate gentrification: from theory to empiricism in Miami-Dade County, Florida. *Environ Res Lett*. Published online April 23, 2018. https://dash.harvard.edu/handle/1/37373268
35. Rigolon A, Németh J. Green gentrification or 'just green enough': do park location, size and function affect whether a place gentrifies or not? *Urban Stud*. 2020;57(2):402–420. doi:10.1177/0042098019849380
36. Cushing LJ, Ju Y, Kulp S, Depsky N, Karasaki S, Jaeger J, Raval A, Strauss B, Morello-Frosch R. Toxic tides and environmental injustice: social vulnerability to sea level rise and flooding of hazardous sites in coastal California. *Environ Sci & Technology*. 2023;57(19):7370–7381. doi:10.1021/acs.est.2c07481
37. Zhuang J, Cox J, Cruz S, Dearing JW, Hamm JA, Upham B. Environmental stigma: resident responses to living in a contaminated area. *Am Behav Sci*. 2016;60(11):1322–1341. doi:10.1177/0002764216657381
38. Schmitt HJ, Calloway EE, Sullivan D, et al. Chronic environmental contamination: a systematic review of psychological health consequences. *Sci Total Environ*. 2021;772:145025. doi:10.1016/j.scitotenv.2021.145025
39. Maantay JA, Maroko AR. 'At-risk' places: inequities in the distribution of environmental stressors and prescription rates of mental health medications in Glasgow, Scotland. *Environ Res Lett*. 2015;10(11):115003. doi:10.1088/1748-9326/10/11/115003
40. Sullivan D, Schmitt HJ, Calloway EE, et al. Chronic environmental contamination: a narrative review of psychosocial health consequences, risk factors, and pathways to community resilience. *Soc Sci Med*. 2021;276:113877. doi:10.1016/j.socscimed.2021.113877
41. ATSDR. CDC/ATSDR Social Vulnerability Index (SVI). November 16, 2022. Updated February 23, 2024. https://www.atsdr.cdc.gov/placeandhealth/svi/index.html
42. EJScreen: EPA's environmental justice screening and mapping tool (version 2.2). U.S. Environmental Protection Agency. Accessed June 17, 2024. https://ejscreen.epa.gov/mapper/
43. Agency for Toxic Substances and Disease Registry. Environmental Justice Index. Centers for Disease Control and Prevention. August 10, 2022. Updated March 15, 2024. https://www.atsdr.cdc.gov/placeandhealth/eji/
44. Agency for Toxic Substances and Disease Registry. Environmental Justice Index indicators. Centers for Disease Control and Prevention. September 7, 2022. Updated May 31, 2023. https://www.atsdr.cdc.gov/placeandhealth/eji/indicators.html

45. National Center for Environmental Health. Radon toolkit for public health professionals. Centers for Disease Control and Prevention. January 10, 2022. https://www.cdc.gov/radon/toolkit/shareable_images.html
46. Bourgois P, Holmes SM, Sue K, Quesada J. Structural vulnerability: operationalizing the concept to address health disparities in clinical care. *Acad Med J Assoc Am Med Coll*. 2017;92(3):299–307. doi:10.1097/ACM.0000000000001294
47. US EPA. EPA's response to Hurricane Ida. September 25, 2021. https://storymaps.arcgis.com/stories/3c0d86c01bb14f7898ae22251e4f5f1b
48. US EPA. EPA and LDEQ announce story map resource. September 13, 2021. https://www.epa.gov/newsreleases/epa-and-ldeq-announce-story-map-resource
49. Harvard Chan-NIEHS Center for Environmental Health. Environmental racism at the neighborhood level. ArcGIS StoryMaps. July 15, 2022. https://storymaps.arcgis.com/stories/1ae25711737f4f379e77331b1d428894
50. Sieber R. Public participation geographic information systems: a literature review and framework. *Ann Assoc Am Geogr*. 2006;96(3):491–507. doi:10.1111/j.1467-8306.2006.00702.x
51. Brown G, Reed P, Raymond CM. Mapping place values: 10 lessons from two decades of public participation GIS empirical research. *Appl Geogr*. 2020;116:102156. doi:10.1016/j.apgeog.2020.102156
52. Verplanke J, McCall MK, Uberhuaga C, Rambaldi G, Haklay M. A shared perspective for PGIS and VGI. *Cartogr J*. 2016;53(4):308–317. doi:10.1080/00087041.2016.1227552
53. iWitness pollution map. Louisiana Bucket Brigade. 2022. Accessed June 17, 2024. https://labucketbrigade.org/pollution-tools-resources/iwitness-pollution-map/
54. Real-time air quality map. PurpleAir. 2023. https://map.purpleair.com/1/mAQI/a10/p604800/cC0#10.87/42.3428/-71.1189
55. Wilson SM, Murray RT, Jiang C, Dalemarre L, Burwell-Naney K, Fraser-Rahim H. Environmental justice radar: a tool for community-based mapping to increase environmental awareness and participatory decision making. *Prog Community Health Partnersh Res Educ Action*. 2015;9(3):439–446. doi:10.1353/cpr.2015.0066
56. Dalemarre L, Wilson SM, Campbell D, Fraser-Rahim H, Williams EM. Summary on the Charleston area pollution prevention partnership environmental justice conference and summit. *Environ Justice*. 2014;7(3). doi:10.1089/env.2014.0007

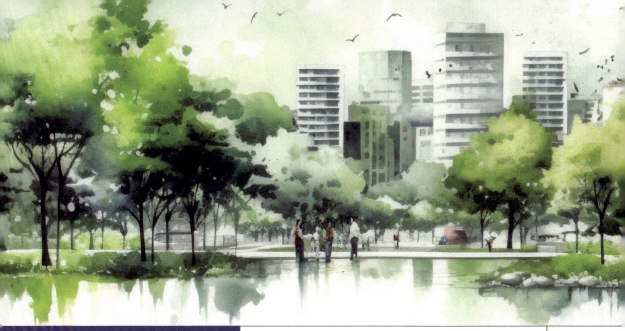

SECTION III

Interconnected: Energy, Air, Water, Food, and Waste

PFAS WHERE WE LIVE, WORK, AND PLAY

In this episode, hosts Natalie Conti and Anchal Malh meet with Sandy Wynn-Stelt of the Great Lakes PFAS Action Network to discuss where per- and polyfluoroalkyl substances (PFAS) show up in our everyday life and how they impact human health. During their conversation, they discuss PFAS in the places we live, work, and play, and what solutions scientists are coming up with to remediate the presence of these forever chemicals in our environment. Tune in to unearth where PFAS may be lurking in your environment and the steps you can take to reduce your exposure.

Access the podcast via the QR code or http://connect.springerpub.com/content/book/978-0-8261-8353-8/chapter/ch00

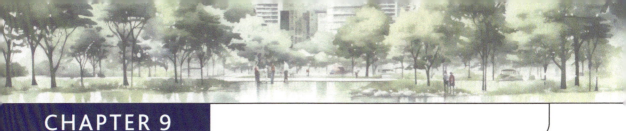

CHAPTER 9

Energy and Health

Carina J. Gronlund, Anchal Malh, Parth Vaishnav, Gibran Washington, Bruce Tonn, Amy J. Schulz, and Marie S. O'Neill

LEARNING OBJECTIVES

- Identify different sources of energy and describe how they impact environmental health.
- Explain the key processes and concepts related to energy infrastructure and policy.
- Highlight the ways that energy use relates to climate change and health.
- Provide case examples of energy injustice and describe the ways that society can work toward energy justice.
- Discuss the strategies for a just transition to renewable energy sources that can better support environmental health globally.

KEY TERMS

- energy burden
- energy democracy
- energy justice
- energy poverty
- Energy Use Intensity (EUI)
- just transition
- life cycle impact assessment
- redlining
- toxicants
- weatherization
- Weatherization Assistance Program (WAP)

OVERVIEW

Energy production is critical for human survival and is essential for basic needs such as heating and cooking. In recent times, energy has also become necessary for refrigeration, air conditioning (AC), transportation, and many methods of communication. Moreover, energy plays an indirect yet crucial role in enabling and supporting medical care by facilitating communication, transportation to medical facilities, and the delivery of medical care itself. In fact, it is challenging to think of a health-related outcome that is not influenced or impacted by energy use in some way. Of course, in many wealthier areas of the world, fossil-fuel-generated energy is used nearly nonstop for nonessential needs too, including entertainment or other luxuries.

The production and use of energy have a long-standing history of health trade-offs. For instance, while it is important to consider the health benefits of warmth and cooking provided by a fire, it is also important to acknowledge the potential adverse health consequences of the smoke and embers it generates. Further, different populations do not experience equal exposure to toxins emitted by coal power plants, tailpipes, and indoor cooking. This unequal exposure leads to health inequities.

In this chapter, we explore the link between energy and health, as well as health inequities. In doing so, we present the concept of **energy justice** which calls on society to recognize who benefits and who is burdened by systems of energy extraction, transport, processing, and use. We examine an example of energy injustice, and discuss interventions aimed at reducing

ENERGY'S IMPACTS ON HEALTH: PAST AND PRESENT

Energy production has likely impacted health since the Paleolithic Period, when the hominid ancestors of modern-day humans began using fire for light, warmth, and cooking.[1] The burning of wood and other biomass, including peat, dung, grasses, and crop waste, emits particulate matter (PM), or fine particles small enough to enter the trachea and lungs. As discussed in more detail in Chapter 10, "The Air We Breathe," these particles are made up of carbon as well as toxins such as volatile organic compounds (VOCs; including benzene, formaldehyde, and acrolein) and polycyclic aromatic hydrocarbons (PAHs), and cause a variety of health issues.[2,3] This heat generation is essential for survival, and there is evidence that we have special genetic mutations to enable our bodies to more rapidly detoxify smoke from biomass burning to help limit the health damage.[4] However, evolutionary adaptations to biomass burning have not made humans immune to the health impacts. Even today, biomass burning still accounts for a large portion of deaths and health problems globally.[5]

Despite the health costs, biomass burning remains vital to providing many communities with heat for cooking and warmth throughout the world. Household air pollution from cooking is a major cause of disease.[6] About a third of the global population, or 2.3 billion people, use open fires or stoves indoors that use kerosene, wood, animal dung, crop waste, or coal as fuels.[5] The burning of biomass also emits greenhouse gases, but the carbon emitted into the atmosphere from burning biomass is part of the "above ground" carbon already present in our current carbon cycle. It is arguably less problematic for climate change than burning fossil fuels. This is especially true if the amount of biomass burned is replaced by new biomass (e.g., trees) that will capture carbon as it grows.[7]

Today, in addition to biomass burning, we rely on many energy sources. These sources and their uses can be loosely categorized as seen in Table 9.1, which focuses particularly on household energy use. Coal, natural gas, liquefied petroleum gases (LPGs), and fuel oils are all fossil fuels that have been buried underground for millions of years. They are extracted in

TABLE 9.1. ENERGY SOURCES AND THEIR COMMON HOUSEHOLD USES

	SPACE HEATING	HOT WATER HEATING	COOKING	ELECTRICITY GENERATION (WHICH CAN BE USED FOR SPACE HEATING, HOT WATER HEATING, AND COOKING)
Coal	X			X
Natural gas	X	X	X	X
Liquefied petroleum gasses	X	X	X	X
Fuel oils	X	X	X	X
Biomass (e.g., wood, peat, dung, crop waste, etc.)	X	X	X	
Solar and Geo-thermal	X	X		X
Wind				X
Hydro-electric				X
Nuclear				X

various ways. Then, through the process of combustion and subsequent processes, energy is converted to forms useful to humans. Through combustion, these fossil fuels contribute to the emission of new greenhouse gasses.

Figure 9.1 shows some of the toxicants produced by each of the energy sources shown in Table 9.1, as well as their health impacts. **Toxicants** include heavy metals, particulate air pollution, gaseous air pollutants, radon, radioactive waste, and even noise. We can also think of carbon dioxide (CO_2) as a toxicant when we consider that it is a greenhouse gas contributing to climate change, and climate change has numerous health effects. The toxicants may

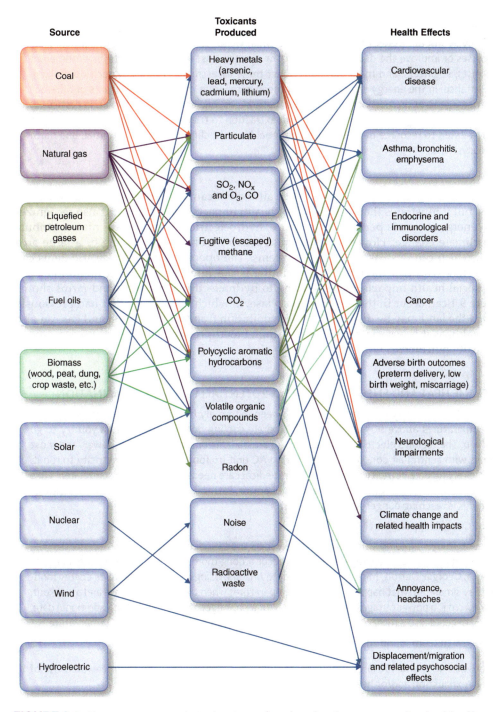

FIGURE 9.1. Energy sources, main toxicants produced, and major corresponding health effects.

be produced at different stages of the energy source's life cycle. For example, exposures to heavy metals in solar panels occur primarily in the construction phase, through human contact with the metals during their mining, and in the construction of the solar panels. Exposure also occurs in the recycling phase, where solvents used to separate the silicon and rare metal elements may produce toxic gasses.[8] For fossil fuels and biomass, much of the human exposure to toxicants comes from burning during the use phase. Of note, all of the energy sources require transportation in some way, and the emissions from the vehicles used to transport them also factor into their total impact across their life cycles.

> ### IN OTHER WORDS: LIFE CYCLE IMPACT ASSESSMENT
>
> A **life cycle impact assessment** can be done when we want to compare different products or processes or improve the design of a product or process. Sustainability experts, environmental scientists, engineers, and many others conduct these assessments to inform decision-making. For instance, in the energy sector, this may mean comparing the life cycle impacts of different electricity generation methods, such as coal, natural gas, nuclear, wind, and solar. In particular, the assessment might consider impacts from extraction to transport to use to waste, including those related to resource depletion, occupational hazards, climate change potential, and harm to ecosystems.

Figure 9.1 is not a comprehensive list of all the toxicants and health impacts of energy sources, but it illustrates that the breadth of health impacts is substantial. It also recognizes that no energy source is perfect. For instance, hydroelectric energy sources may contribute less to climate change. However, dam construction involves the flooding of a large area of land, which can destroy existing ecosystems. The operation of hydroelectric dams can also interfere with fish migration, and windmills can interfere with bird migration.[9] The psychosocial health impacts corresponding to hydroelectric dams and wind farms shown in Figure 9.1 can occur in the construction phase, in which households that had previously occupied the land may be displaced.[10] Noise pollution from drilling for oil and gas can also harm health, as it is associated with stress, high blood pressure, and heart disease, among other health outcomes.

> ### EXTREME HEAT AND ENERGY OUTAGES: A POTENTIALLY DEADLY COMBINATION
>
> Imagine that your city or neighborhood has been extremely hot for days. You are on day five of temperatures above 90° Fahrenheit. It is barely cooling down at night when you try to go to sleep. The region's electrical grid is stressed and fails. Thousands have lost power, and most homes with central air conditioning (AC) or an AC unit no longer have the electricity to run it. People relying on electricity to support their medical care needs are without essential items like their oxygen machine—unless they have a generator. Extreme heat both inside and outside of buildings is reaching dangerously high levels.
>
> **What Could Happen Next?**
>
> A recent study[11] explored this scenario. Researchers used models to estimate excess deaths (i.e., more than the expected average) that could occur among more than 2.8 million residents across Atlanta, Georgia; Detroit, Michigan; and Phoenix, Arizona. Using climate and building energy models, they simulated what happens to indoor temperatures when there is a heat wave and a blackout. (A *blackout* is a power outage of a whole region for a prolonged timeframe.) Using additional data, the team could also estimate the risk of death for each degree increase of indoor temperature.
>
> The research team found that:
>
> - Between 68% and 100% of the urban populations would be exposed to an elevated risk of heat exhaustion and/or heat stroke if they stayed in or near their homes.

(continued)

- In Detroit, the combined heat wave/blackout event would result in 200 excess deaths. If the power stayed on during the heat event, the toll would be closer to 100 deaths.
- In Phoenix, the combined heat wave/blackout event would result in 13,000 excess deaths. If the power stayed on during the heat event, the toll would be closer to 20 deaths.

These differences are likely due to the fact that Detroit has generally milder temperatures and, with the power on, most Phoenix residents would be likely to maintain more comfortable indoor temperatures during high heat given the higher underlying rate of AC use.[12]

IMPACTS OF ENERGY EXTRACTION

The mining, or extraction, of fossil fuels impacts human and ecological health. Coal and gas mining present dangers and health impacts to the workers and surrounding communities.[13] The impacts to the environment and health of the communities include water pollution from strip mining and mountaintop mining removal methods, as well as the destruction and fragmentation of wildlife habitats.[14] Underground mines can also pollute groundwater if they collapse. Occupational hazards include physical trauma from workplace injuries or mine collapses and lung damage related to the inhalation of coal dust.[15] Miners are particularly susceptible to lung diseases known as pneumoconiosis, including "black lung disease," caused by inhaling coal dust.[16]

Natural gas is extracted from conventional gas wells or via hydraulic fracturing (fracking) and then transported to power plants and home heating through pipelines, processing plants, and storage facilities.[17] During the mining and transportation of natural gas, leaks can occur. In a recent estimate,[18] these leaks result in 2.6% of the mined gas being lost. Natural gas is mostly made up of methane. Because methane is a much stronger greenhouse gas than CO_2, the climate effects from the leakages may be similar to those from the CO_2 emitted when natural gas is burned.[18]

The extraction of solar, nuclear, or wind power energy is not without harm. Although solar and wind power produce virtually no air pollution in their use phase, some systems include batteries, particularly in off-grid applications. The extraction of the materials for the batteries used to store solar- and wind-generated power has health impacts. For example, in heavy metal mining, the erosion of the compounds can lead to the contamination of rivers and streams. Depending on the form of the chemical, the chemical can be released from the sediment and into bodies of water.[19] The runoff from heavy metal mines can further affect human health.[20] Therefore, after mining expeditions are completed, it is necessary that abandoned mines be properly drained and sealed off. If the contaminated water comes into contact with humans through ingestion, it can lead to complications in brain, liver, kidney, and other organ functions.

CASE STUDY 9.1: Cobalt Mining in the Democratic Republic of Congo

As technology advances, the demand for lithium and battery material mining has increased. Lithium, cobalt, and other minerals are commonly found in laptops, cell phones, electric vehicles, and other battery-operated devices. These products are used on a daily basis as our way of life becomes more dependent on electronics. About 90% of the world's lithium can be found in Australia, Chile, and China.[21] Pure cobalt cannot be found on Earth, but cobaltlike minerals are primarily found in Kinshasa (the Democratic Republic of Congo).[22] Miners in Congo are *artisanal miners*, or freelance miners who are put in extreme physical danger for work, but only receive a few dollars of pay per day. They use pickaxes, shovels, and their hands to go deep into the mines to find the minerals used in electronic devices. The age of artisanal miners can vary and can include children, pregnant people, and the elderly. Most are not provided with proper protective equipment or devices used to extract minerals.[23]

These workers are exposed to polluted air, water, and land. Constant exposure to cobalt, uranium, and gaseous pollutants ultimately leads to heart, lung, and blood disorders.[24,25] Poorly ventilated mineshafts and exposure to minerals stored in homes for long periods of time leads to exposure to gaseous radon, a byproduct of uranium's radioactive decay. Long-term exposure to gaseous radon can lead to neurotoxic (damage to the nervous system) and nephrotoxic (rapid kidney deg-

(continued)

> **CASE STUDY 9.1: Cobalt Mining in the Democratic Republic of Congo** (*continued*)
>
> radation) effects.[26] Cobalt has also been found in the soil, vegetation, and wildlife in mining regions.[27] Human exposure can occur through the ingestion of foods grown in contaminated soil. Furthermore, a study published in 2020[28] suggests that birth defects, such as spina bifida and limb abnormalities, are most common in children who have a parent that works in the mines.
>
> Even though the world is shifting to prioritize a cleaner and more energy-efficient environment, the populations most negatively impacted by technological advancements may be the least likely to reap the benefits of those advancements.
>
> **REFLECTION QUESTIONS**
>
> *1. The demand for electric vehicles and portable electronic devices continues to grow. What can be done to protect workers, as cobalt mining is likely to continue?*
>
> *2. Initiatives such as the Responsible Cobalt Initiative and Responsible Cobalt Reporting have been established to promote responsible sourcing. As a consumer, what information do you want when purchasing a device? How would having this information affect your purchasing decisions, if at all?*

ENERGY AND HEALTH EQUITIES

The benefits and burden of our global energy infrastructure are not experienced equally.[29] Many lower- and middle-wealth countries have less adequate or reliable energy sources compared to wealthier nations.[30,31] Within countries, there can also be significant disparities, particularly between rural and urban areas. Rural areas are more likely to lack reliable access to electricity and rely on less efficient energy sources.[32] Furthermore, poor access to energy may hinder economic growth, limiting the resources available for healthcare infrastructure and disease prevention. In general, energy poverty is closely linked to overall poverty. Lack of access to modern energy services limits opportunities for education, economic development, and improved living standards—social determinants of health that are crucial.[33,34]

Another disconnect between benefits and burden can be found in Ogoniland, a region of the Niger River Delta in Southern Nigeria. The region is 385 square miles—smaller than many U.S. counties. The British petroleum company Shell has operated in the region since the 1930s, when oil was first discovered. In recent years, local leaders estimate that there have been thousands of oil spills, including those from fires and damaged pipelines.[35] In 2009, at the Nigerian government's request, the United Nations Environment Programme (UNEP) assessed the impact of contamination from oil across the Ogoni region. The report, released in 2011, found extremely high levels of PAHs in the drinking water and damage to farmland and mangrove swamps, and called for a massive cleanup.[36] Shell no longer extracts oil in the region, but the company's pipeline still runs through the area. The area remains contaminated, and spills from the pipeline have continued since 2011, blamed in part on armed groups bombing the pipeline to suppress oil production and distribution.[37–40]

In the United States, millions of families are energy burdened or experience energy poverty, and disproportionately they are low-wealth families of color.[41] **Energy burden** means that households spend 6% or more of their income on home utility bills. Consider two households, Household A and Household B, with different income levels and energy consumption patterns. Household A has a household income of $30,000 and spends about $3,200 (or 10.7% of their income) on energy expenses annually. Household B has a household income of $80,000 and spends about $4,000 (or 5% of their income) on energy expenses annually. A higher energy burden means that a higher portion of the household's income is allocated to energy expenses, leaving less money for other essential needs, such as food, healthcare, and education. Energy burden is not necessarily the same as **energy poverty**. *Energy poverty* is broader. It could mean that a household does not have access to reliable electricity or electricity at all. It could mean that it has fewer light bulbs or appliances. It could also mean that these households are too hot in the summer and too cold in the winter because of energy costs and/or inadequate housing. Energy poverty can also lead to the "heat or eat dilemma," whereby households must choose between paying utility bills or buying food, medicine, and other basic necessities each month. Estimates of households in energy poverty vary but, according to the Residential Energy Consumption Survey, one in five American households reported forgoing food or medicine to pay utility bills.[42]

In the United States, structural racism has led to housing inequality, which is inextricably linked to patterns of energy burden and poverty. In the early 1900s, the Home Owners' Loan Corporation (HOLC) in the United States instituted lending practices that reinforced long-standing practices of housing segregation, with marginalized racial and ethnic groups relegated to distinct neighborhoods, often in less desirable locations. As discussed in several chapters, **redlining** refers to a mid-20th century practice that used HOLC scoring criteria to classify the quality of neighborhoods for investment and lending practices based on housing stock and demographics. Neighborhoods in urban communities were color-coded and mapped, with those classified as "lower quality" neighborhoods colored yellow (grade C) and red (grade D, hence the origin of "redlining"; see Figure 9.2 for an example of HOLC scores in Detroit, Michigan).

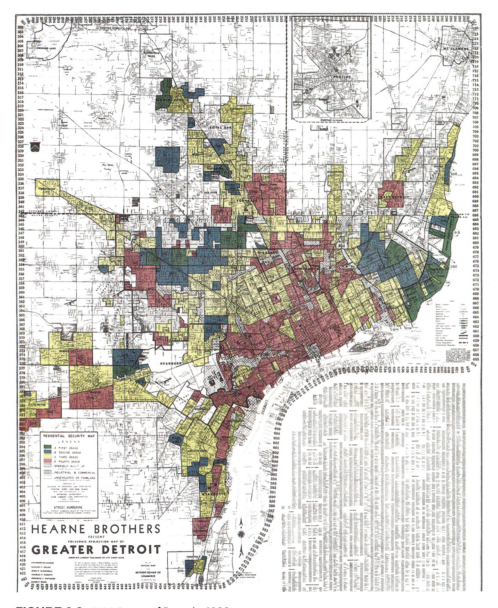

FIGURE 9.2. HOLC map of Detroit, 1939.

HOLC, Home Owners' Loan Corporation.

Source: University of Richmond. Mapping Inequality: Redlining In New Deal America. Creative Commons.

Neighborhoods with existing or growing Black, immigrant, or other ethnic group populations were classified as "low" or "declining" quality, and were systematically denied mortgages and loans for home upgrades. "High-quality" neighborhoods, typified by affluent, majority White populations, received easy access to credit. This practice exacerbated racial segregation and economic inequities by reducing opportunities for investment in redlined neighborhoods. Even though the practice was outlawed in 1968, there is substantial evidence of ongoing adverse health impacts for today's residents of formerly redlined communities.[43,44]

Aside from creating or exacerbating inequities in housing quality, redlining further concentrated fossil-fuel power plants near neighborhoods of color. According to Figure 9.3, before 1940, about 2% of grade-D neighborhoods had one or more power plants within five kilometers (km) upwind (or in a location where the power plant's air pollution usually blows into the neighborhood). Power plant proximity has increased for all neighborhoods over different time periods, but as time progressed, grade-D neighborhoods had a disproportionate increase in the presence of upwind power plants. Specifically, the increase among grade-D neighborhoods was greater than among grade A neighborhoods (17% vs. 10%, respectively).[45] Oil and gas wells are also more likely to be located in redlined neighborhoods in the United States.[46]

To reduce energy poverty, households are often encouraged to make weatherization and energy-efficiency modifications and basic home upgrades to their homes, but these upgrades are generally costly. **Weatherization** refers to housing modifications that improve the building envelope—locking in heat in the winter and cool air in the summer—and includes air sealing, wall and attic insulation, and replacement of windows and doors with more energy-efficient products.[47] Energy-efficiency upgrades include the replacement of appliances, including furnaces, air conditioners, hot water heaters, and refrigerators, with more energy-efficient models.[48] These upgrades can result in substantial savings on utility bills. Households that cannot afford such improvements may have relatively higher energy use per square foot of their home, which further worsens inequities.

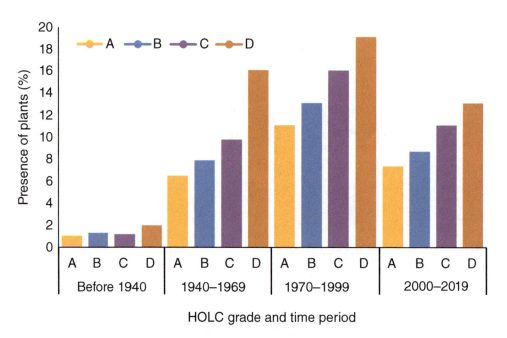

FIGURE 9.3. Percentage of HOLC-graded neighborhoods with one or more upwind power plant(s) within 5 km.

HOLC, Home Owners' Loan Corporation.

Source: Cushing LJ, Li S, Steiger BB, Casey JA. Historical red-lining is associated with fossil fuel power plant siting and present-day inequalities in air pollutant emissions. *Nat Energy.* 2023;8:52–61. doi:10.1038/s41560-022-01162-y.

CASE STUDY 9.2: Energy Justice in Southeast Michigan

Detroit has a long history of housing segregation and unfair mortgage lending practices, which has made poverty and housing issues worse in certain areas.[49] People in these areas are more likely to face health problems. Additionally, especially in Southwest Detroit, the urban heat island effect contributes to extreme heat, and residents often don't have access to central air conditioning (AC)—one of electricity's major benefits. This area also deals with high levels of air pollution from various sources, including an oil refinery, steel mills, and a power plant.[50]

Several years ago, environmental advocates began organizing to address concerns around energy injustice in Southeast Michigan. Leaders of the Michigan Environmental Justice Coalition (MEJC) worked in conjunction with the Great Lakes Environmental Law Center and Soulidarity to understand this energy burden and its impacts in the region. Researchers at the University of Michigan's School of Public Health joined the effort by helping to specifically investigate the health impacts.

Together, the community–academic team used several measures and examined how they were related:

- **Energy use:** The team used Residential Energy Consumption Survey data to model residential energy use and Energy Use Intensity (EUI)—a measure of energy poverty—by household characteristics. Then, the team used census-tract-level information on household characteristics from the American Community Survey to model energy use and EUI at the census-tract level.
- **Air pollution from power plants:** To estimate the health impacts of air pollution, the team used estimates of emissions of major pollutants from the smokestacks of coal and natural gas power plants owned by DTE Energy. (Some of these data came from an Integrated Resource Plan [IRP] assessment case. IRPs, required by the Michigan Public Service Commission of Michigan's utilities, describe how the utility will meet their customers' energy demands, including what plans the utility has for new power plants and decommissioning old plants.) The team used a tool called the CalPUFF dispersion model to estimate the annual average level of particulate matter 2.5 ($PM_{2.5}$) in each census tract based on wind direction, weather, the emissions from the smokestacks, and the chemical reactions these emissions can undergo.
- **Lack of AC:** The team used estimates they had previously made—from American Housing Survey data—of the percentage of residents in a census tract who had AC.
- **Cost of health impacts:** The team then used the U.S. Environmental Protection Agency's (EPA's) BenMAP software to combine the estimates of an individual's risk of experiencing $PM_{2.5}$ and lack of AC with estimates of the risk of related health effects. These could include premature death, heart attack, or asthma attacks.

When looking for correlations among these variables, the team found that low-income, predominantly Black and Hispanic or Latino communities in Southeast Michigan are more likely to be located downwind of power plants,[51] *use less energy* generated by those power plants, and *experience greater health costs* from power-plant air pollution exposure and from heat associated with lack of AC (Figure 9.4).

Electricity generation, use, and segregation in Southeast Michigan provide a striking example of energy injustice. Closing coal-fired power plants is one step toward substantially reducing these energy injustices. Encouragingly, DTE Energy has now changed their proposed closure of all coal plants from a deadline of 2040 to 2032, in part owing to strong advocacy from environmental leaders, as well as increasing scientific evidence of the associated health harms.[52] The health benefits of these closures will be realized much more quickly.

The transition depends on increasing the use of natural gas-powered plants. Although natural gas-powered plants burn much more efficiently, emitting far less carbon dioxide (CO_2) per kilowatt-hour (kWh) than coal, while also emitting far less $PM_{2.5}$ at the point of energy generation, these plants also have many health harms associated with the extraction process,

(continued)

CASE STUDY 9.2: Energy Justice in Southeast Michigan (continued)

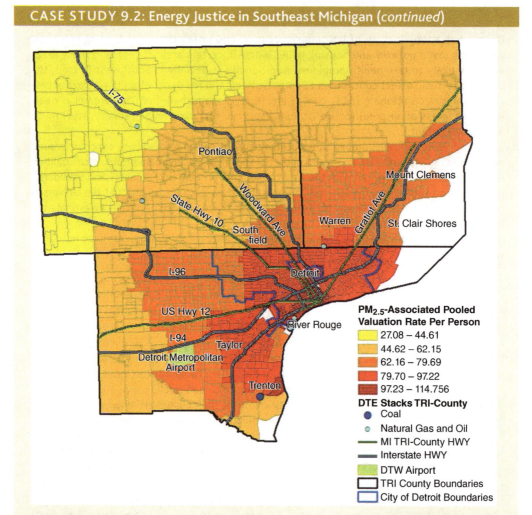

FIGURE 9.4. Health costs associated with PM$_{2.5}$ exposure from power plants in the tri-county Detroit metropolitan area, 2018. These costs are the dollars per person per year attributable to PM$_{2.5}$ exposure from power plants.

HWY, highway; PM$_{2.5}$, particulate matter 2.5.

Source: Gronlund C, Reames T, Martinez M, Schulz A. Energy equity: health impact assessment of DTE's integrated resource plan. Presentation for the M-LEEaD Center. University of Michigan School of Public Health Lifestage Environmental Exposures and Disease Center. March 9, 2021. https://mleead.umich.edu/files/SLIDES_20210309 _HealthImpactAssessmentsAsAToolForEnergyAndPublicPlanning.pdf

which shifts some of the burden of energy harms to communities proximate to hydraulic fracturing (fracking) extraction. Continued advocacy is necessary to ensure that utilities across the United States continue to move vigorously to increase the amount of clean renewable energy in the energy mix.[53]

REFLECTION QUESTIONS

1. As coal plants are shut down, what energy injustice issues might be addressed? What issues might remain unresolved?

2. AC is protective in extreme heat events, especially for populations with underlying health issues. In our changing climate, what policies or actions can help to reduce the increased air pollution from AC use? Meanwhile, how might we address health inequities related to inequitable AC ownership and use?

WORKING TOWARD ENVIRONMENTAL HEALTH AND JUSTICE

As referenced in other chapters, the United Nations' (UN's) Sustainable Development Goals (SDGs) are a set of 17 global goals adopted by all UN member states in 2015 as part of the 2030 Agenda for Sustainable Development. The SDGs are aimed at ending poverty, protecting the planet, and ensuring prosperity for all; in particular, Goal 7 aims to ensure affordable and clean energy. With regard to how these goals can be accomplished, the UN states, "[W]e must accelerate electrification, increase investments in renewable energy, improve energy efficiency and develop enabling policies and regulatory frameworks."[54(para10)]

However, we must think critically, as many proposed solutions can create new challenges or actually worsen inequities, which Chapter 4 ("Environmental Health Policies and Protections: Successes and Failures") explains further. For instance, some industries are beginning to use carbon capture and storage methods, which—as it sounds—means capturing emissions to store underground. Yet, this approach may be costly and create new environmental risks associated with storage, while failing to reduce fossil fuel use. Another example is the use of food crops like corn or sugarcane to generate biofuels. Many environmentalists are concerned that this practice would lead to unsustainable agricultural practices, deforestation, and increased food prices.

Effective policies and programs are needed to ensure affordable and clean energy in the United States, particularly as climate change remains a pressing issue layered on top of related inequities. There is concern that the United States must more rapidly update its aging power grid infrastructure to enhance resilience against natural disasters, cyber threats, and other emergencies. Some relevant policies and programs are referenced in Chapter 4, which examines the U.S. environmental policy landscape, including recent large federal investments in energy infrastructure: the Bipartisan Infrastructure Law (also known as the Infrastructure Investment and Jobs Act) of 2021 and the Inflation Reduction Act of 2022. In particular, the Inflation Reduction Act supports clean energy installation, promotes wind and solar energy, and creates supply chains for critical minerals and battery manufacturing. In this legislation, $100 billion was allocated to the Department of Energy (DOE) to catalyze energy transition. Next, we look at some of the strategies that are underway or under consideration to improve energy systems in ways that protect public health and promote environmental justice (EJ).

TRANSITIONING TO RENEWABLE ENERGY AND A REGENERATIVE ECONOMY

A shift toward healthier energy sources is underway in the United States. No new coal power plants have been built in the continental United States since 2015.[55] To address the air pollution generated by coal power plants, the U.S. Congress amended the Clean Air Act in 1990 (discussed in Chapter 4, "Environmental Health Policies and Protections: Successes and Failures," and in Chapter 10, "The Air We Breathe," in detail), and further regulation of emissions has been accomplished through EPA initiatives, such as the Acid Rain Program and the National Ambient Air Quality Standards. A major driver of the decline in coal power is the high price of coal in comparison to other fuel sources. Coal is expensive not only to mine—particularly from underground mines such as those in the Appalachian region of the United States—but also to transport to power plants.[56]

Many nations, including the United States, are investing heavily in renewable energy and decentralized energy infrastructure to reduce their reliance on fossil fuels like coal and natural gas. Many nations have set targets and established policies to incentivize utilities and households to make these shifts. This approach requires integrating renewable energy into existing power grids where energy can flow in and out and be stored in a decentralized way, as shown in Figure 9.5. To do this, agencies, utilities, and communities must reimagine the energy sector together. To this end, the U.S. DOE coordinates the Clean Energy for Low-Income Communities Accelerator, which can support placing small power sources, like solar panels, on roofs or in neighborhoods. Technology is rapidly advancing, as costs for wind, solar, and hydroelectric energy sources decrease. This change means that renewable energy is becoming more competitive with natural gas in the energy economy.

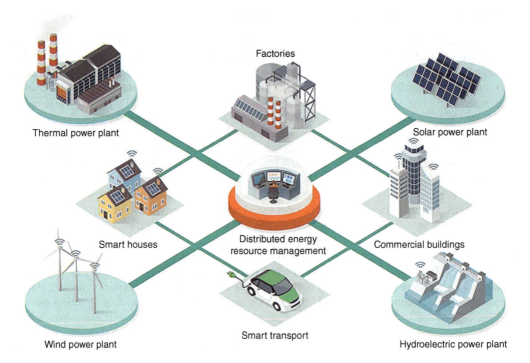

FIGURE 9.5. Distributed energy resource management systems.
Source: Distributed energy resource management systems. National Renewable Energy Laboratory. Accessed June 17, 2024. https://www.nrel.gov/grid/distributed-energy-resource-management-systems.html

In recent years, there has also been a movement toward community-owned and -managed renewable energy systems. As described earlier, we have long relied on a comprehensive infrastructure managed by public and private partners. In community-owned energy projects, the local community or a cooperative of residents collectively owns the energy infrastructure. Community ownership has many challenges, including financing, barriers within current regulatory structures, and technical difficulties connecting to the existing infrastructure. Yet, there are an increasing number of examples in the United States and globally of what community control looks like. For example, on the island of Eigg, Scotland, islanders have established a combination of wind, solar, and hydroelectric power sources, collectively known as the Eigg Electric Grid.[57] They have control over energy production, reducing their reliance on external sources.

EJ advocates have long called for a **just transition**, as described by the Climate Justice Alliance, "a vision-led, unifying, and place-based set of principles, processes, and practices that build economic and political power to shift from an extractive economy to a regenerative economy. This means approaching production and consumption cycles holistically and waste-free."[58(para1)] This framework calls for energy democracy using a multipronged approach that involves communities in decision-making, particularly those communities most burdened by energy's health impacts.

ELECTRIFICATION

In the United States, the heavier use of electricity for heating and cooling can put a lot of pressure on the power grid, especially during busy times. To address this concern, there are programs that encourage people to use less electricity when demand is high by charging more money during those times. For example, the cost of electricity might be increased when a lot of people are using AC. However, studies have found that this pricing strategy can negatively affect the health of households with disabled or low-wealth residents, as they may be more impacted by higher costs and warmer temperatures. Low-wealth households also tend to wait longer before using AC, putting them at risk of higher heat exposure. While higher wealth households overall have higher electricity demands, a study of electricity-demand response has demonstrated that low-wealth households are more responsive to price-based incentives.[59]

In the United States, there is widespread support for the electrification of heating. Using electric heat pumps can save money, especially in new buildings. Heat pumps extract heat from a nearby source, such as surrounding air or water or from geothermal energy stored underground, and amplify and transfer this heat. But upgrading existing buildings in cold areas from natural gas to electric heat pumps may increase energy bills. This increase could exacerbate energy access inequities, especially because lower wealth families often live in less efficient homes and have reduced access to efficient technologies. There is also a bias toward cheaper and less efficient upgrades for heating and cooling systems in low-wealth areas when homeowners have to pay for replacements themselves. A survey even showed that energy-efficient LED bulbs are harder to find and more expensive in areas with high poverty.[60]

In addition to supporting energy-efficient households, the United States and many other nations are navigating the transition from internal-combustion engine vehicles to electric vehicles. Some individuals, local governments, and corporations are among the earlier adopters. For instance, in early 2023, New York City used $10.1 million in federal grants to replace nearly 925 fossil-fuel-powered fleet vehicles with electric vehicles and to install 315 new chargers across the city.[61] Much work is underway to incentivize car companies to produce electric vehicles and for states to build the charging infrastructure necessary to scale up their use in our daily lives.[62] As the cost of electric vehicles decreases, technology advances, and perceptions shift, electric vehicles may be the norm in the United States within a few decades.

IMPROVING ENERGY EFFICIENCY THROUGH WEATHERIZATION

Weatherization is a way to make homes more efficient and reduce energy bills. Weatherization may include adding insulation; sealing drafts; and repairing heating, ventilation, and air conditioning (HVAC) systems. Studies show that weatherization programs can significantly reduce energy consumption and bills, helping to address energy inequality.[63–65] Combining weatherization with solar and electrification programs can have even greater benefits, reducing greenhouse gas emissions and providing financial savings.

Many of these interventions may be too costly for low- or middle-wealth households, but low-wealth households can get support through programs like the DOE's Weatherization Assistance Program (WAP). Such weatherization programs install energy-efficient measures in homes for free to qualified households. One national evaluation of WAP found that the program reduced consumption of natural gas by almost 19% in single family homes heated with natural gas.* Electricity consumption was also reduced in these homes by weatherization. Reduced energy bills reduce energy burdens.

However, some argue that WAP has major limitations. It can be inflexible as it limits the kinds of repairs that are allowable. Many benefits are probably best achieved through comprehensive weatherization programs that address multiple problems all at once. For example, reducing fire risk can be accomplished through furnace upgrade, insulation, and electrical repairs.[67] Another example is that of AC, which is increasingly necessary to maintain safe indoor temperatures in the summer in many climates. The use of AC may become affordable to households when accompanied by air sealing, insulation, and the installation of an energy-efficient air-conditioning system. In contrast, the installation of an AC system without upgrades to the building envelope may leave families still unable to afford the cost of running the unit.

Weatherization not only saves energy, but also has nonenergy impacts on health and well-being (Figure 9.6).[68–76] It improves indoor conditions, reduces the risk of fire and carbon monoxide poisoning, and enhances air quality. Financial benefits from reduced bills can alleviate stress and improve overall health. Comprehensive weatherization programs can address

---

*A summary of recent evaluations of the WAP, containing estimates for both energy-costs savings and energy savings for single-family homes, mobile homes, and multifamily buildings that heat with a variety of fuels and are located across the United States can be found in Tonn et al.[66]

multiple issues, such as fire risk and the need for AC. Research indicates that weatherization positively impacts the quality of life by improving general health, mental health, social well-being, indoor air quality, thermal comfort, and reducing noise and financial stress. Overall, weatherization is a holistic approach that goes beyond just energy savings, making homes healthier and more comfortable for residents.

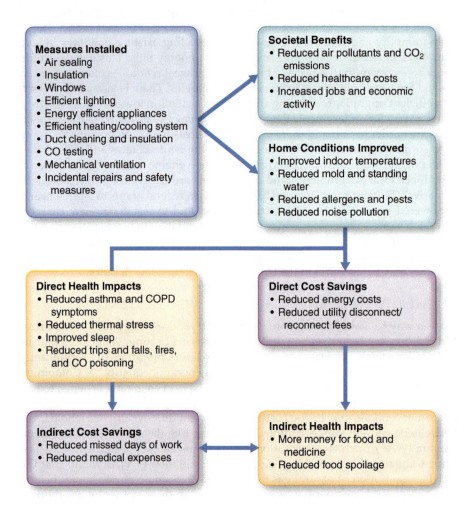

FIGURE 9.6. How weatherization can produce nonenergy benefits.
CO, carbon monoxide; CO_2, carbon dioxide; COPD, chronic obstructive pulmonary disease.

IN OTHER WORDS: HOW DOES NORTH AMERICA'S ELECTRICITY CURRENTLY REACH HOUSEHOLDS?

For those privileged enough to live in places with semireliable or reliable energy systems, we flip a light switch, drive our car, or plug in our devices, and things generally work for us. Are we relying on coal, natural gas, or other sources of energy for these daily activities? Many of us do not know exactly how electricity works and who controls it in our communities.

In simple terms, electricity is generated at power plants and may come from a variety of energy sources, including coal, natural gas, nuclear energy, or renewable energy. Electricity is transported primarily through high-voltage transmission lines across the United States to substations. These substations manage the flow and send electricity out to our homes, businesses, schools, workplaces, and so forth through low-voltage transmission lines to power our lives.

(continued)

IN OTHER WORDS: HOW DOES NORTH AMERICA'S ELECTRICITY CURRENTLY REACH HOUSEHOLDS? (*continued*)

More specifically, in North America, 10 regional transmission organizations (RTOs) operate our electric power systems (Figure 9.7). RTOs are nonprofit organizations that work to ensure reliability and respond to demands for wholesale electric power. In the United States, RTOs manage about 60% of the power supplied to utilities. In other parts of the country, electricity systems are operated by individual utilities. Utilities are generally for-profit companies, but they are regulated as part of the public service infrastructure. RTOs are responsible for purchasing power from generators and reselling it to utilities, who then resell it again to end-use customers, including households, municipalities, and businesses. RTOs post electricity prices for thousands of locations, with updates occurring as often as every 5 minutes.[77]

How much of this energy is distributed to households, and how are we using it? According to the U.S Environmental Protection Agency (EPA), residential energy accounts for 21% of total U.S. consumed energy. Electricity and gas energy are the two most common forms of energy used in a home.[78,79] Furthermore, 52% of a household's annual energy consumption is directed toward air conditioning and space heating. This means that households across the country are spending most of their home's energy to heat and cool the space, depending on where they live.

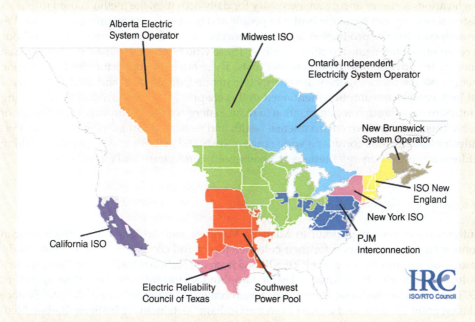

FIGURE 9.7. The 10 RTOs in North America.

ISO, independent system operator; PMJ, Pennsylvania-New Jersey-Maryland; RTOs, regional transmission organizations.

Source: U.S. Energy Information Administration. About 60% of the U.S. electric power supply is managed by RTOs. April 4, 2011. https://www.eia.gov/todayinenergy/detail.php?id=790

MAIN TAKEAWAYS

In this chapter we learned that:

- Energy production and use impacts health in a variety of ways.
- Energy extraction impacts the health of workers around the world who are often treated unfairly and exposed to harsh physical and chemical conditions.

- Redlined neighborhoods tend to be in close proximity to energy production centers (e.g., coal plants), and houses in these neighborhoods often fail to protect residents from toxicants and high energy costs.
- A transition toward renewable energy requires decentralized and distributed energy pathways and upgraded infrastructure.
- Weatherization programs can have positive impacts by reducing energy poverty and improving household health.
- Energy justice is needed in communities experiencing a heavy exposure to toxicants while using a relatively smaller fraction of energy, and efforts toward a stronger energy democracy can benefit environmental health for all.

SUMMARY

This chapter recognizes the interplay between society's energy use and our environmental health. Once again in this textbook, we must consider the historical factors that shape these issues today—from our early days of primarily burning biomass to our modern-day culture that drives fossil fuel consumption. By design, our economy continues to rely heavily on fossil fuels. Although various forms of energy are necessary for daily activities, the methods used to extract and distribute energy can harm the health of people and our environment on a global scale. We have examined what the production and use of energy means for local communities and our global community with regard to climate justice. Those who benefit the most are often the least burdened by the adverse health impacts and costs. There are many opportunities to reimagine our energy systems, including the ways energy is generated, distributed, and used. Solutions to combat high energy consumption mentioned in this chapter include electrification, improving home infrastructure through weatherization to reduce energy costs, and an increase in the use of renewable energy. To achieve environmental health and justice, community, agency, academic, and industry leaders must consider a wide range of costs and benefits in energy policy making and address inequitable energy burdens at a household, community, and global scale.

ACKNOWLEDGMENTS

The authors are extremely grateful to Michelle Martinez and Bridget Vial of the Michigan Environmental Justice Coalition for their coleadership of and contributions to the case study. The case study was funded by grant P30ES017885 from the National Institute for Environmental Health Sciences. We also acknowledge Dr. Gronlund's funding from the following grants: R01ES032157 from the National Institute for Environmental Health Sciences, National Science Foundation grant 1952038, and a grant from the Graham Sustainability Institute Carbon Neutrality Acceleration Program. We also thank Brittni Delmaine for her contributions and editing.

END-OF-CHAPTER RESOURCES

DISCUSSION QUESTIONS

1. Describe some of the major EJ issues related to energy use. How might we begin to address them in the United States? How might we begin to address them globally?
2. After reading this chapter, what challenges and opportunities do you see as we work to transition the United States to a regenerative economy?
3. The proceeding chapters discuss issues related to air pollution; water quality and access; food safety, security, and sovereignty; and waste management. In considering these interconnected topics, how do you think energy relates to each one?

4. Have you ever calculated your carbon footprint? If not, there are many online tools to try if you do a quick search. Reflect on what you learn about your own energy consumption. Many argue that this tool is useful for individuals or institutions to reflect on their environmental impacts, but it can also shift attention away from the fossil-fuel industry's role in climate change. In your opinion, how are carbon footprint calculators useful?

LEARNING ACTIVITIES
THE TIME IS NOW

In Case Study 9.1, Michigan residents leaned on community–academic research to inform advocacy efforts. The team called on the Michigan Public Service Commission to consider energy justice in their decision-making process. This commission approves IRPs put forth by companies like DTE Energy and Consumers Energy. IRPs include information about how each utility company will set rates, increase infrastructure investments, and address issues related to service quality and reliability, as well as the breakdown of energy sources (e.g., percentage of natural gas and the percentage of renewable energy) they will rely on.

Each state has its own Public Utility Commission or Public Service Commission (the names may vary by state). These commissions are responsible for regulating utilities within their respective states.

Do some research. Some questions you might investigate:

- What is your state's commission called?
- Who sits on the commission? Are the members appointed (by whom) or elected? (How members are chosen varies by state.)
- Does the commission consider environmental health and justice in their oversight of energy providers?
- Who are the major energy providers in your state? What is their energy portfolio? (In other words, what percentage of their electricity comes from fossil fuels compared to renewable sources?) Where is their major infrastructure located?

If you have concerns about what you learn, reach out to your state's commissioners and advocate for addressing them.

IN REAL LIFE

Factors such as geographic location, climate, and household size are all considerations when understanding household energy use. Although many of the changes needed to achieve a just energy transition require policy changes, it is helpful for individuals and households to learn more about their energy use.

Begin by looking at your household's utility bill. Does it tell you what types of energy are supporting your household?

Next, here are some energy-efficiency exercises you might try to monitor home energy use and reduce your energy consumption:

- The DOE's Do-It-Yourself Home Energy Assessment: www.energy.gov/energysaver/do-it-yourself-home-energy-assessments
- Energy Savers: Tips on Saving Money and Energy at Home: www.energy.gov/sites/prod/files/2013/06/f2/energy_savers.pdf

Some of these efforts may be costly or require additional approvals, for example, from landlords, homeowner associations, or local governments. Others may be affordable and relatively simple. For instance, basic weatherization tactics such as insulating windows and sealing drafts can be helpful to keep cold air out during the winter months. Installing white window shades and using white curtains during the summer can reflect heat. Solutions to reduce your energy bill that do not involve changes to the home's infrastructure include:

- using energy-saving lightbulbs,
- using ENERGY STAR products like refrigerators and laundry machines,
- unplugging phone chargers and electronics when not at home, and
- washing only full loads of clothes and dishes.

A robust set of instructor resources designed to supplement this text is located at http://connect.springerpub.com/content/book/978-0-8261-8353-8. Qualifying instructors may request access by emailing textbook@springerpub.com.

REFERENCES

1. Stepka Z, Azuri I, Horwitz LK, Chazan M, Natalio F. Hidden signatures of early fire at Evron Quarry (1.0 to 0.8 Mya). *Proc Natl Acad Sci U S A*. 2022;119(25):e2123439119. doi:10.1073/pnas.2123439119
2. U.S. Environmental Protection Agency. Smoke from residential wood burning. Indoor Air Quality (IAQ). December 2, 2014. Updated January 30, 2024. https://www.epa.gov/indoor-air-quality-iaq/smoke-residential-wood-burning
3. U.S. Environmental Protection Agency. Wood smoke and your health. Burn wise. May 28, 2013. Updated April 9, 2024. https://www.epa.gov/burnwise/wood-smoke-and-your-health
4. Hubbard TD, Murray IA, Bisson WH, et al. Divergent Ah receptor ligand selectivity during hominin evolution. *Mol Biol Evol*. 2016;33(10):2648–2658. doi:10.1093/molbev/msw143
5. World Health Organization. Household air pollution. December 15, 2023. https://www.who.int/news-room/fact-sheets/detail/household-air-pollution-and-health
6. United States Environmental Protection Agency. Indoor air quality. November 2, 2017. Updated July 14, 2023. https://www.epa.gov/report-environment/indoor-air-quality
7. Biomass energy basics. National Renewable Energy Laboratory. Accessed June 17, 2024. https://www.nrel.gov/research/re-biomass.html
8. Xu Y, Li J, Tan Q, Peters AL, Yang C. Global status of recycling waste solar panels: a review. *Waste Manag*. 2018;75:450–458. doi:10.1016/j.wasman.2018.01.036
9. Can wind turbines and migrating birds coexist? Max Planck Society. Updated April 20, 2022. https://phys.org/news/2022-04-turbines-migrating-birds-coexist.html
10. Mejía-Montero A, Jenkins KEH, van der Horst D, Lane M. An intersectional approach to energy justice: individual and collective concerns around wind power on Zapotec land. *Energy Res Soc Sci*. 2023;98:103015. doi:10.1016/j.erss.2023.103015
11. Stone B, Mallen E, Rajput M, et al. Compound climate and infrastructure events: how electrical grid failure alters heat wave risk. *Environ Sci Technol*. 2021;55(10):6957–6964. doi:10.1021/acs.est.1c00024
12. Stone B, Gronlund CJ, Mallen E, et al. How blackouts during heat waves amplify mortality and morbidity risk. *Environ Sci Technol*. 2023;57(22):8245–8255. doi:10.1021/acs.est.2c09588
13. Coal and the environment. U.S. Energy Information Administration. Updated April 17, 2024. https://www.eia.gov/energyexplained/coal/coal-and-the-environment.php
14. Fossil fuels: the dirty facts. Natural Resources Defense Council. June 1, 2022. https://www.nrdc.org/stories/fossil-fuels-dirty-facts
15. Centers for Disease Control and Prevention. Pneumoconioses. May 23, 2023. https://www.cdc.gov/niosh/topics/pneumoconioses/default.html
16. Miner health matters. Mine Safety and Health Administration. Accessed June 17, 2024. https://www.msha.gov/miner-health-matters
17. U.S. Energy Information Administration. Natural gas explained. December 27, 2022. https://www.eia.gov/energyexplained/natural-gas/
18. Alvarez RA, Zavala-Araiza D, Lyon DR, et al. Assessment of methane emissions from the U.S. oil and gas supply chain. *Science*. 2018;361(6398):186–188. doi:10.1126/science.aar7204

19. American Geosciences Institute. How can metal mining impact the environment? November 13, 2014. https://www.americangeosciences.org/critical-issues/faq/how-can-metal-mining-impact-environment
20. Concas A, Ardau C, Cristini A, Zuddas P, Cao G. Mobility of heavy metals from tailings to stream waters in a mining activity contaminated site. *Chemosphere*. 2006;63(2):244–253. doi:10.1016/j.chemosphere.2005.08.024
21. Tedesco M. The paradox of lithium. state of the planet. January 18, 2023. https://news.climate.columbia.edu/2023/01/18/the-paradox-of-lithium/
22. Cobalt. Geology and Mineral Resources. Virginia Department of Energy. Accessed June 16, 2024. https://energy.virginia.gov/geology/Cobalt.shtml
23. Gross T. How "modern-day slavery" in the Congo powers the rechargeable battery economy. NPR. February 1, 2023. https://www.npr.org/sections/goatsandsoda/2023/02/01/1152893248/red-cobalt-congo-drc-mining-siddharth-kara
24. Paustenbach DJ, Tvermoes BE, Unice KM, Finley BL, Kerger BD. A review of the health hazards posed by cobalt. *Crit Rev Toxicol*. 2013;43(4):316–362. doi:10.3109/10408444.2013.779633
25. Lison D. Cobalt. In: Nordberg GF, Fowler BA, Nordberg M, eds. *Handbook on the Toxicology of Metals*. Vol 2. Elsevier; 2015:743–763.
26. Banza Lubaba Nkulu C, Casas L, Haufroid V, et al. Sustainability of artisanal mining of cobalt in DR Congo. *Nat Sustain*. 2018;1(9):495–504. doi:10.1038/s41893-018-0139-4
27. Davey C. The environmental impacts of cobalt mining in Congo. Earth.org. March 28, 2023. https://earth.org/cobalt-mining-in-congo/
28. Brusselen DV, Kayembe-Kitenge T, Mbuyi-Musanzayi S, et al. Metal mining and birth defects: a case-control study in Lubumbashi, Democratic Republic of the Congo. *Lancet Planet Health*. 2020;4(4):e158–e167. doi:10.1016/S2542-5196(20)30059-0
29. International Energy Agency. SDG7: Data and Projections. September 2023. https://www.iea.org/reports/sdg7-data-and-projections
30. United Nations Conference on Trade and Development. Over half of the people in least developed countries lack access to electricity. July 1, 2021. https://unctad.org/topic/least-developed-countries/chart-july-2021
31. World Bank. Report: Universal Access to Sustainable Energy will Remain Elusive without Addressing Inequalities. June 7, 2021. https://www.worldbank.org/en/news/press-release/2021/06/07/report-universal-access-to-sustainable-energy-will-remain-elusive-without-addressing-inequalities
32. Access to electricity, urban vs. rural, 2021. Our World in Data. Accessed June 16, 2024. https://ourworldindata.org/grapher/access-to-electricity-urban-vs-rural
33. Almeshqab F, Ustun TS. Lessons learned from rural electrification initiatives in developing countries: insights for technical, social, financial and public policy aspects. *Renew Sustain Energy Rev*. 2019;102:35–53. doi:10.1016/j.rser.2018.11.035
34. Hernández D. Understanding "energy insecurity" and why it matters to health. *Soc Sci Med*. 2016;167:1–10. doi:10.1016/j.socscimed.2016.08.029
35. Nigerian Oil Spill Monitor. Accessed June 16, 2024. https://nosdra.oilspillmonitor.ng/
36. United Nations Environment Programme. Environmental Assessment of Ogoniland. January 17, 2011. http://www.unep.org/resources/report/environmental-assessment-ogoniland
37. Owolabi T. Nigeria investigates Shell's Trans Niger pipeline spill. *Reuters*. June 26, 2023. https://www.reuters.com/business/energy/nigeria-investigates-shells-trans-niger-pipeline-spill-2023-06-26/
38. Saint E. Timeline: half a century of oil spills in Nigeria's Ogoniland. *Aljazeera*. December 21, 2022. https://www.aljazeera.com/features/2022/12/21/timeline-oil-spills-in-nigerias-ogoniland
39. Uguru H, Faula M. Militants bomb Nigerian state-owned Trans Forcados pipeline. *AP News*. November 2, 2016. https://apnews.com/article/153df3990df54393842122c638dd8625
40. Obida CB, Blackburn GA, Whyatt JD, Semple KT. Counting the cost of the Niger Delta's largest oil spills: satellite remote sensing reveals extensive environmental damage with >1 million people in the impact zone. *Sci Total Environ*. 2021;775:145854. doi:10.1016/j.scitotenv.2021.145854
41. American Council for an Energy-Efficient Economy. Report: Low-income Households, Communities of Color Face High "Energy Burden" Entering Recession. September 10, 2020. https://www.aceee.org/press-release/2020/09/report-low-income-households-communities-color-face-high-energy-burden

42. About the Residential Energy Consumption Survey (RECS): table HC1.1 fuels used and end uses in U.S. homes by housing unit type, 2015. U.S. Energy Information Administration. May 2018. https://www.eia.gov/consumption/residential/data/2015/hc/php/hc11.1.php
43. Mehdipanah R, McVay KR, Schulz AJ. Historic redlining practices and contemporary determinants of health in the Detroit metropolitan area. *Am J Public Health*. 2023;113(S1):S49–S57. doi:10.2105/AJPH.2022.307162
44. Swope CB, Hernández D, Cushing LJ. The relationship of historical redlining with present-day neighborhood environmental and health outcomes: a scoping review and conceptual model. *J Urban Health*. 2022;99(6):959–983. doi:10.1007/s11524-022-00665-z
45. Cushing LJ, Li S, Steiger BB, Casey JA. Historical red-lining is associated with fossil fuel power plant siting and present-day inequalities in air pollutant emissions. *Nat Energy*. 2023;8(1):52–61. doi:10.1038/s41560-022-01162-y
46. Gonzalez DJX, Nardone A, Nguyen AV, Morello-Frosch R, Casey JA. Historic redlining and the siting of oil and gas wells in the United States. *J Expo Sci Environ Epidemiol*. 2023;33(1):76–83. doi:10.1038/s41370-022-00434-9
47. Weatherization. U.S. Department of Energy. Accessed June 16, 2024. https://www.energy.gov/energysaver/weatherization
48. Appliances and electronics. U.S. Department of Energy. Accessed June 16, 2024. https://www.energy.gov/energysaver/appliances-and-electronics
49. Sugrue TJ. *The Origins of the Urban Crisis*. Princeton University Press; 2014. https://press.princeton.edu/books/paperback/9780691162553/the-origins-of-the-urban-crisis
50. Gronlund CJ, Berrocal VJ. Modeling and comparing central and room air conditioning ownership and cold-season in-home thermal comfort using the American Housing Survey. *J Expo Sci Environ Epidemiol*. 2020;30(5):814–823. doi:10.1038/s41370-020-0220-8
51. Martenies SE, Milando CW, Williams GO, Batterman SA. Disease and health inequalities attributable to air pollutant exposure in Detroit, Michigan. *Int J Environ Res Public Health*. 2017;14(10):1243. doi:10.3390/ijerph14101243
52. James JD. Michigan regulators approve DTE plan to cut pollution, close Monroe plant. *Bridge Michigan*. July 26, 2023. https://www.bridgemi.com/michigan-environment-watch/michigan-regulators-approve-dte-plan-cut-pollution-close-monroe-plant
53. SB-100 California Renewables Portfolio Standard Program: emissions of greenhouse gases: Chapter 312. September 10, 2018. https://leginfo.legislature.ca.gov/faces/billNavClient.xhtml?bill_id=201720180SB100
54. Ensure access to affordable, reliable, sustainable and modern energy. Sustainable Development Goals. United Nations. Accessed June 17, 2024. https://www.un.org/sustainabledevelopment/energy/
55. Henneman LRF, Rasel MM, Choirat C, Anenberg SC, Zigler C. Inequitable exposures to U.S. coal power plant–related PM$_{2.5}$: 22 years and counting. *Environ Health Perspect*. 2023;131(3):37005. doi:10.1289/EHP11605
56. U.S. Energy Information Administration. Coal prices and outlook. Coal Explained. October 27, 2022. Updated Apri 17, 2024. https://www.eia.gov/energyexplained/coal/prices-and-outlook.php
57. Eigg Electric. The Isle of Eigg. Accessed June 16, 2024. http://isleofeigg.org/eigg-electric/
58. Just transition: a framework for change. Climate Justice Alliance. Accessed June 16, 2024. https://climatejusticealliance.org/just-transition/
59. Hansen AR, Leiria D, Johra H, Marszal-Pomianowska A. Who produces the peaks? Household variation in peak energy demand for space heating and domestic hot water. *Energies*. 2022;15(24):9505. doi:10.3390/en15249505
60. Reames TG, Reiner MA, Stacey MB. An incandescent truth: disparities in energy-efficient lighting availability and prices in an urban U.S. county. *Appl Energy*. 2018;218:95–103. doi:10.1016/j.apenergy.2018.02.143
61. Mayor Adams announces nearly 1,000 new electric vehicles. NYC.gov. January 4, 2023. http://www.nyc.gov/office-of-the-mayor/news/003-23/mayor-adams-nearly-1-000-new-electric-vehicles-replace-fossil-fuel-powered-city-fleet
62. The White House. Fact sheet: Biden-Harris administration announces new private and public sector investments for affordable electric vehicles. April 17, 2023. https://www.whitehouse.gov/briefing-room/statements-releases/2023/04/17/fact-sheet-biden-harris-administration-announces-new-private-and-public-sector-investments-for-affordable-electric-vehicles/

63. Tonn B, Hawkins B, Rose E, Marincic M. Income, housing and health: poverty in the United States through the prism of residential energy efficiency programs. *Energy Res Soc Sci*. 2021;73:101945. doi:10.1016/j.erss.2021.101945
64. Hernández D. Energy insecurity: a framework for understanding energy, the built environment, and health among vulnerable populations in the context of climate change. *Am J Public Health*. 2013;103(4):e32–e34. doi:10.2105/AJPH.2012.301179
65. Hernández D, Phillips D. Benefit or burden? Perceptions of energy efficiency efforts among low-income housing residents in New York City. *Energy Res Soc Sci*. 2015;8:52–59. doi:10.1016/j.erss.2015.04.010
66. Tonn B, Rose E, Hawkins B. Evaluation of the U.S. Department of Energy's weatherization assistance program: impact results. *Energy Policy*. 2018;118:279–290. doi:10.1016/j.enpol.2018.03.051
67. Rose EM, Hawkins BA, Tonn BE. *Exploring Potential Impacts of Weatherization and Healthy Homes Interventions on Asthma-Related Medicaid Claims and Costs in a Small Cohort in Washington State*. Oak Ridge National Lab (ORNL); 2015. doi:10.2172/1354644
68. Tonn B, Rose E, Hawkins B, Marincic M. Health and financial benefits of weatherizing low-income homes in the southeastern United States. *Build Environ*. 2021;197:107847. doi:10.1016/j.buildenv.2021.107847
69. Tang J, Chen N, Liang H, Gao X. The effect of built environment on physical health and mental health of adults: a nationwide cross-sectional study in China. *Int J Environ Res Public Health*. 2022;19(11):6492. doi:10.3390/ijerph19116492
70. Baker E, Lester L, Mason K, Bentley R. Mental health and prolonged exposure to unaffordable housing: a longitudinal analysis. *Soc Psychiatry Psychiatr Epidemiol*. 2020;55(6):715–721. doi:10.1007/s00127-020-01849-1
71. Kang S. The cumulative relationship between housing instability and mental health: findings from the Panel Study of Income Dynamics. *J Soc Distress Homelessness*. 2022;31(2):191–203. doi:10.1080/10530789.2021.1925038
72. Rolfe S, Garnham L, Godwin J, Anderson I, Seaman P, Donaldson C. Housing as a social determinant of health and wellbeing: developing an empirically-informed realist theoretical framework. *BMC Public Health*. 2020;20(1):1138. doi:10.1186/s12889-020-09224-0
73. Brown MA, Soni A, Lapsa MV, Southworth K. *Low-Income Energy Affordability: Conclusions from a Literature Review*. Oak Ridge National Lab (ORNL); 2020. doi:10.2172/1607178
74. Shrubsole C, Macmillan A, Davies M, May N. 100 unintended consequences of policies to improve the energy efficiency of the UK housing stock. *Indoor Built Environ*. 2014;23(3):340–352. doi:10.1177/1420326X14524586
75. Skumatz LA. Non-Energy Benefits/Non-Energy Impacts (NEBs/NEIs) and their role & values in cost-effectiveness tests: State of Maryland. Energy Efficiency for All. March 31, 2014. https://www-new.energyefficiencyforall.org/resources/non-energy-benefits-non-energy-impacts-nebs-neis-and-their-role-and-values/
76. Willand N, Ridley I, Maller C. Towards explaining the health impacts of residential energy efficiency interventions—a realist review. Part 1: pathways. *Soc Sci Med*. 2015;133:191–201. doi:10.1016/j.socscimed.2015.02.005
77. United States Energy Information Administration. About 60% of the U.S. electric power supply is managed by RTOs. April 1, 2011. https://www.eia.gov/todayinenergy/detail.php?id=790
78. Use of energy explained: Energy use in homes. U.S. Energy Information Administration. Updated December 18, 2023. https://www.eia.gov/energyexplained/use-of-energy/homes.php
79. U.S. Department of Energy. Energy savers: tips on saving money & energy at home. Office of Energy Efficiency and Renewable Energy. 2011. https://www.energy.gov/sites/prod/files/2013/06/f2/energy_savers.pdf

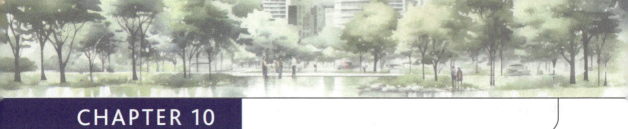

CHAPTER 10

The Air We Breathe

Beto Lugo Martinez and Shir Lerman Ginzburg

LEARNING OBJECTIVES

- Describe various types and sources of indoor and outdoor air pollution, as well as the many different effects of air pollution on human health.
- Describe a few major air pollution events in history.
- Demonstrate the successes and limits of current federal, state, and local responses to air pollution, particularly describing ways that environmental justice is not adequately addressed.
- Recognize the importance of community-led environmental health research.
- Highlight the importance of prioritizing and working with frontline communities in decision-making for policies and investments earmarked to improve air quality for all.
- Underline the ways that many people have responsibility for improving air quality, including public health practitioners; researchers; government staff at the local, state, and federal levels; elected officials; industry leaders; community advocates; and professionals in other sectors (e.g., in planning, housing, and education).

KEY TERMS

- air pollution
- ambient air pollutants
- community science
- cumulative impacts
- environmental justice (EJ)
- fenceline communities
- sensitive receptors

OVERVIEW

The World Health Organization (WHO) estimates that air pollution is among the top five leading causes of death worldwide.[1] A large majority, more than 90%, of these deaths occur in low- and middle-income countries, primarily in Southeast Asia and the Western Pacific.[1] In particular, indoor air pollution was responsible for approximately 3.2 million deaths in 2020, including the deaths of over 237,000 children under the age of 5.[2]

Air pollution is the modification and contamination of indoor or outdoor environments by any physical, chemical, or biological agent in the air that interferes with human health.[3,4] The most common sources of air pollution are:

- the burning of fossil fuels in electricity generation,
- transportation,
- forest fires,
- household combustion devices (e.g., vehicles that burn diesel or oil, gas stoves), and
- industrial combustion (e.g., coal burners, commercial boilers).

These varied sources emit pollutants such as particulate matter (PM), carbon monoxide, ozone, nitrogen dioxide, and sulfur dioxide, as well as other hazardous chemicals into the air.[5] Many air pollutants are also greenhouse gasses that contribute to climate change, with the most common including carbon dioxide, methane, nitrous oxide, and fluorinated gasses. Our air is a vital part of our global ecosystem.

Although there have been pollutants in the air for longer than humans have existed, it is important to recognize the overall staggering increases that have occurred over the past century from both slight increases over time and urgent air pollution events.[6] This chapter discusses how air pollution is a widespread problem that affects everyone, although some are burdened more than others. We interweave a firsthand account of growing up in a community harmed by redlining and environmental racism and an example of community-based participatory research (CBPR) that was used to address air pollution and related health inequities. After completing this chapter, the reader will see that much work remains, and that there is a need for ongoing efforts to reduce air pollution through regulatory standards, rule making, and legislation that tackle the underlying causes of environmental injustice in our changing climate.

HISTORY OF AIR POLLUTION

The earliest recorded account of air pollution dates to around 400 BCE, when Hippocrates published a book titled *Airs, Waters, and Places* that documented a variety of illnesses thought to be associated with unclean air, such as having a hoarse voice from living in cities with damp westerly winds.[7] The ancient Romans referred to the smog in Rome as *gravioris Caeli* ("heavy heaven") and *infamis aer* ("infamous air"); the philosopher Seneca remarked in 61 BCE that his health immediately improved upon leaving behind the poisonous fumes, clouds of ash, and oppressive atmosphere of Rome.[7]

Multiple air-pollution-related incidents occurred in the 20th century that led to legislation to improve air quality. In October 1948, a deadly phenomenon hit the town of Donora, Pennsylvania, just in time for Halloween. A lethal blanket of gray smog encased the town for five days, causing such poor visibility that people could not see far enough ahead to leave town despite the strong urgings of the town's doctor. By the time the smog dissipated, 20 people had died, another 6,000 of the town's 14,000 residents were experiencing such severe respiratory and cardiovascular problems that the region's hospitals were overflowing, and the community center had been converted into a morgue.[8] It was later determined that two factories in the region, the American Steel and Wire Plant and Donora Zinc Works, were emitting a dangerous combination of poisonous gasses, heavy metals, and fine PM into the air, all of which were trapped under a pocket of warm air in the narrow valley surrounding Donora.[8,9] The Donora Smog, as the event came to be known, is the deadliest air pollution crisis in the United States to date.

Likewise, the Great Smog that smothered London for five days in December 1952 was attributed to an anticyclone that passed over London, in which pollution was trapped under a pocket of warm air, much like what occurred in Donora.[10] Owing to trapped gas emissions from nearby factories and coal burning to heat homes during unseasonably cold temperatures, there were anywhere from 3,500 to 4,000 deaths and more than 100,000 ill people, although more recent estimates place the total death rate at around 12,000 people.[11]

More recently, the Bhopal Gas Tragedy was a chemical accident that occurred in Bhopal, India, in December 1984. Over 40 tons of methyl isocyanate gas spilled from the Union Carbide pesticide plant, immediately killing over 3,800 people, and causing significant illness for many more people at both the pesticide plant and in the surrounding villages.[12] The Indian government initially tried to distance itself from one of the worst industrial accidents on record. However, the government eventually reached a settlement with Union Carbide in 1989 through the Indian Supreme Court and paid more than $470 million in damages to the over 500,000 survivors.[13] Even then, Union Carbide continued to deny responsibility, no cleanup has been done, and no one has ever been brought to justice for their role in the disaster.

THE BASICS OF AIR POLLUTION

Air pollution takes many forms. It is typically classified by whether it is indoor or outdoor and by its chemical composition. However, it is sometimes difficult to know the chemical composition or determine the "speciation" of pollutants, such as with PM that may be composed of various chemicals (Figure 10.1).

INDOOR AIR POLLUTANTS

Americans spend roughly 90% of their time indoors, and WHO estimates that 3.2 million people worldwide die every year from harmful indoor air quality. Many different indoor air pollutants are found in our homes, workplaces, schools, and other places we frequent. Without a properly sealed structure or effective heating, ventilation, and air conditioning, cooling (HVAC) and filtration, some outdoor air pollution makes its way inside. For instance, homes and schools near trucking routes or industry may have worse indoor air quality than those in areas with fewer pollution sources. Much indoor air pollution occurs as a result of human activity and products, including: [14-16]

- smoking;
- household cleaning products;
- scented products (e.g., air fresheners, candles);
- fossil fuel stoves and heating;
- common building materials and carpet installation;
- burning wood, fuel, or coal for heating or cooking; and
- appliances with hydrofluorocarbons (e.g., air conditioners, refrigerators).

Mold and pollen may also affect indoor air quality with implications for health. Naturally occurring radon can also seep into buildings via cracked foundations or minor cracks or pores in the structure.

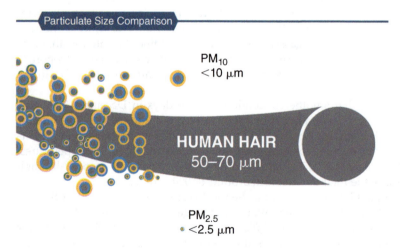

FIGURE 10.1. Comparison of PM sizes.

PM sizes vary from $PM_{2.5}$ (PM that is 2.5 micrometers or less in diameter) to PM_{10} (PM that is 10 micrometers or less); $PM_{2.5}$, or fine PM, is considered especially dangerous because of its small size, which makes it easier to penetrate the alveoli of the lungs and enter the bloodstream.

PM, particulate matter.

Source: Inhalable particulate matter and health ($PM_{2.5}$ and PM_{10}). California Air Resources Board. 2023. https://ww2.arb.ca.gov/resources/inhalable-particulate-matter-and-health

The changes needed to reduce indoor air pollution are not always accessible or affordable, of course. For instance, many communities on the frontline of multiple pollution sources consist of multifamily-dwelling rental households who may have little to no power or resources to address housing conditions as they relate to building materials, HVAC, or appliances. Given the amount of time humans spend indoors and the number of deaths associated with indoor air pollution, urgency is needed to hold fossil fuel, petrochemical, and utility industries, as well as landlords and government leaders, accountable for inaction on this major public health issue.[17,18]

CASE STUDY 10.1: Out of Gas, In With Justice

Burning fossil fuels in residential buildings, particularly using gas stoves for cooking and heating, poses a major threat to environmental health. Gas stoves release pollutants like nitrogen oxide and carbon monoxide, which can lead to respiratory and cardiovascular illnesses.

This problem disproportionately affects communities that are of low wealth and communities of color already burdened by air pollution, rising energy costs, poor housing, and climate change. In New York, for instance, gas stoves are responsible for 19% of childhood asthma cases, predominantly impacting Black and Hispanic or Latino children and young adults.

New York's Climate Leadership and Community Protection Act, passed in 2019, commits the state to achieve 100% zero-emission electricity by 2040. This transition to electric buildings and appliances powered by renewable energy is crucial for reducing greenhouse gas emissions and improving air quality.

The "Out of Gas, In With Justice" pilot study by WE ACT for Environmental Justice examined the feasibility and benefits of transitioning from gas to electric stoves in New York City Housing Authority apartments.[19] The study focused on indoor air quality improvements and resident satisfaction. It involved air-quality monitoring during daily activities, controlled cooking tests, and stove-usability focus groups.

Participants in the study overwhelmingly preferred induction stoves for their ease of use, time-saving benefits, and safety. They felt relieved as safety concerns about gas stoves were eliminated with induction stoves. No household requested their gas stove back at the study's end.

In the controlled cooking test, gas stoves produced high nitrogen dioxide levels, averaging 197 parts per billion (ppb), exceeding the U.S. Environmental Protection Agency's (EPA's) "Unhealthy for Sensitive Groups" threshold. Induction stoves maintained 14 ppb, similar to background levels. Nitrogen dioxide concentrations in gas stoves were on average 190% higher than in induction stoves during a standardized meal. Over 10 months, households with induction stoves saw a 35% reduction in daily nitrogen dioxide levels. However, other sources still impacted indoor air quality.

Overall, the pilot study's results offer insights for policy makers and housing providers on cooking electrification and its impact on indoor air quality, social acceptance, and infrastructure challenges.

REFLECTION QUESTIONS

1. In light of the findings from the pilot study, what are the key considerations for policymakers in implementing widespread electrification of residential buildings, particularly in low-wealth and communities of color?

2. How can these policies address both environmental health concerns and social equity issues effectively?

OUTDOOR (AMBIENT) AIR POLLUTANTS

Ambient air pollutants come either from human industrial activity, like industrial emissions, air travel, road traffic, or agriculture, or from natural hazards such as earthquakes, tsunamis, forest fires, and volcanic eruptions.[14] Anthropogenic, or human-produced, sources of outdoor air pollution are of interest because of the potential to decrease the root causes of these pollutants. While outdoor air pollution is decreasing in Western Europe, the air quality in the Western United States has grown markedly worse in the past decade and is also surging in Asian, African, and South American countries that are experiencing rapid urbanization and industrialization.[14,20] Examples of air pollutants are covered in Table 10.1.

TABLE 10.1. EXAMPLES OF AIR POLLUTANTS[15,20,21]

AIR POLLUTANT	DESCRIPTION
Particulate matter (PM)	Composed of either liquids or solids and comprises a wide range of materials from dust and volcanic ash to diesel exhaust, pesticides, and aerosols. Produced from the biomass burning of wood, leaves, crops, and forests; also in industrial sources and vehicle emissions (both highway and off road, including air, rail, and marine vehicles).
Carbon monoxide (CO)	Produced by vehicle emissions, coal-fired power generation, industrial sources, and biomass burning.
Sulfur oxides (SO_x)	Produced by coal-fired power generation, vehicle emissions, and emissions from oil/gas wells, flaring, fields, and refineries.
Nitrogen oxide (NO_x)	Produced by vehicle emissions, coal-fired power generation, and by the oxidation of nitrogen fertilizers and is also an important ozone precursor.
Ozone (O_3)	Formed as a secondary pollutant from volatile organic compounds (VOCs), NO_2, and CO. O_3 plays a vital role as part of the stratosphere in blocking out harmful ultraviolet light from the sun, but when it is close to the ground, it is toxic to humans.
Lead	A toxic heavy metal that can be an air pollutant, its sources include leaded gasoline, industrial emissions, and lead-based paint. Inhalation of lead particles can lead to severe health issues, especially in children, causing developmental and cognitive problems.
Traffic-related air pollution (TRAP)	A mixture of gasses and particles, mostly ground-level ozone, carbon compounds, nitrogen oxide, sulfur oxides, and motor-vehicle emissions from fossil fuel combustion.

AIR POLLUTION AND HEALTH

Air pollution has negative multisystem health outcomes. The exact physiological response depends on the dose and length of exposure and the composition of the pollutants.[22] Air pollution can contribute to health problems throughout the body, such as asthma and heart disease (Figure 10.2), and other impacts like attention deficit hyperactivity disorder (ADHD), Alzheimer disease, Parkinson disease, and learning disabilities.[4,14,23] Studies have long documented that urbanization, rapid population growth, living near busy roadways, and burning biomass fuel are major contributors to air-pollution-related health problems.[23,24]

Women and children, who tend to bear more responsibility for household chores such as cooking and cleaning, are disproportionately affected by indoor air pollution.[25] In lower income areas, these effects can be greater from indoor stoves fueled by natural gas, kerosene, coal, or biomass such as dung.[26] Children can also be more affected by outdoor air pollution because of their still-developing immune systems, smaller size, and the fact that their breathing rates are higher than those of adults, resulting in higher exposure levels per unit of body weight.[27] Garcia and colleagues reported that decreases in ambient nitrogen dioxide and $PM_{2.5}$ were significantly associated with lower asthma levels among children in California who played outdoors,[28] suggesting that efforts to reduce air pollution's health effects are possible.

Older adults, people with preexisting health conditions, and people who work or are active outside are more prone to developing air-pollution-related health problems with prolonged exposure.[29] Older adults are especially susceptible to the health effects of air pollution, as age-related physiological degeneration increases toxin susceptibility, and the chronic conditions that are more prevalent later in life, such as cardiovascular disease, increase the risk that pollutants pose to health.[30]

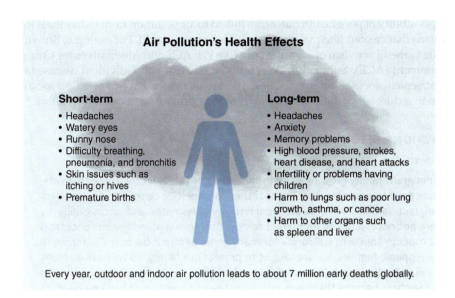

FIGURE 10.2. Health effects of air pollution.
Source: Adapted from Air pollution and health infographics. University of Southern California Environmental Health Centers; 2022. Accessed July 11, 2023. https://envhealthcenters.usc.edu/infographics

AIR POLLUTION AND ENVIRONMENTAL JUSTICE

Air pollution in the United States disproportionately impacts communities of color, low-wealth populations, recent immigrants, and other underserved or marginalized populations, leading to significantly disparate health outcomes for these communities.[31,32] Patel and colleagues found that a Black child in the United States is eight times more likely to die of an asthma attack than a White child due to structural factors, such as poverty and housing discrimination, that contribute to geographic health disparities.[31] As explained several times in this textbook, industrial and chemical plants, hazardous waste facilities, and other toxic facilities are commonly located in communities of color and of low wealth.[33,34] Underserved neighborhoods in urban areas also face high levels of air pollution from nearby busy roadways, an overabundance of cheap heating fuels and building materials, and residential overcrowding.[35,36] For example, the Bronx, which is the least affluent of New York City's five boroughs, has a dense network of busy roadways, waste disposal industries, and power-generating facilities, all the while struggling with low household-income rates, high poverty rates, and low educational attainment.[37]

Research on air pollution as a matter of **environmental justice (EJ)** is increasing globally in countries such as India,[38] New Zealand,[39] and Chile.[40] Verbeek's research in Ghent, Belgium, found that air pollution was more pervasive in neighborhoods with lower household incomes, higher unemployment rates, newer immigrants, and more rental properties.[36] Ribeiro and colleagues simultaneously collected similar data in São Paulo, Brazil, finding that lung cancer rates were higher among lower-income neighborhoods that experienced frequent traffic congestion.[41] Sovacool found that political coalitions that included multinational for-profit companies with cobalt-mining contracts in the Democratic Republic of the Congo overlooked the needs of local communities who relied on this natural-resource mining. They received no economic benefits while experiencing overmining, worsening air quality, and harms to their health under corrupt schemes.[42]

In low- and middle-income countries, the rapid industrialization and an overuse of crude fuels contributes to decreased air quality and worsening health outcomes.[43] In South Asia and Sub-Saharan Africa, household air pollution from crude fuels accounts for the primary risk factors for disease burden; of the 2.6 million air pollution-related deaths in 2016, 75% occurred in Asia and 22% occurred in Africa and the Middle East.[44] For example, Tefera and colleagues found that Ethiopia had a high prevalence of acute respiratory illnesses among children living in households using crude biomass fuels, and these households also experienced higher levels of indoor carbon monoxide than U.S. recommended regulatory levels.[45]

Shifting the responsibility of poor health outcomes linked to air pollution from individuals to the societal conditions that created unequal exposure is also a matter of EJ. For example, Brown et al. found that due to the EJ activism of organizations like WE ACT and Alternatives for Community and Environment (ACE), asthma has been transformed from an individual disease to a broader social movement focused on inequalities. The organizations have focused on social and political action to reduce air pollution, thereby promoting primary prevention of asthma.[46]

AUTHOR REFLECTIONS: BETO'S STORY

Beto Lugo Martinez

As a son of an immigrant family growing up within minutes of the California/Mexico divide, I learned to endure environmental racism. In the rather conservative county where we lived, children of immigrant families were treated unjustly by classmates and occasionally by teachers. We were not necessarily an immigrant family; Chicanos and Indigenous ancestors have always had roots in Southern California for many years before it became California. In most Chicano or Hispanic families, we are taught to protect our family, so we have a strong sense of responsibility for both each other and each other's choices. In my family, the choices made by family members became their own to celebrate—and sometimes became burdens to carry.

Our family's first residence was a two-bedroom apartment in an alley behind a neighborhood grocery store. Then we moved to substandard housing with a huge yard with plenty of space to play. Then a few years later came the best surprise of our lives. With the help of a local nonprofit, my parents had applied for assistance for low-income, rural farmworkers in our county, and we were going to get our own house.

There were strings attached, however. My family had to put in some "sweat equity" and be actively involved in building the house. This requirement was an added burden for my dad, who had a full-time job working in industrial agriculture, and for my mom, who was responsible for raising my sister, myself, and my two younger twin brothers, as well as cleaning homes to make ends meet.

We built our first home, and so did our new neighbors. We all supported one another. Because we were all from low-income families, parents brought their kids to the worksite, and I got to meet the future neighborhood kids. Even the youngest of kids contributed to building the homes. I remember children helping with pouring concrete and framing, roofing, and painting the homes. There were no child workforce protection laws, and if there were, they did not apply to us. We were all kids with similar struggles and all very happy to have a house.

This was a time of joy for us, but there is a dark side to this history. These aid programs are intended to help Brown, Black, immigrant, low-income, and rural communities. However, the essence of empowerment obscures local, state, and federal agencies' practices that are discriminatory and damaging, and perpetuate environmental racism. Discriminatory housing policies known as "redlining" and land-use zoning practices intentionally put people of color in harm's way. Additionally, many people who live in federally assisted housing in the United States are at risk of being poisoned by dangerous toxic contamination. These injustices have happened for generations, all over the United States.

My parents never considered the environmental health hazards that we would face for the rest of our lives. Our house was built about 100 steps from a Unocal/Chevron subsidiary, called PureGro (yes, a greenwashed name for a petrochemical facility). The PureGro Company produced pesticides, agro-chemicals, and fertilizers for industrial agriculture operations. The facility had been in operation since the 1940s and was a well-known manufacturer of dichlorodiphenyltrichloroethane (DDT). By the time we moved in, DDT had already been banned in the United States because of its adverse environmental effects and human health risks. We know, though, that corporate farmers continued to spray and store these chemicals for decades to come. Research has continued to support the relationship between human DDT exposure and reproductive health effects. For example, people who were exposed to these chemicals in utero or as children, have a higher risk of breast cancer, while their mothers

(continued)

have higher rates of gestational diabetes and preeclampsia.[47,48] In addition to breast cancer, diabetes, and preeclampsia, studies link elevated exposure to DDT to other types of cancer, infertility, and developmental delays. Most recently, research also showed that a parent's exposure to DDT can be passed to a second generation, as the pesticide can travel through the placenta to a fetus and can be delivered to a nursing infant via breast milk.[48,49] DDT is called a *legacy pesticide*, which refers to a pesticide that was once used in the United States but is now banned because of health risks to humans or the environment. The legacy these pesticides leave behind is their long-lived persistence in the environment and damage to humans and animals.

During the time I was growing up, my family and our neighbors were exposed to the toxic chemical releases coming from this facility for decades. In 2000, after many years of community-organizing efforts about the dangers of historical violations, explosions, and disregard for public health and the environment, the facility was closed, but the damage was already done. Now in 2023 we are still dealing with the unjust burden. In 2013, the state regulators labeled the facility a hazardous waste site, adding it to the group of Superfund sites.[50] Although only a few community members have been able to prove that their health problems are directly linked to living near this facility, the health and medical literature on the subject matter supports our beliefs that DDT is still ubiquitous, showing up in food, water, and nearly everyone's blood, even though it was banned in most countries more than 40 years ago.

THE CLEAN AIR ACT

As introduced in Chapter 4, "Environmental Health Policies and Protections: Successes and Failures," the Clean Air Act (CAA) requires the U.S. Environmental Protection Agency (EPA) to establish National Ambient Air Quality Standards (NAAQS) and to monitor the six "criteria" air pollutants: ground-level ozone, $PM_{2.5}$, CO, lead, SO_2, and NO_2 throughout the United States (see Box 10.1). These pollutants are referred to as *criteria pollutants* because the EPA regulates them by establishing allowed levels based on human health and environmental criteria or science-based guidelines. There are also a series of monitoring networks maintained by state, local, and Tribal monitoring agencies, which measure ambient air pollution. In some locations, these networks have been shown to be insufficient for the measuring of local and short-term spikes in air pollution.

BOX 10.1. SCIENCE SHAPING POLICY: A CLOSER LOOK AT $PM_{2.5}$

One type of air pollution, particulate matter 2.5 ($PM_{2.5}$), is especially dangerous for health owing to the miniscule size of the particles, which aids them in penetrating deep into the lungs, entering the bloodstream, and traveling to other organs to cause systemic damage.[24] The Six Cities study, a prospective cohort study run by researchers at the Harvard School of Public Health, followed adults in six U.S. cities with varying levels of ozone, fine PM, and aerosol acidity. The study identified a clear association between fine PM and mortality, finding that life expectancy was 2 to 3 years lower in cities with high levels of fine PM.[51] This study paved the way for strengthened U.S. regulations that have significantly decreased the $PM_{2.5}$ levels over the past 30 years.

The U.S. Clean Air Act, which was enacted in 1963 and was amended in 1970 when the U.S. Environmental Protection Agency (EPA) was established, was the first environmental law to provide the federal government with major regulatory oversight of air pollution control policy.[52,53] The EPA used the findings from the Six Cities study as the foundation for the 1997 regulations on $PM_{2.5}$—the first time that this pollutant had ever been federally regulated.[55]

(continued)

> **BOX 10.1. SCIENCE SHAPING POLICY: A CLOSER LOOK AT PM$_{2.5}$** *(continued)*
>
> Periodically, the EPA announces proposals to strengthen the National Ambient Air Quality Standards (NAAQS) to better protect communities. For instance, in 2024, the agency lowered the primary (health-based) annual PM$_{2.5}$ standard from 12 micrograms per cubic meter to 9 micrograms per cubic meter. This adjustment is based on the latest health data and scientific evidence.[52-54]
>
> When revising the NAAQS, it is crucial for the EPA to use more accurate risk estimation methods, and a thorough review can help prioritize emission reductions in the most heavily overburdened communities. Importantly, any standards and regulations without equally powerful enforcement will continue to perpetuate environmental injustices.

The CAA also regulates hazardous air pollutants (HAPs), or air toxics or toxic air pollutants (TAPs). According to the EPA, some air toxics include dioxin, asbestos, toluene, and metals, such as cadmium, mercury, chromium, and lead compounds. There are over 187 hazardous air pollutants which are known or suspected to cause cancer or other serious health effects, such as reproductive effects or birth defects, or adverse environmental effects, and there are no standards to regulate those emissions.[55] Research shows that exposure to methyl bromide (bromomethane)—a chemical primarily utilized for aerial pesticide application near **sensitive receptors**, or specific populations or environments that are particularly susceptible to adverse effects from pollutants (e.g., workers or communities near heavy industrial agriculture operation)—may cause damage to the brain and nervous system including poor vision, mental confusion, hallucination, tremors, problems with speech and physical coordination, and loss of balance.[55,56]

Community members and EJ activists are frequently told by the EPA that nearby emissions comply with CAA regulations. However, the EPA and other state environmental agencies that are tasked with protecting public health cannot truly protect all communities because of loopholes in the law, inadequate monitoring, and a failure to enforce environmental violations. Even if companies and governments comply, many communities still experience the harmful levels of pollutants.

> **IN OTHER WORDS: PUBLIC NOTICES AND AIR-QUALITY PERMIT APPLICATIONS**
>
> Have you ever seen a public notice for an industrial facility that is looking to increase or change its air pollution emissions in your community? These notices can be hard to access, understand, or act on. Figure 10.3 depicts an example from Illinois.
>
> Review some examples of public notices and air-quality-permit applications on your state environmental agency's website. How might agencies use plain language so that communities can meaningfully engage in decision-making related to air pollution? Questions you might ask about the public notice:
>
> - What makes sense? What is confusing?
> - Where is this facility located?
> - Are there already pollution sources nearby that impact air quality? (Would this lead to cumulative impacts?)
> - Which pollutants does the facility plan to emit?
> - How do these pollutants affect health?
> - Who can you contact to ask questions or submit comments?

(continued)

> **IN OTHER WORDS: PUBLIC NOTICES AND AIR-QUALITY PERMIT APPLICATIONS** (*continued*)
>
> Practice "translating" the notices into plain language for a general audience.
>
> ---
>
> **Illinois Environmental Protection Agency**
>
> Public Notice
> Renewal of the Federally Enforceable State Operating Permit
> True Value Manufacturing in Cary
>
> True Value Manufacturing has applied to the Illinois Environmental Protection Agency to renew the federally enforceable state operating permit (FESOP) regulating air emissions from its facility located at 201 Jandus Road in Cary. The facility is a paint manufacturing plant. The Illinois EPA has reviewed the application and made a preliminary determination that the application meets the standards for issuance and has prepared a draft permit for public review and comment.
>
> The Illinois EPA is accepting written comments on the draft permit. Comments must be received by 11:59 PM on March 20, 2022. If sufficient interest is expressed in the draft permit, a hearing or other informational meeting may be held. Requests for information, comments, and questions should be directed to Cassandra Metz, Office of Community Relations, Illinois Environmental Protection Agency, 1021 N. Grand Ave East, PO Box 19506, Springfield, Illinois, 62794-9506, phone 217/785-7491, TDD phone number 866/273-5488, Cassandra.Metz@Illinois.gov.
>
> The repositories for these documents and the application will be made available at the Illinois EPA's offices at 9511 West Harrison in Des Plaines, 847/294-4000 and 1021 North Grand Avenue East, Springfield, 217/785-7491 (please call ahead to assure that someone will be available to assist you). The draft permit and other documents may also be available at http://bit.ly/2SiUSql. Copies of the documents may also be obtained upon request to the contact listed above.
>
> The 1990 amendments to the Clean Air Act require potentially major sources of air emissions to obtain federally enforceable operating permits. A FESOP permit allows a source that is potentially major to take operational limits in the permit so that it is a non-major source. The permit will contain federally enforceable limitations that restrict the facility's emissions to non-major levels. The permit will be enforceable by the USEPA, as well as the Illinois EPA.
>
> **FIGURE 10.3.** Illinois EPA public notice.
> EPA, Environmental Protection Agency.
> *Source:* Illinois Environmental Protection Agency.

ENFORCEMENT

The Clean Air Act requires emissions standards and technology controls for facilities releasing hazardous air pollutants, but these rules mean very little without enforcement, and enforcement is difficult. The EPA is mandated to consider the effects of individual chemicals on fenceline communities one at a time in its risk analyses. **Fenceline communities** are those communities and populations living directly adjacent to industrial facilities, such as factories, chemical plants, or refineries. Fenceline community monitoring is not required for most types of polluting facilities, which means that communities typically have no way of knowing what type of or how much chemical exposure they are experiencing. Even when companies are meeting the standards, the cumulative impact and exposure to many different facilities and chemicals are not considered in the context of the EPA's current regulatory approach.[33,57]

Many times, regulatory agencies state that they do not have enforcement capability; in such situations, they should not issue permits or allow new polluting facilities in overburdened communities without a robust public participation engagement plan that is transparent and thorough and that acknowledges community expertise in the decision-making. Additional tools that may be needed for a robust engagement plan are public engagement and environmental impact statements or reports, required by the National Environmental Policy Act (NEPA) and the California Environmental Quality Act (CEQA).[58] Furthermore, federal, state, and local agencies should be required to conduct occasional unannounced inspections, and robust multimedia approaches (in which soil, water, and air discharges are all measured and assessed) should be encouraged to identify other potential health risks to fenceline communities.

REGULATORY AIR POLLUTION MONITORING AND COMMUNITY AIR MONITORING

As part of the CAA requirements, the EPA collaborates with state officials to place air monitors to determine ambient background pollution levels. However, these monitors often fail to capture local neighborhood conditions, especially in communities already overburdened with multiple environmental exposures. Since the goal of the CAA is to protect public health, it is important that the air monitors are placed near sensitive receptor locations, where at-risk populations such as children, older adults, individuals with underlying health conditions, and others at a higher risk of negative health impacts reside.[59]

The current networks of federal- and state-operated air-quality monitors have significant geographic gaps, particularly in communities near major sources of air pollution.[60] Fenceline communities often do not have adequate agency air-quality monitoring nearby; when they do, the monitors are often not properly maintained, or they fail to adequately capture industrial emissions like smoke plumes, flaring, fires, explosions, or other fugitive emissions because of where the monitors are placed or their ability to monitor only certain pollutants. Even when functioning monitors are available, often state regulators prioritize monitor placement to serve the needs of industry over local public health concerns.[61,62] Regulatory air monitors also have a longer reporting period, measuring ambient air pollution, and reporting it in either 12-hour or 24-hour periods. These monitors do not show peaks in pollution and are ineffective in addressing short-term emission spikes.[63]

In contrast, low-cost sensors can be deployed more broadly and cost between $100 and $7,000. Although they often cannot be calibrated to provide the same level of specificity as agency monitors, they can help communities to validate concerns or identify hot spots, for instance. They are also available as either mobile or stationary units and can be placed to assist community members in capturing hyperlocal neighborhood air pollution data. Low-cost sensors also update the data continuously and display the average air quality every few minutes. The availability of lower cost air pollution sensors allows for community scientists to take ownership of and use the data in ways they choose; however, it is more challenging to understand, access, and effectively use the data sets when many academics and governing bodies exclude communities from the decision-making processes.[64,65] Low-cost sensors can be used to build spatially dense community-monitoring networks, which can be deployed by community members to support community engagement and increase health literacy, as well as an understanding of local, state, and federal land-use policies that ideally improves overall civic engagement. One potential benefit of hyperlocal monitoring is the ability to discern episodes of increased air pollution, rather than seeing only average levels over space and time. In this context, communities can identify pollution exceedances in higher risk areas where they would otherwise be unaware of risks and, unfortunately, often uninformed. Additionally, hyperlocal monitoring fills the spatial data gaps by collecting data in locations that have not been identified by the government as high risk. When these networks are built and owned by the community, the data and knowledge tend to serve the community's needs. With high-resolution, real-time neighborhood air pollution data, public health warnings and overall protections for overburdened communities could be improved.

CUMULATIVE AIR POLLUTION EXPOSURES

Cumulative impacts are the totality of pollution exposures and environmental health hazards that overburdened and fenceline communities face and that have a direct impact on their well-being and quality of life outcomes. The CAA fails to address cumulative impacts to protect communities that are exposed to pollution from multiple sources. Even if companies and governments comply, these communities still experience harmful levels of pollutants. Environmental epidemiologic research tends to correlate residential proximity to polluting facilities with health outcomes rather than with specific chemical exposures, as the exposure data are often inadequate.[66]

Several U.S. states have passed cumulative impact laws, or are considering similar laws, that would prohibit industrial projects whose environmental and health impacts are higher in EJ communities than in non-EJ communities. See Table 10.2 for more information.

> **AUTHOR REFLECTIONS: BETO'S STORY, CONTINUED**
>
> My childhood neighborhood was built adjacent to an industrial chemical plant that produced known toxic substances. My neighbors and my family members continue to have substantial environmental health concerns because of the hazards from living near what is now an Environmental Protection Agency (EPA)-designated Superfund site. This injustice led me to lead air-monitoring efforts in California and organize alongside a local social justice organization. Our organization, in partnership with the California Tracking and the Public Health Institutes, was awarded a National Institute of Environmental Health Sciences (NIEHS) community-based participatory research (CBPR) grant for air monitoring during 2014 and 2018. Through this work, we built what would become the largest community-owned air-monitoring network in the country and, at the time, in the world.
>
> One purpose in this study was to assess the accuracy of the low-cost sensors. The sensors were calibrated against regulatory air monitors. When hyperlocal pollution episodes occurred (where particulate matter [PM] hourly average concentrations were equal to or greater than the National Ambient Air Quality Standards [NAAQS]), they were identified and corroborated with other sites in the network and assessed against the small number of government monitors in the region. During a period of five months, over 100 exceedance episodes were identified and corroborated by six government monitors in the study region; however, more than 10 times as many episodes were identified by the community air monitors.[67]
>
> In other words, around 90% of the pollution-level exceedance episodes were not captured by the government monitors but were identified by monitors in the community network. These findings suggested that the dense network of community air monitors could address the limitations in the spatial coverage of government air monitoring. The findings also highlighted a lack of properly maintained federal monitors, resulting in the government's inability to provide real-time warnings of high-pollution episodes to at-risk populations and the necessary regulation of industrial polluters. This real-time air-monitoring network was designed by the community for the community, and the fact that this project was developed as CBPR project was a huge advantage.[68]

TABLE 10.2. CUMULATIVE IMPACT LAWS IN SELECT STATES

STATE	BILL/LAW	SUMMARY	CURRENT STATUS
Connecticut	SB1147 (Environmental Justice Program)	A tool that measures existing environmental and health stressors in a community will be developed to help applicants for new permits to assess whether cumulative impact thresholds would be exceeded if the permit was approved. Permits can be denied if a project's cumulative environmental and health impacts are higher in an EJ community than in non-EJ communities.	Signed into law in May 2023

(continued)

TABLE 10.2. CUMULATIVE IMPACT LAWS IN SELECT STATES (*continued*)

STATE	BILL/LAW	SUMMARY	CURRENT STATUS
Illinois	SB1823/HB5013	Would require the Illinois EPA to annually review data that would be used to determine whether a community qualifies as an EJ community. Requires industrial facilities to submit an EJ assessment identifying the environmental impacts to the areas near the project.	With the Illinois Senate (as of June 2024)
Maryland	HB24/SB96 (Environmental Justice Evaluation of Environmental Permit Applications)	Aims to prevent environmental racism by requiring state agencies to assess the health and environmental impacts of potentially polluting projects on marginalized communities and prioritize these communities for public protection.	With the Maryland House (as of June 2024)
Minnesota	HF637 (Frontline Communities Protection Act)	Requires the Pollution Control Agency to deny facility permits if it adds to cumulative adverse environmental stressors in an EJ area.	Signed into law May 2023 as part of HF2310
New Jersey	The EJ Rules	The rules require enhanced upfront community engagement before pollution-generating facilities are proposed in the state's overburdened communities. Also directs permit applicants to avoid and minimize environmental and public health stressors and enables the DEP to establish permit conditions that better protect at-risk communities.	Adopted in April 2023
New York	S8830	Prevents the approval and reissuing of permits for actions that would increase disproportionate and/or inequitable pollution burdens on disadvantaged communities.	Signed into law in December 2022
Rhode Island	SB2535 (Environmental Justice Act)	Establishes requirements that would have to be met by facilities prior to the issuing of permits for activities that have an environmental impact on an EJ area.	With the Rhode Island Senate (as of June 2024)

DEP, Department of Environmental Protection; EJ, environmental justice; EPA, Environmental Protection Agency

WORKING TOWARD ENVIRONMENTAL HEALTH AND JUSTICE

Many of the health inequities discussed in this chapter might have been prevented had the concept of EJ been prioritized. Fenceline communities often have limited recourse. EJ embodies several principles: that all people are equal partners at every level of decision-making, including that of needs assessment, planning, implementation, enforcement, and evaluation, which affirms the fundamental right to political, economic, cultural, and environmental self-determination of all peoples.[33,57] Beyond informing policies or practice, EJ advocates for community-driven approaches not only identify harmful air pollution exposure(s), but also reduce health disparities through community-centered approaches aimed at mitigating harmful exposures.

COMMUNITY SCIENCE

Given their real-world, on-the-ground experience, local communities have critical insights into how environmental hazards affect the health of their inhabitants and which measures might prove most useful in studying exposure to these hazards.[69-71] As referenced in Chapter 5, "Environmental Health Science for the People," terms such as **community science**, *crowdsourced science, citizen science, street science,* and *civic tech* are methods for capturing data or information. These methods can be useful to assist overburdened communities that need hyperlocal environmental and health data to fill gaps that are not included in multiple environmental screening tools provided by academic and government institutions. These tools are used to identify federal investment opportunities to address environmental injustice, data and funding. However, funding primarily supports academic researchers and government employees, creating an inequitable, colonialist approach that perpetuates environmental injustice.[64,72] The body of knowledge around the impacts of pollution on health continues to grow without application of this knowledge to effectively improve the health of those impacted.[73]

As described in Chapter 5, "Environmental Health Science for the People"; Chapter 7, "Understanding the Environment and How It Relates to Health Using Toxicology and Epidemiology Research Methods"; and Chapter 8, "Mapping Environmental Health and Justice Issues," there are numerous potential benefits to effectively engaging community members. Through collaboration, communities can cocreate and participate in environmental health research, policy development, planning and permitting processes, and environmental enforcement efforts where they live.[74,75] This inclusive and equitable approach is invaluable for advancing health protections in overburdened communities.

In air pollution research, for example, teams can engage in a systematic process to design and develop air-monitoring networks. This process involves training community scientists who are already part of the local neighborhood. Seen in this light, community members become the leaders of this movement, sharing their expertise and knowledge of local injustices, while academics and other participants work to support this process. All participants work together to utilize the data to inform decision makers and regulatory agencies about broad systems change.[76] Additionally, these community-engaged projects provide a mechanism for communities to advocate for protections and address harmful air pollution and environmental health risks in EJ communities. When both community members and academic researchers work together, they can ask or demand that local and federal authorities inspect monitoring stations across the country, many of which were installed decades ago, and embrace community participation in running tests and calibrations to ensure that the regulatory monitor readings are accurate. This process creates an opportunity for a more transparent and robust approach in the placement of monitors, and better conveys what other types of pollutants to measure.

Because government-operated air-quality monitoring already exists in many communities across the United States, some may argue that there would be little added value in supplementing this data with community-monitoring data. Additionally, community monitoring has historically been challenging due to the high costs involved, but the emergence of low-cost sensors has provided new opportunities.[77] Overburdened communities also are motivated to conduct their own air monitoring because the process of working together as an EJ community validates their lived experiences.[78] Placing the monitors in their neighborhood and homes acknowledges the importance of localized exposures and the environmental health inequities the communities face. It also allows for greater civic engagement and public participation in decision-making spaces.[72] Community members can inform local and state decision makers using scientific data to help them to make decisions that will protect their community. Furthermore, as Chapter 5 discusses, community data, regardless of the sensor technology or open-sourced capabilities, should belong to the community and shared only and when there are agreements in place that articulate how the data will be used and shared.

AUTHOR REFLECTIONS: BETO'S STORY, CONTINUED

After moving to Kansas City in 2019 and becoming the executive director of CleanAirNow, an environmental justice (EJ) organization, I continued to work to develop a community-air-monitoring network utilizing a mix of low-cost sensors and other higher cost sensors that measure black carbon, ozone (O_3), and nitric oxide and nitrogen dioxide (NO_x). The network was deployed through the use of successful environmental health workshops and community hazard-mapping activities.

While leading CleanAirNow, I understood that community data accessibility and ownership were important for building community power.[73] An online dashboard was developed together with a trusted academic partner who engaged with organizers by continuously asking participants what they wanted to see from the project. Interactive data visualization provided a powerful outlet to present data to the communities, building power among those affected to advocate for themselves. The data visualization itself has become a tool for education, allowing people to connect with each other.

Simultaneously, a start-up reached out to CleanAirNow regarding testing the performance of a new air monitor (which was like the particulate matter 2.5 [$PM_{2.5}$] sensors used by our organization). We politely declined, but continued to keep tabs on their work and attended meetings when we were informed about them. At the meetings, the organizers referred to their work as a community-engaged project. The people in their group were from academic institutions, the EPA, and a large and influential planning organization. The start-up group claimed that their project was novel, but as the executive director of CleanAirNow, I had already built the largest community-owned and -developed air-monitoring network in the country before commercialized sensors had become well known. Additionally, I clearly articulated that these researchers were not permitted to use our air-monitoring network data for comparison or analyses without expressed consent from our organization. Though no justification should have been needed, our project was designed by the community, and I believed that the data, therefore, should belong to the community.

A year later I attended a workshop at which this start-up group was presenting their project and findings to the public. On the screen I saw the location of their own monitors and all of the CleanAirNow monitors on display. The data that they did not have permission to use was being appropriated.

COMMUNITY-DIRECTED POLICIES

Fenceline communities continue to suffer adverse health effects, while regulations lag behind scientific advancements. Furthermore, findings from federally funded research that support academic institutions are seldom, if ever, translated into practical measures that safeguard the health of both these overburdened communities and society at large. Because the *precautionary principle* (not approving products for use until they are known to be safe) is not part of the decision-making processes of the U.S. government, in land-use policies or in health assessments, communities are often left to fend for themselves. They often have to prove they are being unjustly exposed to toxins or to prove that their health outcomes are disproportionately worse than other similar populations because of hazardous exposures.[77–80] However, there are examples in which the utilization of community-led research has been able to inform policies from the ground up to effectively serve and support fenceline communities.

AUTHOR REFLECTIONS: BETO'S STORY, CONTINUED

One of the key findings from the community-based air-monitoring project in California was identified by a community member scientist completing her PhD. She determined that the federal monitors did not capture exceedances above a certain level. We agreed that the resulting data reports were misleading and potentially risky for community members; this finding led to ongoing conversations with the EPA, and the agency replaced the outdated monitors with more accurate equipment. The limitations of these monitors were already known by our academic partners, but not taken into account in the same manner. This example highlights how

(continued)

communities perceive and approach data and knowledge very differently from people studying or governing the community.

The largest air-monitoring network built in Southern California through CBPR allowed for greater involvement in government processes and for community members to be involved in decision-making processes. This project and associated partnerships were a major accomplishment that ultimately led to the passage of the California Legislature Assembly Bill 617 (AB617), which mandated the development of a state community-air-protection program to reduce air pollution and improve health in impacted communities. EJ organizations played a direct role in informing the implementation of AB617.

Similarly, in 2021, CleanAirNow, produced the Environmental Justice Recommendations on the Armourdale General Plan, a long term land use and development plan. Community concerns were directly embedded in the document; fenceline-community expertise based on lived experience was supported by their own data and the data reported by the federal government. The report was added as an Appendix to the City's Master Plan and is used as a living document for accountability and continuing investments in the community.

ClearAirNow's direct contribution to the plan has changed the way decision makers view the community and the organization. CleanAirNow has a seat at the table and collaborates with the public health and planning departments and the mayor's office. CleanAirNow's efforts directly contributed to the city plan, increased access to decision makers, and used community data to inform government efforts, and drafted legislation to benefit community health.[81]

MAIN TAKEAWAYS

In this chapter, we learned that:

- Air pollution has negative multisystem health outcomes. Certain groups of people, such as children, older adults, and members of marginalized communities, are more at risk of developing air-pollution-related health problems due to prolonged exposure.
- Environmental epidemiologic research tends to correlate residential proximity to polluting facilities with health outcomes rather than with specific chemical exposures.
- Federal, state, and local governments are charged with protecting environmental public health, although how successful they are is highly debated.
- Fenceline communities live in the shadows of industrial pollution facilities and suffer from the environmental injustices associated with bad land use and zoning decisions.
- There are many benefits to effectively engaging communities in community science and other environmental health efforts.
- Following the principles of EJ allows for robust community engagement, health indicators, and other relevant community-level data to ensure that there is no continued harm for already overburdened populations.
- Community-led research can inform policies from the ground up to effectively protect not only EJ communities' health, but also society's health in general.

SUMMARY

Air pollution is a global public health issue that affects everyone, but affects some of us more than others. Many advocates, academics, government scientists, and policy makers continue to push for stronger protections, while many are complacent with the status quo. As the narrative throughout this chapter highlights, much more work is needed to confront the root causes of environmental racism that drive patterns of air pollution and resulting health inequities. Members of fenceline communities—those closest to the exposures and experiencing the cumulative impacts—have largely been the ones leading the efforts to eliminate air pollution and holding air polluters accountable. These communities cannot continue to be sacrificial zones and should be valued as leaders in shaping science and policy solutions toward cleaner air for all.

END-OF-CHAPTER RESOURCES

DISCUSSION QUESTIONS

1. What do you know about air quality in your community? Are there any major sources that concern you? How is the air quality today? Do you know where to look to find out?
2. Think about the indoor places where you spend much of your time. How is air quality protected indoors in these places, if at all?
3. How does past and present zoning impact the distribution of air pollution in the United States? How does zoning perpetuate environmental injustice? Do you think zoning should be used to achieve EJ?

LEARNING ACTIVITIES

THE TIME IS NOW

Does your state have a policy to protect against cumulative impacts related to air pollution? If the answer is yes, how effective is it? If not, reach out to agency staff and elected leaders to learn more, educate them about existing policies in other states, and advocate for change. You might begin by looking to see if any local environmental or EJ organizations are working on this issue in your state or region already.

- For a list of regional EPA offices: www.epa.gov/aboutepa/regional-and-geographic-offices
- To find your state and district representatives: www.house.gov/representatives/find-your-representative

IN REAL LIFE

How do your daily activities contribute to air pollution?[82]

1. First, gather your materials: a clean large jar; water; red, blue, and yellow food coloring; a spoon/other stirrer.
2. Brainstorm a list of the sources of air pollution, and organize the list into categories (e.g., gasoline-burning vehicles and engines, electricity from fossil fuels).
3. Create a simple model of the atmosphere. Use food coloring to model air pollutants in the atmosphere throughout the day.
    - Red: pollution from burning gasoline,
    - Blue: pollution from burning fossil fuels like coal, and
    - Yellow: pollution from products that release chemicals into the air
4. Write down your schedule for a typical day, divided into one-hour blocks. For instance:
    6:00 a.m.: Wake up and shower.
    7:00 a.m.: Prepare breakfast.
    8:00 a.m.: Drive/take the bus/walk to school or work . . .
5. For each one-hour block, identify the various sources of pollutants you might encounter from your daily activities. For example, you use hot water for a shower that is heated by a water heater that uses natural gas. Maybe your coffeemaker and microwave all use electricity. (You may have to do some research.)
6. For each hour, add one drop of the appropriate food colors.

7. Take a close look at your jar after going through 24 hours of your day. Which colors do you see in your jar? What would happen if the "air" (the water in the jar) had been moving?
8. Use the spoon to stir the air pollutants. Which colors do you see in your jar now?
9. Write or discuss your reflections about which air pollutants you release into the atmosphere on a typical day.

 A robust set of instructor resources designed to supplement this text is located at http://connect.springerpub.com/content/book/978-0-8261-8353-8. Qualifying instructors may request access by emailing textbook@springerpub.com.

REFERENCES

1. World Health Organization. Ambient (outdoor) air pollution. December 19, 2022. https://www.who.int/news-room/fact-sheets/detail/ambient-(outdoor)-air-quality-and-health
2. World Health Organization. Household air pollution. December 15, 2023. https://www.who.int/news-room/fact-sheets/detail/household-air-pollution-and-health
3. Vallero DA. *Fundamentals of Air Pollution*. 5th ed. Elsevier; 2014.
4. World Health Organization. Air quality, energy and health. 2022. Accessed November 19, 2023. https://www.who.int/teams/environment-climate-change-and-health/air-quality-and-health/health-impacts
5. NIEHS. Air pollution and your health. National Institutes of Health. 2020. https://www.niehs.nih.gov/health/materials/air_pollution_and_your_health_508.pdf
6. Fowler D, Brimblecombe P, Burrows J, et al. A chronology of global air quality. *Philos Trans A: Math Phys Eng Serv*. 2020;378(2183):20190314. doi:10.1098/rsta.2019.0314
7. Morrison J. Air pollution goes back way further than you think. *Smithsonian Magazine*. 2016. https://www.smithsonianmag.com/science-nature/air-pollution-goes-back-way-further-you-think-180957716/
8. Jacobs ET, Burgess JL, Abbott MB. The Donora smog revisited: 70 years after the event that inspired the clean air act. *Am J Public Health*. 2018;108(suppl 2):S85–S88. doi:10.2105/ajph.2017.304219
9. Berger RE, Ramaswami R, Solomon CG, Drazen JM. Air pollution still kills. *N Engl J Med*. 2017;376(26):2591–2592. doi:10.1056/nejme1706865
10. Bell M, Davis DL. Reassessment of the lethal London fog of 1952: novel indicators of acute and chronic consequences of acute exposure to air pollution. *Environ Health Perspect*. 2001;109(suppl. 3):389–394. doi:10.1289/ehp.01109s3389
11. Polivka BJ. The Great London Smog of 1952. *Am J Nurs*. 2018;118(4):57–61. doi:10.1097/01.naj.0000532078.72372.c3
12. Broughton E. The Bhopal disaster and its aftermath: a review. *Environ Health*. 2005;4(1):6. doi:10.1186/1476-069X-4-6
13. Izarali MR. Globalization and the Bhopal disaster: a criminogenic inquiry. *Int J Soc Inq*. 2013;6(1): 91–112.
14. Kim D, Chen Z, Zhou LF, Huang SX. Air pollutants and early origins of respiratory diseases. *Chronic Dis Trans Med*. 2018;4(2), 75–94. doi:10.1016/j.cdtm.2018.03.003
15. Tran VV, Park D, Lee YC. Indoor air pollution, related human diseases, and recent trends in the control and improvement of indoor air quality. *Int J Environ Res Public Health*. 2020;17(8):2927. doi:10.3390/ijerph17082927
16. NIEHS. Indoor air pollution quality. National Institutes of Health. 2022. Updated March 11, 2024. https://www.niehs.nih.gov/health/topics/agents/indoor-air/index.cfm
17. Indoor air exposure and characterization research. United States Environmental Protection Agency. 2023. Updated July 14, 2023. https://www.epa.gov/report-environment/indoor-air-quality
18. World Health Organization. Household air pollution. December 15, 2023. https://www.who.int/news-room/fact-sheets/detail/household-air-pollution-and-health
19. Out of Gas, In With Justice. WE ACT. Accessed November 19, 2023. https://www.weact.org/campaigns/out-of-gas/

20. Laumbach RJ, Cromar KR. (2022). Personal interventions to reduce exposure to outdoor air pollution. *Annu Rev Public Health*. 2022;43:293–309. doi:10.1146/annurev-publhealth-052120-103607
21. Inhalable particulate matter and health ($PM_{2.5}$ and PM_{10}). California Air Resources Board. 2023. Accessed July 12, 2023. https://ww2.arb.ca.gov/resources/inhalable-particulate-matter-and-health#:~:text=Those%20with%20a%20diameter%20of,comprises%20a%20portion%20of%20PM10
22. Manisalidis I, Stavropoulou E, Stavropoulous A, Bezirtzoglou E. Environmental and health impacts of air pollution: a review. *Front Public Health*. 2020;8:4. doi:10.3389/fpubh.2020.00014
23. Tessari L, Angriman M, Díaz-Román A, Zhang J, Conca, A, Cortese, S. Association between exposure to pesticides and ADHD or autism spectrum disorder: a systematic review of the literature. *J Atten Disord*. 2020;26(1):48–71. doi:10.1177/1087054720940402
24. Public Health Service, U.S. Department of Health and Human Services. National Toxicology Program. NTP monograph on the systematic review of traffic-related air pollution and hypertensive disorders of pregnancy. NTP Monograph 07. December 2019. https://ntp.niehs.nih.gov/ntp/ohat/trap/mgraph/trap_final_508.pdf
25. Ali MU, Balal Yousaf YY, Mujtaba Munir MA. Health impacts of indoor air pollution from household solid fuel on children and women. *J Hazard Mater*. 2021;416:126127. doi:10.1016/j.jhazmat.2021.126127
26. Agrawal S, Yamamoto S. Effect of indoor air pollution from biomass and solid fuel combustion on symptoms of preeclampsia/eclampsia in Indian women. *Indoor Air*. 2015;25(3):341–352. doi:10.1111/ina.12144
27. Karimi B, Shokrenizhad, B. Air pollution and mortality among infant and children under five years: a systematic review and meta-analysis. *Atmos Pollut Res*. 2020;11(6): 61–70. doi:10.1016/j.apr.2020.02.006
28. Garcia E, Berhane KT, Islam T, et al. Association of changes in air quality with incident asthma in children in California, 1993–2014. *JAMA*. 2019;321(10):1906–1915. doi:10.1001/jama.2019.5357
29. MassDEP. Commonwealth of Massachusetts, Department of Environmental Protection. Health & environmental effects of air pollution. 2022. https://www.mass.gov/doc/health-environmental-effects-of-air-pollution/download
30. Ailshire J, Brown, LL. The importance of air quality policy for older adults and diverse communities. *Public Policy Aging Rep*. 2021;31(1), 33–37. doi:10.1093/ppar/praa036
31. Patel L, Friedman E, Johannes SA, Lee SS, O'Brien HG, Schear SE. Air pollution as a social and structural determinant of health. *J Clim Change Health*. 2021;3:100035. doi:10.1016/j.joclim.2021.100035
32. Salas RN. Environmental racism and climate change—missed diagnoses. *N Engl J Med*. 2021;385(11):967–969. doi:10.10156/NEJMp2109160
33. Anderson CM, Kissel KA, Field CB, Mach KJ. Climate change mitigation, air pollution, and environmental justice in California. *Environ Sci Technol*. 2018;52(18):10829–10838. doi:10.1021/acs.est.8b00908
34. Montague D. Systematic environmental racism exposed. *Nat Sustain*. 2022;5:462–463. doi:10.1038/s41893-022-00875-y
35. Rickenbacker H, Brown F, Bilec M. Creating environmental consciousness in underserved communities: implementation and outcomes of community-based environmental justice and air pollution research. *Sustain Cities Soc*. 2019;47:101473. doi:10.1016/j.scs.2019.101473
36. Verbeek T. Unequal residential exposure to air pollution and noise: a geospatial environmental justice analysis for Ghent, Belgium. *SSM Popul Health*. 2019;7:100340. doi:10.1016/j.ssmph.2018.100340
37. Orellana RE, Moradeyo I, Uzodinma P. Decades in crisis: adapting a social-ecological framework to assess structural elements impacting asthma rates in the South Bronx. *Soc Med*. 2022;15(1):21–31.
38. Saha S, Pattanayak SK, Sills EO, Singha, AK. Under-mining health: environmental justice and mining in India. *Health and Place*. 2011;17(1):104–148. doi:10.1016/j.healthplace.2010.09.007
39. Pearce J, Kingham S. Environmental inequalities in New Zealand: a national study of air pollution and environmental justice. *Geoforum*. 2008;39(2):980–993. doi:10.1016/j.geoforum.2007.10.007
40. Rose-Pérez R. Environmental justice and air quality in Santiago de Chile. *Revista de Salud Pública*. 2015;17(3):337–350. doi:10.15446/rsap.v17n3.38465
41. Ribeiro AG, Downward GS, Umbelino de Freitas C, et al. Incidence and mortality for respiratory cancer and traffic-related air pollution in São Paulo, Brazil. *Environ Res*. 2019;170:243–251. doi:10.1016/j.envres.2018.12.034
42. Sovacool BK. The precarious political economy of cobalt: balancing prosperity, poverty, and brutality in artisanal and industrial mining in the Democratic Republic of the Congo. *Extr Ind Soc*. 2019;6(3):915–939. doi:10.1016/j.exis.2019.05.018

43. Kaufman JD, Elkind MSV, Bhatnagar A, et al. Guidance to reduce the cardiovascular burden of ambient air pollutants: a policy statement from the American Heart Association. *Circulation*. 2020;142:e432–e447. doi:10.1161/cir.0000000000000930
44. Mocumbi AO, Stewart S, Patel S, Al-Delaimy WK. Cardiovascular effects of indoor air pollution from solid fuel: relevance to Sub-Saharan Africa. *Curr Environ Health Rep*. 2019;6:116–126. doi:10.1007/s40572-019-00234-8
45. Tefera W, Asfaw A, Gilliland F, et al. Indoor and outdoor air pollution-related health problem in Ethiopia: review of related literature. *Ethiop J Health Dev*. 2016;30(1):5–16.
46. Brown P, Mayer B, Zavestoski S, Luebke T, Mandelbaum J, McCormick S. The health politics of asthma: environmental justice and collective illness experience in the United States. *Soc Sci Med*. 2003;57(3):453–464. doi:10.1016/s0277-9536(02)00375-1
47. Jones DP, Cohn BA. A vision for exposure epidemiology: the pregnancy exposure in relation to breast cancer in the child health and development studies. *Reprod Toxicol*. 2020;92:4–10. doi:10.1016/j.reprotox.2020.03.006
48. Varshavsky J, Smith A, Wang A, et al. Heightened susceptibility: a review of how pregnancy and chemical exposure influence maternal health. *Reprod Toxicol*. 2020;92:14–56. doi:10.1016/j.reprotox.2019.04.004
49. Schlanger Z. The DDT of this generation is contaminating water all over the US and Australia. *Quartz*. September 7, 2018. https://qz.com/1381593/the-ddt-of-this-generation-is-contaminating-water-all-over-the-us-and-australia
50. Lewis R. California toxics: out of state, out of mind. Cal Matters. January 25, 2023. http://calmatters.org/environment/2023/01/california-toxic-waste-dumped-arizona-utah/
51. Dockery DW, Pope CA, Xu X, et al. An association between air pollution and mortality in six U.S. cities. *N Engl J Med*. 1993;329(24):1753–1759. doi:10.1056/NEJM199312093292401
52. Currie J, Walker R. What do economists have to say about the clean air act 50 years after the establishment of the environmental protection agency? *J Econ Perspect*. 2019;33(4):3–26. doi:10.1257/jep.33.4.3
53. Schmalensee R, Stavins RN. Policy evolution under the Clean Air act. *J Econ Perspect*. 2019;33(4):27–50. doi:10.1257/jep.33.4.27
54. U.S. Environmental Protection Agency. Final Rule to Strengthen the National Air Quality Health Standard for Particulate Matter. February 7, 2024. https://www.epa.gov/system/files/documents/2024-02/pm-naaqs-overview.pdf
55. Park MG, Hong YS, Park CG, Gu DC, Mo HH. Variations in methyl bromide concentration with distance and time during quarantine fumigation. *Environ Monit Assess*. 2021;193:397. doi:10.1007/s10661-021-09154-3
56. Gharibi H, Entwistle MR, Schweizer D, Tavallali P, Thao C, Cisneros R. Methyl-bromide and asthma emergency department visits in California, USA from 2005 to 2011. *J Asthma*. 2020;57(11):1227–1236. doi:10.1080/02770903.2019.1645167
57. Coburn J. Concepts for studying urban environmental justice. *Curr Environ Health Rep*. 2017;4(1):61–67. doi:10.1007/s40572-017-0123-6
58. National Environmental Policy Act review process. United States Environmental Protection Agency. 2022. Updated October 3, 2023. https://www.epa.gov/nepa/national-environmental-policy-act-review-process#:~:text=Environmental%20Impact%20Statements%20(EIS),the%20requirements%20for%20an%20EA
59. Sensitive receptor assessment. California Air Resources Board. 2023. Accessed July 11, 2023. https://ww2.arb.ca.gov/capp-resource-center/community-assessment/sensitive-receptor-assessment#:~:text=Sensitive%20receptors%20are%20children%2C%20elderly,are%20considered%20sensitive%20receptor%20locations
60. McLaughlin T, Kearney L, Sanicola L. Special report: U.S. air monitors routinely miss pollution—even refinery explosions. Reuters. 2020. Accessed February 21, 2023. https://www.reuters.com/article/usa-pollution-airmonitors-specialreport/u-s-air-monitors-routinely-miss-pollution-even-refinery-explosions-idUSKBN28B4RT
61. deSouza P, Kinney PL. On the distribution of low-cost $PM_{2.5}$ sensors in the US: demographic and air quality associations. *J Expo Sci Environ Epidemiol*. 2021;31:514–524. doi:10.1038/s41370-021-00328-2
62. Evolution of the Clean Air Act. United States Environmental Protection Agency. 2022. Updated November 21, 2023. https://www.epa.gov/clean-air-act-overview/evolution-clean-air-act

63. Agarwal AK, Mustafi NN. Real-world automotive emissions: monitoring methodologies and control measures. *Renew Sustain Energy Rev.* 2021;137:110624. doi:10.1016/j.rser.2020.110624
64. Davis LE, Ramirez-Andreotta MD, McLain JET, Kilungo A, Abrell L, Buxner S. Increasing environmental health literacy through contextual learning in communities at risk. *Int J Res Public Health.* 2018;15(10):2203. doi:10.3390/ijerph15102203
65. Proma RA, Sumpter M, Lugo H, Friedman, E, Huq KT, Rosen P. CleanAirNowKC: building community power by improving data accessibility. 2021 IEEE Workshop on Visualization for Social Good. IEEE Computer Society Digital Library. 2021. https://www.computer.org/csdl/proceedings-article/vis4good/2021/136600a001/1yNiR2p5vBC
66. Solomon GM, Morello-Frosch R, Zeise L, Faust JB. Cumulative environmental impacts: science and policy to protect communities. *Annu Rev Public Health.* 2016;37:83–96. doi:10.1146/annurev-publhealth-032315-021807
67. English PB, Amato H, Bejarano E, et al. Performance of a low-cost sensor community air monitoring network in imperial county, CA. *Sensors.* 2020;20(11):3031. doi:10.3390/s20113031
68. Boston PQ, Strouble B, Balogun, A, et al. Community voices on the experiences of community-based participatory research in the environmental justice movement. *Soc Sci.* 2023;12(6):358. doi:10.3390/socsci12060358
69. Lerman Ginzburg S, Dimitri NC, Araujo Brinkerhoff C, Angali England S, Haque S, Sprague Martinez, LS. Exploring intergroup conflict and community-based participatory research partnerships over time. *Res All.* 2022;6(1):16. doi:10.14324/RFA.06.1.16
70. Lochotzki H, Williams KP, Colen CG, et al. A framework for interfacing and partnering with environmental justice communities as a prelude to human health and hazard identification in the vulnerable census tracts of Columbus, Ohio. *Int J Environ Res Public Health.* 2022;19:13846. doi:10.3390/ijerph192113846
71. Mitchell FM, Billiot S, Lechuga-Peña S. Utilizing photovoice to support Indigenous accounts of environmental change and injustice. *Genealogy.* 2020;4(2):51. doi:10.3390/genealogy4020051
72. Sánchez V, Sanchez-Youngman S, Dickson E, et al. CBPR implementation framework for community-academic partnerships. *Am J Community Psychol.* 2021;67(3–4):284–296. doi:10.1002/ajcp.12506
73. LaVeaux D, Simonds VW, Picket V, Cummins, J, Calkins E. Developing a curriculum for change: water & environmental health literacy in a Native American community. *Prog Community Health Partnersh.* 2018;12(4):441–449. doi:10.1353/cpr.2018.0069
74. Sprague-Martínez LS, Zamore W, Finley A, Reisner E, Lowe L, Brugge D. CBPR partnerships and near-roadway pollution: a promising strategy to influence the translation of research into practice. *Environments.* 2020;7(6):44. doi:10.3390/environments7060044
75. Lugo H. Comment letter: DTSC draft remedial action plan and mitigated negative declaration for the former PureGro facility property in Brawley, CA. California Environment Protection Agency. 2019. https://dtsc.ca.gov/wp-content/uploads/sites/31/2019/11/PureGro-Brawley-Community-Update-RAP-Mitigated-Neg-Dec.pdf
76. Varaden D, Leidland E, Lim S, Barratt B. "I am an air quality scientist"—using citizen science to characterise school children's exposure to air pollution. *Environ Res.* 2021;201:111536. doi:10.1016/j.envres.2021.111536
77. English PB, Olmedo L, Bejarano E, et al. The imperial county community air monitoring network: a model for community-based environmental monitoring for public health action. *Environ Health Perspec.* 2017;125(7):074501. doi:10.1289/EHP1772
78. IAP2. Public participation pillars. 2023. https://cdn.ymaws.com/www.iap2.org/resource/resmgr/Communications/A3_P2_Pillars_brochure.pdf
79. Carruthers DV. Environmental justice and the politics of energy on the US-Mexico border. *Environ Polit.* 2007;16(3):394–413.doi:10.1080/09644010701251649
80. Fowlie MR, Walker R, Wooley D. Climate policy, environmental justice, and local air pollution. Economic Studies at Brookings. October 20, 2020. https://www.brookings.edu/research/climate-policy-environmental-justice-and-local-air-pollution/
81. CleanAirNow. CleanAirNow environmental justice recommendations: comments on the Armourdale general plan. May 2021. https://www.docdroid.net/3ghe2XL/5-20-final-armourdalegeneralplan-docx-pdf#page=2
82. Gardinar L. Whirling, swirling, air pollution. UCAR Center for Science Education. 2023. Accessed August 25, 2023. https://scied.ucar.edu/activity/whirling-swirling-air-pollution

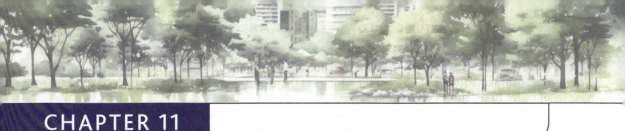

CHAPTER 11

Clean Water for All

Margaret J. Eggers, Mary Grant, Marcela González Rivas,
Anne K. Camper, James Olson, John Doyle, and Monica Lewis-Patrick

LEARNING OBJECTIVES

- Describe the water cycle and explain the sources and routes of human-caused contamination.
- Explain why climate change is primarily a water crisis through worsening floods, rising sea levels, shrinking ice fields, and more frequent wildfires and droughts—and how these events affect human health.
- Describe the basics of water treatment and municipal and private wastewater treatment systems
- Name and describe three major U.S. water laws and explain the National Primary Drinking Water Regulations.
- Explain the human right to water, water as a public commons, and why privatization and commoditization of water threatens both rights.
- Describe key issues facing public water supplies across urban, rural, and Tribal communities.
- Describe the United Nation's Sustainable Development Goal 6, and list five global measures to assess progress on this goal.

KEY TERMS

- disinfection by-products (DBP)
- harmful algal blooms (HABs)
- microplastics (MPs)
- per- and polyfluoroalkyl substances (PFAS)
- Public Water Commons
- Sustainable Development Goals (SDGs)
- water stress

"Everything is connected, and the deeper we understand that, the better we will all be. When it comes to water, all living things—including us—are close neighbors. We are all upstream from others, including the natural life who live with us. We are their voice—if we don't speak on their behalf, they are left out. We are responsible for our neighbors—we shouldn't create a bad situation they cannot fix. The Earth is alive, too."

—John Doyle, Apsáalooke Elder

OVERVIEW

All of life depends on water. To achieve environmental health for all, we must recognize and honor the ways in which water is essential for the continuation of life and the well-being of the planet. In recent decades, however, the harmful impacts of human activities on both water quantity and quality have become notably global in scope. How have we stressed our ecosystems? What are the many ways humans have contaminated our waterways and oceans?

How does the current management of our water resources protect public health and perpetuate health inequities? This chapter addresses these questions and delves into the critical role of water in sustaining life on Earth.

Since ancient societies, humans have created and managed water systems. In the American Southwest, the Hohokam and Anasazi people developed irrigation systems in the first millennium,[1] and large water storage basins have been found dating back to as early as 700 BCE.[2] Early European colonists who occupied New England relied on collecting rainwater in cisterns, dipping buckets in rivers, and digging shallow wells. The first colonial water works in our country were built of wooden pipes in Boston in the mid-1600s.[3] Until the mid-1800s, private companies owned nearly every water system and served the wealthy, excluding poor households and tenements.[3] From 1850 to 1920, following deadly cholera and other disease outbreaks, as well as destructive fires, thousands of cities assumed public ownership of their water supplies.[4] Public health was the main driver.[3] To prevent the spread of disease, cities made large improvements, built new treatment facilities, and extended water lines to low-income and Black communities, in particular, that had been excluded by private companies.[4] Notably, public ownership of water systems in the South reduced waterborne diseases in Black populations significantly, while making more minor improvements in White populations,[5] who already had better access to safe water.

A century later, this chapter addresses the ways in which we must work with our existing water infrastructure and create policies and plans to address inequities that move us toward a more sustainable future. We begin by revisiting the basic science of the water cycle and the far-reaching effects of climate change. We discuss the intricate interplay between water, human activities, and health. Next we discuss the governance, systemic disparities and challenges around water and water supplies. Lastly, we focus on public and private water supplies and wastewater treatment, including wastewater technologies, laws, regulations, and water quality. We recognize the global human right to water and water challenges, and some of the cutting-edge methods and technologies in the field of water and health are described.

THE WATER CYCLE AND CLIMATE CHANGE

Although almost three quarters of the Earth's surface is covered by water, 97% of global water is salty, 2% is freshwater locked up in Arctic and Antarctic ice, and only 1% is freshwater circulating through the atmosphere, land, and sea. At some depth below the ground surface, soil and rocks are saturated with water. The upper surface of this zone is called the water table and water below this surface is called groundwater. Groundwater feeds springs, rivers, and lakes. These bodies of water lose water through evaporation that eventually becomes rain to either replenish the groundwater or make its way to the ocean. During dry periods, the base flows of streams are maintained by groundwater discharges. Groundwater is replenished by rainfall and snowmelt infiltrating where the ground surface is porous or by wetlands that slow the flow of water and allow it to soak in. In places where buildings, pavement, and hard surfaces cover these recharge areas or where wetlands have been destroyed, groundwater cannot be easily replenished (Figure 11.1).

Water is in constant movement, and wherever it travels it can pick up contaminants and carry them along—from agricultural chemicals in fields to microplastics, pharmaceuticals and more. These pollutants can move through the water cycle, including into groundwater and surface water, and back into our drinking water supplies. Contaminants in water also affect agriculture, ranching, fisheries, recreation, and the health of the ecosystems essential to all of life on Earth. However we impact the water cycle, it will come back to affect our health.

CLIMATE CHANGE

According to the United Nations, "Climate change is primarily a water crisis. We feel its impacts through worsening floods, rising sea levels, shrinking ice fields, wildfires and droughts. However, water can fight climate change."[6(para1-2)] To reduce carbon emissions and build resilience, effective water management is essential.

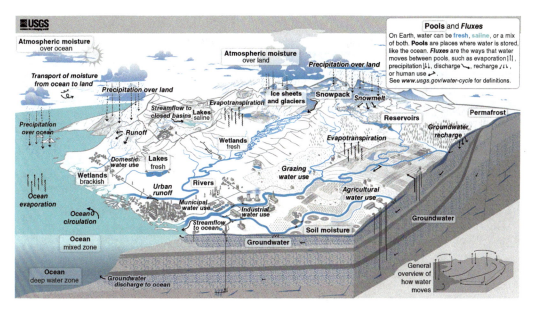

FIGURE 11.1. The water (or hydrologic) cycle and how humans impact it.

The water cycle describes how freshwater continuously circulates from the land to the sea to the atmosphere and back again. Water precipitates as rain or snow, runs off into rivers and lakes or infiltrates into the soil. Soil moisture evaporates, is transpired by plants back into the atmosphere, or percolates down to recharge the groundwater.

Source: U.S. Geological Survey. Water cycle diagrams. October 3, 2022. https://www.usgs.gov/special-topics/water-science-school/science/water-cycle-diagrams

As detailed in Figure 11.2 and in Chapter 3, "Confronting the Realities of Climate Change," the interactions between climate change, water cycles and water quality are complex, as are the implications for human health. The following list contains just a few brief examples of the complex interactions between water and health emerging in our changing climate:

- **Flooding:** Scientists project increased frequency and intensity of climate-related flooding in many areas,[7] and research suggests that flooding will lead to more diseases.[8] Communities already overburdened by environmental injustice are more at risk for harmful impacts from flooding.[9]
- **Droughts:** As expected, associations have been made between the increased frequency and intensity of droughts with decreased access to water and food but also with cardiovascular disease, infectious diseases, and worsening mental health, including suicide.[10,11]
- **Infectious disease:** Due to warming ocean waters, pathogens are now living in new regions, exposing more people to possible infection.[12] The bacteria *Vibrio cholera* causes cholera, outbreaks of which can occur any time water supplies are contaminated, like after flooding, in conflict zones, or after earthquakes. *Vibrio vulnificus*, a warm-water bacterium, causes wound infections that can be fatal, especially in people with underlying conditions like diabetes.[13]
- **Subsistence resources:** For people whose livelihoods are directly tied to the land, the effects of climate change on water resources impact not only physical and economic health, but also emotional and spiritual well-being.[14,15] These effects are particularly true for those who subsistence hunt, fish, and gather, and especially for Indigenous Peoples for whom the sacredness of water is central to their worldview and culture.

The toll of environmental disruption on human health due to climate change is profound, with many of the true costs yet to be determined.

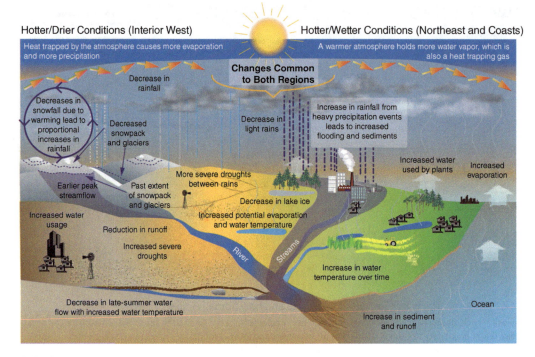

FIGURE 11.2. How climate change impacts the water cycle.
Source: Karl TR, Melillo JM, Peterson TC. Water cycle changes. In: *Global Climate Change Impacts in the United States*. U.S. Global Change Research Program; 2009. https://nca2009.globalchange.gov/water-resources/index.html#Water_Cycle_Changes

WATER AND HUMAN HEALTH

An assessment of *water stress* provides a perspective on the degree to which humans put our own health at risk via the changes we are causing in the water cycle and ecosystems. **Water stress** is not only the degree of water shortage for meeting our direct needs, it is more broadly the level of pressure that human activities exert over natural freshwater resources, indicating the environmental sustainability of the use of water resources. It is a measure of how much freshwater is being withdrawn by all economic activities, compared to the total renewable freshwater resources available. Water stress also takes into account the quantity and timing of freshwater flows and levels necessary to sustain aquatic ecosystems that, in turn, support human cultures, economies, sustainable livelihoods, and well-being.[16] As discussed later in the chapter, aquatic and terrestrial ecosystems and human well-being are also stressed by the deterioration of water quality through many types of contamination.

PUBLIC WATER AND WASTEWATER TREATMENT

About 85% of Americans receive their drinking water from one of the approximately 50,000 community water systems. U.S. public water suppliers provide about 39 billion gallons of water per day, with about 61% of this coming from surface water sources and the remainder from groundwater.[17] The source of the water dictates the type of treatment and the specific processes required to meet drinking water standards and protect public health.

Drinking-water treatment plants are designed to meet federal and state regulations. State requirements may be more stringent than federal regulations but not less. These plants have multiple treatment strategies that provide protection from regulated contaminants so that the processed, "finished" water is safe to drink. Federal drinking water regulations can be found on the U.S. Environmental Protection Agency (EPA) website and require that water systems test for:

- turbidity (i.e., clarity or cloudiness of the water),
- certain microbes (e.g. total coliform bacteria, *Giardia, Legionella*, and viruses),
- a limited number of inorganic and organic compounds in the finished water, and
- the impact the water may have on the corrosion of pipes, which can affect lead and copper levels at the tap.

Treatment plants may also be designed to remove tastes, odors, or excessive hardness (i.e., water with high mineral content). Public water system customers can obtain information about the levels of contaminants in their drinking water by requesting a copy of the Consumer Confidence Report from their local water supplier. This report explains whether their water supply meets EPA and state drinking-water standards.[18]

Surface water treatment plants extract water from rivers, lakes, and reservoirs. A surface water treatment plant may include preliminary disinfection, coagulation to consolidate colloidal materials, flocculation to increase particle size, sedimentation to remove the coagulated particles, filtration to further remove particulate matter, additional disinfection to provide a residual disinfectant in the distribution system, and corrosion control to reduce lead and copper leaching in household plumbing (Figure 11.3). Unfortunately, some types of disinfectants react with organic matter in the water to create hazardous chemicals referred to as **disinfection by-products (DBPs)**. For example, in the case of the Flint Water Crisis (described in Chapter 4, "Environmental Health Policies and Protections: Successes and Failures," and in Chapter 15, "Preparing for and Recovering From Disasters in Our Changing Climate"), excessive amounts of chlorine were added to address the corrosion of lead pipes. However, the use of chlorine triggered chemical reactions resulting in an increase of the DBP trihalomethane, a known carcinogen that is also associated with negative developmental and reproductive health issues. An alternative is to use ozone or ultraviolet light instead of chlorine for a primary disinfectant and chloramines as a secondary disinfectant to provide a "residual" in the distribution system to suppress microbial growth.

Groundwater treatment plants draw water from below the water table. Groundwater quality is likely to be different from surface water quality. Groundwater often has higher levels of metals and other inorganic contaminants, while surface water typically has more turbidity and may have higher levels of microbial contamination. Treatment of groundwater may require water softeners to remove dissolved minerals, filtration to remove microbes, or other technologies to remove organic chemicals like solvents, pesticides, and disinfectants.[19]

WASTEWATER TREATMENT

Humans generate runoff and wastewater with daily activities such as flushing toilets, using dishwashers and washing machines, and driving cars. Our commercial, industrial, and agricultural systems also contribute to runoff that may contain pesticides, animal waste, chemicals, heavy metals, or other pollutants (Figure 11.4).

The maintenance of public health demands that sewage and wastewater be collected and treated before it is returned to water bodies, spread over the land surface, or reused. Untreated water can carry pathogens that cause illnesses such as cholera, typhoid, pneumonia, and many other protozoans, bacteria, and viruses. Most of these organisms cause gastrointestinal diseases, but a few are associated with respiratory infections or other illnesses. Several are regulated and appear on the EPA's National Primary Drinking Water Regulations (NPDWR) list, and several more pathogens are found on the EPA's current Contaminant Candidate List 5 (CCL5).[20] The CCL5 contains contaminants of concern that may become regulated in the future and is updated periodically (Table 11.1). Public health agencies are on guard to respond, particularly if there is a sudden increase in cases of these specific illnesses.

Water Treatment Plant

Follow a drop of water from the source through the treatment process. Water may be treated differently in different communities depending on the quality of the water which enters the plant. Groundwater is located underground and typically requires less treatment than water from lakes, rivers, and streams.

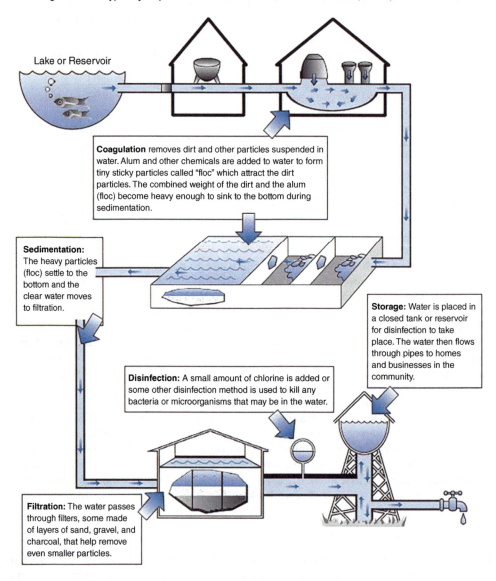

FIGURE 11.3. Diagram of a water treatment plant.

Source: U.S. Environmental Protection Agency. *Water on Tap: What You Need to Know.* EPA 816-K-09-002. National Service Center for Environmental Publications; December 2009.

Most American cities and towns have two separate sewer systems: one to collect and treat the sewage and wastewater, and another to collect and discharge stormwater. Systems collecting both wastewater and stormwater are termed *combined sewers*. Modern construction of combined sewers is rare because of risks of sewage overflows and the widely varied water quality they may deliver to the treatment plant. However, about 860 older cities like Detroit, Michigan; Pittsburgh, Pennsylvania; and Baltimore, Maryland, still have combined sewer systems.[21] More than 850 billion gallons of raw sewage were spilled from combined sewer systems into

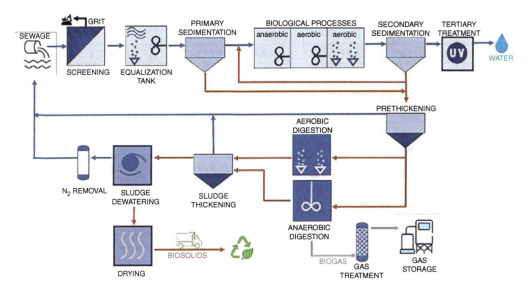

FIGURE 11.4. Wastewater treatment system.

A typical municipal wastewater treatment plant will include grit removal and screening to remove larger materials, a primary clarifier to settle out organic matter, aeration to encourage microbes to degrade into more organic and inorganic compounds, a secondary clarifier to further remove particles, and disinfection. The material collected in the primary and secondary clarifiers is called sludge and requires further treatment before disposal.

Source: Jazbec M, Turner AJ. *Wastewater Gas Recovery Opportunities in a Circular Economy*. Institute for Sustainable Futures, University of Technology Sydney; January 2020.

TABLE 11.1. WATERBORNE PATHOGENS OF MOST CONCERN FOR PUBLIC AND PRIVATE DRINKING WATER SUPPLIES

MICROORGANISM	CATEGORY	HEALTH EFFECTS	SOURCE
Protozoans			
Cryptosporidium	Regulated	Gastrointestinal illness	Human and animal fecal material
Giardia lamblia	Regulated	Gastrointestinal illness (giardiasis)	Human and animal fecal material
Naegleria fowleri	CCL5	Primary amebic meningoencephalitis, rare disease	Naturally occurring in warm waters
Bacteria			
Campylobacter jejuni	CCL5	Gastrointestinal illness	Human and animal fecal material
Escherichia coli (O157)	CCL5	Gastrointestinal illness, kidney failure	Human and animal fecal material
Fecal coliform and *E. coli*	Regulated	Indicators of fecal contamination, may cause disease	Human and animal fecal material
Helicobacter pylori	CCL5	Gastrointestinal ulcers	Human and animal fecal material
Heterotrophic plate count	Regulated	None, analytical method for general microbial quality	Naturally occurring

(continued)

TABLE 11.1. WATERBORNE PATHOGENS OF MOST CONCERN FOR PUBLIC AND PRIVATE DRINKING WATER SUPPLIES (*continued*)

MICROORGANISM	CATEGORY	HEALTH EFFECTS	SOURCE
Bacteria			
Legionella	Regulated	Respiratory disease	Naturally occurring
Legionella pneumophila	CCL5	Respiratory disease	Naturally occurring
Mycobacterium abscessus and *M. avium*	CCL5	Respiratory disease	Naturally occurring
Pseudomonas aeruginosa	CCL5	Pneumonia, infections	Naturally occurring
Total coliforms	Regulated	Indicators of contamination	May be naturally occurring
Shigella sonnei	CCL5	Gastrointestinal illness	Human and animal fecal material
Viruses			
Adenoviruses	CCL5	Respiratory disease, gastrointestinal illness	Human and animal fecal material
Caliciviruses (including Norovirus)	CCL5	Gastrointestinal illness	Human and animal fecal material
Enteric viruses	Regulated	Gastrointestinal illness	Human and animal fecal material
Enteroviruses	CCL5	Respiratory disease	Human sources

CCL, contaminant candidate list

waterways in 2004, per the latest EPA estimate.[22] The siting of combined sewer outfalls can disproportionately impact low-wealth and communities of color. While improvements have been made, outdated infrastructure combined with climate-change-fueled storms continue to cause raw sewage to back up into basements, flood onto streets, and spill into rivers, lakes, and streams.[23] Thousands of people become sick each year just from exposure to sewage-contaminated recreation areas. Hepatitis, gastroenteritis, and infections of the skin, lungs, and ears are concerns with sewage-polluted waters.[24] See Table 11.1 for more information on the most concerning waterborne pathogens. For further information and diagrams, see the EPA's "Combined Sewer Overflow Basics."[25]

As with drinking water treatment, municipal wastewater treatment processes are designed around the characteristics of the local wastewater and the regulations governing the quality of the final treated wastewater or the effluent (i.e., the liquid waste or sewage discharged into waterways). Federal and state requirements regulate the amounts of organic carbon, nitrogen, and microbial loads in the effluent or final treated wastewater. For instance:

- Too much organic carbon can lead to higher bacteria activity and depleted oxygen levels that can kill fish or cause other damage to the ecosystem.
- Too much nitrogen or phosphate can cause excessive algal growth that can be a source for toxins and also lead to decreases in oxygen.
- Microbes can harm recreational users and downstream drinking water supplies.

PRIVATE WATER SUPPLIES: WELLS AND SEPTIC SYSTEMS

Public water and wastewater services are not available in many rural areas. People must rely instead on individual water systems consisting of personal wells and septic systems. Research in 2021 estimated that over 23 million U.S. households relied on personal, private systems.[26] Water systems consist of the well, pump, pressure tank, and household plumbing.

Getting home well water tested and, if needed, treated to remove local groundwater contaminants, is essential for protecting health. If water quality is poor, homeowners may install softeners to remove hardness and iron, home chlorination or ultraviolet (UV) systems for disinfection, or reverse-osmosis filtration systems to remove chemical and microbial contaminants, which may be particularly costly.

For many of the same households, wastewater is typically treated and disposed via septic systems, also called decentralized or on-site systems (Figure 11.5). In most areas, a permit is required for the installation of a septic system. The system consists of a septic tank (often buried) where the solids collect, the organics are digested by natural bacteria, and the oils and greases float. After passage through the tank, the effluent is discharged into buried perforated pipes called the leach field or drain field. Alternatively, constructed wetlands containing plants such as sedges and rushes can help to treat effluent with their associated microbial communities, which is an important treatment option for rural areas and less developed areas around the world.[27] Periodically, the septic tank must be pumped to remove accumulated solids, or the drainfield will be clogged and septage will back up into the home. Installing, protecting, maintaining, and repairing home wells and septic systems are solely the responsibility of the homeowner and, again, can be quite costly over time.

Private wells are not regulated by federal laws. Well installation and water-quality testing are not federally mandated either.[28] Because there are no federal laws governing private wells, regulations vary by state. Most states have standards for the location and installation of new wells, as well as limits on the amount of water that can be withdrawn from the aquifer. After a well is installed, many states require a basic water test to ensure the absence of total coliform bacteria before the well can be used.[29] Private well owners are responsible for testing and protecting the quality of their well water. Wells can be contaminated by agricultural, industrial, mining, and military practices, as well as landfills, leaking underground storage tanks, septic tank discharge, livestock, floodwaters, firefighting foam, transportation and pipeline accidents or spills, naturally occurring minerals, and more. Many states also have laws regarding private-well septic systems, which require inspection, correction, or replacement before the sale of property. These laws have contributed to a significant reduction in

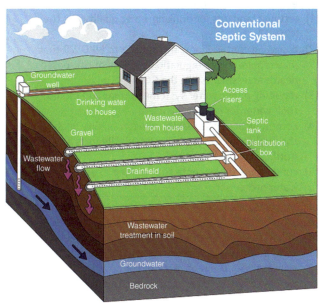

FIGURE 11.5. Home well and septic system.

Source: Types of septic systems. U.S. Environmental Protection Agency. 2022. Updated August 7, 2023. https://www.epa.gov/septic/types-septic-systems#septictank

contamination from nutrients and *Escherichia coli*, particularly near rivers and lakes. However, many homeowners are unaware of the processes for testing private wells, interpreting the results, and managing septic systems, highlighting the need for educational programming for households.

LAWS AND REGULATIONS AFFECTING WATER SUPPLIES

Introduced in Chapter 5, "Environmental Health Science for the People," the 1972 Clean Water Act (CWA) and the 1974 Safe Drinking Water Act (SDWA), as amended, are two critical U.S. water quality laws. The CWA helps to restore and maintain the integrity of water bodies nationwide. The SDWA protects public health by regulating public water supplies, protecting groundwater, and conducting source water assessments. More recently, to help us meet the standards in the CWA and SDWA, the 2021 Infrastructure Investment and Jobs Act invested almost $55 billion in water infrastructure across the United States (Table 11.2).

TABLE 11.2. KEY U.S. FEDERAL WATER LAWS

LAW	GOAL(S)	PRIMARY METHODS OF PROTECTING WATER QUALITY AND PUBLIC HEALTH
1972 Clean Water Act (CWA)	Restore and maintain the chemical, physical, and biological integrity of the nation's waters	Helps to restore and maintain the integrity of water by (1) regulating pollutant discharge from point sources; (2) setting water quality standards for surface waters; (3) developing programs for the control of pollution from nonpoint sources, like stormwater management; and (4) developing programs for funding water-treatment infrastructure.
1974 Safe Drinking Water Act (SDWA)	Protect sources of drinking water and ensure that public water systems provide safe drinking water for public health protection	Protects public health drinking water by: (1) setting standards for drinking water quality like the NPDWR; (2) assessing contaminants not subject to NPDWR that may require future regulation because of risk-based health assessments like the CCL; (3) requiring public water systems to treat and monitor their water for contaminants; (4) communicating the results of water quality analysis to the public via Consumer Confidence Reports and public notification; and (5) conducting assessments and working to ensure source water protection.
2021 Infrastructure Investment and Jobs Act	Expand access to clean drinking water, tackle the climate crisis, and advance environmental justice, among other goals	Includes a focus on water-quality improvements across the United States, investing almost $55 billion, including $15 billion for lead service line removal projects and $2 billion to address contaminants like PFAS; state and local governments can use recovery funds from the American Rescue Plan toward water-quality improvement projects

CCL, Contaminant Candidate List; HAs, Health Advisories; NPDWR, National Primary Drinking Water Regulations; PFAS, per- and polyfluoroalkyl substances.

Among other things, the SDWA sets the National Primary Drinking Water Regulations (NPDWR) for public water supplies, including:

- *Maximum Contaminant Level Goal* (MCLG), defined as "the level of a contaminant in drinking water below which there is no known or expected risk to health. MCLGs allow for a margin of safety and are nonenforceable public health goals,"[30(para3)] and
- *Maximum Contaminant Level* (MCL), defined as, "The highest level of a contaminant that is allowed in drinking water [see Table 11.3]. MCLs are set as close to the MCLG as feasible using the best available analytical and treatment technologies and taking cost into consideration. MCLs are enforceable standards."[31(pvi)]

For instance, the MCLG for arsenic is 0 mg/L, as any detectable amount of arsenic in drinking water increases various health risks. However, it is not feasible to remove all arsenic from

TABLE 11.3. SELECT CONTAMINANTS COVERED BY THE EPA'S NPDWR

CONTA-MINANT	MCLG (MG/L)	MCL OR TT (MG/L)	POTENTIAL HEALTH EFFECTS	SOURCES OF CONTAMINANT IN DRINKING WATER
Inorganic Chemicals				
Arsenic	0	0.01	Increased risk of lung, bladder, and skin cancer; neurological effects; vascular and respiratory abnormalities; skin lesions; diabetes; neurodevelopmental risks for children; adverse pregnancy outcomes; and mortality.	Erosion of natural deposits; runoff from orchards and from glass and electronics production wastes; arsenical pesticides, including wood preservatives
Asbestos (fiber > 10 μm)	7 million fibers/L	7 MFL	Increased risk of developing benign intestinal polyps	Decay of asbestos cement in water mains; erosion of natural deposits; some evidence that migration from waste sites through soil is possible
Chromium (total)	0.1	0.1	Allergic dermatitis; hexavalent chromium: stomach irritation, ulcers; likely gastrointestinal carcinogen; effects on the liver, blood, and lower respiratory tract; developmental toxicity. May affect immune and reproductive systems	Discharge from steel and pulp mills and a wide variety of other industrial activities; erosion of natural deposits
Copper	TT = 1.3	TT = 1.3	Acute: gastrointestinal distress. Chronic: liver or kidney damage. People with Wilson disease are more vulnerable.	Corrosion of household plumbing systems; erosion of natural deposits

(continued)

TABLE 11.3. SELECT CONTAMINANTS COVERED BY THE EPA'S NPDWR (*continued*)

CONTA-MINANT	MCLG (MG/L)	MCL OR TT (MG/L)	POTENTIAL HEALTH EFFECTS	SOURCES OF CONTAMINANT IN DRINKING WATER
Inorganic Chemicals				
Fluoride	4	4	Bone disease (pain, tenderness, and fragility of the bones); Children may get mottled teeth.	Water additive that promotes strong teeth; erosion of natural deposits; discharge from fertilizer and aluminum factories
Lead	zero	TT = 0.015	Infants and children: delays in physical or mental development; deficits in attention span and learning abilities. Adults: kidney problems; high blood pressure	Corrosion of household plumbing and distribution infrastructure systems; erosion of natural deposits
Mercury (inorganic)	0.002	0.002	Kidney damage	Coal burning; discharge from refineries and factories; runoff from landfills and croplands; erosion of natural deposits
Nitrate (measured as Nitrogen)	10	10	Infants who drink water containing nitrite above the MCL could become seriously ill and, if untreated, may die. Symptoms include shortness of breath and blue baby syndrome. Associated with colorectal and bladder cancers, neural tube defects, and thyroid disease.	Runoff from fertilizer use; leaking from septic tanks, sewage, livestock manure; erosion of natural deposits
Selenium	0.05	0.05	Hair or fingernail loss; numbness in fingers or toes; circulatory problems	Discharge from petroleum and metal refineries; erosion of natural deposits; discharge from mines
Thallium	0.0005	0.002	Hair loss; changes in blood; kidney, intestine, or liver problems	Leaching from ore-processing sites; discharge from electronics, glass, and drug factories; coal burning and smelting
Manganese - *Health-Based Screening Levels (HBSLs)*		0.3	Poorer attention, memory, and other neurological effects	Industrial emissions and pollution; erosion of natural deposits

(*continued*)

TABLE 11.3. SELECT CONTAMINANTS COVERED BY THE EPA'S NPDWR (*continued*)

CONTA-MINANT	MCLG (MG/L)	MCL OR TT (MG/L)	POTENTIAL HEALTH EFFECTS	SOURCES OF CONTAMINANT IN DRINKING WATER
Radionuclides				
Radium 226 and Radium 228	zero	5 pCi/L	Increased risk of bone, liver, and breast cancer	Coal burning; uranium and hard rock mining; waste piles; erosion of natural deposits
Uranium	zero	30 ug/L	Increased risk of cancer, kidney toxicity, osteotoxicity; DNA repair inhibition in human embryonic kidney cells. Linked to diabetes	Uranium mining and milling; waste piles; nuclear testing; contaminant of fertilizer; erosion of natural deposits
Organic Chemicals				
Disinfection By-Products (DBPs): More than 700 have been identified; only 11 are regulated by the EPA.				
Bromate	zero	0.01	Increased risk of cancer	By-product of drinking water disinfection
Chlorite	0.8	1	Anemia in infants and young children; nervous system effects	By-product of drinking water disinfection
Haloacetic acids (HAA5)	variable	0.06	Increased risk of cancer	By-product of drinking water disinfection
Total trihalomethanes (TTHMs)	variable	0.08	Liver, kidney, or central nervous system problems; increased risk of bladder cancer	By-product of drinking water disinfection
Per- and polyfluoroalkyl substances (PFAS)	0–10 ppt (or ng/L)	4–10 ppt	Reproductive harm, hormone disruption, immune system dysfunction, and increased risk of cancer	Human-made chemicals used in industry and consumer products

EPA, U.S. Environmental Protection Agency; L, liter; MCL, maximum contaminant level; MCLG, maximum contaminant level goal; MFL, million fibers per liter; MG, milligram; ng, nanogram; NPDWR, National Primary Drinking Water Regulations;[32] pCi, picocuries; ppt, part per trillion; TT, treatment technique action levels; μg, microgram; μm, micrometer.

Source: U.S. Environmental Protection Agency. National primary drinking water regulations. 2009. Updated January 2, 2024. https://www.epa.gov/ground-water-and-drinking-water/national-primary-drinking-water-regulations; Per- and polyfluoroalkyl substances (PFAS): Final PFAS National Primary Drinking Water Regulation. *Safe Drinking Water Act*. U.S. Environmental Protection Agency. Updated June 17, 2024. https://www.epa.gov/sdwa/and-polyfluoroalkyl-substances-pfas

public drinking water, so treatment plants are only required to reduce arsenic to its MCL of 0.010 mg/L. Lead and copper have treatment technique action levels (TTs) instead of MCLs, or the processes that must be implemented to reduce the level of each contaminant in drinking water.[32]

As is evident from the EPA's NPDWR discussed earlier and as explained in Chapter 4, "Environmental Health Policies and Protections: Successes and Failures," and Chapter 6, "Understanding (Unequal and Cumulative) Risks in Our Daily Environment," regulatory efforts in the United States are typically focused on assessing human health risks from exposure to *individual* chemicals and pathogens. More recently, risk-assessment techniques that address the combined risk from exposure to multiple chemical and nonchemical stressors have been and are being developed.[33] This approach, called *cumulative risk assessment* (CRA), acknowledges that we are exposed to complex mixtures of contaminants through drinking water, food, air, and other sources each day. CRA also acknowledges that marginalized populations often face increased morbidity and mortality because of combined exposures to environmental, psychosocial, and economic stressors.[34] An example of CRA is the additive approach used by the U.S. Geological Survey (USGS) and other organizations to estimate the cumulative risk from drinking water contaminants, which have indicated substantial risks to the most vulnerable populations, such as infants, children, pregnant persons, and older adults, and immune-compromised populations.[35]

OTHER COMMON CONTAMINANTS IN WATER

Altogether, the U.S. EPA has defined more than 90 MCLs for organic and inorganic contaminants, 6 MCLs for per- and polyfluoroalkyl substances (PFAS; see the following section), 430 nonenforceable Human Health Benchmarks for Pesticides (HHBP), and 100-plus nonenforceable drinking water Health Advisories (HAs). In addition, the USGS has defined 174 nonenforceable Health-Based Screening Levels (HBSLs), primarily for organic chemicals. Collectively, these standards only cover about 0.2% of the more than 350,000 chemicals and chemical mixtures currently registered for production and use.[36] Thousands of chemicals with known health risks are unregulated or underregulated.

Per- and Polyfluoroalkyl Substances

PFAS are a class of millions of compounds that pose a public health concern owing to their prevalence and persistence, toxicity, and human exposure through water and food.[37] PFAS can be found in many products, such as nonstick cookware; water-resistant fabrics; grease-resistant food packaging; personal care products, such as dental floss, nail polish, eye makeup, and shampoo; and innumerable other products (Figure 11.6).[38] These substances are commonly

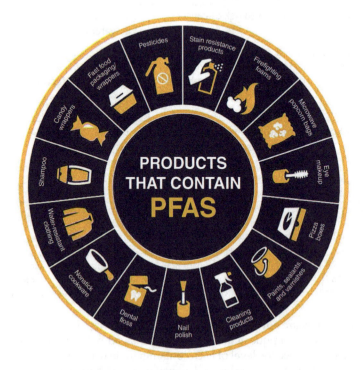

FIGURE 11.6. Products that contain PFAS.

PFAS, per- and polyfluoroalkyl substances.

Source: PFAS. City of Riverside Public Utilities. Accessed June 14, 2024. https://www.riversideca.gov/utilities/residents/our-water/pfas

detected in human blood and can be transferred from mother to child before and after birth. They have been associated with developmental, metabolic, and immune disorders.[39] PFAS are found worldwide in surface and groundwater drinking water supplies, and potential pathways are diverse and well documented.[38]

In the United States, regulations regarding PFAS in drinking water have been changing rapidly, with increasingly strict guidelines established over the past 20 years.[40] In April 2024, the EPA released the first national MCLs for 6 different PFAS at levels between 4 and 10 parts per trillion (ppt) and MCLGs for perfluorooctanoic acid (PFOA) and perfluorooctane sulfonate (PFOS) at 0 ppt, indicating growing concerns about PFAS exposure through drinking water.[41] The information currently available on PFAS in drinking water mainly comes from regulated public water supplies prior to distribution, but there are limited data on unregulated private well users at the point of exposure. Approximately 45% of the drinking water samples collected in the United States have been found to contain at least one PFAS, with no differences between public and private water supplies.[41] The detection of PFAS in drinking water combined with the lack of information on health risks highlight the ongoing need for monitoring, particularly in unmonitored private wells and in underserved communities relying on small community water supplies.

Disinfection By-Products From Drinking Water Treatment

The public health benefits of drinking-water disinfection for the prevention of historical, high-mortality waterborne diseases are unarguable, but the public-health trade-offs of disinfection are of increasing concern.[42] An estimated 90%, 80%, and 50% reductions in outbreaks of cholera, typhoid, and amoebic dysentery, respectively, in the United States in the early 20th century can be attributed to the widespread adoption of drinking-water disinfection.[43] With decreasing waterborne outbreaks and our collective fading memories of historic epidemics of previous centuries, the public may question the value of some disinfection efforts. Public attention has increasingly focused on the chlorine taste and odor of treated drinking water and the health risks of DBP.

First reported in 1974, DBP are types of compounds formed from the reactions of chemical disinfectants with natural organic matter (NOM) or algal organic matter (AOM) in source waters.[44] Epidemiologic studies have documented associations of various DBP with adverse human health effects, including bladder cancer, colorectal cancer, miscarriage, and birth defects.[45] Only 11 DBP are currently regulated, which limits their concentrations in public drinking water. However, more than 700 have been identified to date.[44] Many unregulated DBP, including the nitrogenous and iodinated (iodine-containing) forms, are more toxic than the regulated DBP, hence they are important drivers of drinking-water toxicity.[46] DBPs commonly exceed one or more EPA MCLGs, both in public water supplies and in bottled water sourced from purified tap water.[47] These incidents illustrate the dire need for better understanding of the health risks of exposures to individual and combined regulated and unregulated DBP. Additionally, it is vital that we improve source-water pretreatment technologies to reduce concentrations of the organic matter precursors to DBP.

Pesticides

There are 500 to 600 active pesticide ingredients in use in the United States, with more than a billion pounds used annually. In a 2021 study testing over 1,200 wells from aquifers representing 70% of the drinking water supply, 41% were positive for pesticides or pesticide residues.[48]

- Traditional public drinking water treatment does little to reduce pesticide concentrations. Only nine pesticides in current use have MCLs and, of these, the herbicides alachlor, atrazine, and simazine are most commonly found to seasonally exceed their MCLs in water samples.[49]
- Seventy-two of the agricultural pesticides in use in the United States are banned or are being completely phased out in the European Union.[50]

- Four hundred thirty pesticides lack an MCL or HA, but now have nonenforceable EPA HHBP owing to their health effects when consumed in drinking water.[51]
- The two most commonly used pesticides are atrazine and glyphosate; atrazine may impact human reproduction.[52] Although the EPA has not found glyphosate to cause cancer when used according to labeling instructions, the World Health Organization's International Agency for Research on Cancer reviewed approximately 1,000 studies of glyphosate and subsequently listed the herbicide as a "probable carcinogen."[53] For further information, see the USGS website "Pesticides and Water Quality."[54]

Pharmaceuticals

Of the more than 4,000 human and livestock pharmaceuticals used in the United States, many enter the environment from pharmaceutical plants, as well as through humans and livestock as waste. These pharmaceuticals can bioaccumulate and biomagnify, harming humans and wildlife such as birds, fish, and insects. This happens when chemicals or toxins build up in humans or animals over time. Instead of being quickly broken down or expelled, they stay in our tissues or organs. For example, perch that consume damselfly larvae contaminated with the antianxiety drug oxazepam exhibit decreased caution and leave their protective schools more frequently.[55]

Even when passed through surface waters, many wastewater treatment systems do not break pharmaceuticals down. Mixtures of pharmaceuticals are widely reported in rivers that typically receive wastewater effluent. However, a recent USGS study found that 75% of smaller streams without wastewater effluent also commonly have pharmaceutical mixtures, which can reach concentrations likely to have effects on vertebrates. Pharmaceutical contamination is a nationwide issue needing mitigation to reduce surface-water contamination.[56]

Volatile Organic Compounds

Volatile organic compounds (VOCs) are defined by the EPA as "organic chemical compounds whose composition makes it possible for them to evaporate under normal indoor atmospheric conditions of temperature and pressure."[57(para5)] Although VOCs are both indoor and outdoor air pollutants, they also persist and migrate in groundwater, and hence can contaminate well water. Produced in huge quantities, they are found in many different commercial and household products, including gasoline, paints, cleaners, plastics, glues, carpets, fumigants, degreasers, refrigerants, dry cleaning fluids, personal care products, pharmaceuticals, pesticides and more. There are also many industrial uses for VOCs in manufacturing. The EPA is required to monitor some VOCs in our water systems, but their ubiquitous and long-term use raises concerns about both environmental and human health.[58]

Harmful Algal Blooms and Cyanotoxins

Harmful algal blooms (HABs) are composed of aquatic cyanobacteria, which are unicellular photosynthetic organisms that, when exposed to high concentrations of inorganic nutrients under favorable conditions, can produce cyanotoxins.[59] In the past several decades, bloom frequency and intensity has increased dramatically.[60] Climate change and human-caused increased nutrient abundance promote HAB development.[59] HABs generally prefer warmer waters since hotter temperatures reduce the mixing of water, allowing the cyanobacteria to grow faster and thicker, creating more blooms. However, HABs also occur in cold waters where temperatures are below 15°C (59°F), with some living in ice-covered conditions.[61]

HABs can have negative impacts on ecosystems, water quality, and human and animal health, as well as the economic health of coastal communities reliant on tourism or recreational activities. Nontoxic HABs can also damage ecosystems by depleting oxygen, blocking sunlight, harming aquatic animals, and forming brown tides. Human health effects include abdominal pain, vomiting, diarrhea, fever, headache, sore throat, and, in rare circumstances, death. Exposure routes include inhalation, ingestion of contaminated water or seafood, or direct contact with a water source containing cyanotoxins.[60]

Cyanotoxins are not yet federally regulated drinking water contaminants, therefore, it is the responsibility of individual public water suppliers to voluntarily monitor for cyanotoxins.

Since there is no EPA requirement for testing, analytical methods vary among states.[62] Cyanotoxins can also be difficult to remove because conventional water treatment can usually remove cyanobacterial cells and low levels of cyanotoxins but is less effective during severe bloom outbreaks.[63]

Microplastics

Microplastics (MPs), defined as plastic particles less than 5 mm in size, are an emerging contaminant of environmental concern. Like many other contaminants mentioned previously, they are long-lived and ubiquitous in our environment, having been found in 93% of drinking-water sources tested across 11 countries.[64] Much attention has been paid to the presence of MPs in surface water environments with less attention paid to them in groundwater sources and in the atmosphere, soils, seabed, and terrestrial lifeforms.[65] Humans are exposed through food ingestion, inhalation, and dermal absorption, with effects on our digestive, respiratory, immune, neurologic, hepatic, dermal and reproductive systems.[66] There is a critical need to characterize and reduce MPs in public water supply systems, our food supply, and in ecosystems worldwide.[67]

REAL PEOPLE AND PLACES: BOOKS AND MOVIES ABOUT INDUSTRIAL WATER CONTAMINATION

There are a number of well-known cases of serious health effects from industrial contamination of community water sources in the United States whose stories you can learn through popular books or movies, such as those listed in the following.

- The 2014 Pulitzer Prize-winning, best-selling nonfiction book *Toms River: A Story of Science and Salvation* discusses the contamination of the water supply in Toms River, New Jersey, by industrial chemicals that led to elevated numbers of leukemia and brain and central nervous system cancers.[68]
- The poisoning of the Woburn, Massachusetts, aquifer with the industrial solvent trichloroethylene (TCE) in the 1980s and the deaths of a dozen children from leukemia is documented in the book *A Civil Action* and in a 1998 film of the same name.[69]
- The book *A Terrible Thing to Waste: Environmental Racism and Its Assault on the American Mind* details how environmental exposures to untested chemicals and heavy metals such as lead (in both water and paint), diminish IQ and impact health in multigenerational ways.[70] One case described is the poisoning of people in Anniston, Alabama, by Monsanto Chemical Corporation's releases of polychlorinated biphenyls (PCBs) into air and water.
- The Pacific Gas and Electric Corporation discharged wastewater contaminated with hexavalent chromium—a cancer-causing heavy metal—into unlined ponds in Hinkley, California, resulting in groundwater pollution.[71] Pacific Gas and Electric was sued and in 1996 settled the case for $333 million. The movie *Erin Brockovich*, starring Julia Roberts, tells the story.

PUBLIC WATER SUPPLIES: GOVERNANCE

Sewage management relied on privy vaults and cesspools (holes in the ground) until the mid-1800s. The early sewers were used as storm drains. While most major cities had a sewer system by the early 1900s, more than 95% of cities released untreated wastewater to waterways.[72] Many of the nation's wastewater treatment plants were built or improved with the federal dollars provided by the Clean Water Act of 1972, one of the largest public works programs in United States history (see Table 11.4).[23]

Currently, the United States has about 50,000 community water systems—defined as a system providing water to at least 15 households or at least 25 people. A utility is the entity that provides water and charges households, and a utility can own one or more water systems. Most people receive their water service from their local government, but there are many small

TABLE 11.4. FORMS OF PUBLIC WATER SUPPLY GOVERNANCE AND OPPORTUNITIES FOR PUBLIC ENGAGEMENT

UTILITY OWNER	DESCRIPTION	DECISION-MAKING
Public or governmental ownership model		
Local government	Municipalities (e.g., city, town, village) and counties usually have water departments or divisions that provide service within, and often outside of, their jurisdiction. Counties can serve unincorporated areas within their borders and can own more than one water system.	Local elected officials
Public districts	Public districts are separate governmental entities established to provide water service, usually with the same powers as local government, such as the power to use eminent domain, issue revenue bonds, and collect user fees.	Elected board of commissioners
Regional or local authority	Local authorities are typically established to serve one jurisdiction and can serve multiple jurisdictions. Regional authorities are created to serve multiple municipalities, and can be direct-service providers and/or bulk water providers, which treat and supply water to other water systems for distribution.	Board of directors, with members appointed by participating governments
State	State facilities, such as prisons, colleges, and mental health hospitals.	State government
Federal	they are often military bases, many of which are privatized under concession agreements.	Federal agencies, such as the Department of Defense
Tribal systems	These include Tribal government, the Bureau of Indian Affairs (BIA), and the Indian Health Service (IHS), with some Tribes assuming BIA and/or IHS responsibilities.	Complicated and varies by Tribe and by state.
Private or nongovernmental ownership model		
Investor-owned utilities	For-profit water corporations are called investor-owned utilities and own about 20% of privately owned systems. A handful of large corporations own many of these systems.	Corporate executives with economic regulation by the state's Public Utility Commission
Nonprofit systems	About 40% of private systems are owned by not-for-profit entities, including homeowners associations (HOAs) and cooperatives.	HOA board or membership
Ancillary services	About 40% of private systems are ancillary systems (typically very small), wherein the primary business is not water service, but water service is a necessary part of the primary business. These systems are mostly manufactured home parks.	Owners and managers of ancillary systems

Source: Safe Drinking Water Information System (SDWIS) Federal Reporting Services. U.S. Environmental Protection Agency. 2022. Updated March 14, 2024. https://www.epa.gov/ground-water-and-drinking-water/safe-drinking-water-information-system-sdwis-federal-reporting

private-ancillary or nonprofit systems. As of 2022, 87% of the U.S. population connected to a community water system received service from a publicly owned system.[73]

Water services are perfect examples of "natural monopolies"; it is more efficient to have one provider instead of multiple ones owing to the prohibitively high cost of building multiple networks of water pipes and sewers in the same place. Because of the way in which water services are structured, most states regulate the rates of investor-owned water systems through public utility commissions or public service commissions, but it is challenging to regulate natural monopolies when corporate providers have more resources and power than regulatory agencies.

PUBLIC WATER SUPPLIES: KEY ISSUES AND CHALLENGES

Despite advancements in water treatment, about 24 million people were served by community water systems with health-based water quality violations in 2021. Since 2000, on average, 8% of the population connected with community water systems received water that violated health-based standards.[74] As exemplified by many recent major water crises, water quality problems in large cities disproportionately harm majority Black and Hispanic or Latino communities.[75] Systemic issues drive this inequity, including:

- poor planning,
- economic inequality and poverty,
- racism,
- housing instability,
- climate change,
- White population and wealth flight from majority Black cities that left water systems without the customer base to support necessary improvements,[76] and
- decades of federal and state austerity and disinvestment in water infrastructure.

A recent analysis of water hardship across the United States found that nearly 490,000 households lack complete plumbing, 1,165 public water systems are in serious violation of the SDWA, and more than 21,000 permittees are in significant noncompliance with the CWA. Incomplete plumbing is more common for Indigenous communities and is also significantly associated with poverty, older populations, lower education, and living in very rural areas.[77]

Affordability Challenges

Just as water is recognized as a **public water commons** where water is available for all (Box 11.1), water-service provision should also be treated as a public good. However, even with public ownership, water affordability is a national challenge, in part, because public water supply is among the most capital-intensive industries. These essential services require large investments for building, maintaining, and periodically upgrading costly infrastructure, as water is heavy to transport and expensive to treat.

Water rates increased nationally by 5% from 2014 to 2018, while median household income increased by 2.74% over that period, contributing to an affordability gap.[79] Increases in water bills are due to aging and increasingly costly infrastructure, more stringent regulations, diminished federal funding, and climate change, among other factors.[80] Privatization is also contributing to the affordability crisis. When a water service is privately owned, it operates under the business model of profit maximization, which is in direct conflict with the central aspect of the UN Resolution to guarantee access to affordable and safe water for all.[81] An estimated 1 in 10 households in the United States face unaffordable water bills, exceeding 4.5% of their household income, with disparate impacts on Black and low-wealth populations.

Two collection practices used by utilities for unpaid water bills are tax liens on properties, which can lead to tax-sale foreclosures, evictions, and service shut-offs.[82] In 2016, an estimated 15 million people experienced a shut-off for nonpayment of water bills.[83] Shut-off rates are higher in communities of color.[84] Water shut-offs pose risks to human health, particularly for the elderly, pregnant people, children, and people with diabetes and other illnesses, as underscored by the COVID-19 pandemic, when water shut-off moratoria were shown to be

BOX 11.1. A LEGAL PERSPECTIVE ON WATER RIGHTS, WATER COMMONS, AND THE PUBLIC TRUST

James Olson, JD, LLM

WATER AS A COMMONS AND PUBLIC TRUST

Common and Public Trust Water: As courts often say, "no one owns the water." Generally, water is considered a public resource. While states may not own water like they do land, they do have the responsibility to manage the water within their jurisdiction for the benefit of their residents. Water management includes lakes and streams that are navigable under the public trust doctrine. For example, in 1892, the U.S. Supreme Court stopped Illinois from giving nearly one-square mile of Lake Michigan to a railroad company for a private industrial harbor. The Court ruled that navigable waters and the lakebed are owned and held by the state in public trust for the rights of citizens, including navigation, fishing, bathing, and sustenance.[78] Any significant interference or sale of these public trust rights is illegal. Courts have also extended these rights to groundwater that is connected to lakes and streams. If a state fails to consider the effects of a water diversion on the public trust and the public's rights, the approval of the diversion can be stopped. Public-trust law limits property rights to use, divert, privatize, or commodify water.

USE OF WATER AS PROPERTY RIGHT

Surface water: The owner of land that touches a lake or stream is a *riparian owner*. While a riparian owner does not own the water of the lake, the owner has a property right to reasonable use of the water commons to benefit the owner's land, such as domestic water supply, hydroelectric power, or irrigation for food production. A reasonable use is determined by balancing the rights and lawful uses of other riparian owners on the same lake. Riparian rights also include the right to anchor or dock a boat or to reach deeper water for navigation and commerce.

Groundwater: Like the surface water law, a landowner has a right to use the groundwater moving beneath the land on and in connection with the overlying land, according to the property and water law of each state. Although the standards differ in each state, the use of groundwater must be reasonable and not unreasonably harm the use of water from the same aquifer by neighboring landowners. Groundwater uses include domestic activities, such as food production, and other artificial or commercial-type uses. However, similar to a landowner's rights regarding surface water, groundwater cannot be severed and diverted for use off-tract if it diminishes the flow or level of a lake, stream, creek, pond, or wetland.

SUMMARY

Water rights govern the right to use water, not sell it. It is important that diversions, exports, or investments in water be governed carefully by common law principles, particularly those that protect water as public trust or a commons as in the public trust doctrine. If states and citizens fail to protect water, their right to protect and access water for human health and well-being may end up being jeopardized by these private interests. (For additional resources and model legislation, see https://forloveofwater.org, the Water Justice Toolkit at http://blueplanetproject.net, and Cornell's case law public access site at www.law.cornell.edu.)

an effective public health intervention.[85] Shut-offs can also have cascading impacts on families and communities. Lack of running water at home can be considered child neglect in 21 states, causing children to be taken from their homes under child protection laws.[82] Water shut-offs can force families to move, negatively impacting children's education, and causing trauma.[86]

Rural Public Water Supplies: Key Issues and Challenges

Recent studies have shown that rural areas in the United States, particularly Black, Hispanic or Latino, and Indigenous communities, have less reliable access to clean drinking water compared to urban and suburban areas.[87] The disparity is arguably driven by three interconnected factors. First, rural industries like agriculture, mining, forestry, and tourism can degrade water quality, but addressing these environmental damages conflicts with economic trade-offs.[88] Second, the development of water infrastructure is challenging in rural regions owing to small and scattered populations, resulting in higher costs per user that often exceed the financial capacity of local governments.[89] Third, rural communities often lack the resources and expertise to fully benefit from state and federal safe-drinking-water assistance programs. These programs may have criteria that disadvantage small and economically marginalized communities, including minimum population requirements and the need for local institutions to match funding.[90] Communities of color in rural areas may face deep disadvantages because of historic barriers, unaffordable water rates, and exclusionary program eligibility requirements.[91] In conclusion, rural drinking water injustices are complex issues that affect racial groups unevenly, encompassing environmental, economic, infrastructural, social, and structural factors.

Tribal Public Water Supplies: Key Issues and Challenges

Reservation communities face challenges that are similar to those of rural communities, but also have additional issues due to Federal Indian law and Tribes' unique legal status. In 2007–2008, health-based violations were found in 16% of tribally owned public-water-supply systems, compared to 7% nationally.[92] To effectively manage their public water supplies and protect community health, Tribal communities face several key issues in water and law policy that need to be addressed:

- the difficulty acquiring Rights of Way (ROW) for distribution system lines across non-Tribal lands due to the lack of authority for Tribes, complexities of mixed jurisdictions, and fractionated land ownership (where multiple heirs own land together);
- legal conflicts regarding federal Tribal Workforce Protection law and Tribal sovereign immunity, making the establishment of water districts to govern and finance public-water supply systems difficult;
- inadequate infrastructure planning and poor environmental enforcement, resulting in challenges and increased costs for infrastructure improvements; and
- challenges in staff training and certification due to state laws not applying on reservations, making it difficult to acquire the necessary training skills within driving distance and Tribal budgets[93]

Private Wells: Key Issues and Challenges

In the absence of federal well-water quality and well-installation standards, rural families with private wells are more vulnerable to exposure to groundwater contamination, compared to people served by regulated public water supplies. A nationwide USGS survey of well-water quality found that 22% of home wells in 62 major U.S. aquifers sampled had at least one chemical contaminant exceeding an EPA health standard (MCL or HBSL), most often manganese, arsenic, radon, strontium, uranium and/or nitrate.[94] Of these common, hazardous inorganic contaminants, only manganese causes poor taste and water discoloration—the other five are tasteless and colorless. Hence, well owners often assume that their clear, great-tasting well water is safe to drink and does not need testing. People with private wells have been found to have higher inorganic arsenic and lead body burdens than those receiving municipal water, even after controlling for housing age and condition (to eliminate lead paint as a contributing factor).[95] Exposures to toxic metals in home well water have been linked to adverse health effects, including hearing loss, neurodevelopmental effects, and birth defects.[96] The potential health risks from long-term exposure to these contaminants could be significant, and the nationwide burden is unknown. Furthermore, research shows that public water and sewers are not equally extended to communities of color and low-wealth communities, resulting in increased exposure to toxic metals from home well water, compared to those on community water systems.[97]

For many families with limited financial resources, the costs of testing and remediating their home well are barriers, and purchasing all drinking and cooking water can be unaffordable, so they consume even awful-tasting well water. In a Tribal community in Montana, 86% of home wells had salty/metallic-tasting water due to very high total dissolved solids, yet only approximately 2% of people had installed water treatment, and 80% of families were still consuming their well water. Almost half of these wells subsequently tested unsafe owing to metals and/or nitrate.[35] As a Tribal member explains:

> *As a country, we may imagine our citizens have universal access to safe drinking water—but for millions of rural residents with poor quality well water, and who cannot afford cisterns, treatment systems, or all the bottled water they might want—this simply is not the case. In our communities, people are cooking with poor tasting, contaminated water, and living with the health consequences.*[98]

CASE STUDY 11.1: Addressing Disparities in Safe Public Drinking Water on the Apsáalooke Nation (Crow Tribe) Reservation in Montana, USA

The Apsáalooke (Crow) community primarily resides in south-central Montana on ancestral lands. With a total membership of around 11,000 individuals, approximately 7,900 live on the Reservation. The primary towns within the Reservation—Crow Agency, Lodge Grass, Wyola, and Pryor—are predominantly Native American, with populations ranging from 80% to 95% Indigenous. Crow Agency, the largest town on the Reservation, houses essential governmental facilities, such as the Crow Tribe's headquarters, the Indian Health Service Hospital (IHS), Bureau of Indian Affairs (BIA) offices, the Tribal College (Little Big Horn College [LBHC]), and other vital services.

The water and sewage infrastructure in Crow Agency was constructed over a century ago to serve a population that was less than half of its current size. At the turn of the century, there had been no significant updates or improvements made to the distribution system or the sewage lagoon. As chapter coauthor and Crow Tribal member John Doyle explains:[93]

> *The municipal water treatment plant in Crow Agency draws surface water from the Little Bighorn River. As Crow Tribal members, we have always lived along the Little Bighorn River; we spent our childhoods playing, swimming, fishing, hunting, and berry picking along the river. Our families always drew water directly from the river for both household and ceremonial consumption, and some of those practices continue today. Given our close ties to the river, we observed and remember that water quality began visibly deteriorating in the late 1970s, with the intensification of both ranching and farming, and a growing population. Our reports of evident water quality problems to the federal authorities, including leakage from municipal sewage lines directly into the river, went unresolved. We realized that the aging municipal water and wastewater infrastructure was deteriorating and inadequate to serve the growing population, and that we had to address these issues ourselves. Several of us formed the Apsáalooke Water and Wastewater Authority (AWWWA), volunteering to take on the responsibility for Tribal water and wastewater infrastructure.*

Over the last few decades, the AWWWA successfully secured nearly 50 grants from federal, state, county, and Tribal sources, alongside multiple loans, amassing a total exceeding $20 million. The AWWWA has successfully upgraded much of their local water and wastewater infrastructure. These upgrades included replacing their sewage lagoon, replacing 75% of their wastewater lines and half of the water lines, installing new water infrastructure connecting to local schools, and replacing 19 fire hydrants, as well as implementing a "water salesman" system to provide water at a minimal cost to any community member.

They have reflected on and written about the opportunities and challenges they faced, including the following:[93]

(continued)

> **CASE STUDY 11.1: Addressing Disparities in Safe Public Drinking Water on the Apsáalooke Nation (Crow Tribe) Reservation in Montana, USA** (*continued*)
>
> - Learning about and implementing community-based participatory research (CBPR) with academic partners have been essential in acquiring the water-quality data needed to both plan and secure funding for the infrastructure.
> - Updating municipal water and wastewater infrastructure is a tremendously complicated and multiyear job, requiring substantial experience and institutional memory—hence the long-term stability of staffing is vital; it helps to have a Water Authority independent of Tribal elections.
> - Legal counsel has been essential, as there are policy and regulatory challenges created by overlaps, conflicts, and gaps in mixed Tribal/federal/state/county jurisdiction on reservations, further complicated by intersecting responsibilities of the Tribe, the county, the IHS, the BIA, and the EPA.[93]
>
> To read more about this process see Doyle JT, Kindness L, Realbird J, Eggers MJ, Camper AK. Challenges and opportunities for Tribal waters: addressing disparities in safe public drinking water on the Crow Reservation in Montana, USA. *Int J Environ Res Public Health*. 2018;15(4). doi:10.3390/ijerph15040567
>
> **REFLECTION QUESTIONS**
>
> *1. The AWWWA needed water quality data in order to plan a course of action and apply for grant funding for water and wastewater infrastructure. To accomplish this task, Doyle and his colleagues Lefthand, Young, Eggers, and others, formed the Crow Environmental Health Steering Committee and followed the principles of CBPR in partnering with LBHC and Montana State University to conduct research in an equitable and effective way. What do you think the principles of collaborative research should include to ensure that it is carried out in a good way?*

THE HUMAN RIGHT TO WATER AND GLOBAL WATER CHALLENGES

We face many global challenges related to water quality, sustainability, governance, and access. For example, over 85% of the planet's wetland ecosystems have been lost over the past 300 years.[99] Further, in 2018, 3.6 billion people faced inadequate access to water at least one month per year.[100] Water does not recognize borders, and 60% of global freshwater supplies are found in transboundary basins shared by 153 countries.[101] Therefore, it is easy to see that while water challenges are rooted locally, they also take place on a global scale.

These problems are not experienced equally around the world. Some countries of the world are more impacted than others: Almost 30% of the global population live in countries with water stress (Figure 11.7). However, looking at data at aggregated levels, such as at the country level, can mask inequitable access to water and sanitation within countries. Even in wealthy countries, where most of the population enjoys access to water and sanitation, some communities lack even the most basic infrastructure for these important services.[87] For example, in the United States approximately 2 to 4 million people lack access to water and sanitation infrastructure.[102] It is very critical to have information at finer levels to have a greater understanding of the causes and effects of water stress, supporting the policy choices of the relevant authorities and communities.

The human right to water and sanitation is a framework stating that clean drinking water and sanitation are universal human rights because they are essential to the actualization of all human rights. In 2010, this right was recognized in Resolution 64/292 by the United Nations General Assembly, which is the main deliberative, policy-making and representative organ of the United Nations that includes all 193 Members.[103] The Resolution calls upon States and international organizations to provide financial resources, capacity-building and technology transfer to help low-income countries provide safe, clean, accessible and affordable drinking water and sanitation for all. The recognition of the human right to water and sanitation within the UN General Assembly is considered a major milestone for water justice.

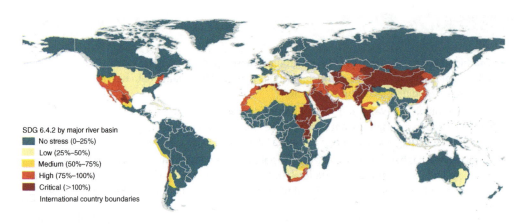

FIGURE 11.7. Global map of the level of water stress by major basin, with country boundaries, 2018.
SDG, Sustainable Development Goal.

Source: Food and Agriculture Organization of the United Nations. *Progress on Level of Water Stress. Global Status and Acceleration Needs for SDG Indicator 6.4.2, 2021.* FAO, United Nations Water (UN Water); 2021. https://www.unwater.org/publications/progress-level-water-stress-2021-update

Although the United States has not recognized the human right to water, California law does, and the state has allocated funding to provide safe drinking water to all residents. California is now the first state to have a framework for measuring the state's progress on realizing the human right to water.[104]

However, scholars and activists have also expressed concerns over this recognition of our right to water. One concern relates to the variety of values people hold about water, like water being considered an economic good. For many Indigenous groups around the world their relationship with water is spiritual as well, as water—and nature more generally—is the source of all life.[14] As such, the human right to water framework is anthropocentric because it is centered on the right for humans, and not the rights of all living things and of ecosystems.[14]

WORKING TOWARD ENVIRONMENTAL HEALTH AND JUSTICE

Many countries have agreed to work on global water challenges as part of the United Nations' 2030 Agenda for Sustainable Development (described in Chapter 4, "Environmental Health Policies and Protections: Successes and Failures"), which aims to tackle the most pressing global issues expressed in development goals. Sustainable Development Goal 6 (SDG6) aims to "Ensure access to water and sanitation for all."[105(parai)] SDG6 is comprehensive, in addressing safe drinking water, sanitation, the sustainable management of water resources, wastewater, and ecosystems but also in recognizing the importance of creating an enabling environment to implement sustainable water policies. Countries have committed to engage in a systematic follow-up and review of progress toward the **Sustainable Development Goals (SDGs)** and their targets, using a set of global indicators. There are 11 global indicators to track progress toward SDG6, reflecting how water security is interrelated with everything else, from human health and ecosystems to governance and economics. These indicators also tell us that the world is not on track to achieving the Goals by 2030.[106] Experts have called for governments to make commitments in all dimensions of water-related challenges, including strengthening the public sector, committing to water sector financing, and enabling public participation.

ENSURING WATER ACCESS

Much more work is needed to ensure that water is accessible and affordable. Public water systems were initially created to protect public health, and the use of water shut-offs for those who cannot afford their water is both immoral and counterproductive.

A fundamental shift in the principles that guide our water policies is likely necessary. There is a need for collaborative action at federal, state, and local levels to implement equitable and affordable billing structures and ensure that there are strong support systems for those struggling with water expenses. Affordable billing also involves rethinking how rates are set and bills are collected.

IN OTHER WORDS: WATER ASSISTANCE VERSUS WATER AFFORDABILITY

When talking about public water systems, the terms *affordability program* and *assistance program* are often used interchangeably. They are not the same.

Water **assistance** programs help customers to pay their water bills.

Water **affordability** programs help lower the cost of water so that a household's bills are lower. Water affordability means that water bills are less than or equal to about 2% of a household's income. For a household with an annual income of $30,000, this cost is about $600 a year.

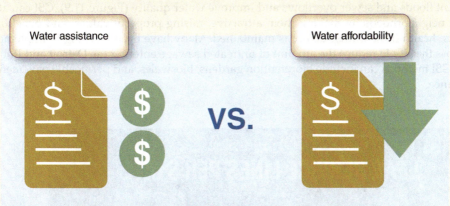

Why Do These Programs Matter?

Average water and sewer bills have increased by about 50% in the past decade and by much more in some states. For many households, assistance programs are inadequate to address both debt and incoming bills, and they likely will not prevent the long-term realities of unaffordable water. Water affordability programs, sometimes referred to as percentage-of-income payment plans, are uncommon but a few do exist.

REDUCING WATER CONTAMINATION

There are countless efforts to reduce water contamination that we can look to for inspiration. We discuss a few of these programs, including programs that involve participatory research and infrastructure investments.

Nitrate is among the most common contaminants from human sources found in groundwater.[107] For infants, consumption of water with high nitrate can cause blue baby syndrome (methemoglobinemia), a potentially fatal condition. Nitrate exposure is also associated with colorectal and bladder cancers, neural tube defects, and thyroid disease (see Table 11.3). In rural settings, farming is commonly a dominant land use, and nitrate loss to groundwater in these settings is controlled by the interaction of land management with soils and weather.[108] For example, in the Judith Watershed of central Montana, well-drained soils are necessary for growing wheat and barley crops, but the soil's limited ability to hold water results in nitrate leaching to shallow aquifers that many farming communities rely on for drinking water. Approximately 5% to 10% of wells in the area are over the 10 mg/L drinking-water standard for nitrate nitrogen.[109] Farming is the primary source of nitrate in the shallow groundwater of the Judith Watershed, and the Judith River Nitrogen Project engaged farmers in a participatory research approach over a 4-year period, discovering through a postproject survey that 85% of farmers in the area were considering nitrate leaching in farm-management decisions, up from 35% before the project.[110]

For infants and children, lead exposure can cause delays in physical or mental development, deficits in attention span, and learning disabilities. For adults, lead exposure increases the risks of kidney problems and high blood pressure (see Table 11.3). Lead contamination of drinking water disproportionately impacts economically depressed cities and communities of color.[111] An estimated 15 to 22 million people in the United States receive their tap water through a full or partial lead service lines, and more than one-third of public-school districts have found elevated lead levels in school drinking water (Figure 11.8).[22] The 2021 Bipartisan Infrastructure Law helps to address this issue by focusing on water-quality improvements across the United States, investing almost $55 billion, with the largest targeted investment being $15 billion for lead service line removal projects.[112]

Many cities with combined-sewer overflow systems are rethinking nature-based solutions like green stormwater infrastructure (GSI) while making investments to address aging infrastructure and climate change. For instance, Detroit, Michigan, has had several extreme rain events that have led to flooding throughout the city.[113] GSI manages rainwater where it lands to prevent floods and sewer overflows and improve water quality (Figure 11.9). GSI can also support neighborhoods by making them attractive, raising property values, and benefiting residents' health if the infrastructure is maintained. Many have been working to implement GSI across the city to reduce the amount of untreated sewage entering the Detroit and Rouge Rivers. GSI methods can include bioretention gardens, bioswales, and permeable pavements, for instance.

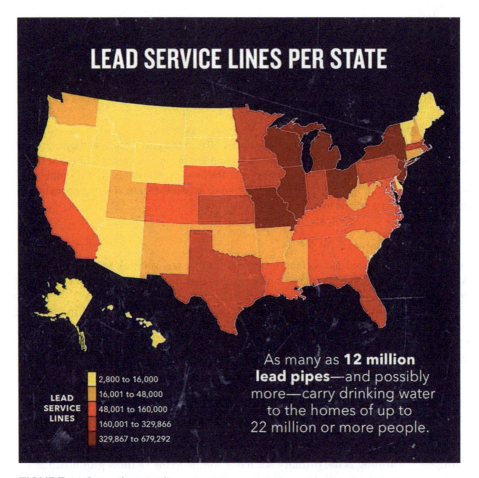

FIGURE 11.8. Lead service lines per state.
Source: Olson ED, Stubblefield A. Lead pipes are widespread and used in every state. Natural Resources Defense Council. July 8, 2021. https://www.nrdc.org/resources/lead-pipes-are-widespread-and-used-every-state

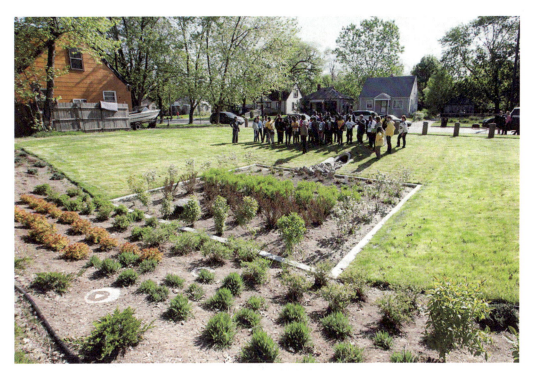

FIGURE 11.9. A bioretention garden designed to capture and hold stormwater in a subsurface layer of gravel, while beautifying the Cody Rouge area on Detroit's west side as part of a partnership between city, community, and academic partners.
Source: Photograph courtesy of the City of Detroit.

CASE STUDY 11.2: Addressing Disparities in Safe Public Drinking Water in Detroit, Michigan

"We are the opportunity in our crises."

—*Detroit poet and activist, Tawanna "Honeycomb" Petty*

We the People of Detroit (WPD) was cofounded in 2008 by Chris Griffith, Aurora Harris, Monica Lewis-Patrick, Cecily McClellan, and Debra Taylor in response to the emergency-management takeover of the local government of Detroit and the Detroit Public Schools.

To deal with the city's financial struggles, the state appointed unelected emergency managers to take over local government operations, essentially replacing elected officials. Emergency management not only undermined the democratic process by disregarding the voices of the city's predominantly Black population but also exacerbated systemic racial disparities. The decisions made by these appointed emergency managers often prioritized austerity measures and budget cuts, leading to severe reductions in public services, including education, healthcare, and basic utilities like water.

One of the most glaring examples was the Detroit water crisis, in which the Detroit Water and Sewerage Department (DWSD) initiated widespread water shut-offs owing to unpaid bills, disproportionately affecting low-wealth communities, which were predominantly Black. Nearly 40% of Detroit residents lived below the poverty line, and many faced difficulties paying their water bills. The water shut-offs resulted in tens of thousands of households losing access to clean and affordable water, raising significant public health concerns and intensifying the hardships faced by vulnerable communities.

(continued)

CASE STUDY 11.2: Addressing Disparities in Safe Public Drinking Water in Detroit, Michigan (*continued*)

As Monica Lewis-Patrick, one of the authors of this chapter, explains: "Communities are . . . figuring out ways to get each other water. Detroiters . . . were running water hoses from house to house to make sure that their neighbors had access to water so they could keep their dignity, keep their jobs, and so their children could go to school. One man who lived on my block went into his pension fund and paid the water bills for 22 houses in our neighborhood: tens of thousands of dollars, because he knew that each one of those houses who couldn't pay their water put us all in jeopardy. This just gives you an idea of the benevolence, of the love, of the genius and the belovedness of Detroiters to really go beyond." In response to these water shut-offs, WPD has worked persistently, mobilizing volunteers to provide water to residents and advocate for a sustainable water future. Through door-to-door canvassing, information dissemination, managing a water hotline, overseeing water stations, and delivering water to households in need, WPD strives to address this crisis. Collaborating with grassroots organizations, WPD pushes for fair water-payment plans, emphasizing water as a fundamental human right. In tandem with activists, academics, researchers, and designers, the WPD Community Research Collective uses data to highlight the impacts of austerity policies in Detroit. WPD has worked to counter mainstream narratives with advocacy and in publishing reports such as, "Mapping the Water Crisis: The Dismantling of African American Neighborhoods in Detroit" and "Cumulative Total and Rate of COVID-19 Cases per ZIP Code."

REFLECTION QUESTIONS

1. Who in your community or state lacks equitable access to safe drinking water? What are some local examples of health inequity that involve water?

EMERGING RESEARCH METHODS AND TECHNOLOGIES

Environmental health is a tremendously interdisciplinary field, and there are multiple disciplines across the natural and social sciences that are helpful in working on water justice, security, and quality. Here are just a few examples of emerging and exciting methods, technologies, and research from the fields of geography, biology, engineering, environmental science, and community health—all of which are contributing to water research and action.

GEOGRAPHIC INFORMATION SCIENCE

As described in Chapter 8, "Mapping Environmental Health and Justice Issues," geographic information science (GISc) and geospatial technologies provide a set of tools to locate, analyze, manage, and visualize water resources information. GISc is especially useful for its capacity to aid in organizing information and to facilitate linkages among distinct data sets. There are many examples of water data portals with geospatial components, including The National Map Viewer,[106] the Navajo WaterGIS,[114] Chesapeake Bay Open Data Portal,[115] and the Santa Barbara Channelkeeper Stream Team Data Portal.[116] These resources and many others illustrate how GISc tools may facilitate the visualization and analysis of community-based data-collection initiatives to support a dialogue between regulatory agencies, decision makers, and community members, and to support community-led efforts to address exposures that diminish health and well-being.

METAGENOMICS

Our ability to isolate, identify, and track the sources of pathogens and hazardous algae in water used to be extremely limited. Since 2000, technological advancements in DNA sampling and analysis have revolutionized biosurveillance capabilities, especially in aquatic ecosystems. This new field, *metagenomics*, allows for the direct genetic analysis of genomes contained in an environmental sample.[117] Now, robotic DNA samplers are collecting biological samples from rivers, lakes, and oceans around the clock and analyzing their DNA.[118] The USGS is placing these robots in stream gages on several rivers to integrate water quality and genetic data.[119] While challenges to widespread implementation remain, there is tremendous potential for using these technologies to better understand, manage, and restore aquatic ecosystems and protect public health. For instance, we can not only identify pathogens in water bodies, but also track the source of the fecal contamination. Metagenomics and wastewater surveillance were used for monitoring community-wide transmission of SARS-CoV-2 during the COVID-19 pandemic.[113]

SENSOR TECHNOLOGIES, SYNOPTICS, AND REMOTE SENSING

Advances in sensor technology are revolutionizing our ability to characterize and understand patterns in Earth systems over space and time, including patterns in water quality.[120] In addition to increasing the number of environmental variables that can be measured, new technologies are rapidly increasing the spatial resolution and temporal frequency with which we can characterize environmental signals. *Environmental variables* refers to the properties of water and other environmental systems that sensor technologies are designed to measure, and *environmental signals* are patterns in those variables over space or time that tell us how Earth systems function.[121] The collection of environmental data for research, education, and public-health monitoring efforts using these technologies is becoming more affordable.[122] For example, new hyperspectral camera technology and image-processing techniques are being developed to characterize the abundance of harmful algal blooms in oceans, lakes, and rivers, based on aerial imagery of reflected solar radiation and laser light.[121]

BIOMONITORING WITH COMMUNITIES

Exposures to chemicals may affect our health in ways that we cannot immediately perceive and may not manifest for decades—for instance, as cancer in later life. However, there is a solution: Often our immune system will be affected by such chemical exposures in ways that can be readily measured. Such measured responses may occur at the molecular, cellular, physiological, or functional level and collectively are called *biomarkers* of exposure. This study of toxic effects of chemicals (or physical agents such as radiation) on the immune system is called *immunotoxicology*, and can be used in risk assessment.[123] Communities concerned that their exposures to environmental contaminants may be impacting their health can investigate by partnering with an immunotoxicologist through CBPR.[124] CBPR could allow for the integration of local expertise with toxicological and risk-assessment findings (covered in more detail in Chapter 6, "Understanding (Unequal and Cumulative) Risks in Our Daily Environment") to rigorously examine and mitigate water-related health disparities. Combining applied immunotoxicology with our deep understanding of environmental injustices will help us protect public health.

MAIN TAKEAWAYS

In this chapter, we learned that:

- Communities all across the United States face water-contamination challenges from mining, industry, agriculture, the energy sector, logging, transportation, urbanization, Superfund sites, extreme climate events, and more.
- Climate change is a water crisis, causing drastic environmental disruption; the resulting toll on human health will be profound, with the true costs yet to be determined.
- Current standards for public drinking water quality often only consider one contaminant at a time, even though we always consume mixtures of them. Initial cumulative health-risk assessments by the USGS are finding that for the great majority of both public and private drinking water supplies sampled, cumulative-risk calculations

- indicated substantial risks of human health effects, notably to the health of most susceptible subpopulations (e.g., infants, children, pregnant people, older adults, and those who are immune-compromised).
- Historically, the development of public water supplies greatly reduced waterborne diseases and dramatically improved public health. Microbial contaminants in water are a key consideration for municipal drinking water and wastewater treatment-plant design and operation.
- Water is essential and has unique characteristics. Provision of water can become a natural monopoly and requires resource-intensive management. It also holds economic, public, and spiritual values. Therefore, water-service governance models must consider these aspects. Scarcity is driving the privatization and commercialization of water, which runs counter to the fundamental nature of water as a human right.
- There are racial, ethnic and socioeconomic disparities in water quality, security, and affordability driven by systemic inequities in multiple aspects of water access.
- Communities, nonprofit organizations, and researchers are partnering to address water contamination and injustice issues, often through community-engaged participatory research.
- The UN General Assembly has formally recognized the human right to water, and although the United States as a country has not, California has model laws recognizing the human right to water
- The global availability of water and related water challenges are experienced differently across the world, but local action should be considered in the global context, because it is all interrelated.

SUMMARY

Water sustains all life on Earth. Recognizing it as a fundamental human right is vital, as clean water and sanitation are essential for upholding all human rights. Despite assumptions to the contrary, about half a million people in marginalized communities in the United States lack complete household plumbing, perpetuating disparities in water quality, accessibility, and affordability based on race, ethnicity, and economic status. These inequities stem from systemic issues in infrastructure, funding, and management, exacerbated by decades of neglect by federal and state authorities. Additionally, only a fraction of chemicals on the market in the United States have health standards, leaving the full extent of drinking water risks unknown. Multiple threats like unregulated chemicals, climate change impacts, water privatization, and stress on ecosystems affect water security. Preserving water as a public asset is crucial for both public health and ecosystem well-being, given its interconnectedness and vital role in the global cycle of life. Because of water's interconnectedness and its importance to all life, comprehensive approaches in water law and management must safeguard it as a public resource, essential for both human and ecosystem health.

ACKNOWLEDGMENTS

The authors wish to acknowledge the contributions of the following individuals in the writing of this chapter: **Elliott Barnhart, PhD**, Research Hydrologist (Microbiologist), Wyoming Montana Water Science Center, Helena, Montana; **Paul Bradley, PhD**, Research Ecologist/Hydrologist, South Atlantic Water Science Center, Columbia, South Carolina; **Robert Byron, MD, MPH, FACP**, Internist, Vice Chair, Montana Health Professionals for a Healthy Climate, Cochair, Citizens Climate Lobby Health Team; Chapter Author, *Fifth National Climate Assessment*, Hardin, Montana; **Michael DeGrandpre, PhD**, Professor, Chemistry Department, University of Montana, Missoula, Montana; **Esther Erdei, M. Sc. Hons, MED, MPH, PhD**, Research Assistant Professor, Health Sciences Center, University of New Mexico, Albuquerque,

New Mexico; **Christine Foreman, PhD**, Professor and Associate Dean, Norm Asbjornson College of Engineering, Montana State University, Bozeman, Montana; **Grete Gansauer**, PhD candidate, Department of Earth Sciences, Montana State University, Bozeman, Montana; **Julia Haggerty, PhD**, Associate Professor, Earth Sciences Department, Montana State University, Bozeman, Montana; **Joseph Hoover, MA, PhD**, Assistant Professor, Department of Environmental Science, University of Arizona, Tucson, Arizona; **Madeleine Martinelli**, Honors College/Land Resources Environmental Science Department, Montana State University, Bozeman, Montana; **Robert Payn, MS, PhD**, Associate Professor, Land Resources and Environmental Sciences Department, Montana State University, Bozeman, Montana; **Adrienne Phillips, MS, PhD**, Associate Professor, Civil Engineering, Montana State University, Bozeman, Montana; **Adam Sigler, MS, PhD**, Assistant Professor and Extension Water Quality Specialist, Land Resources and Environmental Sciences, Montana State University, Bozeman, Montana; and **Kelly Smalling, MS**, Research Hydrologist (Environmental Organic Chemist), New Jersey Water Science Center, Lawrenceville, New Jersey.

END-OF-CHAPTER RESOURCES

DISCUSSION QUESTIONS

1. When we say "water is a public commons," what does this mean?
2. Management of our drinking and wastewater systems is complex in the United States. What did you learn that surprised you? What topics do you think are particularly relevant for your own city or community?
3. An estimated 1 in 10 households in the United States face unaffordable water bills, exceeding 4.5% of their household income. What strategies should be used to address this issue and ensure all that communities have access to safe, affordable water?
4. We have discussed cumulative risk assessment in several chapters. Why is it important in the context of water issues and environmental justice?

LEARNING ACTIVITIES

IN REAL LIFE

The U.S. EPA requires community water systems to create an annual Consumer Confidence Report, commonly known as drinking water quality reports. These reports should include: (a) information about where your drinking water comes from (e.g., aquifer, local watershed), (b) a list of regulated chemical or infectious contaminants and the level at which they are detected, (c) potential health effects of these contaminants, and (d) how your community's levels of contaminants compare to national standards.

Do a quick search to see if you can find an annual drinking-water quality report for your community. It will likely turn up if you simply search "<your city's name>" and "drinking-water quality report" or "consumer confidence report."

Note: If your household relies on a well rather than a municipal water source, you may not be able to find this information. If this is the case, choose a nearby community of your choice.

Ask yourself these questions:

- What are some of the exposures (e.g., chemical or infectious agents) reported on?
- Is there anything surprising, concerning, or interesting that you learned when reviewing the report?
- Is the report helpful? Do you understand it? Do you trust it? Which aspects of the report are effective at communicating environmental health risks? What suggestions would you make for improving the report?

THE TIME IS NOW

Talk to your state's decision makers! Ask your representatives, senators, and public service commissioners:

- What is the average cost for water and sewer bills in our state? On average, is it affordable for residents?
- Do we have water-assistance programs funded in our state? Do we have water-affordability programs in our state? (Teach them the difference if they don't know!)
- Have you considered implementing a water-affordability program? Encourage them to use financial tools to understand the impacts of potential or current plans for customers, such as those available through the EPA's Environment Finance Centers: www.epa.gov/waterfinancecenter/efcn.

A robust set of instructor resources designed to supplement this text is located at http://connect.springerpub.com/content/book/978-0-8261-8353-8. Qualifying instructors may request access by emailing textbook@springerpub.com.

REFERENCES

1. The Hohokam. Arizona Museum of Natural History. Accessed April 23, 2023. https://www.arizonamuseumofnaturalhistory.org/plan-a-visit/mesa-grande/the-hohokam
2. Salzman J. Thirst: a short history of drinking water. *Yale J Law Humanit*. 2006;17:94–121.
3. Kempe M. Drinking water in the early days, in New England water supplies—a brief history. *J N Engl Water Works Assoc*. 2006;120(3):4–22.
4. Spar D, Bebenek K. To the tap: public versus private water provision at the turn of the twentieth century. *Bus Hist Rev*. 2009;83(4):675–702.
5. Troesken W. Race, disease, and the provision of water in American cities, 1889–1921. *J Econ Hist*. 2001;61(3):750–776.
6. Water and climate change. United Nations. Accessed February 10, 2023. https://www.unwater.org/water-facts/water-and-climate-change
7. Reidmiller DR, Avery CW, Easterling DR, et al, eds. *Impacts, Risks, and Adaptation in the United States: Fourth National Climate Assessment*. U.S. Global Change Research Program; 2018:1515.
8. Lo Iacono G, Armstrong B, Fleming LE, et al. Challenges in developing methods for quantifying the effects of weather and climate on water-associated diseases: a systematic review. *PLoS Negl Trop Dis*. 2017;11(6):e0005659. doi:10.1371/journal.pntd.0005659
9. Tate E, Rahman MA, Emrich C, Sampson CC. Flood exposure and social vulnerability in the United States. *Na Hazards*. 2021;106(1):435–457. doi:10.1007/s11069-020-04470-2
10. Ebi KL, Bowen K. Extreme events as sources of health vulnerability: drought as an example. *Weather Clim Extrem*. 2016;11:95–102. doi:10.1016/j.wace.2015.10.001
11. Stanke C, Kerac M, Prudhomme C, Medlock J, Murray V. Health effects of drought: a systematic review of the evidence. *PLoS Curr*. 2013;5. doi:10.1371/currents.dis.7a2cee9e980f91ad7697b570bcc4b004
12. Watts N, Amann, M, Arnell N, et al. The 2020 report of The Lancet Countdown on health and climate change: responding to converging crises. *Lancet*. 2021;397(10269):129–170. doi:10.1016/S0140-6736(20)32290-X
13. Baker-Austin C, Trinanes J, Gonzalez-Escalona N, Martinez-Urtaza J. Non-cholera *Vibrios*: the microbial barometer of climate change. *Trends Microbiol*. 2017;25(1):76–84. doi:10.1016/j.tim.2016.09.008
14. Cozzetto K, Chief K, Dittmer K, et al. Climate change impacts on the water resources of American Indians and Alaska Natives in the US. In: Maldonado JK, Colombi B, Pandya R, eds. *Climate Change and Indigenous Peoples in the United States: Impacts, Experiences and Actions*. Springer; 2014:61–76.
15. Howard M, Ahmed S, Lachapelle P, Schure MB. Farmer and rancher perceptions of climate change and their relationships with mental health. *J Rur Mental Health*. 2020;44(2):87–95. doi:10.1037/rmh0000131

16. Food and Agriculture Organization of the United Nations. *Progress on Level of Water Stress. Global Status and Acceleration Needs for SDG Indicator 6.4.2, 2021.* FAO, United Nations Water (UN Water); 2021.
17. U.S. Geological Survey. Groundwater use in the United States. June 18, 2018. https://www.usgs.gov/special-topics/water-science-school/science/groundwater-use-united-states
18. Basic information about your drinking water. U.S. Environmental Protection Agency. 2023. Updated January 2, 2024. https://www.epa.gov/ground-water-and-drinking-water/basic-information-about-your-drinking-water
19. Drinking water technologies. U.S. Environmental Protection Agency. 2023. Updated February 6, 2024. https://www.epa.gov/ground-water-and-drinking-water/drinking-water-technologies
20. Contaminant candidate list 5—CCL 5. U.S. Environmental Protection Agency. 2022. Updated January 4, 2024. https://www.epa.gov/ccl/contaminant-candidate-list-5-ccl-5
21. Combined sewer overflow frequent questions. National Pollutant Discharge Elimination System, U.S. Environmental Protection Agency. 2021. Updated June 1, 2023. https://www.epa.gov/npdes/combined-sewer-overflow-frequent-questions
22. U.S. Environmental Protection Agency. Report to congress: impacts and control of combined sewer overflows and sanitary sewer overflows. August 2004. https://www.epa.gov/sites/default/files/2015-10/documents/csossortc2004_full.pdf
23. American Society of Civil Engineers. 2021 report card for America's infrastructure. 2021. Accessed June 20, 2023. https://infrastructurereportcard.org/
24. National enforcement initiative: keeping raw sewage and contaminated stormwater out of our nation's waters. U.S. Environmental Protection Agency. 2017. Accessed March 16, 2023. https://19january2017snapshot.epa.gov/enforcement/national-enforcement-initiative-keeping-raw-sewage-and-contaminated-stormwater-out-our_.html
25. Combined sewer overflow basics. U.S. Environmental Protection Agency. 2023. Updated October 5, 2023. https://www.epa.gov/npdes/combined-sewer-overflow-basics
26. Murray A, Hall A, Weaver J, Kremer F. Methods for estimating locations of housing units served by private domestic wells in the United States applied to 2010. *J Am Water Resour Assoc.* 2021;57(5):828–843. doi:10.1111/1752-1688.12937
27. Wu H, Zhang J, Ngo HH, et al. A review on the sustainability of constructed wetlands for wastewater treatment: design and operation. *Bioresour Technol.* 2015;175:594–601. doi:10.1016/j.biortech.2014.10.068
28. Private drinking water wells. U.S. Environmental Protection Agency. 2023. Updated May 9, 2024. https://www.epa.gov/privatewells
29. Types of Septic Systems. U.S. Environmental Protection Agency. 2022. Updated August 7, 2023. https://www.epa.gov/septic/types-septic-systems#septictank
30. Drinking Water Health Advisories (HAs). U.S. Environmental Protection Agency. Accessed April 29, 2024. https://www.epa.gov/sdwa/drinking-water-health-advisories-has
31. U.S. Environmental Protection Agency. 2018 Edition of the Drinking Water Standards and Health Advisories. March 2018. https://www.epa.gov/system/files/documents/2022-01/dwtable2018.pdf
32. U.S. Environmental Protection Agency. National Primary Drinking Water Regulations. 2009. Updated January 2, 2024. https://www.epa.gov/ground-water-and-drinking-water/national-primary-drinking-water-regulations
33. U.S. Environmental Protection Agency. Framework for cumulative risk assessment. EPA/630/P-02/001F. May 2003. https://www.epa.gov/sites/default/files/2014-11/documents/frmwrk_cum_risk_assmnt.pdf
34. Sexton K, Linder SH. The role of cumulative risk assessment in decisions about environmental justice. *Int J Environ Res Public Health.* 2010;7(11):4037–4049. doi:10.3390/ijerph7114037
35. Eggers MJ, Doyle JT, Lefthand MJ, et al. Community engaged cumulative risk assessment of exposure to inorganic well water contaminants, Crow Reservation, Montana. *Int J Environ Res Public Health.* 2018;15(1):76. doi:10.3390/ijerph15010076
36. Wang Z, Walker GW, Muir DCG, Nagatani-Yoshida K. Toward a global understanding of chemical pollution: a first comprehensive analysis of national and regional chemical inventories. *Environ Sci Technol.* 2020;54(5):2575–2584.

37. Schymanski EL, Zhang J, Thiessen PA, Chirsir P, Kondic T, Bolton EE. Per- and polyfluoroalkyl substances (PFAS) in PubChem: 7 million and growing. *Environ Sci Technol*. 2023;57(44):16918–16928. doi:10.1021/acs.est.3c04855
38. Evich MG, Davis MJB, Mccord JP, et al. Per- and polyfluoroalkyl substances in the environment. *Science*. 2022;375(6580):eabg9065. doi:10.1126/science.abg9065
39. Fenton SE, Ducatman A, Boobis A, et al. Per- and polyfluoroalkyl substance toxicity and human health review: current state of knowledge and strategies for informing future research. *Environ Toxicol Chem*. 2021;40(3):606–630. doi:10.1002/etc.4890
40. Drinking water health advisories for PFOA and PFOS. U.S. Environmental Protection Agency. 2022. Updated May 16, 2024. https://www.epa.gov/sdwa/drinking-water-health-advisories-pfoa-and-pfos
41. Per- and polyfluoroalkyl substances (PFAS): Final PFAS National Primary Drinking Water Regulation. *Safe Drinking Water Act*. U.S. Environmental Protection Agency. Accessed June 17, 2024. https://www.epa.gov/sdwa/and-polyfluoroalkyl-substances-pfas
42. Hrudey SE. Chlorination disinfection by-products, public health risk tradeoffs and me. *Water Res*. 2009;43(8):2057–2092. doi:10.1016/j.watres.2009.02.011
43. Cutler D, Miller G. The role of public health improvements in health advances: the twentieth-century United States. *Demography*. 2005;42(1):1–22. doi:10.1353/dem.2005.0002
44. Richardson SD, Postigo C. Drinking water disinfection by-products. In: Barceló D, ed. *Emerging Organic Contaminants and Human Health*. Springer; 2012:93–137.
45. Li X-F, Mitch WA. Drinking water Disinfection Byproducts (DBPs) and human health effects: multidisciplinary challenges and opportunities. *Environ Sci Technol*. 2018;52(4):1681–1689. doi:10.1021/acs.est.7b05440
46. Allen JM, Plewa MJ, Wagner ED, et al. Drivers of disinfection byproduct cytotoxicity in U.S. drinking water: should other DBPs be considered for regulation? *Environ Sci Technol*. 2022;56(1):392–402. doi:10.1021/acs.est.1c07998
47. Bradley PM, Romanok KM, Smalling KL, et al. Bottled water contaminant exposures and potential human effects. *Environ Int*. 2023;171:107701. doi:10.1016/j.envint.2022.107701
48. Bexfield LM, Belitz K, Lindsey BD, Toccalino PL, Nowell LH. Pesticides and pesticide degradates in groundwater used for public supply across the United States: occurrence and human-health context. *Environ Sci Technol*. 2021;55(1):362–372. doi:10.1021/acs.est.0c05793
49. U.S. Geological Survey. Pesticides in surface waters. U.S Geological Survey Fact Sheet FS-039-97. March 4, 2014. https://water.usgs.gov/nawqa/pnsp/pubs/fs97039/sw4.html
50. Donley N. The USA lags behind other agricultural nations in banning harmful pesticides. *Environ Health*. 2019;18(1):44. doi:10.1186/s12940-019-0488-0
51. U.S. Environmental Protection Agency. Human health benchmarks for pesticides: updated 2021 technical document. August 2021. https://www.epa.gov/system/files/documents/2021-07/hh-benchmarks-technical-document-2021.pdf
52. Agency for Toxic Substances and Disease Registry (ATSDR). Public health statement Atrazine. U.S. Department of Health and Human Services. September 2003. https://www.atsdr.cdc.gov/toxprofiles/tp153-c1-b.pdf
53. International Agency for Research on Cancer. IARC monographs volume 112: evaluation of five organophosphate insecticides and herbicides. World Health Organization. January 26, 2017. https://publications.iarc.fr/Book-And-Report-Series/Iarc-Monographs-On-The-Identification-Of-Carcinogenic-Hazards-To-Humans/Some-Organophosphate-Insecticides-And-Herbicides-2017
54. U.S. Geological Survey. Pesticides and water quality. March 1, 2019. https://www.usgs.gov/mission-areas/water-resources/science/pesticides-and-water-quality
55. U.S. Geological Survey. Pharmaceuticals in water. June 6, 2018. https://www.usgs.gov/special-topics/water-science-school/science/pharmaceuticals-water
56. Bradley PM, Journey CA, Button DT, et al. Multi-region assessment of pharmaceutical exposures and predicted effects in USA wadeable urban-gradient streams. *PLoS One*. 2020;15(1):e0228214. doi:10.1371/journal.pone.0228214
57. Technical overview of volatile organic compounds. U.S. Environmental Protection Agency. 2022. Updated March 5, 2024. https://www.epa.gov/indoor-air-quality-iaq/technical-overview-volatile-organic-compounds

58. U.S. Geological Survey. Volatile organic compounds (VOCs). February 27, 2019. https://www.usgs.gov/mission-areas/water-resources/science/volatile-organic-compounds-vocs#overview
59. Khan RM, Salehi B, Mahdianpari M, Mohammadimanesh F. A meta-analysis on harmful algal bloom (HAB) detection and monitoring: a remote sensing perspective. *Remote Sens.* 2021;13(21):4347. doi:10.3390/rs13214347
60. Lad A, Breidenbach JD, Su RC, et al. As we drink and breathe: adverse health effects of microcystins and other harmful algal bloom toxins in the liver, gut, lungs and beyond. *Life.* 2022;12(3):418. doi:10.3390/life12030418
61. Climate change and harmful algal blooms. U.S. Environmental Protection Agency. 2022. Updated March 4, 2024. https://www.epa.gov/nutrientpollution/climate-change-and-harmful-algal-blooms
62. American Water Works Association. Cyanotoxins in US drinking water: occurrence. Case studies and state approaches to regulation. September 2016:1–56. https://www.awwa.org/Portals/0/AWWA/Government/201609_Cyanotoxin_Occurrence_States_Approach.pdf?ver=2018-12-13-101832-037
63. Summary of cyanotoxins treatment in drinking water. U.S. Environmental Protection Agency. 2022. Updated March 1, 2024. https://www.epa.gov/ground-water-and-drinking-water/summary-cyanotoxins-treatment-drinking-water
64. World Health Organization. Microplastics in drinking-water [Technical document]. August 28, 2019. https://www.who.int/publications/i/item/9789241516198
65. Zhang Y, Gao T, Kang S, Sillanpää M. Importance of atmospheric transport for microplastics deposited in remote areas. *Environ Pollut.* 2019;254(Pt A):112953. doi:10.1016/j.envpol.2019.07.121
66. Rahman A, Sarkar A, Yadav OP, Achari G, Slobodnik J. Potential human health risks due to environmental exposure to nano- and microplastics and knowledge gaps: a scoping review. *Sci Total Environ.* 2021;757:143872. doi:10.1016/j.scitotenv.2020.143872
67. Koelmans AA, Redondo-Hasselerharm P, Hazimah A, De Ruijter VN, Mintenig S, Kooi M. Risk assessment of microplastic particles. *Nat Rev Mater.* 2022;7(2):138–152. doi:10.1038/s41578-021-00411-y
68. Fagin D. *Toms River: A Story of Science and Salvation.* Bantam; 2013.
69. Ebert R. Review: a civil action. January 8, 1999. https://www.rogerebert.com/reviews/a-civil-action-1999
70. Washington HA. *A Terrible Thing to Waste: Environmental Racism and Its Assault on the American Mind.* Hachette; 2019.
71. Soderbergh S. *Erin Brockovich.* DVD; 2000.
72. Lofrano G, Brown J. Wastewater management through the ages: a history of mankind. *Sci Total Environ.* 2010;408(22):5254–5264. doi:10.1016/j.scitotenv.2010.07.062
73. Center for Sustainable Systems, University of Michigan. U.S. water supply and distribution factsheet. Pub. No. CSS05-17. 2023. https://css.umich.edu/publications/factsheets/water/us-water-supply-and-distribution-factsheet
74. U.S. Environmental Protection Agency. Report on the environment, in population served by community water systems with no reported violations of health-based standards. 2022. https://cfpub.epa.gov/roe/indicator.cfm?i=45
75. McDonald YJ, Jones NE. Drinking water violations and environmental justice in the United States, 2011–2015. *Am J Public Health.* 2018;108(10):1401–1407. doi:10.2105/AJPH.2018.304621
76. Brown J, Acey CS, Anthonj C, et al. The effects of racism, social exclusion, and discrimination on achieving universal safe water and sanitation in high-income countries. *Lancet Glob Health.* 2023;11(4):e606–e614. doi:10.1016/S2214-109X(23)00006-2
77. Mueller JT, Gasteyer S. The widespread and unjust drinking water and clean water crisis in the United States. *Nat Commun.* 2021;12(1):3544. doi:10.1038/s41467-021-23898-z
78. Sax JL. The public trust doctrine in natural resource law: effective judicial intervention. *Michigan Law Rev.* 1970;68(3):471.
79. Patterson LA, Doyle MW. Measuring water affordability and the financial capability of utilities. *AWWA Water Sci* 2021;3(6):e1260.
80. U.S. Environmental Protection Agency. Drinking water infrastructure needs survey and assessment: sixth report to congress. Office of Water. March 2018. https://www.epa.gov/sites/default/files/2018-10/documents/corrected_sixth_drinking_water_infrastructure_needs_survey_and_assessment.pdf
81. United Nations Human Rights Office of the High Commissioner Special Rapporteur on the human rights to safe drinking water and sanitation. Human rights and the privatization of water and

sanitation services. 2020. https://www.ohchr.org/sites/default/files/Documents/Issues/Water/10anniversary/Privatization_EN.pdf
82. Amirhadji J, Anvid T, Burcat L, et al. Tapped out: threats to the human right to water in the urban United States. 2013. https://www.law.georgetown.edu/human-rights-institute/wp-content/uploads/sites/7/2017/07/Tapped-Out.pdf
83. Food and Water Watch America's secret water crisis: national shutoff survey reveals water affordability emergency affecting millions. 2018. https://affordablewater.mit.edu/americas-secret-water-crisis-national-shutoff-survey-reveals-water-affordability-emergency-affecting
84. U.S. Government Accountability Office. Water infrastructure: information on selected midsize and large cities with declining populations. September 15, 2016. https://www.gao.gov/products/gao-16-785
85. Zhang X, Warner ME, Grant M. Water shutoff moratoria lowered COVID-19 infection and death across US states. *Am J Prev Med*. 2022;62(2):149–156. doi:10.1016/j.amepre.2021.07.006
86. Gaber N, Silva A, Lewis-Patrick M, Kutil E, Taylor D, Bouier R. Water insecurity and psychosocial distress: case study of the Detroit water shutoffs. *J Public Health*. 2020;43(4):839–845. doi:10.1093/pubmed/fdaa157
87. Roller Z, Gasteyer S, Nelson N, Lai W, Shingne M. Closing the water access gap in the United States: a national action plan. Dig Deep & US Water Alliance. 2019. https://uswateralliance.org/wp-content/uploads/2023/09/Closing-the-Water-Access-Gap-in-the-United-States_DIGITAL.pdf
88. Hayter R, Barnes TJ, Bradshaw MJ. Relocating resource peripheries to the core of economic geography's theorizing: rationale and agenda. *Area*. 2003;35(1):15–23. doi:10.1111/1475-4762.00106
89. Gansauer G, Haggerty J. Beyond city limits: infrastructural regionalism in rural Montana, USA. *Terri Politic Gov*. 2021:1–19. doi:10.1080/21622671.2021.1980428
90. McFarlane K, Harris LM. Small systems, big challenges: review of small drinking water system governance. *Environ Rev*. 2018;26(4):378–395. doi:10.1139/er-2018-0033
91. Baskaran P. Thirsty places. *Utah Law Rev*. 2021;2021(3):501. doi:10.26054/0d-6zb6-r05v
92. U.S. Environmental Protection Agency. Providing safe drinking water in America: 2007–2008 National Public Water Systems compliance report. Office of Enforcement and Compliance Assurance. June 3, 2010. https://www.epa.gov/sites/default/files/2014-04/documents/sdwacom2007.pdf
93. Doyle JT, Kindness L, Realbird J, Eggers MJ, Camper AK. Challenges and opportunities for Tribal waters: addressing disparities in safe public drinking water on the Crow Reservation in Montana, USA. *Int J Environ Res Public Health*. 2018;15(4):567. doi:10.3390/ijerph15040567
94. DeSimone LA. Quality of water from domestic wells in principal aquifers of the United States, 1991–2004. U.S. Geological Survey Scientific Investigations Report 2008-5227. 2009:139. http://pubs.usgs.gov/sir/2008/5227
95. Gibson JM, Fisher M, Clonch A, MacDonald JM, Cook, PJ. Children drinking private well water have higher blood lead than those with city water. *Proc Natl Acad Sci U S A*. 2020;117(29):16898–16907. doi:10.1073/pnas.2002729117
96. Sanders AP, Desrosiers TA, Warren JL, et al. Association between arsenic, cadmium, manganese, and lead levels in private wells and birth defects prevalence in North Carolina: a semi-ecologic study. *BMC Public Health*. 2014:14(1):955. doi:10.1186/1471-2458-14-955
97. Balazs CL, Ray I. The drinking water disparities framework: on the origins and persistence of inequities in exposure. *Am J Public Health*. 2014;104(4):603–611. doi:10.2105/AJPH.2013.301664
98. Eggers MJ, Lefthand MJ, Young SL, Doyle JT, Plenty Hoops A. 2013. When it comes to water, we are all close neighbors. EPA Blog It All StartsWith Science. June 6, 2013.
99. United Nations. *The Sustainable Development Goals Report 2022*. July 2022.
100. UNFAO. Progress on level of water stress—2021 update, in global status and acceleration needs for SDG indicator 6.4.2. 2021. Accessed June 13, 2024. https://www.unwater.org/publications/progress-level-water-stress-2021-update
101. United Nations. Economic Commission For Europe. *Guidance on Water and Adaptation to Climate Change*. Vol. 9. United Nations; 2009.
102. Almazán-Casali S, Puga BP, Lemos MC. Who governs at what price? Technocratic dominance, ways of knowing, and long-term resilience of Brazil's water system. *Front Water*. 2021;3:735018. doi:10.3389/frwa.2021.735018
103. United Nations Water Decade Programme on Advocacy and Communication (UNW-DPAC). The human right to water and sanitation milestones. 2014. Accessed June 13, 2023. https://www.un.org/waterforlifedecade/pdf/human_right_to_water_and_sanitation_milestones.pdf

104. OEHHA. The human right to water in California. January 28, 2021. https://oehha.ca.gov/water/report/human-right-water-california
105. Goal 6: Ensure access to water and sanitation for all. United Nations Sustainable Development. https://www.un.org/sustainabledevelopment/water-and-sanitation/
106. U.S. Geological Survey. The National map viewer. November 3, 2022. https://www.usgs.gov/tools/national-map-viewer
107. Abascal E, Gómez-Coma L, Qrtiz I, Ortiz A. Global diagnosis of nitrate pollution in groundwater and review of removal technologies. *Sci Total Environ*. 2022;810:152233. doi:10.1016/j.scitotenv.2021.152233
108. Sigler WA, Ewing SA, Jones CA, et al. Water and nitrate loss from dryland agricultural soils is controlled by management, soils, and weather. *Agric Ecosyst Environ*. 2020;304:107158. doi:10.1016/j.agee.2020.107158
109. Sigler WA, Ewing SA, Jones CA, et al. Connections among soil, ground, and surface water chemistries characterize nitrogen loss from an agricultural landscape in the upper Missouri River Basin. *J Hydrol*. 2018;556:247–261. doi:10.1016/j.jhydrol.2017.10.018
110. Jackson-Smith D, Ewing SA, Jones C, Sigler A, Armstrong A. The road less traveled: assessing the impacts of farmer and stakeholder participation in groundwater nitrate pollution research. *J Soil Water Conserv*. 2018;73(6):610–622. doi:10.2489/jswc.73.6.610
111. Butler LJ, Scammell MK, Benson EB. The Flint, Michigan, water crisis: a case study in regulatory failure and environmental injustice. *Environ Justice*. 2016;9(4):93–97. doi:10.1089/env.2016.0014
112. The White House. Updated fact sheet: Bipartisan Infrastructure Investment and Jobs Act. August 2, 2021. https://www.whitehouse.gov/briefing-room/statements-releases/2021/08/02/updated-fact-sheet-bipartisan-infrastructure-investment-and-jobs-act/
113. Larson PS, Gronlund C, Thompson L, et al. Recurrent home flooding in Detroit, MI 2012–2020: results of a household survey. *Int J Environ Res Public Health*. 2021;18(14):7659. doi:10.3390/ijerph18147659
114. Hoover JH, Coker E, Barney Y, Shuey C, Lewis J. Spatial clustering of metal and metalloid mixtures in unregulated water sources on the Navajo Nation–Arizona, New Mexico, and Utah, USA. *Sci Total Environ*. 2018;633:1667–1678. doi:10.1016/j.scitotenv.2018.02.288
115. Chesapeake Bay open data portal. Chesapeake Bay Program Partners. Accessed June 10, 2023. https://data-chesbay.opendata.arcgis.com/
116. Santa Barbara Channelkeeper. Stream team data portal. Accessed June 13, 2024. https://www.sbck.org/our-work/field-work/stream-team/stream-team-data-portal/
117. Thomas T, Gilbert J, Meyer F. Metagenomics—a guide from sampling to data analysis. *Microb Inform Exp*. 2012;2(1):3. doi:10.1186/2042-5783-2-3
118. Yamahara KM, Preston CM, Birch J, et al. In situ autonomous acquisition and preservation of marine environmental DNA using an autonomous underwater vehicle. *Front Mar Sci*. 2019;6:373. doi:10.3389/fmars.2019.00373
119. Sepulveda AJ, Hoegh A, Gage JA, et al. Integrating environmental DNA results with diverse data sets to improve biosurveillance of river health. *Front Ecol Evol*. 2021;9. doi:10.3389/fevo.2021.620715
120. Hampton SE, Jones MB, Wasser LA, et al. Skills and knowledge for data-intensive environmental research. *BioScience*. 2017;67(6):546–557. doi:10.1093/biosci/bix025
121. Rolim SBA, Veettil BK, Vieiro AP, Kesssler AB, Gonzatti C. Remote sensing for mapping algal blooms in freshwater lakes: a review. *Environ Sci Pollut Res Int*. 2023;30(8):19602–19616. doi:10.1007/s11356-023-25230-2
122. Ighalo JO, Adeniyi AG, Marques G. Internet of things for water quality monitoring and assessment: a comprehensive review. In: Hassanien AE, Bhatnagar R, Darwish A, eds. *Artificial Intelligence for Sustainable Development: Theory, Practice and Future Applications*. Springer International Publishing; 2021:245–259.
123. Germolec D, Luebke R., Rooney A, Shipkowski K, Vandebriel R, van Loveren H. Immunotoxicology: a brief history, current status and strategies for future immunotoxicity assessment. *Curr Opin Toxicol*. 2017;5:55–59. doi:10.1016/j.cotox.2017.08.002
124. Pool EJ, Magcwebeba TU. The screening of river water for immunotoxicity using an in vitro whole blood culture assay. *Water Air Soil Pollut*. 2009;200:25–31. doi:10.1007/s11270-008-9890-x

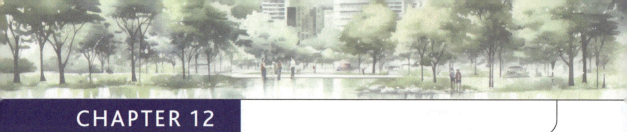

CHAPTER 12

Food Safety, Security, and Sovereignty

Sara El-Sayed, Sandra M. Long, and Benjamin Ryan

LEARNING OBJECTIVES

- Provide an overview of the history of food policy.
- Understand how our food system and ecosystems influence each other.
- Learn and apply key concepts when understanding our food environment, including food security, sovereignty, regenerative food systems, and industrial food systems.
- Explore the ways industrialized food systems harm the environment and perpetuate health inequities.
- Further explore the concept of One Health and how it can improve human, nonhuman, and environmental health.

KEY TERMS

- ecosystem services
- food
- food apartheid
- food safety
- food security
- food sovereignty
- food systems
- foodborne outbreak
- One Health

OVERVIEW

Food and the environment are intricately interwoven. Our **food system** includes complex systems of production, processing, distribution, consumption, and disposal of **food**, or any nutritious substance consumed to provide energy and overall health. Our food system reflects our cultural, aesthetic, spiritual, and economic values as a society. To provide sufficient, accessible, equitable, nutritious, culturally appropriate, and flavorful food for humans, it is essential to work toward an understanding of our environment and the ecosystem services it provides, while learning from the communities that have coevolved with it.[1] **Ecosystem services** can include all of the benefits, like food, water, and raw materials, that humans get from ecosystems. They can also include the ability of the ecosystem to regulate climate, water quality, and control of diseases and populations in ways that greatly impact human and planetary health.

Today's industrialized food system harms our planet in many ways. Conceived during the Green Revolution in the 1950s to address global hunger, it has led to:

- soil depletion,
- water pollution,
- diminished biodiversity (the diversity of species and genetic diversity within species),
- increased greenhouse gas emissions,
- displacement of small-scale farmers and other food producers,
- increased consumption of nutrient-poor foods, and
- a strong and necessary reliance on stringent food safety regulations.[2-4]

Paradoxically, this system perpetuates both malnourishment and hunger among the populations it was intended to sustain. The industrialized food system's reliance on chemical fertilizers, heavy machinery, and long-distant (often global) supply chains has contributed 25% to 30% of greenhouse gasses, thus being one of the primary causes of climate change.[5] This food system has created a reinforcing feedback loop where human activities lead to droughts, floods, heat waves, and other extreme weather conditions, which damages our environment and further decreases crop yields.

As this chapter explores, a paradigm shift in the global food system is needed to ensure environmental health and justice for all. Many argue that it is necessary to reverse the ongoing issues of worsening climate change, food insecurity, and food-safety outbreaks.[6] After briefly examining the history of food and food policy, we look at the ways food is a matter of environmental health. Moving beyond food security, we explore how to also achieve food sovereignty, in which communities can seek out food systems that reflect their values and culture and feed everyone. There are indeed many examples and communities to learn from. As described later, these systems may look like supporting small-scale farmers, local markets, and cooperatives, as well as local food production and consumption and reduction of food waste. As discussed, regenerative agriculture and a One Health framework may help society to honor the linkages between people, animals, plants, and environmental health.

A HISTORY OF FOOD AND FOOD POLICY

From ancient civilizations to modern societies, food policies have evolved in response to challenges, including food scarcity, food contamination, and changing dietary patterns. One of the earliest recorded instances of food policy dates back to ancient civilizations such as Mesopotamia and Egypt, which flourished for millennia. In these civilizations, the stability of the food supply was linked to health and prosperity owing to a heavy emphasis on agriculture and trade. To ensure a stable food supply, there were policies focused on management of agricultural resources, establishment of irrigation systems, and storage of food stocks to serve as reserves during times of famine or drought.[7]

During the Middle Ages, food policy was heavily influenced by social hierarchies and religious beliefs. European monarchs enacted laws to regulate the types of food consumed by different social classes. These laws aimed to maintain social order but, at the same time, led to unequal access to nutritious food and health inequities.[8] Meanwhile, in the precolonial period in the Americas, Indigenous societies developed intricate food systems rooted in cultural, ecological, and spiritual traditions. Unlike much of Europe, their food policy was not governed by central institutions. Instead, it was shaped by communal practices and traditional knowledge passed down from one generation to the next.[9]

Colonization of the Americas brought various food safety challenges. There were often food shortages due to an unfamiliarity with local crops and a disruption of traditional food systems. Additionally, the establishment of settlements often led to the concentration of populations in areas where poor sanitation, lack of access to clean water, and overcrowding facilitated the spread of foodborne illnesses among both colonists and Indigenous Peoples. One notable example in the early 1600s was the Jamestown colony, which is thought to have failed as a result of typhoid fever, a bacterial infection transmitted through contaminated food and water.[10]

Modern food-policy development has been shaped by pivotal events and legislative acts that addressed food safety, public health, and consumer protection. Upton Sinclair's *The Jungle* was published in 1906, and it raised concerns about unsanitary and hazardous conditions in the meatpacking industry. As Sinclair wrote, "There would be meat stored in great piles in rooms; and the water from leaky roofs would drip over it, and thousands of rats would race about on it. It was too dark in these storage places to see well, but a man could run his hand over these piles of meat and sweep off handfuls of the dried dung of rats."[11(p161)] Once Sinclair exposed these conditions, labor organizers, workers, and the general public called for reform, and the Pure Food and Drug Act of 1906 was enacted to protect consumers.[12] This legislation laid the foundation for modern food safety regulation and led to the establishment of the U.S. Food and Drug Administration (FDA).

TABLE 12.1. FEDERAL FOOD POLICY IN THE UNITED STATES

POLICY	DESCRIPTION	IMPACT ON HEALTH
Pure Food and Drug Act (1906)	Prohibited the sale of adulterated or misbranded food and drugs, leading to improved food-safety standards and increased consumer confidence	Reduced the risk of foodborne illnesses and exposure to harmful substances
Federal Food, Drug, and Cosmetic Act (1938)	Established comprehensive regulations for food, drugs, cosmetics, and medical devices	Enhanced consumer protection and safety through improved labeling, product safety standards, and regulatory oversight of food and pharmaceutical products
Food Safety Modernization Act (2011)	Implemented preventive controls for food facilities, enhancing food import safety and improving traceability of foodborne illnesses	Reduced the incidence of foodborne illnesses by implementing preventive measures throughout food supply chain
Farm Bill (first created 1933, renewed approximately every 5 years)	Comprehensive legislation addressing agriculture and food policy, including nutrition assistance, crop insurance, and conservation initiatives	Influences agricultural practices, supporting food access and affordability and promoting sustainable food systems

Subsequent federal policies, such as the Federal Food, Drug, and Cosmetic Act, the Food Safety Modernization Act, and the Farm Bill have further strengthened food safety standards, expanded regulatory oversight, and enhanced protection of public health. These policies and their impact on health are covered in Table 12.1.

In the United States, the Farm Bill sets policies that have major implications for our food system. Past Farm Bills involved hundreds of billions of dollars in funding, and the next one may exceed 1 trillion dollars.[13] The cost is high because it addresses many vital agricultural and food-related issues, such as nutrition programs, crop subsidies, conservation efforts, rural development, and agricultural labor safety. One of the primary areas funded by the Farm Bill are nutrition programs like the Supplemental Nutrition Assistance Program (SNAP) and the Emergency Food Assistance Program, among others. These programs aim to provide millions of Americans with access to nutritious food. Crop subsidies are also covered in the bill and play a significant role in determining which foods are grown, how they are produced, and ultimately, what ends up on consumers' plates. Conservation initiatives are another crucial component of the Farm Bill, focusing on preserving soil, water, and wildlife habitat by providing voluntary financial and technical support to private and Tribal landowners, farmers, and ranchers.[14] The Farm Bill is typically up for reconsideration by Congress every 5 years, and many people engage in ongoing advocacy efforts to ensure it is designed to support a healthy food system.

CASE STUDY 12.1: Learning From the Dust Bowl

In the United States, many high school and university students are assigned to read *The Grapes of Wrath*. In it, author John Steinbeck tells the story of the Joads, a sharecropping family from Oklahoma who head to the Salinas Valley in California in the early 1930s during the Dust Bowl. The story shares a fictional glimpse of the Joads trying to survive in the larger context of

(continued)

CASE STUDY 12.1: Learning From the Dust Bowl (continued)

environmental, economic, and social crises during the Great Depression. At the time, approximately 500,000 people left the Great Plains region and headed to California in search of a better life. What many experienced instead was discrimination and unsafe working and housing conditions.

The Dust Bowl was a time of severe and persistent drought and dust storms over several years. It led to crop failures owing to the lack of water, soil depletion, and damage from the blowing dust. Looking back, many who have studied the event recognized that unsustainable agriculture was also a major contributing factor. Farmers were intensively plowing the Great Plains and planting the same crop season after season, known as monoculture farming. These approaches led to severe erosion of the soil.

As told by *The Grapes of Wrath* narrator:

> In the morning the dust hung like fog, and the sun was as red as ripe new blood. All day the dust sifted down from the sky, and the next day it sifted down. An even blanket covered the earth. It settled on the corn, piled up on the tops of the fence posts, piled up on the wires; it settled on roofs, blanketed the weeds and trees.[15(p2)]

These events influenced advocacy efforts and the creation of new policies, including:

- The Soil Conservation Act of 1935: This act established the Soil Conservation Service (now the Natural Resources Conservation Service) within the U.S. Department of Agriculture (USDA) to provide technical assistance and financial incentives to farmers for implementing soil conservation practices.
- The Agricultural Adjustment Act (AAA) of 1938: This act provided financial incentives to farmers who implemented conservation measures and participated in soil conservation programs.
- Civilian Conservation Corps (CCC) and the Works Progress Administration (WPA): As part of the President Franklin D. Roosevelt's New Deal, these programs employed thousands of people to undertake soil conservation projects, such as tree planting, erosion control, and building terraces and windbreaks.
- New Deal policies, such as the Farm Bill, addressed overproduction and its contribution to the Dust Bowl. By managing the supply of easily storable crops like wheat, corn, and soy, these policies controlled the agricultural market. They bought crops at low prices to reduce oversupply and later resold them at higher prices when supplies were lower. This approach reduced price fluctuations, benefiting farmers and consumers.

Many have reflected on these events and drawn parallels to some of the natural and human-made disasters within our food system today.

REFLECTION QUESTIONS

1. What parallels do you see between the events of the Dust Bowl and today's food system? After briefly learning about the Dust Bowl, what lessons do you think we learned as a society from these events? What lessons may have been lost on us?

2. Activist, farmer, founder of Soul Fire Farm, and author of *Farming While Black: Soul Fire Farm's Practical Guide to Liberation on the Land*, Leah Penniman, speaks and writes about a sacred ancestral relationship of Black people to the soil. As she describes in her essay "Black Gold": "[T]his black gold has high concentrations of calcium and phosphorus, as well as 200 to 300 percent more organic carbon than soils typical to the region. Today, community elders measure the age of their towns by the depth of the black soil, since every farmer in every generation participated in its creation."[16(p390)] Think about the role of soil in our food system. When was the last time you touched soil or had dirt in your fingernails from digging in the ground?

FROM FOOD SECURITY TO FOOD SOVEREIGNTY

The U.S. Department of Agriculture (USDA) defines **food security** as having access to enough food for an active, healthy life at all times.[17] The World Food Summit in 1996 described it as all people having both the physical and economic ability to obtain sufficient, safe, and nutritious food that meets their dietary needs and preferences for a healthy and active life.[18] Food security encompasses various components such as food production, nutrition, trade, and the ways in which individuals and nations maintain access to food during times of stress.[19] There are four main components considered for achieving food security:

- availability,
- accessibility,
- stability, and
- utilization.

Availability refers to the level of food production, trade, and stock levels, while *accessibility* relates to physical aspects (transport and infrastructure) and the economic means (purchasing power).[20] *Stability* is crucial for food security because it ensures adequate access over time, and *utilization* focuses on food's nutritional value and safety.[21] The path to food security is circular, as there is a feedback loop from utilization to availability, emphasizing the importance of optimal nutrition in agriculture and all production sectors.[20]

Levels of food security can fluctuate over time for individuals, communities, and nations. Fluctuations can range from high food security, where households have no problems accessing food, to marginal, low, and very low food security, where the eating patterns of one or more household members are disrupted due to a lack of money or other resources.[22] In the United States, 10.2% of households were food insecure (very low security, 3.8%, and low security, 6.4%) at some time during 2021.[22] Those most at risk for food insecurity are the poorest households, which often spend about 70% of their income on food and are particularly vulnerable to sudden changes in household income.[23] During the COVID-19 pandemic, food insecurity increased in the United States from 11% in 2018 to 38% in March 2020 because of disruptions in food access and an increased instability of food prices.[23,24] Poor access to transportation, lack of resources, and inadequate infrastructure can all contribute to food insecurity.

When looking at food insecurity in specific places, the USDA defines food deserts as areas characterized by access to poor, unhealthy, and unaffordable food, which may result in social disparities in diet and diet-related health outcomes, such as cardiovascular disease and obesity.[25,26] The term *food deserts* has been the subject of much attention and research since the early 1990s[27]; however, the term is increasingly recognized as problematic. Geographer Ashanté Reese discusses how food deserts are associated with a deficit model, that refers to areas where access to healthy and affordable food is limited.[28] Instead, she and other scholars recommend that we use the term **food apartheid**, which refers to a shift from the visual image of desolate barren spaces, and instead centers on the systematic sociocultural and political injustices that lead to lack of food resources.[27,28] However, many governmental agencies still use the term food deserts.

> **CASE STUDY 12.2: Texas Food Deserts**
>
> Texas has more than three million people living in food deserts that mostly consist of Black and Latino or Hispanic populations. To address the issue of access to safe and nutritious food, the state of Texas has implemented several initiatives.
>
> The first initiative supports existing federal programs like the Supplemental Nutrition Assistance Program (SNAP), previously known as the Food Stamp Program.[29] SNAP is the largest federally funded nutrition program and serves as a household-supporting infrastructure for individuals facing food insecurity.[30] Through SNAP, eligible low-income individuals and families receive benefits via an Electronic Benefits Transfer card, similar to a debit card, which they can use to purchase eligible food in authorized food stores. However, there are some concerns about the SNAP program. For example, the program is restrictive in terms of what food communities are eligible to consume; many

(continued)

CASE STUDY 12.2: Texas Food Deserts (continued)

culturally based foods are not available since they may cost more and since the ideal of a balanced diet is based on a Eurocentric food model.[31]

The Texas Department of Agriculture has launched the Food Access and Nutrition Network (FANN) and the Healthy Corner Store Initiative. FANN aims to create healthier communities by improving and strengthening awareness about healthy food and nutrition. It works to educate and provide collaboration between local businesses, farmers, and food banks to ensure that food-insecure communities can access healthy foods. The Healthy Corner Store Initiative provides funding to local convenience stores and markets to stock their shelves with produce and other healthy food items.

Other initiatives include the Healthy Food Financing Initiative, which provides grants and loans to help small businesses and entrepreneurs open or expand grocery stores in food deserts. Through this initiative, communities across the state are working with local organizations to provide programs and services to help food-insecure communities access healthy food. These programs include nutrition education, food pantries, and other services for families to access nutritious food.

The state is also working with organizations to provide job training and career development opportunities for people to help them gain the skills needed to secure employment in the food industry. By working with local businesses, farmers, and other organizations, the state of Texas is working to address food insecurity in communities statewide.

REFLECTION QUESTIONS

1. How can some of the initiatives mentioned above move toward a food sovereignty model?
2. Why are some scholars encouraging us to use terms like food apartheid rather than food deserts?

In addition to food security, La Via Campesina, an international movement founded in 1993 by peasant organizations of small and medium-sized food producers worldwide, calls for centering the concept of **food sovereignty**.[32] *Food sovereignty* has been defined in many ways, with the most recent being, "the right of peoples to healthy and culturally appropriate food produced through ecologically sound and sustainable methods, and their right to define their own food and agriculture systems. It puts those who produce, distribute and consume food at the heart of food systems and policies rather than the demands of markets and corporations."[33(para1)] Some of the principles of food sovereignty include:

- people's right to self-governance and democracy,
- supporting local production and economies, and
- valuing agricultural systems based on agroecology.

Food security is focused on access to food and is embedded in a system that prioritizes increased production and supports transnational agribusiness with governance at the national and international levels.[34] In contrast, the food sovereignty concept emerges from civil society and nongovernmental organizations; it rejects a deficit model[35] and aligns with social justice ideals that center the rights of people.[34] Food sovereignty prioritizes the needs and preferences of communities over market forces to promote access to nutritious, culturally appropriate food, while ensuring the rights of farmers, fishers, and Indigenous Peoples.[36] By supporting access to nutritious food, food sovereignty has a dramatic impact on health. Poor nutrition is one of the leading contributors of deaths, leading to over half a million deaths each year in the United States and an estimated 11 million deaths worldwide.[37]

IN OTHER WORDS: AGROECOLOGY

Agroecology is about farming in a way that works with nature, not against it. Instead of using lots of chemicals, like fertilizers and pesticides, the practice focuses on natural ways to grow food, such as with composting. The focus is on making sure farms are sustainable and do not harm the environment. Agroecology also values the knowledge of local farmers and their communities, helping them grow food that is healthy for people and the environment (Figure 12.1).

(continued)

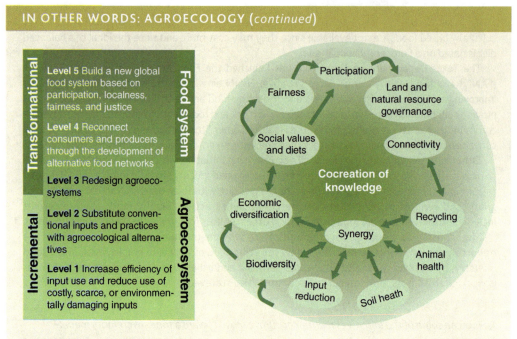

FIGURE 12.1. Transition levels toward sustainable food systems and related consolidated principles of agroecology.

Source: Wezel A, Herren BG, Kerr RB, Barrios E, Gonçalves ALR, Sinclair F. Agroecological principles and elements and their implications for transitioning to sustainable food systems: a review. *Agron Sustain Dev.* 2020;40(6). doi:10.1007/s13593-020-00646-z.

INDUSTRIALIZED VERSUS REGENERATIVE FOOD SYSTEMS

Despite some initial good intentions, industrialized food systems have put humanity on a concerning trajectory. The system is based on efficiency and profits, and the use of monocultures, mass production, extractive processes, and chemical-based farming. By default, societies have been forced to enact very strict food safety rules to control mass production, which has harmed people and the environment in many ways. It has also made it difficult for other food systems, such as regenerative systems, to gain a foothold due to competition, often from multinational corporations. Regenerative food systems are based on agroecological practices, with net-positive impacts on the environment; they are often decentralized systems that empower small and medium-scale producers.

INDUSTRIAL FOOD SYSTEMS

The roots of the industrial food system started during the Green Revolution, when scientists such as Borlaug, Haber, and Bosch began processes like grain intensification and the production of synthetic fertilizers to increase food production to address growing hunger.[38,39] Over time, this system created a path dependency on large corporations, based largely on monocultures, synthetic fertilizers, pesticides, and genetically modified crops, leading to depleted soils, polluted water sources, and the inability of small-scale producers to compete in the global market.[1-3,40] Today, despite its initial intentions of curbing hunger, populations worldwide remain largely hungry and undernourished. Additionally, these food systems often contribute to land degradation, biodiversity loss, and greenhouse gas emissions, worsening environmental health inequities.

This industrialized food system has in many ways removed people from their food. In past generations, people were closer to the land, perhaps as farmers themselves, or living and working closely with farmers, ranchers, pastoralists, or fisherfolk. Today, with an industrialized food system whose main purpose is efficiency and mass production, people purchase foods at large grocery stores, eat at restaurants, and use microwavable meals. Many people are not cooking at home.[41,42] Removing people from their food's production and making it cheaper has, in turn, created a new problem: unhealthy eating habits. At the same time, in some places where food apartheid exists, food-related chronic diseases are on the rise owing to the overavailability of cheap, unhealthy foods.

Industrialized food systems have also disproportionately burdened marginalized communities. Environmental hazards include pesticide exposure, water pollution, and air pollution from food production, processing, and transportation. For instance, in areas of California where agriculture dominates, predominantly Hispanic or Latino communities face higher rates of pesticide exposure because they are in proximity to agricultural fields where pesticides are used.[43] Exposure to pesticides can lead to adverse health outcomes that include neurological disorders, respiratory issues, eye and skin irritation, hormone disruption, and cancer.[44] Furthermore, pollution generated by industrial food production, processing, and transportation disproportionately affects low-wealth communities living near industrial zones and transportation corridors. In Chicago's South Side, for example, communities near meatpacking plants experience elevated levels of air pollution owing to the release of particulate matter and other contaminants during food processing. These communities of predominantly Black residents face disproportionate and rising levels of pollution stemming from systemic racism practices like redlining that have resulted in a dense concentration of industrial facilities.[45] (The StopGeneralIron campaign is a recent example of an environmental justice fight in this area that is covered in more detail in Chapter 19, "Organizing for Environmental Health and Justice: Lessons From #StopGeneralIron.")

An example of a food system that exacerbates environmental health inequities is Concentrated Animal Feeding Operations (CAFOs), also known as factory farms, which contribute to water pollution in rural areas of the United States. CAFOs are often located near low-wealth communities and communities of color. These farms produce meat and dairy products to meet growing demand. However, these intensive livestock production systems also generate large volumes of animal waste that can contaminate nearby water sources and cause air pollution.[46] CAFOs generate greenhouse gas emissions and are significant contributors to climate change. For example, the methane produced by flatulating ruminant animals, such as cows, and their manure is a potent greenhouse gas with a much higher warming potential than carbon dioxide. Additionally, CAFOs can contribute to deforestation by requiring the large-scale production of feed crops for the animals like soybeans and corn.[47] Deforestation caused by this type of animal agriculture, as well as other forms of agriculture, further exacerbates climate change.

INDUSTRIALIZED FOOD SYSTEM, FOOD SAFETY, AND ANTIBIOTIC RESISTANCE

Concentrated Animal Feeding Operations (CAFOs) and other large farms often administer antibiotics to their livestock as a preventive measure, even when animals are not sick. This practice, known as *prophylactic use*, is intended to prevent diseases that can arise from the crowded and unsanitary conditions in which animals are kept. However, the excessive and inappropriate use of antibiotics in this manner significantly contributes to the emergence and spread of antibiotic-resistant bacteria, posing a serious threat to human health (Figure 12.2). In response to this concern, various governmental efforts are underway to promote the responsible use of antibiotics in both animals and humans. These efforts include regulations, technical assistance, education, and training.

(continued)

280 ■ III INTERCONNECTED: ENERGY, AIR, WATER, FOOD, AND WASTE

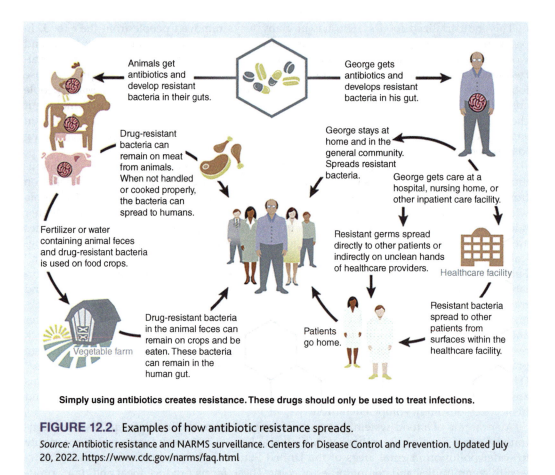

FIGURE 12.2. Examples of how antibiotic resistance spreads.
Source: Antibiotic resistance and NARMS surveillance. Centers for Disease Control and Prevention. Updated July 20, 2022. https://www.cdc.gov/narms/faq.html

Another example of the shortcomings of the industrialized food system is the ease with which infectious diseases can spread with large-scale farming productions. In 2021, the FDA and state and local regulatory officials traced an outbreak of *Escherichia coli* O157:H7 reported in six states to romaine lettuce from 23 farms and 36 fields in the Yuma growing region of Arizona. The FDA, along with the Centers for Disease Control and Prevention (CDC) and state partners, started an environmental assessment in the Yuma growing region and collected samples of water, soil, and manure. CDC laboratory testing identified the outbreak strain of *E. coli* O157:H7 in water samples taken from a canal in the Yuma region. Whole genome sequencing (WGS) showed that the *E. coli* O157:H7 found in the canal water was closely related genetically to the *E. coli* O157:H7 from ill people. The FDA is working with the lettuce industry to improve the safety of leafy greens. In the Yuma region, there are thousands of acres of farmland all dedicated to leafy greens, making it the winter salad capital. It is no surprise that contamination of such an enormous industrial production led to a large foodborne outbreak. Indeed today, the Yuma region has implemented strict protocols on traceability to respond to potential outbreaks; however, part of the compromise is also a huge aspect of potential food loss in case of infections.

WHO IS RESPONSIBLE FOR MANAGING AND ADDRESSING FOODBORNE OUTBREAKS?

About 1 in 6, or 48 million people, in the United States contract foodborne illnesses each year.[48] Norovirus is the main culprit behind most foodborne outbreaks, with other common pathogens including *Salmonella, Clostridium perfringens, Campylobacter, Escherichia coli,* and *Staphylococcus aureus.*[49] If two or more people get sick from contaminated food or drink, the event is called

(continued)

an outbreak. The foods associated with the most outbreaks in the United States include chicken, pork, beef, fruits, and vegetable row crops like lettuce and spinach.

Environmental health specialists, epidemiologists, microbiologists, and other public health professionals are involved in investigating a foodborne outbreak and implementing preventative measures during and after the outbreak. The responsibility for investigating foodborne illness typically rests with local health departments, who may also seek the expertise of state health departments. Once an outbreak emerges, federal agencies step in to provide additional support and track the spread across state lines. Depending on the source of the outbreak, the Centers for Disease Control and Prevention (CDC) the U.S. Food and Drug Administration (FDA), and the U.S. Department of Agriculture (USDA) may all be involved. The CDC plays a crucial role in monitoring and tracking outbreaks nationwide through its Foodborne Disease Outbreak Surveillance System (FDOSS), while the FDA has the Coordinated Outbreak Response and Evaluation (CORE) Network to help find, stop, and prevent foodborne illness.[50] Along with the FDA, the USDA is responsible for regulating and inspecting food production facilities to ensure compliance with food safety standards.

The spread of COVID-19 at the beginning of 2020 in the United States and across the globe, was an example of an external disruption that revealed many shortcomings of our globalized food system. The severity of spread of COVID-19 and the requirements for lockdown led to a breakdown in the food value chain and as a result disrupted food access, shifting some consumers toward cheaper foods with low nutritional value.[24] Social-distancing measures, such as quarantines and school closures, that led to trade restrictions, failures in transportation, and other disruptions showcased the vulnerability of large-scale industrial food systems. The industrial food system is reliant on transporting food from far away, including from overseas. In some places, there was a need to increase reliance on local production, intensifying the burden on local food-supply chains.[51] Tight lock-in mechanisms, shaped by a system developed for efficiency and just-in-time delivery, limited consumers' ability to access some staples, such as fresh produce, flour, and beans.[52-54] COVID-19 revealed the ways in which this large industrialized system is not resilient and nimble.

REGENERATIVE FOOD SYSTEMS

"Regenerative agriculture provides answers to the soil crisis, the food crisis, the climate crisis, and the crisis of democracy."

—Vandana Shiva

A regenerative food system remains aspirational, yet it embraces complexity, is based on positive impact, and is built on reciprocity, restoration, and life promotion.[55-57] El-Sayed and Cloutier, define a regenerative food system as "a whole-system approach to food that uses place-based education, integrates traditional agroecological knowledge with modern practices, and adopts nature-inspired solutions, while being engaged civically and economically. It is a system that produces both flavorful and culturally appropriate food, which is ecologically net positive, and which aims at intergenerational and interspecies justice."[1(p30,32)] *Regenerative farming practices* are practices that look at nature for inspiration and often Indigenous practices to find ways to farm that are in tune with the environment. In this conceptual framework, once a regenerative food system is established, growth happens slowly from the bottom up, as complex communities are nested within and benefit one another, while developing together to create a complex and interdependent society. When put into practice, this framework may ensure a more resilient food system in the face of unforeseen circumstances or environmental threats.

Examples of Regenerative Farming Practices in the Desert

Desert ecosystems are dryland systems with intense sun exposure, nutrient-poor soils, and little rainfall.[58] In these ecosystems, it is often believed hard to grow food. However, traditional communities across the world have adapted and even thrived in these environments through deep observations of the land, spiritual connection, and systems that are nature inspired and well adapted to place. Some of the practices developed by several Indigenous communities that have enabled them to be regenerative in harsh environments include the following:[1]

- **Supporting soil-across seasons:** Many desert ecosystems can sustain multiple growing seasons, sometimes as many as three per year. There are various practices that help the soil recover between seasons, such as planting nitrogen-fixing plants, using mulch, or incorporating cover crops. In these systems, it is common to rotate drought-tolerant grain varieties like barley or sorghum with nitrogen-fixing crops like clover, alfalfa, or tepary beans. Soil fertility can be improved by rotating animals, such as goats, which leave behind manure, and by adding mulch.
- **Use of polycultures:** Another technique is to grow crops in polycultures, such as the "three-sisters" method, in which corn, beans, and squash are planted in succession to mutually benefit each other. These plants involve a cover crop, a nitrogen fixer, and a stalk to support growth, among other benefits.
- **Water-diversion systems:** To make the most of scarce rainfall, different types of water diversion systems, like dykes or lower basins, can be built to attract water and retain water. Subterranean irrigation systems, such as clay bowls, as well as growing crops along water channels are also used.[58]
- **Seed selection and preservation:** Seed selection and preservation, often done by women, plays a crucial role in adapting crops to desert ecosystems. For instance, Hopi corn is planted one foot deep in the ground to optimize the crop's chances of survival and productivity in the challenging environmental conditions.

Alongside these practices, songs, stories, dances, ceremonies, and gifts are given as offerings to the land, plants, and organisms, creating a strong feedback loop and strengthening the connection between people and the land.[59]

CASE STUDY 12.3: The Pueblo Food Experience

The Pueblo Food Experience was run by a group of Indigenous People from Tewa Pueblo, New Mexico, giving us a glimpse of what it looks like to embrace food sovereignty and regenerative food practices. The experiment was initiated by Roxanne Swentzell, cofounder of the Flowering Tree Permaculture Institute. Her premise is that it is important to center food sovereignty. She suggests we are not only what and where we eat, but we are what and where our ancestors ate. Swentzell states how we can make it as easy as possible for those interested in their cultural preservation and health to convert over to our original diet.[60] The purpose of the project is to promote healing and balanced ways of eating by returning to the original foodways of the Pueblo peoples.

Before the contact of the Spanish in the 1540s, known as the precontact period, the Indigenous diet emphasized chemical-free meat, fowl, fish, and a wide variety of whole grains, nuts, seeds, fruits, and vegetables. The Pueblo Food Experience brought together 14 volunteers of Pueblo descent of different ages, some of whom were healthier than others. All participants agreed to be tested for different health metrics and would eat, for three months, only the foods available to their ancestors in the precontact period. The purpose was to try and address issues of obesity that the community was suffering from.[61]

The results were wildly successful and significantly decreased fast food's negative health impacts on the Pueblo volunteers, such as obesity and high cholesterol, triglycerides, and blood sugar. The experience gave the participants the necessary push to continue to valorize their traditional and culturally appropriate foods and, thus, a desire to cultivate historic Pueblo crops.

(continued)

> **CASE STUDY 12.3: The Pueblo Food Experience** (*continued*)
>
> Sponsor Five and other community members have begun growing various precontact crops, including blue corn, sweet corn, Hopi purple string beans, squash, wild asparagus, and watermelon. They produce the food using traditional Tewa agricultural practices and sell it at a local farmer's market for the community's consumption. Eating and growing these traditional foods are positive steps toward making the Pueblo a healthier community connected to its food heritage, and a move toward their food sovereignty.[61]
>
> **REFLECTION QUESTIONS**
>
> 1. How does the Pueblo Food Experience challenge conventional notions of diet and health, and what lessons can be drawn from the participants' return to traditional food?
>
> 2. Consider the broader implications of the Pueblo Food Experience beyond individual health outcomes. How does the cultivation and consumption of traditional Pueblo crops contribute to community resilience, cultural preservation, and the assertion of food sovereignty?

WORKING TOWARD ENVIRONMENTAL HEALTH AND JUSTICE

Food systems that prioritize food sovereignty and regenerative practices offer a pathway toward environmental health for all. Environmental health practitioners and researchers can engage in these efforts by supporting communities in controlling their own food systems and by promoting sustainable agricultural practices that enhance ecosystem and human health. There are many examples of local food systems to learn from where leaders are improving access to healthy, culturally appropriate food, while mitigating environmental harms. Two great examples of these systems include the Detroit Black Community Food Sovereignty Network (DBCFSN) and the Alabama Sustainable Agriculture Network (ASAN).

Founded in 2006, DBCFSN's mission is to foster self-reliance, food security, and justice within Detroit's Black community by promoting community-based urban agriculture, cooperative buying, and youth leadership development. They have launched several initiatives to increase access to fresh and healthy food for Detroiters, including urban gardening and farming projects, farmers' markets, food distribution and education programs, and advocacy efforts to promote an equitable food system. Major activities include the operation of D-town farm and the Detroit Food Commons, which includes a Black-led, community-owned grocery store.[62]

In another example, ASAN works to promote sustainable agricultural practices that prioritize environmental health, particularly in rural areas where communities face disproportionate environmental burdens. ASAN focuses on creating a more equitable food system in Alabama by supporting small-scale farmers, advocating for policy changes, and educating the community about the benefits of sustainable agriculture. ASAN also works to increase access to healthy, locally produced food in underserved communities, which often face disproportionate exposure to environmental hazards and lack access to fresh, nutritious food. One of the members of the network, Hvrvnrvcukwv Ueki-honecv Farm (Hummingbird Springs Farm), is an Indigenous food forest, nonprofit teaching farm, and future land trust in Florala, Alabama. They focus on forming an intentional community that centers communities of color, particularly Southeastern Indigenous communities, to promote Indigenous sovereignty, provide community access to nutritious food, and foster native plant biodiversity, among other initiatives.[63,64]

PARADIGM SHIFT TOWARD ONE HEALTH

As described in Chapter 1, "Fundamentals of Environmental Health and Justice," **One Health** is an approach that considers the health of people, animals, plants, and the environment together. This framework may be useful in improving our food system. The One Health approach is not suggesting a return to a more agrarian system, in which humans were more closely connected to their food as they may have been a few generations ago, and in which many people were farmers, ranchers, pastoralists, or fisherfolk. Instead, it assumes that we come together and prioritize One Health throughout the food system. It is also necessary to view the food system as a whole. This shift in mindset requires prioritizing the land and enabling it to provide ecosystem services, as well as managing the resources it has in a regenerative manner.[65] For example, it is important to focus on soil building rather than soil depletion, to prioritize animal health through welfare programs, and to promote people's health by incentivizing the consumption of healthy foods and access to fresh produce through policies and programs.

Because regenerative farming practices either mimic nature's strategies or are inspired by practices and Indigenous knowledge that have been passed down through generations, they can contribute positively to producing ecosystem services.[66] Valued at $33 trillion dollars per year across the globe, ecosystem services can include the regulation of the atmosphere and water, and support for food production, animal habitats, raw materials, and waste treatment, as well as cultural services like educational and spiritual uses.[67] The desert ecosystem example discussed earlier illustrates how regenerative farming practices can have a positive impact on ecosystem services. By rotating crops that include legumes, nutrients, including nitrogen, are cycled back into the earth, supporting the cycling of nutrients rather than depleting them. Furthermore, adding mulch and manure to the soil improves it over time, enhancing the ecosystem services of soil formation and nutrient cycling. This practice contrasts with the more conventional farming practices that deplete the soil over time with the use of chemical fertilizers and tilling that destroys topsoil, degrades soil health, and erodes the land. No-tillage practices and adaptive multipaddock grazing practices, which involve rotating cattle in a rapid manner that mimics the movement of bison, also contributes to improving and stabilizing soil. These practices create deep root systems, increase soil biodiversity, enhance the soil's ability to capture and store carbon, and attract more biodiversity, including pollinators, birds, and beneficial insects.[68] All of these practices enhance regulating, supporting, and provisioning ecosystem services.

Our industrialized food system, and the abundance of food, has meant that in the past 100 years, our demand for more animal products has increased. This demand has led to intensified livestock production and an explosion of zoonotic pathogens, or pathogens of animal origin. Like farming systems, animal systems also need to be diversified and more regenerative. Raising animals in CAFOs often means that animals are weaker owing to uniform genetics, that disease spreads faster, that inhumane practices are used, and that, ultimately, the animals produce less nutritious food.[69] In addition to reducing the amount of animal protein consumed, especially by Americans, and focusing on a plant-forward, but not necessarily vegetarian, diet, the way animals are raised needs to be more regenerative. Practices might include *silvopasture*,[70] a practice in which animals are raised in collaboration with food forests, or systems that include trees as living fences, foraging material, and areas suitable for pasture. Silvopasture creates a mutually beneficial relationship between plants and animals. Another example is *aquaponic systems*, which combine raising fish with hydroponics, or growing plants without food, in a mutually beneficial system wherein fish waste provides nutrients for plants and plants help filter and purify the water.[71]

One Health takes a holistic approach to health and advocates for a system that promotes healthier lifestyles. As part of this approach, it is important to create programs and policies that increase access to nutrient-dense fruits and vegetables, including organic options, and prioritize a plant-forward and whole-grain diet. To achieve this change, it is necessary to make healthier alternatives cheaper, more attractive, and more readily available. Numerous initiatives throughout the United States, for example, are focusing on improving school lunches. These initiatives aim to ensure that students have access to free school lunches and breakfasts that are nutritionally balanced. Additionally, they encourage practices like establishing school gardens, where students can learn about different fruits and vegetables and supplement their diets with fresh produce.

PRINCIPLES FOR A REGENERATIVE FOOD SYSTEMS

What a regenerative food system looks like is still unfolding, but there are some principles that can guide the work. These principles are based on research from many different scholars, but especially from the work of Duncan and colleagues[72] and El-Sayed and Cloutier.[1] Regenerative food systems should:

1. **Acknowledge and include diverse ways of knowing and being, inspired from Indigenous ways of knowing, or Traditional Ecological Knowledge (TEK)**[73-76]: Many communities have built well-adapted ecosystems, based on place-based and intergenerational knowledge of local ecosystems, climate, and local crops. This knowledge has helped communities create diversified diets, while incorporating patterns of self-renewal and spirituality through ritual and ceremony. Ultimately systems are more resilient because of community survivance; the ability to persist; and food traditions passed through stories, songs, and rituals. As a community persists, it evolves and passes this knowledge across generations, adapted to present situations with a forward outlook. In Indigenous traditions, learning and replicating strategies that work and validating them ultimately evolves across seven generations.[76,77]

2. **Think beyond capitalist approaches:** Many industrial corporations are accountable for their profits and bottom lines, which, as a result, does not ensure a balanced relationship between food, people, and the environment. The capitalist approach is driven by profit and efficiency,[6] thus resulting in abundant and cheap food. Unintentionally, the approach has also led to nutrient-poor food that has depleted soil and water, and thus is not driven by community or land needs. Capitalist approaches that are valuable, like entrepreneurial skills, should be geared toward supporting small-scale producers and their local economy, giving value to social capital.

3. **Incorporate place-based knowledge:** Strong cooperative relationships, not just with people, but with plants and animals, support a healthy food system. Therefore, relationships must be reciprocal with nonhumans[75] and the cosmos.[78] These relationships in agriculture are called *agroecological practices*, namely farming practices that are attuned to place, are developed by traditional farmers, and take inspiration from natural systems.[79] Agroecological practices also help reduce the spread of disease vectors and the presence of disease reservoirs. These practices include diversification of crop species, crop rotations, mulching, composting, agroforestry, and more. Many practices help manage pests, from the use of biological controls, such as the introduction of beneficial insects that prey on pests, rather than the use of chemical insecticides or the presence of trees, hedges, and other vegetation to create physical barriers that provide shelter for beneficial organisms. Such local attunement is achieved by understanding nature's cycles and leveraging them by knowing when to grow in tune with the seasons and cycles.

4. **Ensure reciprocity through creating a feedback loop and a cycle of community care**[77]: Reciprocity can be achieved by creating more local economies that also support local access to markets. Many tools exist for this purpose, such as developing public–private partnerships, establishing farmers' cooperatives, and linking farmers to local, regional, and international markets.

IN OTHER WORDS: COMMUNITY SURVIVANCE

Community survivance refers to the ability of a community to not only survive, but also to do well despite facing challenges. It goes beyond simply existing, and focuses on strength and lasting endurance, while keeping alive cultural traditions. Survivance shows how communities can stand up for themselves despite unfair treatment, inequities, or climate change.

MAIN TAKEAWAYS

In this chapter, we learned that:

- The relationship between food, the environment, and health is complex.
- Food policy that works to ensure access to food and improve health has a long history, from ancient civilizations to the present day.
- While food security focuses on ensuring access to sufficient, safe, and nutritious food, food sovereignty emphasizes the right of communities to define and control their own food systems.
- There are major consequences of the industrialized food system such as biodiversity loss and worsened climate change, and these consequences further worsen environmental injustices for low-wealth communities and communities of color.
- A paradigm shift that considers a One Health framework and applies regenerative principles grounded in agroecology and Indigenous knowledge is needed. This may help us to address environmental health and justice issues in our global industrialized food system.
- Environmental health practitioners, advocates, and researchers can support food sovereignty by supporting communities in controlling their own food systems, promoting sustainable agricultural practices, and enhancing ecosystem and human health.

SUMMARY

Food is not just essential for our physical and mental well-being but also symbolizes our unique identities, cultures, and traditions. Throughout history, food policies have been crucial in advancing public health, adapting to challenges like food shortages, food contamination, and changing dietary habits. However, the current industrialized global-food system presents countless obstacles to ensuring a healthy future for our planet—from soil depletion to antibiotic resistance to worsened climate change. By working to advance food sovereignty, we can strive for fairer and more sustainable food systems. Embracing the principles and practices of regenerative food systems, along with frameworks like One Health, provides a pathway to promoting environmental health and justice.

END-OF-CHAPTER RESOURCES

DISCUSSION QUESTIONS

1. How would you design a city to eliminate areas without access to healthy foods?
2. What are the impacts of using the food-sovereignty framework rather than the food security one?
3. Use three words to describe an industrial food system and three words to describe a regenerative food system.
4. Can you think of what regenerative farming practices might look like in your community and ecosystem?
5. Consider the journey your food takes before it reaches your plate. Reflect on the distance traveled, the resources consumed, and the environmental impact incurred. How far have your groceries traveled? What implications do these "food miles" have on sustainability, carbon emissions, and local economies?

LEARNING ACTIVITIES

THE TIME IS NOW

Investigate the U.S. Farm Bill and consider the ways we can continue to improve it. Consider what implications it has for your state or community. Remember that this bill includes policies related to nutrition programs, crop subsidies, conservation efforts, rural development, and agricultural labor safety. In your opinion, what changes would you like to see in the next version? Come up with two to three recommendations for your federal representatives and senators. Then, contact them by email or phone. Find trusted organizations working on these issues and engage in their advocacy efforts.

IN REAL LIFE

According to the USDA, over 44 million individuals reside in neighborhoods lacking convenient access to fresh, affordable, and nutritious food options. This issue impacts children as well as adults and affects residents living in both urban and rural areas. Visit the following link to better understand healthy food access in your community: www.healthyfoodaccess.org/access-101-research-your-community. The interactive map available at the Healthy Food Access Portal helps you understand and describe the food access in communities where you or your family live or work in. Enter a location to find a report that includes information on the food environment of that community and the population living there. Some measures include the number of healthy food retailers, demographics, health information, fruit and vegetable consumption, and federal programs.

A robust set of instructor resources designed to supplement this text is located at http://connect.springerpub.com/content/book/978-0-8261-8353-8. Qualifying instructors may request access by emailing textbook@springerpub.com.

REFERENCES

1. El-sayed S, Cloutier S. Weaving disciplines to conceptualize a regenerative food system. *J Agric Food Syst Community Dev*. 2022;11(5):1–29. doi:10.5304/jafscd.2022.112.003
2. Carlisle L. Making heritage: the case of black Beluga agriculture on the Northern Great Plains. *Ann Am Assoc Geogr*. 2016;106(1):130–144. doi:10.1080/00045608.2015.1086629
3. Patel R. *Stuffed or Starved: The Hidden Battle for the World Food System. Melville House*. 2nd ed. Melville House; 2012.
4. Trauger A. *We Want Land to Live: Making Political Space for Food Sovereignty*. The University of Georgia Press; 2017.
5. Crippa M, Solazzo E, Guizzardi D, Monforti F, Tubiello FN, Leip A. Food systems are responsible for a third of global anthropogenic GHG emissions. *Nature Food*. 2021;2(3):1–12, doi:10.1038/s43016-021-00225-9
6. Rushton J, Barry JM, Wilson ME, Mazet JAK, Shankar B. A food system paradigm shift: from cheap food at any cost to food within a one health framework. *NAM Perspect*. 2021;11:1–5. doi:10.31478/202111b
7. Alcock JP. *Food in the Ancient World*. Greenwood Press; 2003
8. Woolgar CM. *The Culture of Food in England, 1200–1500*. Yale University Press; 2016.
9. Mihesuah D, Hoover E. *Indigenous Food Sovereignty in the United States: Restoring Cultural Knowledge, Protecting Environments, and Regaining Health*. University of Oklahoma Press; 2019.
10. Earle C. Environment, disease and mortality in early Virginia. *J Hist Geogr*. 1979;5(4):365–390. doi:10.1016/0305-7488(79)90224-x
11. Sinclair U. *The Jungle*. Ten Speed; 1905.
12. Kantor AF. Upton Sinclair and the Pure Food and Drugs Act of 1906. "I aimed at the public's heart and by accident I hit it in the stomach." *Am J Public Health*. 1976;66(12):1202–1205. doi:10.2105/ajph.66.12.1202
13. The United States Senate Committee on Agriculture, Nutrition, and Forestry. Minority analysis: the May 2023 Farm Bill scoring baseline. May 15, 2023. https://www.agriculture.senate.gov/newsroom/majority-blog/minority-analysis-the-may-2023-farm-bill-scoring-baseline

14. Farm Bill conservation programs. U.S. Fish and Wildlife Service. Accessed June 14, 2024. https://www.fws.gov/service/farm-bill-conservation-programs
15. Steinbeck J. *The Grapes of Wrath*. Pearson Education; 1939.
16. Penniman L. Black gold. In: Johnson AE, Wilkinson KK. *All We Can Save*. Kindle e-Book. One World; 2020:chap 7.
17. Food security in the U.S.: overview. U.S. Department of Agriculture Economic Research Service. Updated October 25, 2023. https://www.ers.usda.gov/topics/food-nutrition-assistance/food-security-in-the-u-s/
18. World Food Summit. World food summit—final report—part 1. Food and Agriculture Organization of the United Nations. 1996. Accessed June 15, 2024. https://www.fao.org/3/w3548e/w3548e00.htm
19. Ziervogel G, Ericksen PJ. Adapting to climate change to sustain food security. *Wiley Interdiscip Rev Clim*. 2010;1(4):525–540. doi:10.1002/wcc.56
20. Berry EM, Dernini S, Burlingame B, Meybeck A, Conforti P. Food security and sustainability: can one exist without the other? *Public Health Nutr*. 2015;18(13):2293–2302. doi:10.1017/s1368980015000021x
21. Figiel S, Floriańczyk Z, Wigier M. Impact of the COVID-19 pandemic on the world energy and food commodity prices: implications for global economic growth. *Energies*. 2023;16(7):3152. doi:10.3390/en16073152
22. Key statistics & graphics. USDA ERS. Updated October 25, 2023. https://www.ers.usda.gov/topics/food-nutrition-assistance/food-security-in-the-u-s/key-statistics-graphics/#:~:text=The%20prevalence%20of%20very%20low%20food%20security%20in%202022%20(5.1
23. Kakaei H, Nourmoradi H, Bakhtiyari S, Jalilian M, Mirzaei A. Effect of COVID-19 on food security, hunger, and food crisis. *COVID-19 Sustain Dev Goals*. 2022;3(29):3–29. doi:10.1016/b978-0-323-91307-2.00005-5
24. Laborde D, Martin W, Swinnen J, Vos R. COVID-19 risks to global food security. *Science*. 2020;369(6503):500–502. doi:10.1126/science.abc4765
25. Beaulac J, Kristjansson E, Cummins S. A systematic review of food deserts, 1966–2007. *Prev Chronic Dis*. 2009;6(3):A105. https://www.ncbi.nlm.nih.gov/pmc/articles/PMC2722409/
26. Alexis AC. What are food deserts? All you need to know. *Healthline*. June 14, 2021. https://www.healthline.com/nutrition/food-deserts
27. Dickinson M. Black agency and food access: leaving the food desert narrative behind. *City*. 2019;23(4–5):690–693. doi:10.1080/13604813.2019.1682873
28. Reese AM. *Black Food Geographies: Race, Self-Reliance, and Food Access in Washington, D.C.* Chapel Hill University of North Carolina Press; 2019.
29. Gundersen C. Viewpoint: a proposal to reconstruct the Supplemental Nutrition Assistance Program (SNAP) into a universal basic income program for food. *Food Policy*. 2021;101:102096. doi:10.1016/j.foodpol.2021.102096
30. DeWitt E, Gillespie R, Norman-Burgdolf H, Cardarelli KM, Slone S, Gustafson A. Rural SNAP participants and food insecurity: how can communities leverage resources to meet the growing food insecurity status of rural and low-income residents? *Int J Environ Res Public Health*. 2020;17(17):6037. doi:10.3390/ijerph17176037
31. Aluoch A, Broxton M, Gordon Y, et al. A community-driven anti-racist vision for SNAP. The Center for Law and Social Policy. September 2022. https://www.clasp.org/wp-content/uploads/2022/09/2022.9.28_A-Community-Driven-Anti-Racist-Vision-for-SNAP.pdf
32. Rosset P. Food sovereignty: global rallying cry of farmer movements. *Food First*. 2003;9(4):2–4. https://foodfirst.org/wp-content/uploads/2013/12/BK9_4-Fall-2003-Vol-9-4-Food-Sovereignty.pdf
33. Declaration of Nyéléni. Friends of the Earth International, Via Campesina, the World March of Women, Réseau des Organisations Paysannes et de Producteurs de l'Afrique de l'Ouest (ROPPA), World Forum of Fish Harvesters and Fishworkers (WFF), World Forum of Fisher Peoples (WFFP). Nyéléni Village, Sélingué, Mali. February 27, 2007. https://nyeleni.org/en/declaration-of-nyeleni
34. Jarosz L. Comparing food security and food sovereignty discourses. *Dialogues Hum Geogr*. 2014;4(2):168–181. doi:10.1177/2043820614537161
35. Nyborg I, Haug R. Measuring household food security: a participatory process approach. *Forum Dev Stud*. 1995;22(1):29–59. doi:10.1080/08039410.1995.9665988
36. Holt Giménez E, Shattuck A. Food crises, food regimes and food movements: rumblings of reform or tides of transformation? *J Peasant Stud*. 2011;38(1):109–144. doi:10.1080/03066150.2010.538578

37. GBD Compare. Institute for Health Metrics and Evaluation. 2019. Accessed June 14, 2024. https://vizhub.healthdata.org/gbd-compare/
38. Dunn R. *Never Out of Season*. Little, Brown; 2017.
39. Raj P, Moore JW. *A History of the World in Seven Cheap Things: A Guide to Capitalism, Nature, and the Future of the Planet*. University of California Press; 2018.
40. Bausch JC, Eakin H, Smith-Heisters S, et al. Development pathways at the agriculture–urban interface: the case of Central Arizona. *Agric Human Values*. 2015;32(4):743–759. doi:10.1007/s10460-015-9589-8
41. Wolfson JA, Leung CW, Richardson CR. More frequent cooking at home is associated with higher healthy eating index-2015 score. *Public Health Nutr*. 2020;23(13):2384–2394. doi:10.1017/S1368980019003549
42. Reicks, M, Kocher M, Reeder J. Impact of cooking and home food preparation interventions among adults: a systematic review (2011–2016). *J Nutr Educ Behav*. 2018;50(2):148–172. doi:10.1016/j.jneb.2017.08.004
43. Teysseire R, Manangama G, Baldi I, et al. Determinants of non-dietary exposure to agricultural pesticides in populations living close to fields: a systematic review. *Sci Total Environ*. 2021;761:143294. doi:10.1016/j.scitotenv.2020.143294
44. Pesticides. U.S. Environmental Protection Agency. 2020. Updated May 9, 2024. https://www.epa.gov/pesticides
45. Illgner T, Lad N. Data to improve air quality environmental justice outcomes in South Chicago. *Front Public Health*. 2022;10:977948. doi:10.3389/fpubh.2022.977948
46. Donham KJ, Wing S, Osterberg D, et al. Community health and socioeconomic issues surrounding concentrated animal feeding operations. *Environ Health Perspect*. 2007;115(2), 317–320. doi:10.1289/ehp.8836
47. Gerber PJ, Steinfeld H, Henderson B, et al. *Tackling Climate Change through Livestock—A Global Assessment of Emissions and Mitigation Opportunities*. Food and Agriculture Organization of the United Nations (FAO); 2013.
48. Foodborne illness. Healthy People 2030. Office of Disease Prevention and Health Promotion. Accessed June 12, 2024. https://health.gov/healthypeople/objectives-and-data/browse-objectives/foodborne-illness
49. Burden of foodborne illness: findings. Centers for Disease Control and Prevention. Updated November 5, 2018. https://www.cdc.gov/foodborneburden/2011-foodborne-estimates.html
50. US Food and Drug Administration. About the CORE network. FDA. Published online October 1, 2020. https://www.fda.gov/food/outbreaks-foodborne-illness/about-core-network
51. International Panel of Experts on Sustainable Food Systems. COVID-19 and the crisis in food systems: symptoms, causes, and potential solutions. April 2020. https://ipes-food.org/report/covid-19-and-the-crisis-in-food-systems/
52. Hobbs, J E. Food supply chains during the COVID-19 pandemic. *Can J Agric Econ*. 2020;68(2):171–176. doi:10.1111/cjag.12237
53. Reiley, L. The industry says we have enough food. Here's why some store shelves are empty anyway. *Washington Post*. April 14, 2020.
54. Nicola, M, Zaid A, Catrin S, et al. The socio-economic implications of the coronavirus pandemic (COVID-19): a review. *Int J Surg*. 2020;78:185–193. doi:10.1016/j.ijsu.2020.04.018
55. Birkeland I. Cultural sustainability: industrialism, placelessness and the re-animation of place. *Ethics Place Environ*. 2008;11(3):283–297. doi:10.1080/13668790802559692
56. Gibbons LV. Regenerative—the new sustainable? *Sustainability*. 2020;12(13):5483. doi:10.3390/su12135483
57. Rhodes CJ. The imperative for regenerative agriculture. *Sci Prog*. 2017;100(1):80–129. doi:10.3184/003685017x14876775256165
58. Nabhan, G. *Growing Food in a Hotter, Drier Land: Lessons from Desert Farmers on Adapting to Climate Uncertainty*. Chelsea Green Publishing; 2013.
59. Cajete, G. 2018. Native science and sustaining Indigenous communities. In Nelson MK, Shilling D, eds. *Traditional Ecological Knowledge*. Cambridge University Press; 2018:15–26. doi:10.1017/9781108552998.003
60. Home. Flowering Tree Permaculture Institute. https://www.floweringtreepermaculture.org
61. Dunphy H, Fakult J, Romero L, et al. Cultural education platform for Tewa speakers. Worcester Polytechnic Institute. 2017. https://core.ac.uk/download/pdf/212975089.pdf

62. Home. Detroit Black Community Food Sovereignty Network. Accessed June 13, 2024. https://www.dbcfsn.org
63. ASAN Online. Alabama Sustainable Agriculture Network. Accessed January 12, 2024. https://asanonline.org/
64. Rematriating Ancestral Mvskoke Lands. Hvrvnrvcukwv Ueki-honecv (Hummingbird Springs) Farm. Accessed June 12, 2024. https://www.hummingbirdspringsfarm.org/
65. Steger, C, Hirsch S, Evers C, et al. Ecosystem services as boundary objects for transdisciplinary collaboration. *Ecol Econ*. 2018;143:153–160. doi:10.1016/j.ecolecon.2017.07.016
66. Costanza R, D'arge R, De Groot R, et al. The value of the world's ecosystem services and natural capital. *Ecol Econ*. 1998;25(1): 3–15. doi:10.1016/S0921-8009(98)00020-2
67. Costanza R, d'Arge R, De Groot R, et al. The value of the world's ecosystem services and natural capital. *Nature*. 1997;387(6630):253–260. doi:10.1038/387253a0
68. Mubvumba P, DeLaune PB, Hons FM. Enhancing long-term no-till wheat systems with cover crops and flash grazing. *Soil Secur*. 2022;8(10):100067. doi:10.1016/j.soisec.2022.100067
69. Hinchliffe S, John A, Stephanie L, Nick B, Simon C. Biosecurity and the topologies of infected life: from borderlines to borderlands. *Trans Inst Br Geogr*. 2013;38:531–543. doi:10.1111/j.1475-5661.2012.00538.x
70. Gliessman SR. *Agroecology: The Ecology of Sustainable Food*. 2nd ed. CRC Press; 2007.
71. Specht K, Siebert R, Hartmann I, et al. Urban agriculture of the future: an overview of sustainability aspects of food production in and on buildings. *Agric Human Values*. 2014;31:33–51. doi:10.1007/s10460-013-9448-4
72. Duncan J, Carolan M, Wiskerke JSC. *Routledge Handbook of Sustainable and Regenerative Food Systems*. Routledge; 2020.
73. Berkes, F. Traditional ecological knowledge in perspective. In: Inglis TJ, ed. *Traditional Ecological Knowledge: Concepts and Cases*. Museum of Nature and International Development Research Centre; 1993:1–9.
74. Berkes, F. Traditional knowledge systems in practice. In: *Sacred Ecology*. Taylor & Francis; 2008: 71–96. https://www.taylorfrancis.com/books/mono/10.4324/9780203123843/sacred-ecology-fikret-berkes
75. Kimmerer, RW. *Braiding Sweetgrass: Indigenous Wisdom, Scientific Knowledge and the Teachings of Plants*. Milkweed Edition; 2013.
76. Whyte K. On the role of traditional ecological knowledge as a collaborative concept: a philosophical study. *Ecoll Process*. 2013;2(7):1–12. doi:10.1186/2192-1709-2-7
77. Kealiikanakaoleohaililani K, Christian PG. Embracing the sacred: an Indigenous framework for tomorrow's sustainability science. *Sustain Sci*. 2016;11(1):57–67. doi:10.1007/s11625-015-0343-3
78. Wilson S. *Research is Ceremony: Indigenous Research Methods*. Fernwood; 2008.
79. Altieri MA, Nicholls CI, Henao A, Lana MA. Agroecology and the design of climate change-resilient farming systems. *Agron Sustain Dev*. 2015;35(3):869–890. doi:10.1007/s13593-015-0285-2.

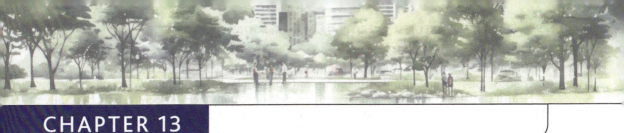

CHAPTER 13

Waste and Sustainability

Denise Patel and Neil Tangri

LEARNING OBJECTIVES

- Define the different types of waste, describing their sources and how they are typically managed.
- Describe how waste systems function on local and global scales.
- Explain how waste systems contribute to environmental injustice and health inequities.
- Explain and compare policies that govern waste systems in the United States and internationally.
- Understand the concept of zero waste as a matter of environmental and social justice and how it can be achieved.

KEY TERMS

- circular economy
- incinerators
- landfill
- sacrifice zones
- waste
- waste colonialism
- waste hierarchy
- waste management
- waste systems
- zero waste

OVERVIEW

The world has never produced as much waste as it does today. Massive waste production came with a cultural shift to the more materialistic, consumer-driven society that emerged after World War II, particularly in high-income countries. In recent decades, the amount of **waste**—material, chemical, or substance that is disposed of or discarded for no further use—that has been generated has grown further in our globalized economy. Some will argue that this pattern is a result of population growth when, in fact, global waste production is expected to grow at *twice* the rate of the global population.[1] The composition of waste we produce has also changed from primarily organic and recyclable materials to more toxic and nonrecyclable materials. Although waste was once primarily a local problem, waste colonialism has taken root, as waste regularly flows across borders, primarily from high-income to low-income countries that lack the resources to properly manage it. Today, high-income countries have nearly universal waste collection systems, whereas open pit dumping occurs more commonly in low-income countries.[1] Over the past century, the patterns of environmental injustice associated with **waste systems** have persisted. Ultimately, the best solution to waste and its related inequities may be to not make it in the first place.[2]

Human health is impacted by waste through many pathways: Landfills and open waste dumps attract rats and other vermin that spread disease, pollute local waterways, and cause foul odors. Even modern landfills, engineered with liners and caps, fail over time. They leach toxins into groundwater, cause fires from concentrated gases, and blow contaminated dust and odors into nearby communities. Burning waste in open pits and incineration facilities pollutes the air and leaves behind toxic ashes. Even so-called "nonhazardous" waste can become hazardous to human health when burned or mixed with hazardous items like batteries and electronics in landfills. Waste transportation leaves a trail of air and water pollutants across hundreds or even thousands of miles by truck, rail, and ocean freight. Methane emissions from landfills and greenhouse gases emitted from incinerators and open-pit burns contribute to climate change.

Health impacts from the waste system are felt unequally across society, and generally those who produce the least waste are the most impacted by it. In 1987, a groundbreaking report commissioned by the United Church of Christ, *Toxic Wastes and Race in the United States*, cataloged toxic waste sites across the United States and found that race is the primary predictor of hazardous waste siting (Figure 13.1).[3] Waste siting is associated with a higher incidence of cardiovascular, respiratory, and neurological disease, improper reproductive development, and cancer. Community-organizing efforts to fight the waste sites documented in the report were the stepping-stones of the environmental justice (EJ) movement of today. Waste processing facilities continue to be located more near communities of color and low-wealth communities than in other areas, which is the case for 79% of municipal solid waste (MSW) incinerators in the United States, according to a 2019 report by the New School (Figure 13.2). These communities are often already burdened with many other environmental exposures.

This chapter provides a broad overview of **waste management** systems (primarily in the United States), the adverse health impacts associated with these systems, and the regulatory measures intended to protect human health. The health and environmental impacts of waste management and siting are determined by the quantity, type, composition, transport, and placement of the waste. This chapter refers to various types of waste, including MSW, industrial nonhazardous and hazardous waste, medical waste, agricultural and animal waste, radioactive waste, construction and demolition (C&D) debris, extraction and mining waste, oil and gas production and combustion waste, and sewage sludge; it also includes a broad

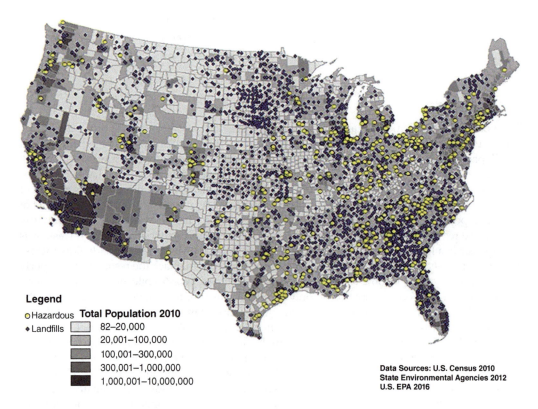

FIGURE 13.1. Types and locations of landfills across the United States.

C&D, construction and demolition; EPA, Environmental Protection Agency.

Source: Cannon C. Intersectional and entangled risks: an empirical analysis of disasters and landfills. *Front Clim.* 2021;3. doi:10.3389/fclim.2021.709439.

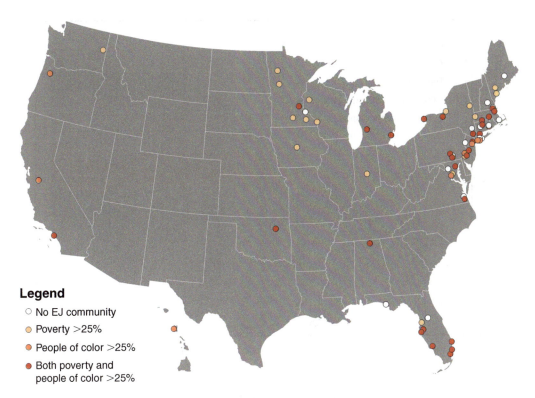

FIGURE 13.2. MSW incinerators in the United States.

EJ, environmental justice; MSW, municipal solid waste.

Source: Baptista AI, Perovich A. U.S. municipal solid waste incinerators: an industry in decline. The New School: Tishman Environment and Design Center. May 2019. https://www.no-burn.org/u-s-municipal-solid-waste-incinerators-an-industry-in-decline

overview of other categories of waste associated with agriculture, energy, and water, which can be found in related chapters. Ultimately, the chapter discusses the need for a Zero Waste Hierarchy and the circularity model as a path to reducing environmental health harms and achieving global EJ.

HISTORY OF WASTE AND WASTE MANAGEMENT IN THE UNITED STATES

Before the introduction of modern waste systems in the early 1900s, most waste in the United States was thrown in open dumps on the outskirts of towns and cities. Primarily composed of biodegradable, quickly decomposing food waste, it caused foul odors and attracted rats that spread disease. The practice of layering soil each day was used to reduce these nuisances but did not prevent runoff and the contamination of local water sources. The growth of cities and concerns over poor sanitation led to changes in waste management practices. By 1960, 94% of waste was dumped in landfills and in waterways or burned in incinerators and in open pits in the United States. A mere 6% was recycled.[4]

As consumerism dominated the culture, Americans began to create more waste per person, and waste composition shifted to an increased use of plastics, electronics, and other materials that are nonrecyclable, slower to decompose, and increasingly likely to contaminate the environment (e.g., microplastics in the food chain and per- and polyfluoroalkyl substances [PFAS]).

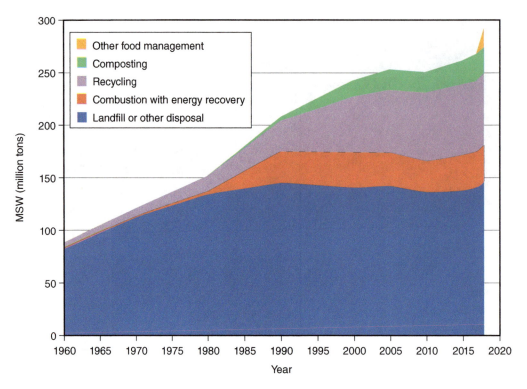

FIGURE 13.3. MSW generation and management in the United States, 1960–2018.
MSW, municipal solid waste.

Source: Data from National overview: facts and figures on materials, wastes and recycling. U.S. Environmental Protection Agency. 2020. Accessed 15 June 2024. https://www.epa.gov/facts-and-figures-about-materials-waste-and-recycling/national-overview-facts-and-figures-materials

Factories were also dumping toxic waste alongside municipal waste. MSW incinerators drew much attention from community groups who filed complaints of foul odors and smokestack emissions. The facilities were also marketed as a way to produce energy, but by 1990, only 12% of waste that was burned was used for energy recovery. Recycling rates and composting steadily increased as more municipalities adopted sustainability measures. Although some waste is recycled, reused, or composted, 62% of waste is still either sent to a landfill or incinerated in the United States (Figure 13.3).[4]

WASTE COLONIALISM TAKES ROOT

The history of waste management is a story of local and global environmental racism. The United States and other wealthier countries have stopped placing some of their waste in their own communities, which has given rise to waste colonialism. **Waste colonialism** is defined as the practice of shipping waste from high-income countries to lower-income nations.

Electronic waste and batteries (also known as e-waste) are a prime example. In 2019, 53.6 million metric tons of e-waste was generated, predominantly in high-income countries, and this number continues to grow (Figure 13.4).[5] More than 80% of that waste was shipped to low- or middle-income countries where it was crudely recycled by waste pickers under extremely poor working and environmental conditions. Heavy metals such as lead, cadmium, zinc, chromium, and nickel have been measured at increased concentrations in soils around open dump sites in India and Nigeria. Health-monitoring studies of female waste pickers have also found that heavy metals transfer from mother to child. In low-income countries where child labor laws are generally nonexistent, child laborers at open dump sites have suffered from impaired development.[1]

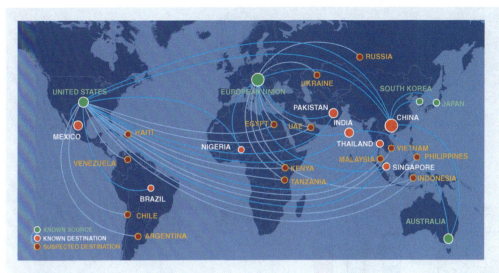

FIGURE 13.4. Global e-waste flow.
Source: Ferronato N, Torretta V. Waste mismanagement in developing countries: a review of global issues. *Int J Environ Res Public Health.* 2019;16(6):1060. doi:10.3390/ijerph16061060.

HEALTH IMPACTS OF WASTE

No matter whether waste is deposited in landfills or burned, it will always be at least as harmful as its most toxic components. Household nonhazardous solid waste from residences, institutions, and commercial sources and industrial nonhazardous solid waste from large-scale manufacturing and goods production include:

- packaging material such as cardboard boxes,
- bottles and cans,
- paper material,
- landscape debris,
- food scraps,
- furniture and fabrics,
- appliances, and
- electronic waste and batteries.

At each point in the waste management system, pollutants from these materials are introduced to the air and water and contribute to respiratory and cardiovascular disease and the risk of ingestion of toxic chemicals from local food and water sources.

Whose health is at risk? Workers at landfills and incinerators experience additional health impacts from skin contact, odors, and facility injuries or accidents, depending on the composition of the waste. Where open-waste dumping and burning is more common, waste pickers are more directly exposed to disease vectors, hazardous chemicals, and cuts and burns.[1] Communities—disproportionately communities of color—near these sites experience exposure to elevated levels of heavy metals, particulate matter (PM), and toxic chemicals that are linked to adverse health outcomes, such as respiratory illnesses and asthma, a higher incidence of cardiovascular disease and hypertension, and impaired reproductive systems.[6] Living in close proximity to landfills and incinerators is also associated with negative mental health effects and higher mortality rates.[6] The nuisance from dust, debris, and odors near communities is a constant reminder of the harms of living near these sites, which add daily stressors to the socioeconomic impacts associated with living at or near the poverty line. These risks are discussed in the following sections as we follow waste through the system (Figure 13.5).

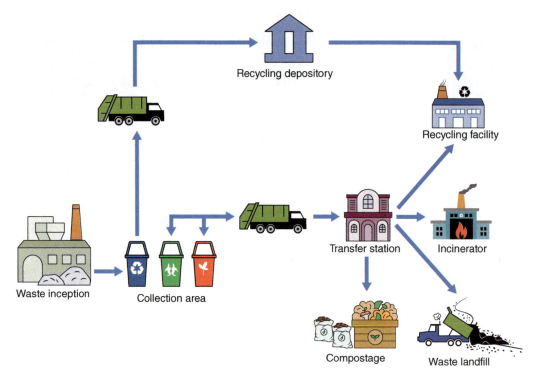

FIGURE 13.5. Waste management life cycle.
Source: Adapted from SafetyCulture Content Team. Waste management system: a guide. SafetyCulture. April 19, 2024. https://safetyculture.com/topics/waste-management-system

THERE IS NO "AWAY"

Waste collection begins in homes and businesses. There it may be sorted into recyclable material and nonrecyclable materials. The waste is often bagged, picked up by a waste truck, and transported away—often through and to communities of color and poor communities. At this point, *most people stop thinking about their trash.* However, the environmental health impacts have just begun. Most waste trucks burn diesel and spew PM, lead, and other pollutants along their route. Truck traffic increases the concentration of pollutants closer to a recycling or processing center or a waste transfer station. Similar to landfills, runoff from open air transfer and storage sites may contaminate local waterways and sewer systems, attract rodents, and cause foul odors. After waste is sorted at the transfer station, the collected waste and associated diesel fumes continue on to a landfill or incinerator.[2]

LANDFILLS

Most of the waste produced in the United States is deposited in one of three types of **landfills**. *Landfills* are sites designated for the burial of solid waste. Once a landfill reaches maximum capacity, it is covered with a permanent cap and may be repurposed in the future if it does not pose a risk to human health or the environment. However, there have been disasters in places where land was repurposed and was not safe.

Types of Landfills

- **MSW landfills:** These receive nonhazardous waste collected from municipalities and counties. A subcategory of MSW landfills are bioreactor landfills, which are engineered to accelerate the breakdown of organic waste and collect methane for fuel.

- **Industrial waste landfills:** These are used to collect commercial and industrial waste, such as C&D debris and coal ash (referred to as coal-combustion residual landfills). Incinerator ash is also disposed of as industrial waste. *Monofills* are landfills that only accept one type of waste and are engineered with specific liners to prevent leaching. For example, an industrial waste landfill that only accepts incinerator ash is a monofill.
- **Hazardous waste landfills:** These are specifically designed to collect hazardous waste and include additional measures engineered to protect human health and the environment. Hazardous waste landfills that contain lead, asbestos, dioxin, radioactive waste, and other chemicals must be closed or abandoned. If they pose a long-term risk to human health, they may be further regulated under the Comprehensive Environmental Response, Compensation, and Liability Act (CERCLA; commonly known as the Superfund) and placed on the Superfund National Priorities List. The Superfund program is funded by a tax on chemical and petrochemical industries, and these funds are used to remediate the most dangerous hazardous waste sites, as described in greater depth in Chapter 4, "Environmental Health Policies and Protections: Successes and Failures."

Anatomy of a Landfill

The structure of a landfill is designed to contain waste and the byproducts of its decomposition (Figure 13.6). When the structure fails, the risk of exposure increases for workers and communities as described in Table 13.1.[7]

Groundwater Contamination

Bottom liners should provide protection from landfill leaks and are typically composed of two layers of thick plastic with a layer of gravel, sand, and clay in between the liners. Rainwater forms leachates as it pulls chemicals and other contaminants from the waste as it flows

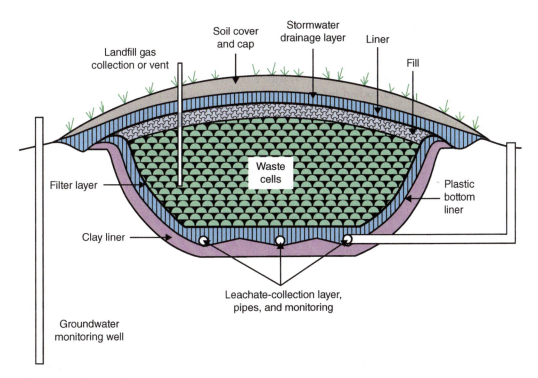

FIGURE 13.6. Landfill diagram.

TABLE 13.1. COMMON FAILURES OF LANDFILL STRUCTURES, CONSEQUENCES, AND ASSOCIATED PATHWAYS OF EXPOSURE

PROTECTIVE STRUCTURE FAILURE	CONSEQUENCES	PATHWAYS OF EXPOSURE
Improper closure of waste cells, soil cover, and caps	Toxic chemicals leaking through to the bottom liner Wind dispersion of debris, particular matter (PM), and odors Increased rodents and pests	Ingestion Inhalation Dermal
Degradation of liners	Toxic chemicals leaking into lower layers, aquifers, and groundwater	Ingestion
Improper collection from stormwater drainage and leachate-collection systems	Contamination of groundwater or local waterways	Ingestion Inhalation Dermal
Landfill gas-collection and leaks	Fires, explosions, and foul odors	Inhalation Dermal
Failed groundwater tests	Leaks	Ingestion

through the landfill. Heavy metals and acids from batteries and electronic waste can corrode plastic liners. Leftover paints, pesticides, pots and pans coated with PFAS, and mattresses or textiles coated with polybrominated flame retardants can leach thousands of persistent, bioaccumulating chemicals. The next protective measure, the leachate-collection system, sends liquid to wastewater treatment plants or to a holding pond. In reality, modern wastewater treatment plants are not designed to remove the many types of chemicals present in waste. Holding ponds use microbacteria to break down some chemicals but may introduce more hazards if the leachate is sprayed into the pond or back over the landfill. Volatile organic compounds (VOCs) evaporate from the ponds. The sludge from processing leachate is laden with a chemical concentrate and must be put into a landfill or incinerated.[8]

Air Pollution and Climate Change

Landfills can take years to decades to fill. Waste cells within the landfill are filled and covered with soil daily to prevent rodent infestation and wind dispersion of PM and debris. Once filled, landfills are capped with 2 to 3 feet of soil, and the area may be repurposed for development. Caps, while protective, also slow the decomposition of waste, allow gasses to form and accumulate, and increase the risk of fires and explosions. Methylmercury can form in landfills, flow out as runoff, leach into groundwater, or be transferred out with landfill gas. Landfill methane gas may be laced with dozens of toxic chemicals, including benzene, vinyl chloride, and chloroform.[9] The burning of landfill gas can release chemicals into the air, especially in an uncontrolled situation. An estimated 80% of landfill gas is released unburned over its lifetime (with only 20% recovered and burned), and it is the greatest source of greenhouse gas emissions from the waste sector.[10]

INCINERATORS

Incinerators are facilities that burn waste in a furnace at high temperatures and are sometimes used to produce heat or electricity. Incineration accounts for 12% of waste disposal in the United States and is far more expensive than landfills.[11] Incineration is the prevalent form of MSW disposal in northern Europe, Japan, South Korea, and China, but is rarely used in low-income countries. Similar to many other polluting industries, incinerators are most (79%) often sited near low-income communities and communities of color.[2] Ten of the 12 incinerators that emit the highest levels of lead or $PM_{2.5}$ are located in EJ communities (Figure 13.7).

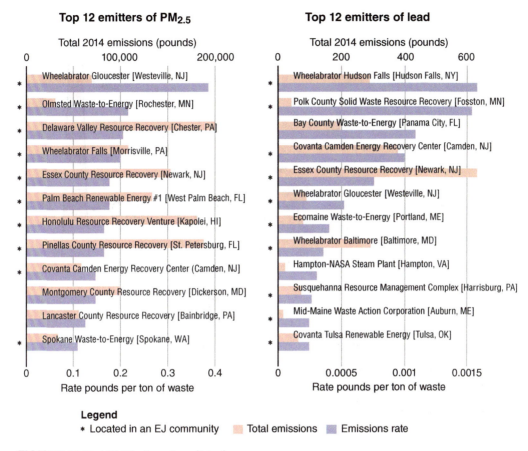

FIGURE 13.7. MSW incinerators dirty dozen.
These charts show the twelve incinerators with the highest emissions for PM$_{2.5}$ (left) and lead (right).
EJ, environmental justice; MSW, municipal solid waste; PM, particulate matter.
Source: Baptista AI, Perovich A. U.S. municipal solid waste incinerators: an industry in decline. The New School: Tishman Environment and Design Center. May 2019. https://www.no-burn.org/u-s-municipal-solid-waste-incinerators-an-industry-in-decline

Types of Incinerators

There are three main types of incinerators:

- **Nonhazardous waste incinerators:** These burn municipal solid waste, medical waste, and biomass.
- **Hazardous waste incinerators:** These burn hazardous materials, such corrosive and reactive materials, and polychlorinated biphenyls (PCBs).
- **Cement kilns:** These burn usually hazardous and industrial waste and use the energy produced in cement production. Cement kilns that accept waste to use as fuel in cement production are increasingly accepting nonrecyclable plastic waste.

Facilities that burn sewage sludge or other specific types of materials are considered subcategories of the three main incinerator types, depending on the material burned on site.

Anatomy of an Incinerator

Incinerators typically have a waste-storage area, a feed-preparation area, a furnace with ash collection, a gas temperature-reduction system used for energy recovery, an air-pollution control system, chemical scrubbers and filters, and a smokestack (Figure 13.8). A combination of toxic and physical hazards impact workers throughout the facility, and emissions from incinerators have long been a concern for community health. These risks are discussed in the following sections and depend on the type of incinerator and waste burned within it.

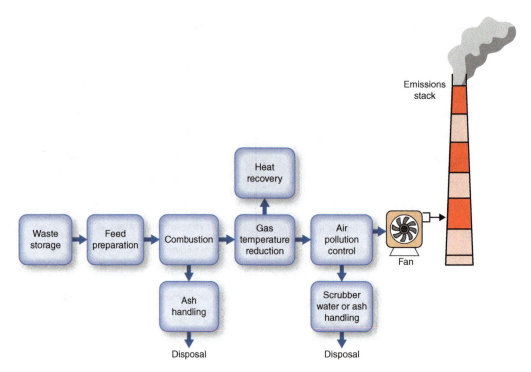

FIGURE 13.8. Site map of incinerator facility.
Source: Adapted from National Research Council, Commission on Life Sciences, Board on Environmental Studies and Toxicology, Committee on Health Effects of Waste Incineration. *Waste Incineration and Public Health*. National Academies Press; 2000. doi:10.17226/5803.

Air Pollution and Climate Change

Air pollution controls are the most critical equipment to prevent fugitive emissions from smokestacks. The high temperatures in incinerators destroy some hazardous materials and induce reactions that create other hazardous chemicals, such as PCBs and dioxins.[11] Incinerator workers face the greatest risk of exposure to chemical and respiratory hazards owing to close proximity and prolonged exposure. Communities downwind of incinerators and ashfills are exposed to fugitive emissions, increased PM, and foul odors. As discussed in Chapter 10, "The Air We Breathe," people can experience a wide range of health effects from exposure to air pollution.

Air pollution controls such as dry electrostatic precipitators, wet scrubbers, and fabric filters (also known as baghouses) are used to remove various pollutants from incinerators, but they may not capture everything. Pollutants can include PM, acidic gases like sulfur oxides and nitrogen oxide, dioxins, mercury, VOCs, and more. Incineration also produces fly ash, which is collected in the baghouse and scrubber water. Scrubber water is usually a mixture of salts, caustic (also known as sodium hydroxide, which effectively removes acidic gases), lime, and the contaminants that have been scrubbed from the smokestack. Local regulations determine if scrubber water must be treated at an on-site wastewater-treatment system or if it can be directly discharged to a municipal sewer. Fly ash and baghouse filters must be disposed of in landfills. Dozens of communities have been exposed to toxic pollution owing to the failure of MSW incinerators to keep up with maintenance, invest in technological upgrades, and receive regular inspections. This failure is largely due to deficiencies in state and federal agencies that should be enforcing the Clean Air Act (CAA).[11]

Metals, such as lead and cadmium, are not destroyed in incinerators and are instead concentrated in the waste ash that is later deposited into landfills. For every ton of waste incinerated, approximately 300 to 500 pounds of ash is produced that must go to a landfill.[12] The amount of pollutants that are released either through the smokestack or in the bottom ash are highly dependent on the composition of the waste and the operation of the air-pollution control equipment. *Bottom ash*, captured under the furnace, is composed of silica, calcium, iron oxide, and aluminum oxide and may contain a concentrate of metals, such as mercury, chromium, arsenic, beryllium, PCBs, and polycyclic aromatic hydrocarbons. Fly ash contains remnants of materials that were not fully combusted, which are called products of incomplete combustion (PICs). PICs may include polycyclic aromatic hydrocarbons, methane, acetylene, benzene, dioxins, and furans.[13]

CASE STUDY 13.1: Shutting Down Detroit's Incinerator

In 1989, Detroit unveiled the world's largest trash-to-energy incinerator, a $438 million project intended to revolutionize waste management. However, it became a financial and environmental nightmare for Detroiters over three decades. The incinerator, emitting air pollution and unbearable odors, triggered health issues for nearby residents and financial losses for the city. In particular, Detroit has long had some of the highest asthma rates in the nation.

Despite protests during the planning stages in the 1970s, city officials proceeded with construction. The incinerator's emission violations, present since its inception, prompted sporadic closures and more protests. Overall, the facility was a financial drain, and the city sold it in 1991 to Detroit Renewable Power. Detroiters, however, paid a hefty $1.2 billion in incinerator debt, contributing to the city's 2013 bankruptcy.

Environmental justice (EJ) groups in the mid-2000s intensified their fight to shut down the incinerator, exposing the facility's impact on marginalized communities. By 2017, the Breathe Free Detroit campaign coalesced, leveraging public hearings and community forums to mobilize residents, and employing a clever tactic of nuisance complaints asking, "What's that smell?" In 2019, the Ecology Center and Environment Michigan dealt a final blow by filing a notice of intent to sue the incinerator's owner, Detroit Renewable Power, forcing its closure. At the time of its closure, the company was burning 5,000 tons of waste daily and hundreds of complaints were reported to the state environmental agency.

Today, like other large cities, Detroit continues to grapple with waste management. In 2015, Detroit became the last major U.S. city to implement waste recycling, largely in response to decades of community mobilization. Many grassroots and city initiatives are taking shape too, including community- and business-composting programs.

REFLECTION QUESTION
1. What were the key factors that led to the shutdown of the Detroit incinerator?

RESEARCHING WASTE AND ITS ENVIRONMENTAL HEALTH AND JUSTICE IMPACTS

Few studies on health impacts from municipal waste incinerators and landfills have been conducted. Most studies have been observational and lack the required investments in long-term community participation and health monitoring. Many of the pollutants of greatest concern emitted by incinerators, such as dioxins and mercury, disperse very widely and bioaccumulate through the food chain; these impacts are not captured in studies of nearby populations.

Also the health impacts attributed to specific waste systems are often confounded by several factors, which makes studying them a challenge. For instance, waste incinerators are often colocated with other industry and heavy vehicle traffic, making it difficult to isolate the incinerator as the source of concern. The collection of on-site monitoring data, particularly in the United States, which has relatively low monitoring requirements, is limited. Tests are often only conducted for specific pollutants, the concentration of pollutants released varies depending on waste composition, and not all air and water monitoring data are collected continuously.

It is clear that many materials entering incinerators and landfills release toxic chemicals and there is scientific consensus about the health impacts of hazardous pollutants on human health. In 2000, the National Research Council (NRC) prepared a report to assess the human health impacts of MSW, medical, and hazardous waste incineration. Although the scope of the study was limited only to hazards of waste burning at a facility, the NRC documented harmful pollutants that could be released to the environment. The NRC did not study the human health impacts from specific incinerator sites but concluded that incinerators contribute to the overall presence of pollutants present in a community.[8] In the case of landfills, the Center for Health, Environment, and Justice similarly found that while the health impacts of siting hazardous-waste landfills have been studied, few studies definitively link MSW landfills with health effects.[8]

The EJ impacts of waste are still understudied as well. After the groundbreaking 1987 report *Toxic Wastes and Race in the United States,* a follow-up report in 2007 showed that little had changed and found that hazardous waste sites in over half of U.S. states were located in communities where over 50% of the population were people of color.[14] More research on where different types of waste are coming from and going to may be helpful to inform interventions to improve EJ.

As waste management evolves, more studies of varying approaches, technologies, and systems are needed as well. A current policy controversy is whether incinerators and landfill-gas capture systems are considered "renewable energy" and required in the fight against climate change, despite their high greenhouse gas and toxic emissions.[15] In the United States, nearly all MSW incinerators have reached their end-of-life stage and are in need of costly repairs in order to properly recover energy and to properly control pollutants; they now cause more good than harm. In the European Union, MSW incinerators have been included for the first time in the Emissions Trading System, indicating that they are major sources of greenhouse gas emissions. In low-income countries cement kilns are being proposed to handle increasing quantities of plastic waste. The environmental health and justice impacts of these approaches and alternatives require further research in our changing climate.

REGULATING THE WASTE SYSTEM

Many U.S. agencies are involved in waste regulation, including, for instance:

- the Department of Transportation, which regulates transportation of waste;
- the Department of Labor, which oversees laws pertaining to worker protection;
- the Centers for Disease Control and Prevention and the Food and Drug Administration, which regulate medical waste; and
- the Department of Energy, which regulates waste from extraction, mining, and oil and gas production.

However, the U.S. Environmental Protection Agency (EPA) is the primary agency responsible for the regulation of landfills and incinerators through its authority under the Resource Conservation and Recovery Act (RCRA) and the CAA. The EPA has oversight authority and must be consulted with regulation of hazardous waste, as described in Chapter 4, "Environmental Health Policies and Protections: Successes and Failures." Although landfills are primarily regulated under the RCRA, the EPA regulates waste incinerators and cement kilns under the CAA (Figure 13.9).

Regulation and enforcement may be further complicated by the funding mechanisms for waste systems. Many municipalities are reliant on revenue bonds that fund transfer stations, landfills, and incinerators, which means they pay for the project with the revenue generated at these sites in the future. Transfer stations, landfills, and incinerators charge municipalities and businesses tipping fees (a fee per ton of waste delivered) for taking waste away. To maximize profit, many municipalities used to only allow waste to be transferred to specific sites within their own boundaries. However, waste began to flow across states' boundaries after the Supreme Court overturned these local flow-control laws in 1994.[16] The result has been that consolidated waste management companies haul waste longer distances to larger landfills, often located near communities of color and low-wealth communities in states with fewer regulations or lower tipping fees.

Landfills and incinerators have a long history of failures, contributing to legacy pollution from toxic dumping prior to the RCRA. Through its authority under the RCRA, the EPA has

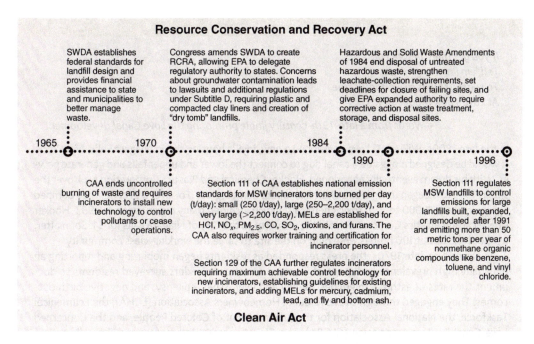

FIGURE 13.9. Waste policy in the United States.
CAA, Clean Air Act; CO, carbon monoxide; EPA, Environmental Protection Agency; HCl, hydrogen chloride; MEL, maximum emission levels; MSW, municipal solid waste; NO$_x$, nitric oxide and nitrogen dioxide; PM$_{2.5}$, particulate matter 2.5; RCRA, Resource Conservation and Recovery Act; SO$_2$, sulfur dioxide; SWDA, Solid Waste Disposal Act.
Source: Denise Patel.

delegated oversight, permitting, and enforcement of waste management regulations to state authorities in 44 states and territories. Delegated authority allows states to regulate specific types of waste sites under more stringent standards. Only a handful of states have set stronger regulations at some waste sites, often following significant efforts by community activists, and many states have failed to adequately protect communities. For example, Long Island, New York, requires landfills to have a double-composite liner system with a primary and secondary leachate-collection system.[17] Since 1984, when Congress expanded the EPA's authority to step in when states failed to protect human health, ground and surface water, and local waterways, the agency has taken corrective actions at over 3,000 sites, including many landfills.

IN OTHER WORDS: WHAT IS A CORRECTIVE ACTION?

According to the Environmental Protection Agency (EPA): *Corrective action is a requirement under RCRA [Resource Conservation and Recovery Act] that facilities that treat, store, or dispose of hazardous wastes investigate and clean up hazardous releases into soil, ground water, surface water, and air. In 1984, Congress passed the Hazardous and Solid Waste Amendments, which granted EPA expanded authority to require corrective action at permitted and non-permitted treatment, storage, and disposal facilities (TSDFs).*

Rather than creating a rigid regulatory framework for corrective action, EPA developed guidance and policy documents to assist facilities conducting cleanups. Some of the resources are broad in scope, while others are more process or media specific.

Corrective action is principally implemented through RCRA permits and orders. RCRA permits issued to TSDFs must include provisions for corrective action as well as financial assurance to cover the costs of implementing those cleanup measures. In addition to EPA, 44 states and territories are authorized to run the Corrective Action program. Corrective action is largely enforced through statutory authorities established by RCRA.[17(para3-5)]

CASE STUDY 13.2: The Love Canal Disaster

If you get there before I do
Tell 'em I'm a comin' too
To see the things so wondrous true
At Love's new Model City.

—Words from a late-19th-century jingle promoting the Love Canal development

In the late 1800s, William T. Love envisioned a new, idyllic housing site in Niagara Falls, New York. It would be designed alongside a canal dug to connect the lower and upper falls and generate power. With his dream eventually abandoned, Hooker Chemical and Plastics Corporation took over the site in 1942 and began using it as a chemical-waste dumping site. For over a decade, they dumped approximately 21,000 tons of toxic chemicals, which included many carcinogens. In 1953, Hooker Chemical and Plastics Corporation sold the property to the City of Niagara Falls for $1. Soon after, a school and about 100 homes were built on the site to serve the working-class community.

In the mid-to-late 1970s, the press responded as residents began mobilizing and reporting an unusually high prevalence and range of illnesses. Grassroots leaders surveyed residents to document the rates of asthma, migraines, kidney and liver issues, epilepsy, and negative birth outcomes. They engaged through the Love Canal Homeowners Association (LCHA), the Ecumenical Taskforce, the National Association for the Advancement of Colored People, and the Concerned Love Canal Renters Association (CLCRA). The CLCRA represented renters and those living in a public housing development, Griffon Manor, many of whom were Black and of low-wealth and were largely ignored by the federal government. Among the most well known of these leaders were Elene Thornton, Vera Starks, Agnes Jones, and Cora Hoffman, who worked with CLCRA; and Lois Gibbs, who worked with LCHA and was a mother whose son's health was severely affected by the chemicals leaching from the ground (Figure 13.10).

Residents were dismissed repeatedly, but eventually their mobilization got the attention of state and federal leaders. This led to air, soil, and water testing, as well as blood testing of residents to assess exposures. Eventually, funds were allocated to New York State to relocate

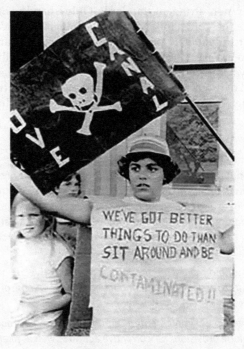

FIGURE 13.10. Protest about the Love Canal contamination by a resident, 1978.
Source: Photograph courtesy of the U.S. Environmental Protection Agency.

(continued)

> **CASE STUDY 13.2: The Love Canal Disaster (*continued*)**
>
> all the residents of Love Canal, including those at Griffon Manor. For decades, residents and environmental leaders worked to advance policies and protections for Love Canal residents and to ensure that the poor government response and outcomes would not be repeated.
>
> In response to Love Canal and similar events, in 1980, Congress established the Comprehensive Environmental Response, Compensation, and Liability Act (CERCLA), more commonly known as the Superfund. The Superfund gives the U.S. Environmental Protection Agency (EPA) the authority to clean up contaminated sites and hold those responsible for contamination financially and legally accountable. The Love Canal Site was removed from the U.S. EPA's Superfund list in 2014—110 years after William T. Love launched the canal project.
>
> **ADDITIONAL READING**
> - Levine AG. *Love Canal: Science, Politics and People.* D.C. Heath and Company; 1982.
> - Newman RS. *Love Canal: A Toxic History From Colonial Times to the Present.* Oxford University Press; 2016.
>
> **REFLECTION QUESTION**
> *1. CERCLA gives the EPA authority to clean up contaminated sites and hold those responsible for the contamination accountable. Which laws are now in place that would prevent a community from being built on contaminated sites?*

HAZARDOUS WASTE INCINERATORS AND CEMENT KILNS

Hazardous waste incinerators (HWIs) are subject to more stringent regulations than MSW incinerators because they burn materials that are flammable, corrosive, reactive, and toxic. For example:

- Incineration of PCBs requires federal permits under the Toxic Substances Control Act.
- Pursuant to CAA Section 112(d), HWIs must limit the emissions of hazardous air pollutants.
- HWIs must continuously monitor emissions, air-pollution control equipment, and pollutant levels across the facility to maintain safe operation.
- Discharges into local waterways require permits under the Clean Water Act (CWA).

Cement kilns, like HWIs, burn at much higher temperatures than MSW incinerators and are fueled by fossil fuels or waste. Cement kilns are exempt from RCRA regulations because it was believed that the temperatures of the kilns were high enough to make the most hazardous materials inert. However, this belief later proved to be untrue. Cement kiln dust (CKD) may contain dioxins and furans, cadmium, lead, and arsenic. Studies have shown that cement kilns that burn hazardous waste, tires, batteries, and increasingly, plastic, produce more dust than cement kilns that burn coal. Some CKD is reincorporated into cement; however, CKD is often too alkaline to be used in cement production and is instead landfilled or mixed with solvents during the equipment-cleaning process, introducing air, water, and water pollutants. Additional regulations have been considered over the past 40 years, but never enacted. The exemption for cement kilns has made them a cheaper option for hazardous waste disposal than other incinerators and landfills.

SPECIAL WASTE CATEGORIES

All waste that is not recycled or reused is eventually are dumped into landfills or incinerated. Some types of waste pose unique hazards. These hazards, and some of the respective regulations that apply to them, are discussed in the following sections.

Medical Waste

Healthcare facilities, medical laboratories, and research centers produce waste material made from paper, plastic, glass, and metals that can be contaminated with bacteria, viruses, human or animal tissue, pharmaceuticals, and toxic chemicals. Medical treatments, such as chemotherapy, may involve the use of toxic chemicals or radiological treatment. Generally, materials contaminated with blood, bodily fluids, or other infectious agents, as well as toxic chemicals or materials used in radiology, are categorized as hazardous. Hazardous medical waste is sent to medical waste incinerators, which have stricter air emissions limits and include more pollutant controls than MSW incinerators do. According to the World Health Organization, only 15% of medical waste is considered hazardous and in need of specialized treatment or disposal methods, and as much as 80% of nonhazardous waste is uncontaminated and could be recycled or treated as nonhazardous waste.[19,20] When medical waste is source separated, some of it can be decontaminated through autoclaving or steam sterilization, resulting in lower volumes of hazardous waste.

Although medical waste is considered its own unique category under EPA policy, it is largely unregulated at the federal level. The Medical Waste Tracking Act of 1988 set federally mandated enforceable standards similar to the RCRA with authority delegated to states. However, it was adopted by few states, and the federal mandate expired after 2 years. Today, only a few states have continued to regulate medical waste.[21]

THE COVID-19 PANDEMIC AND MEDICAL WASTE

Medical waste production accelerated during the COVID-19 pandemic owing to increased testing, vaccination, and treatment from the emergency response actions, as did single-use waste products as people used more masks, gloves, hand sanitizers, and other products to protect themselves before it was understood how the virus spread. The lack of understanding about the virus led many healthcare facilities to consider all medical-care waste infectious, even if it was safe to recycle or process it with other nonhazardous waste. By the end of 2021, medical waste increased by an additional 144,000 tons of waste from glass vials, syringes, needles, and safety boxes used for vaccination. Further, millions of people died during the pandemic, and bodies needed to be disposed of quickly and with dignity in disaster morgues and mass graves in the United States and across the planet.

Chronic prior exposure to particulate matter (PM) acts as a threat multiplier during respiratory pandemics caused by viruses such as SARS-CoV-2. It is well documented that more lives were lost during the pandemic in poor, Black, and Brown communities than in more affluent, White communities.

Construction and Demolition Debris

In 2018, 600 million tons of C&D debris was collected from renovations, demolition, and new construction of buildings, roads, and bridges in the United States. C&D debris has a high rate of recycling and reuse, with only 25% going to landfills. However, 90% of C&D debris consists of older building materials that are health hazards containing VOCs, asbestos, heavy metals, persistent organic compounds, and compounds from paints, varnishes, and solvents.[4] Wood treated for water, fire, and mold resistance contains PCBs. Asbestos, a group of minerals, were widely used for insulation, floor tiles, and other materials due to their ability to resist heat and their durability. It was later discovered that exposure to asbestos fibers is a leading cause of mesothelioma and other respiratory illnesses. Pipes disposed of in landfills risk leaching lead into groundwater.[22]

Despite this combination of materials, the EPA considers most C&D waste to be nonhazardous and, therefore, does not regulate it under the RCRA. Some state regulations require liners and leachate-collection systems, while some do not require any lining under the landfill.[23] The lack of federal regulation and compliance for C&D waste reduces tipping fees and costs and reduces incentives for waste reduction.

Food and Agricultural Waste

Organic waste composes nearly 40% of landfill waste in the United States.[4] Due to its higher water content, organic material also takes longer to incinerate as it must first be dried. Organic material in waste attracts rodents, causes strong odors, and produces leachate and methane gas as it decomposes. Runoff from organic waste and agricultural systems can cause algal blooms and eutrophication of local waterways due to its high nutrient content. Unlike other types of waste, food and agricultural products have a high rate of recyclability as compost, which is discussed further in the "Cities Drive Zero Waste Systems" section on the benefits of source separation later in this chapter.

As of 2023, there are no federal regulations aimed specifically at reducing food waste, although there are a number of proposed bills like the Zero Waste Act and the Compost Food Bill. Some protections exist at the federal level that provide liability protection and tax incentives for those donating food. At the state level, there are regulations in some states against commercial food waste, and in Vermont regulations also extend to individuals.

Sewage and Sewage Sludge

Once it leaves a waste treatment facility, sewage sludge, a mud-like residue containing biosolids, is incinerated (14%), put into a landfill (42%), or used on land applications such as for agriculture and land reclamation (43%). Health impacts from biosolid disposal include foul odors, particularly from ammonia and sulfur, the spread of pathogens from improperly treated waste, and chemical pollutants. These impacts may be experienced by those working with or living nearby facilities or on farms that use biosolids. Over 700 pollutants have been found in biosolids since 1993, when the EPA first began to track them. Chemical pollutants include pharmaceuticals, pesticides, flame retardants, PCBs, dioxins, and PFAS. The health impacts from the presence of these pollutants are dependent on the final application of the biosolids.[24,25] Biosolids are regulated by the EPA as part of the CWA.

Radioactive Waste

Nuclear power plants and military weapons research and development are the greatest source of radioactive waste globally, followed by mining and fossil fuel extraction, and less so from manufacturing, construction, and medicine.[26] The risks of health effects from radioactive waste exposures are highly dependent on:

- the exposure pathway (i.e., ingestion, inhalation, or dermal),
- the type of radiation,
- the length of exposure,
- the rate of metabolism, and
- the duration and location in the body the radionuclides concentrate.[27]

Acute exposures to high doses of radiation can cause radiation sickness. The highest risk of exposure is to workers from accidental handling or rupture of contained waste. Short-term symptoms include nausea and vomiting, skin burns, hair loss, impaired organ function, and fatality, depending on the dose. Low-level exposures over time increase the risk of cancer. Groundwater contamination from leaking storage sites are of great concern. Seismic activity at storage sites increases these risks.[27] Spent fuel from nuclear power plants remains radioactive for tens of thousands of years during which nuclear waste must be secured and isolated. Political pressure on U.S. Congress against local-site proposals has complicated the writing of regulatory policy, resulting in the long-term but temporary storage of over 85,000 metric tons of spent nuclear fuel from power plants at 75 sites in 33 states. An additional 2,000 metric tons are added annually (see Case Study 13.3).[28]

CASE STUDY 13.3: The Fight for Indigenous Rights at Yucca Mountain

"We're going to be voicing our opinion with letters and maybe meeting with both DOE and NRC, talking to them and giving them information that we can have our concerns, and what we, we basically say, we don't want it; we don't like it. We are sending all these papers to all people these are the reasons that the Tribe has issues, which are that we feel is not safe."—Tribal Council Member Kenny Anderson (Zabarte, 2002)

In 1987 Congress determined that Yucca Mountain in Nevada was the only acceptable site for nuclear waste disposal, under the Nuclear Waste Policy Act of 1982 (NWPA). The NWPA also requires the notification and participation of Native American Tribes affected by the siting. The Yucca Mountain site, located 100 miles northwest of Las Vegas, is considered sacred land by two dozen Tribes, including the Southern Paiute and Western Shoshone. Native populations have suffered health impacts from past nuclear-testing contamination and have a valid cause for concern and mistrust about the siting of a nuclear waste repository. The Duckwater Shoshone Tribe and Timbisha Shoshone Tribes sought a designation under the law as an "affected Indian Tribe" to exercise their rights under the law. However, their petitions went unanswered by the Department of the Interior, and they lacked the resources to take the matter further. Tribal concerns included a violation of territorial sovereignty, environmental racism targeting Tribal lands, increased costs due to unfunded monitoring and requirements from the Department of Energy (DOE), increased transportation activity and accidents, and the contamination of land and natural resources used for medicines and subsistence.

Nationally organized groups such as the Indigenous Peoples Network, Honor the Earth, and the National Environmental Coalition of Native Americans seeded resistance to the project with educational forums and political action. The DOE estimated that it was likely that as many as 60 accidents would occur from the transportation of nuclear waste alone. Without rail lines to connect nuclear plants to Yucca Mountain, the proposed truck routes were dubbed the "mobile Chernobyl" plan. Antinuclear activists from across the country joined the effort, holding protests and filing lawsuits against the Environmental Protection Agency (EPA), the National Research Council (NRC) and DOE to stop the proposal. The project has faced so many challenges, including a lawsuit from the state of Nevada, vetoes from state governors, and objections from Nevada's congressional delegation that, in 2010, the DOE finally withdrew its license application to the U.S. Nuclear Regulatory Commission for the Yucca Mountain project. Congress soon stopped funding projects related to the site.

In 2012, the Obama Administration formed the Blue Ribbon Commission and recommended creating a consent-based approach for nuclear-waste siting facilities. The approach was implemented in 2016; however, the project has never received consent from local Tribes. The Trump Administration announced plans to reopen the Yucca Mountain site without consent, going so far as to secretly deliver weapons-grade plutonium to the site. Meanwhile, nuclear power-plant owners have been paid $9 billion over the past half century to keep waste on site at plants and use a variety of technologies to store the spent fuel that will create new challenges when a final disposal site is eventually determined. The Yucca Mountain project is far from dead, and the affected Tribes continue to fight the effort.

REFLECTION QUESTION

1. What do you think should happen to the existing nuclear waste? How would you address health concerns and ensure that community health and the environment are protected near a disposal site?

SOURCES

Zabarte I. *Tribal Concerns about the Yuccan Mountain Repository: An Ethnographic Investigation of the Moapa Band of Paiutes and the Las Vegas Paiute Colony*. Urban Environmental Research, LLC; 2002.

U.S. Government Accountability Office. Commercial spent nuclear fuel: congressional action needed to break impasse and develop a permanent disposal solution. https://www.gao.gov/products/gao-21-603

Slattery R. At Yucca Mountain, united against nuclear waste dump. *Indian Country Today*. September 12, 2018. https://ictnews.org/archive/at-yucca-mountain-united-against-nuclear-waste-dump

Library Guides: Yucca Mountain research collection: 2017–2019: new life for Yucca Mountain? University of Nevada, Reno. 2019. https://guides.library.unr.edu/yuccamountain/timeline2017-present

WORKING TOWARD ENVIRONMENTAL HEALTH AND JUSTICE

Community-led opposition to waste sites during and after the Civil Rights movement gave rise to the EJ movement of today.[29] In 1968, the Memphis Sanitation Strike led by Black workers, supported by Dr. Martin Luther King Jr., emphasized the intersection of labor rights, civil rights, and EJ amid hazardous working conditions. In 1982, a protest for a PCB landfill planned for a poor Black community in Warren County, North Carolina, underscored links between environmental hazards and racial and economic disparities. The publication of the 1987 United Church of Christ's *Toxic Wastes and Race in the United States* was another milestone moment in the early EJ movement.

Communities that are host to waste management facilities have also been a major driver of changes in waste management. The concentration of waste sites in low-wealth communities and communities of color was a deliberate strategy of targeting communities that were perceived to have the least political influence and thus unable to resist undesirable facilities.[30] Resistance to toxic facilities is often derided as NIMBYism ("Not in My Back Yard"), as if these communities were not already exposed to multiple stressors. In fact, local resistance to unsustainable waste facilities is part of a systemic critique that demands larger scale changes in consumption and disposal. The strength of the EJ movement has been crucial in creating the political will to reform the waste management system.

Communities of color and low-wealth communities have long been regarded as **sacrifice zones** that can play host to the environmental costs of unsustainable lifestyles.[31] When these communities gain enough political power to halt environmentally detrimental projects, those projects cannot be built anywhere. This development then creates a need to find better technologies or less-impactful ways of addressing waste and consumption. This dynamic can be clearly seen in California, where the difficulty of siting landfills and incinerators has driven up the costs of waste disposal—both the tipping fee that is paid to the disposal facility and the transport costs, which are substantial. This situation makes innovative programs, such as zero waste (described later), financially attractive in comparison.[32] At the same time, ethical concerns and the concept of EJ have found favor among some legislators, regulators, and the public in general, which has created political space in which cities have stopped using traditional methods of waste management and are experimenting with new approaches, such as zero waste. By defending the most marginalized and vulnerable communities against pollution, EJ activists drive systemic changes, which result in a healthier environment for all communities.

While the sheer magnitude and complexity of modern waste streams may seem daunting, in fact, waste's ubiquitous nature means that everyone can find a constructive role in moving society toward a more sustainable and just system that safeguards environmental health and justice. Indeed, the highly decentralized nature of waste management results in the most consequential decisions being taken at a very small scale and on local levels, which are relatively easier to influence than global systems. This section illustrates a range of positive interventions, beginning at the local level; it is not at all exhaustive.

PRINCIPLES FOR IMPROVING WASTE MANAGEMENT SYSTEMS

Although each waste management system is unique and is tailored to local circumstances, interventions toward environmental health and justice should align with a number of principles that can guide choices and the inevitable trade-offs involved in improving waste management. In addition to the EJ principle and the precautionary principle discussed in previous chapters, additional guiding principles include the following:

- The *proximity principle* explains that waste should be treated in the community in which it is generated rather than being sent to distant locations. It is particularly relevant to the international "trade" in waste, which results in wealthy countries exporting their waste to Africa, Asia, and Latin America for ostensible recycling.[33,34]
- The *polluter pays principle* seeks to assign the financial costs of waste management and its environmental harms to the companies that generate the waste, thus creating a financial incentive to minimize waste. The U.S. Superfund Program is an example of how this principle is applied.[35]

For many decades, the **waste hierarchy** has been the guiding principle behind waste management (Figure 13.11). It prioritizes waste reduction at the source over reuse, which is preferred to recycling. Waste disposal is the last option.[36,37] The **circular economy**, which has now been enshrined into European Union law, seeks to create an economy that practically eliminates waste while also minimizing the demand for raw materials.[38] The most recent principle to be embraced by many cities and companies is **zero waste**, which seeks to incrementally eliminate waste following the waste hierarchy.[39,40] All these principles, along with the EJ principle and the precautionary principle, have been put into effect, to a greater or lesser degree, by various actors around the world; a sampling follows.

> **IN OTHER WORDS: ZERO WASTE HIERARCHY**
>
> Many of us have heard of the 3 Rs—reduce, reuse, recycle. Yet, there is more we can do as a society to create less waste and, when possible, zero waste. The Zero Waste Hierarchy is a good rule of thumb to reduce all environmental harms in the waste system, from greenhouse gas emissions to toxic contamination of the air, water, and soil.

EMPOWERING WORKERS THROUGH ZERO WASTE

Waste pickers are workers who make a living by recovering useful materials, such as paper, glass, metal, and plastic, from trash. An estimated 20 million people worldwide derive their primary income from waste picking, mostly drawn from the poorest populations, including recent rural-to-urban migrants.[41] While waste pickers are primarily associated with poorer countries, they work in every society, including the United States and Europe. In the United States and Europe, many workers in the waste sector are unionized and employed by large waste companies or local governments. As already noted, workers involved with waste management experience higher exposures and are at greatest risk of adverse health impacts.[42] Their health and safety are enshrined in the labor laws in some countries, such as the Occupational Safety and Health Act in the United States, and their wages and benefits may be negotiated through union contracts.

In other parts of the world, most waste pickers are part of the informal economy, where they are not legally recognized as workers, receive no pensions or benefits, and are more likely to experience harassment by police and others. Still, they sell their materials, usually through a series of intermediaries, to established businesses. They form a critical link in the recycling

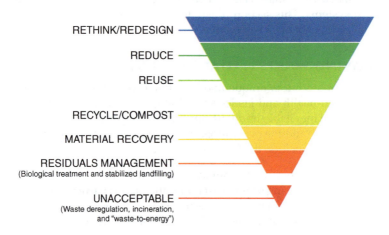

FIGURE 13.11. Zero Waste Hierarchy.

Source: Zero Waste Hierarchy of highest and best use 8.0. Zero Waste International Alliance. Updated May 19, 2022. https://zwia.org/zwh/

chain. In many countries, waste pickers are responsible for the majority of recycling.[43,44] This translates into significant economic benefits—for example, a 30% reduction in the amount of waste that the city of Jakarta has to dispose of, and between $650 million and $1 billion in annual economic activity in the city of Mumbai.[45] With little market power, waste pickers only focus on the most lucrative materials, leaving behind the largest components of the waste stream: organics (such as food waste) and most plastic. In a few locations, such as Pune and Bengaluru, India, the focus is starting to change.

Having organized themselves into cooperatives, unions, and small businesses, the waste pickers now deliver comprehensive waste management services to select neighborhoods.[46] This effort involves teaching individual householders to separate their waste, which avoids cross-contamination and preserves the distinct, recoverable value in each waste stream. Recyclables are sold to industries, while organics are composted or converted into biogas, a renewable fuel. This approach delivers far better environmental outcomes with only a small fraction of waste sent for disposal, but is not financially self-sustaining because waste has inherently low market value.

As with traditional waste hauling and disposal (which is financed through tipping fees), municipalities must provide waste pickers with ongoing financial support in the form of long-term contracts to ensure the viability of these programs. However, the ongoing privatization of waste management in many cities threatens waste pickers' livelihoods and their possibilities of improvement.[47,48] Typically, privatization involves outsourcing waste management to a large, multinational firm, which then asserts ownership of all the waste. These firms rarely conduct source-separated collection, which is more expensive, and thus deliver poorer environmental outcomes. The increasing political organization and influence of waste pickers—as demonstrated by the recent formation of the International Alliance of Waste Pickers, with member organizations in 28 countries[49]—may reverse the trend toward privatization and help to change waste management in ways that improve both environmental and social conditions.

CITIES DRIVE ZERO WASTE SYSTEMS

City governments are critical actors in reforming waste management. Around the world, local governments bear the primary responsibility for managing solid waste, which is usually the largest single budget item at the city level.[11] As such, local governments and large institutions like universities represent the primary agent for potential change in waste management. This is particularly true in the United States, where the ability to issue municipal bonds to raise capital, on the one hand, and the lack of national waste legislation on the other, have created the financial and regulatory freedom to experiment with new models. In many countries, municipal governments are more tightly constrained by financial or regulatory considerations, but still have considerable latitude to devise new systems. Unlike private-sector actors like waste pickers, local governments have both the authority and the mandate to create systemic, holistic solutions to waste. More than 550 municipalities around the world now implement zero waste programs, meaning that they aim to progressively diminish the quantity of waste going to disposal through either incineration or landfill.

The key to zero waste is source separation: once organics, recyclables, household toxics, and nonrecyclable waste are mixed together, they are effectively impossible to separate or to repurpose in any useful way. As source-separated materials, however, the majority of municipal waste has utility. Organics, which includes food, garden, and yard waste, can be composted, converted to biogas, or fed to animals.[50] Sorting out organics not only creates a useful end product, it also avoids sending large quantities of decaying waste to landfills, where they are converted into methane. Methane is an extremely potent greenhouse gas and is responsible for most landfill fires, which pose a major threat to nearby communities. Organic waste in landfills is also responsible for the acidic nature of leachate, the liquid generated in landfills that threatens groundwater supplies. Since organics represent the largest component of municipal waste streams around the world, diverting organics toward compost or other beneficial uses has multiple benefits:

- it dramatically reduces the quantity of waste dumped into landfills, thus extending the working life of the landfill.
- it reduces the cost and environmental impacts of truck traffic through landfill-adjacent neighborhoods.
- it reduces the harms from the landfill itself.

If food waste was a country, it would be the third-largest producer of CO_2 in the world. In low-income countries, 40% of food loss occurs during postharvest and processing. In industrialized countries, more than 40% of loss happens at stores and at home.[51]

Municipalities continue to be challenged by the proliferation of plastic in waste systems at great cost. Concern about plastic is growing so rapidly that in 2022, the United Nations began negotiating a new international treaty to end plastic pollution.[52,53] Meanwhile, many municipalities are taking action on their own by banning the most egregious and unnecessary uses of plastic (e.g., single-use plastic bags, plastic straws, plastic take-out food containers). Conceptually, these bans represent a shift by addressing pollution not through better waste management but through prevention—the highest rung of the waste hierarchy.[54] Plastic is a particularly problematic material whose use is growing at 3.5% to 4% per year.[55] Every stage of the plastic life cycle, from the extraction of its fossil fuel feedstocks, through manufacturing, use, and disposal, creates grave environmental health hazards.[56] Plastic production and disposal (when burned) also generate enormous greenhouse gas emissions.[57] Recycling does not offer a solution. Global recycling rates are stuck around 9% because most plastic cannot be recycled. The chemicals added during manufacturing, including colorants, inks, stiffeners, plasticizers, and flame retardants are effectively impossible to separate from the base polymers.[58] Even plastics that are free of additives and contaminants suffer considerable quality degradation during recycling, making them largely unsuitable for their original use. For example, clear polyethylene terephthalate (PET)—widely used in soda bottles—is typically downcycled into fleece (which sheds microplastics), rather than being put back to its original use.

State and national level governments are generally best situated to implement waste prevention programs. (Although some cities have seen considerable success in pioneering waste prevention programs—Milan, Italy, for example, is lauded for preventing 130 tons of food waste per year.) The modern global economy's long supply chains do not lend themselves to effective local regulation. There are also legal barriers: interstate and international free-trade laws often prevent local regulation of production processes, which could be one way to reduce waste generation at the source. For instance, a U.S. city may have little authority over a global manufacturer's packaging decisions. Waste prevention initiatives vary considerably in nature. Some seek to remove problematic substances or items such as brominated flame retardants, single-use plastics, expanded polystyrene (Styrofoam), and phthalates from the market. Others, such as food-waste prevention programs, aim to address food insecurity while reducing waste and greenhouse gas emissions. In comparison with waste management, waste prevention programs are relatively undeveloped. Although the need for such programs is widely acknowledged—approximately one-third of all food grown is wasted—comprehensive metrics and approaches have yet to be developed.

TAKING ZERO WASTE BEYOND CITY LIMITS

In addition to tackling waste prevention, state and national governments have important roles to play in setting overall waste management policy and in supporting local waste management programs. California has adopted zero waste as a statewide strategy, having required municipalities to implement source separation and collection of organic waste by 2022 and to divert at least 75% of organic waste away from disposal by 2025. The European Union (EU), through its Waste Framework Directive and Landfill Directive, mandates that member countries must reuse or recycle at least 65% of their waste and use landfills for no more than 10% of waste by 2035. Both California and the EU support these targets with grants and other financial incentives to improve source-separated collection and recycling.

Most national governments also have specific protocols for management of hazardous waste, medical waste, nuclear waste, and other particularly problematic waste streams that require special handling. Nevertheless, the constantly changing nature of waste creates a policy lag between the time when significant quantities of waste begin to be generated and the time when effective management systems are implemented. For some waste streams, such as electronics, which manufacturers have made illegal (through trademarking) or impossible to repair, current systems are primarily focused on collection, because no good recycling or disposal options are available. This often results in the export of such waste to low-income countries where they are subject to crude, polluting recycling processes (such as burning circuit boards to extract small quantities of gold and other metals) or used as fuel in cement kilns. This form of waste colonialism can be seen as an internationalization of environmental injustice and has provoked strong reactions from receiving countries. As an alternative, consumer groups are advocating, with some success, for policies such as Right-to-Repair laws to extend the use of electronics, vehicles, and other durable goods.

The drive to change waste management from a process of dumping waste on marginalized communities toward a system that preserves resources, minimizes pollution, and prioritizes equity is a few decades old but rapidly gathering momentum. Waste management is traditionally the preserve of civil engineers, who tend to focus on the last step of the waste hierarchy—waste disposal—with a technical, technology-heavy approach. This process is now being challenged by both activists and a new generation of experts with skills in public health, social work, environmental science, epidemiology, community organizing, climate science, hydrology, and more. All these professions prove useful in designing and implementing better waste management policies and systems in collaboration with the communities they serve.

MAIN TAKEAWAYS

In this chapter, we learned that:

- Health impacts occur along all points of the waste system, and these points are disproportionately sited in low-wealth communities and communities of color and increasingly abroad owing to the practice of waste colonialism.
- Waste composition shifted significantly after World War II as societies in high-income countries shifted toward a more materialistic, consumer-driven culture, consuming more products made with nonrecyclable materials.
- Nonrecyclable materials, such as plastics and electronics, release toxic chemicals that bioaccumulate and persist in the environment as they break down or are incinerated.
- The beginning of the EJ movement was largely focused on waste-related issues, which continue today. Policies and regulations passed in the 1970s, 80s, and 90s are incomplete and outdated, leaving many communities at risk of adverse economic and health impacts of waste.
- In the United States, the EPA is the primary regulator of waste sites with authority under the RCRA and the CAA. The agency has oversight or consultation responsibilities over states and with other agencies responsible for special waste types and waste transport.
- Zero waste systems and the Zero Waste Hierarchy are useful tools to prevent and address waste.
- Cities are successfully addressing waste through policies and systems that provide safer livelihoods for informal workers, while state and national governments focus on banning harmful products to encourage reuse.

SUMMARY

Across the world, communities that have been subjected to the most harmful effects of waste systems are fighting for change. Whether it is a landfill, incinerator, open pit, or waste transfer station, the consequences of waste siting include negative health outcomes for the people who live, work, and play near waste sites, as well as for our global community in our changing climate. Although they have evolved over time, U.S. waste-related policies have largely failed frontline communities, created sacrifice zones, and placed polluting, toxic waste sites in these communities. These communities are not waiting for action. They are leading efforts to manage and implement zero waste systems, reimagining how we look at, use, and manage the end use of products that become waste.

END-OF-CHAPTER RESOURCES

DISCUSSION QUESTIONS

1. This chapter claims that the only real solution to waste and its impacts on humans and the environment is to not make it in the first place. Of course, this is challenging in present-day capitalist societies. What changes would help motivate high-income countries and, in particular, your city or hometown, to embrace a zero waste system?
2. What are the primary waste-related regulations in the United States? How have they been effective? How could they be improved to promote environmental health and justice?
3. How is waste a matter of occupational health and safety? Describe examples of where waste systems have harmed workers. Describe solutions for reducing or eliminating these harms. Refer to Chapter 16, "Ensuring Occupational Health," if necessary.
4. Several different toxicants are mentioned covered in this chapter. Thinking of specific toxins or categories of toxins (e.g., heavy metals, PCBs, VOCs), describe a few different exposure pathways that may affect resident or worker health in the process of waste management.
5. Review Figure 13.5: Waste Management Life Cycle. Compare and contrast how low-, middle-, and high-income countries manage their waste. What types of waste are predominantly produced by their residents? What are the major components of their waste management system? What are the environmental, economic, and social justice issues that arise from their system?

LEARNING ACTIVITIES

THE TIME IS NOW

1. The EPA has required corrective actions at hundreds of waste sites in the United States. Use the EPA website on *Corrective Action Cleanups around the Nation* (www.epa.gov/hwcorrectiveactioncleanups). Pick a waste site and consider the following questions:
    - What are the threats to human health and the environment posed by the waste site?
    - What are the opportunities for community input and action steps needed by the site owner?
    - How is progress toward the corrective actions measured?
    - What happens to material at the site?
    - What other questions do you have?

    Draft bulleted talking points you might use if you were advocating to enforce these corrective actions. Draw on what you learned in this chapter. Try to be evidencebased,

feasible, ethical, and equitable. Be sure to center frontline communities who are most impacted by the waste site, as appropriate.
2. Do a waste audit at your workplace, school, or home. To do this, select a representative sample of waste. With gloves on and a space to audit, sort the waste by its major components (e.g., paper, plastics, glass, metal, compostable organics). Weigh each type. Document the breakdown and use it to track changes over time or to make comparisons. Note if you are reducing waste by recycling and composting when you can.

IN REAL LIFE

Remember there is no "away." Where does your waste go?

- Where are the landfills in your state? Check out the EPA's Project and Landfill Data by State: www.epa.gov/lmop/project-and-landfill-data-state.
- Find out how much MSW is recycled, composted, landfilled, and incinerated in your city, town, or county. Talk with your community's waste management team about the diversion rate. In other words, how much waste is diverted away from landfills and incinerators?
- Visit the facilities that handle your waste. Many landfills and recycling centers have opportunities to tour their facilities.
- Are there any waste prevention programs where you live? For instance, these programs could include food-loss prevention efforts, composting for businesses, or single-use plastic bans. Are there programs you would like to see implemented?

 A robust set of instructor resources designed to supplement this text is located at http://connect.springerpub.com/content/book/978-0-8261-8353-8. Qualifying instructors may request access by emailing textbook@springerpub.com.

REFERENCES

1. Ferronato N, Torretta V. Waste mismanagement in developing countries: a review of global issues. *Int J Environ Res Public Health*. 2019;16(6):1060. doi:10.3390/ijerph16061060
2. Baptista AI, Perovich A. U.S. municipal solid waste incinerators: an industry in decline. The New School: Tishman Environment and Design Center. May 2019. Accessed June 15, 2024. https://www.no-burn.org/u-s-municipal-solid-waste-incinerators-an-industry-in-decline
3. Chavis BF Jr, Lee C. *Toxic Wastes and Race in the United States: A National Report on the Racial and Socio-Economic Characteristics of Communities with Hazardous Waste Sites*. United Church of Christ Commission for Racial Justice; 1987. https://www.ucc.org/wp-content/uploads/2020/12/ToxicWastesRace.pdf
4. U.S. Environmental Protection Agency. Advancing sustainable materials management: 2018 fact sheet. Assessing trends in materials generation and management in the United States. December 2020. https://www.epa.gov/sites/default/files/2021-01/documents/2018_ff_fact_sheet_dec_2020_fnl_508.pdf
5. World Health Organization. *Children and Digital Dumpsites: E-waste Exposure and Child Health*. World Health Organization; 2021.
6. Tait PW, Brew J, Che A, et al. The health impacts of waste incineration: a systematic review. *Aust N Z J of Public Health*. 2020;44(1):40–48. doi:10.1111/1753-6405.12939
7. Siddiqua A, Hahladakis JN, Al-Attiya WAKA. An overview of the environmental pollution and health effects associated with waste landfilling and open dumping. *Environ Sci Pollut Res Int*. 2022;29(39):58514–58536. doi:10.1007/s11356-022-21578-z
8. Center for Health, Environment, and Justice. Landfills: trashing the Earth. April 2016. https://chej.org/publication-landfills-trashing-the-earth

9. U.S. Environmental Protection Agency. RCRA orientation manual. October 2014. https://www.epa.gov/sites/default/files/2015-07/documents/rom.pdf
10. Bogner J, Abdelrafie Ahmed M, Diaz C, et al. Waste management. In: Metz B, Davidson OR, Bosch PR, Dave R, Meyer LA, eds. *Climate Change 2007: Mitigation of Climate Change. Contribution of Working Group III to the Fourth Assessment Report of the Intergovernmental Panel on Climate Change.* Cambridge University Press; 2007.
11. Kaza S, Yao LC, Bhada-Tata P, Van Woerden F. *What a Waste 2.0: A Global Snapshot of Solid Waste Management to 2050.* Urban Development. World Bank; 2018. doi:10.1596/978-1-4648-1329-0
12. Basic information about energy recovery from waste. Municipal Solid Waste, U.S. Environmental Protection Agency. Updated March 30, 2016. https://archive.epa.gov/epawaste/nonhaz/municipal/web/html/basic.html
13. National Research Council, Commission on Life Sciences, Board on Environmental Studies and Toxicology, Committee on Health Effects of Waste Incineration. *Waste Incineration and Public Health.* National Academies Press; 2000. doi:10.17226/5803
14. Mascarenhas M, Grattet R, Mege K. Toxic waste and race in twenty-first century America: neighborhood poverty and racial composition in the siting of hazardous waste facilities. *Environ Soc.* 2021;12(1):108–126. doi:10.3167/ares.2021.120107
15. Tangri N. Waste incinerators undermine clean energy goals. *PLoS Clim.* 2023;2(6):e0000100. doi:10.1371/journal.pclm.0000100
16. McCarthy JE. Flow control of solid waste: issues and options. Congressional Research Service: Report for Congress. May 16, 1995. https://p2infohouse.org/ref/11/10583.htm
17. Solid waste landfills. New York State Department of Environmental Conservation. Accessed June 17, 2024. https://www.dec.ny.gov/chemical/23681.html
18. Learn about corrective action. U.S. Environmental Protection Agency. Updated February 1, 2024. https://www.epa.gov/hw/learn-about-corrective-action
19. World Health Organization. Health-care waste. February 8, 2018. https://www.who.int/news-room/fact-sheets/detail/health-care-waste
20. Kwakye G, Brat GA, Makary MA. Green surgical practices for health care. *Arch Surg.* 2011;146(2):131–136. doi:10.1001/archsurg.2010.343
21. Lichtveld, MY, Rodenbeck, SE, Lybarger, JA. The findings of the Agency for Toxic Substances and Disease Registry Medical Waste Tracking Act report. *Environ Health Perspect.* 1992;98:243–250. doi:10.1289/ehp.9298243
22. Sustainable management of construction and demolition materials. U.S. Environmental Protection Agency. August 22, 2018. Updated January 23, 2024. https://www.epa.gov/smm/sustainable-management-construction-and-demolition-materials
23. U.S. Environmental Protection Agency. RCRA in focus: construction, demolition, and renovation. EPA-530-K-04-005. September 2004. https://www.epa.gov/sites/default/files/2015-01/documents/rif-cd.pdf
24. Basic information about biosolids. U.S. Environmental Protection Agency. July 13, 2016. Updated December 15, 2023. https://www.epa.gov/biosolids/basic-information-about-biosolids#basics
25. Richman T, Arnold E, Williams AJ. Curation of a list of chemicals in biosolids from EPA national sewage sludge surveys & biennial review reports. *Sci Data.* 2022;9(1):180. doi:10.1038/s41597-022-01267-9
26. Deng D, Zhang L, Dong M, Samuel RE, Ofori-Boadu A, Lamssali M. Radioactive waste: a review. *Water Environ Res.* 2020;92(10):1818–1825. doi:10.1002/wer.1442
27. Health effects of radiation. Centers for Disease Control and Prevention. December 7, 2015. Updated August 6, 2021. https://www.cdc.gov/nceh/radiation/health.html
28. Office USGA. Commercial spent nuclear fuel: congressional action needed to break impasse and develop a permanent disposal solution. Published September 23, 2021. https://www.gao.gov/products/gao-21-603
29. Bullard RD. Race and environmental justice in the United States symposium: Earth rights and responsibilities: human rights and environmental protection. *Yale J Int'l L.* 1993;18(1):319–336.
30. Cerrell Associates. *Political Difficulties Facing Waste-to-Energy Conversion Plant Siting.* California Waste Management Board; 1984.
31. Lerner S. *Sacrifice Zones: The Front Lines of Toxic Chemical Exposure in the United States.* MIT Press; 2012.

32. Gokaldas V. Creating a Culture of Zero Waste. In: *On the Road to Zero Waste: Successes and Lessons from around the World*. GAIA;2012:14. https://www.no-burn.org/wp-content/uploads/2023/03/On-the-Road-to-Zero-Waste.pdf
33. Reese M. The proximity principle. In: Faure M ed. *Elgar Encyclopedia of Environmental Law*. Edward Elgar Publishing; 2018:219–233.
34. Global Alliance for Incinerator Alternatives. Discarded: communities on the frontlines of the global plastic crisis. April 2019. https://www.no-burn.org/resources/discarded-communities-on-the-frontlines-of-the-global-plastic-crisis/
35. Munir M. History and evolution of the polluter pays principle: how an economic idea became a legal principle? Published online September 8, 2013. doi:10.2139/ssrn.2322485
36. Gharfalkar M, Court R, Campbell C, Ali Z, Hillier G. Analysis of waste hierarchy in the European waste directive 2008/98/EC. *Waste Manag*. 2015;39:305–313. doi:10.1016/j.wasman.2015.02.007
37. European Commission. Closing the loop: an EU action plan for the circular economy. December 2, 2015. Accessed June 15, 2024. https://eur-lex.europa.eu/resource.html?uri=cellar:8a8e-f5e8-99a0-11e5-b3b7-01aa75ed71a1.0012.02/DOC_1&format=PDF
38. Geissdoerfer M, Savaget P, Bocken NMP, Hultink EJ. The circular economy—a new sustainability paradigm? *J Cleaner Prod*. 2017;143:757–768. doi:10.1016/j.jclepro.2016.12.048
39. Simon JM. A zero waste hierarchy for Europe. Zero Waste Europe. May 20, 2019. https://zerowasteeurope.eu/2019/05/a-zero-waste-hierarchy-for-europe/
40. Zero waste definition. Zero Waste International Alliance. Updated December 20, 2018. http://zwia.org/zero-waste-definition/
41. Cass Talbott T. Extended producer responsibility: opportunities and challenges for waste pickers. In: Alfers L, Chen M, Plagerson S eds. *Social Contracts and Informal Workers in the Global South*. Edward Elgar Publishing; 2022:126–143.
42. Giusti L. A review of waste management practices and their impact on human health. *Waste Manag*. 2009;29(8):2227–2239. doi:10.1016/j.wasman.2009.03.028
43. Dias SM. Waste pickers and cities. *Environ Urban*. 2016;28(2):375–390. doi:10.1177/0956247816657302
44. Linzner R, Lange U. Role and size of informal sector in waste management—a review. *Waste Resour Manag*. 2013;166(2):69–83. doi:10.1680/warm.12.00012
45. Medina M. *The Informal Recycling Sector in Developing Countries: Organizing Waste Pickers to Enhance Their Impact*. World Bank; 2008.
46. Chikarmane P. Integrating waste pickers into municipal solid waste management in Pune, India. Women in Informal Employment: Globalizing and Organizing. 2012. https://www.wiego.org/sites/default/files/publications/files/Chikarmane_WIEGO_PB8.pdf
47. Sandhu K, Burton P, Dedekorkut-Howes A. Between hype and veracity; privatization of municipal solid waste management and its impacts on the informal waste sector. *Waste Manag*. 2017;59:545–556. doi:10.1016/j.wasman.2016.10.012
48. Demaria F, Schindler S. Contesting urban metabolism: struggles over waste-to-rnergy in Delhi, India. *Antipode*. 2016;48(2):293–313. doi:10.1111/anti.12191
49. International Alliance of Waste Pickers. Accessed June 17, 2024. https://globalrec.org/
50. Tangri N, Viella M, Moon D, Naayem N. *Zero Waste to Zero Emissions: How Reducing Waste Is a Climate Gamechanger*. Global Alliance for Incinerator Alternatives; 2022. doi:10.46556/MSTV3095
51. World Food Programme. 5 facts about food waste and hunger. June 2, 2020. https://www.wfp.org/stories/5-facts-about-food-waste-and-hunger
52. United Nations Environment Assembly of the United Nations Environment Programme. End plastic pollution: towards an international legally binding instrument. Published online March 7, 2022. https://wedocs.unep.org/bitstream/handle/20.500.11822/39764/END%20PLASTIC%20POLLUTION%20-%20TOWARDS%20AN%20INTERNATIONAL%20LEGALLY%20BINDING%20INSTRUMENT%20-%20English.pdf?sequence=1&isAllowed=y
53. Global Alliance for Incinerator Alternatives, Environmental Investigation Agency. Global plastics treaty. 2022. Accessed June 17, 2024. https://www.no-burn.org/wp-content/uploads/2022/02/UNEA-publication-packet_plastics-treaty-1.pdf
54. Patel D, Danovitch A, Hubbard S. A tale of five cities: plastic barriers to zero waste. Global Alliance for Incinerator Alternatives. Published online June 17, 2021. doi:10.46556/heoy6222
55. Geyer R, Jambeck JR, Law KL. Production, use, and fate of all plastics ever made. *Sci Adv*. 2017;3(7):e1700782. doi:10.1126/sciadv.1700782

56. Azoulay D, Villa P, Arellano Y, et al. *Plastic & Health: The Hidden Costs of a Plastic Planet*. Center for International Environmental Law; 2019. https://www.ciel.org/plasticandhealth/
57. Cabernard L, Pfister S, Oberschelp C, Hellweg S. Growing environmental footprint of plastics driven by coal combustion. *Nat Sustain*. 2022;5:139–148. doi:10.1038/s41893-021-00807-2
58. Hopewell J, Dvorak R, Kosior E. Plastics recycling: challenges and opportunities. *Philos Trans R Soc Lond B Biol Sci*. 2009;364(1526):2115–2126. doi:10.1098/rstb.2008.0311
59. Yeung P. Milan is winning the fight against food waste. Reasons to Be Cheerful. November 5, 2021. https://reasonstobecheerful.world/milan-italy-zero-food-waste/

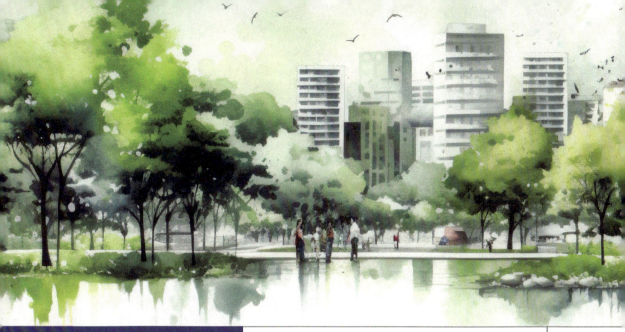

SECTION IV

Reimagining Environmental Health for All

FIREFIGHTERS AND FOREVER CHEMICALS: OCCUPATIONAL EXPOSURE TO PFAS AND HEALTH-RELATED CONSEQUENCES

In this second-to-last episode on per- and polyfluoroalkyl substances (PFAS) in our environment, hosts Natalie Conti and Anchal Malh sit with advocates Ayesha Khan and Jamie Honkawa of the Nantucket PFAS Action Group. During their conversation, they discuss exposure to PFAS in firefighting communities and ways to improve protections for community members. Tune in to learn how certain occupations can lead to increases in exposure to PFAS and related health effects.

HALTING THE PFAS CYCLE AND ITS COSTS ON INDIVIDUALS, COMMUNITIES, AND SOCIETY

In this final episode, hosts Natalie Conti and Anchal Malh wrap up their conversation on PFAS in the environment with Kristin Mello and Christopher Clark of Westfield Residents Advocating for Themselves (WRAFT). They discuss the ways research, policies, and technology can help us to reduce PFAS exposures for all, highlighting the work of current advocacy groups. They also remind us about environmental justice issues related to PFAS. Listeners are left with final takeaways on what the field of environmental health—and all of society—can learn from PFAS. Finally, there is a call-to-action: How can we ensure marginalized communities, particularly communities of color and low-wealth communities, are not experiencing disproportionate impacts from PFAS? Tune in to conclude our case study on PFAS.

Access the podcasts via the QR code or http://connect.springerpub.com/content/book/978-0-8261-8353-8/chapter/ch00

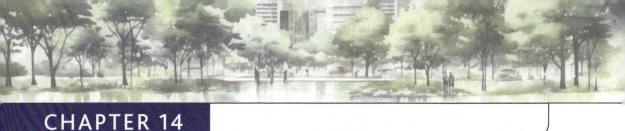

CHAPTER 14

Healthy Communities for All

Kate Robb and Sandra F. Whitehead

LEARNING OBJECTIVES

- Understand how our built environments affect environmental health and justice.
- Discuss historical and current policy and planning decisions that impact land use, housing, transportation, and our food environments.
- Identify the many ways that structural racism and other forms of discrimination contribute to disparities in the built environment and related health outcomes, such as a disproportionate exposure to pollution and limited access to safe, affordable housing.
- Present promising strategies and tools for promoting environmental health and justice through intentional and equitable planning and design, including zoning reforms and co-governance models.
- Identify the ways that environmental health practitioners, researchers, and advocates can work with communities and other sectors toward healthy communities for all.

KEY TERMS

- built environment
- co-governance
- community benefits agreements
- community engagement
- comprehensive plan
- cumulative impacts
- gentrification
- Health Impact Assessments (HIAs)
- Health in All Policies (HiAP)
- infrastructure
- land use
- redlining
- shared or joint-use agreements
- structural racism
- zoning

OVERVIEW

Our health is influenced by multiple factors outside the direct influence of the public health and healthcare sectors. For instance, those working to design and plan the places where we live, work, play, and learn have a responsibility in promoting environmental health and justice. They shape our built environments. The **built environment** comprises the physical structures engineered and designed by people, including buildings, neighborhoods, streets, parks, and transportation systems. Built environments can promote or inhibit health through a variety of pathways, for example, providing or failing to provide access to affordable, healthy food and safe places to exercise, promoting or inhibiting social interaction, and influencing traffic-related fatalities.

Historical and current land use, housing, infrastructure, and transportation policies and investment decisions have long influenced how our environments are developed and, as a result, their impacts on health. For example, some environments contribute to health by promoting an active lifestyle through such approaches as mixed land use and street connectivity, or the pattern of streets, intersections, and their connections to each other. These approaches can entail the strategic and accessible design of road networks and the integration of various types of land uses (e.g., residential, commercial, recreational) in ways that reduce commute time, encourage social interaction, and reduce greenhouse gas emissions. Meanwhile, some other environments, like those with sprawling development, can inhibit health by exposing people to a sedentary lifestyle.[1-3] People living, working, or learning near a source of pollution, such as a highway, power plant, incinerator, or bus depot can experience negative health impacts, like cancers and decreased lung function. A majority of our lives are spent indoors, and how the buildings are built and maintained and where they are placed also impacts our health.

In crafting solutions, we also cannot ignore the ways that structural racism and other types of discrimination underlie these relationships between our built environment and health. Numerous studies have demonstrated the disproportionate placement of emitters primarily in communities of color, which results in disproportionate exposure to pollutants, negatively impacting health.[4-6] Rural areas, lower-wealth communities, and communities of color are less likely to have access to safe places that support active living.[7-9] Inequities in housing access and quality have disproportionately harmed the health of communities of color, those experiencing low wealth, and people with disabilities.[10-14]

Throughout this chapter, we examine how features of the built environment relate to climate change, air pollution, water quality and access, physical injury, and physical and mental health. We outline the promising practices used by government agencies and community leaders to advance planning and design strategies in ways that promote environmental health and justice. These practices may entail reimagining zoning plans, intentionally designing parks and green spaces with equity in mind, and the use of tools such as **community benefits agreements (CBAs)** and **Health Impact Assessments (HIAs)**. Governments can also reduce negative health impacts through investments to our public transit systems and proactive practices, such as housing inspections, that involve communicating the potential health risks of nearby environmental contaminants, for instance. Of course, we discuss the ways that these approaches and tools alone cannot ensure health equity without a commitment to correcting harms from historical injustices and transforming how decisions are made *by* and *with* communities, particularly those on the front line of environmental injustice.

IN OTHER WORDS: DEFINING COMMUNITIES

We all belong to multiple communities and move throughout them. Minkler, Wallerstein, and Hyde provide a summary of the ways that communities are typically defined:

> *Historically, communities have been defined as (1) functional spatial units meeting basic needs for sustenance, (2) units of patterned social interaction, or (3) symbolic units of collective identity (Hunter, 1975). Eng and Parker (1994) added a fourth definition of communities as social units where people come together politically to make change.*[15(p36)]

In this chapter, we use the term *communities* in the first and fourth sense: as specific spatial units within an area where people reside, work, live and play and groups of people who come together to advocate for change.

OUR BUILT ENVIRONMENT: BY DESIGN

The design of our built environments often is the responsibility of our local government, but regional, county, state, and federal decision makers also have a role to play, especially when determining what happens across multiple jurisdictions. For instance, our local government may decide where to place parks, public restrooms, and other amenities within our community. They also may work with county or state planners to make changes to our streetscapes if county or state roads are involved. Additionally, public participation is an integral part of the land-use planning process, ensuring that decisions align with community needs and assets and the priorities of residents. Given the intricate relationship between planning and public health, all of these partners have a role to play in promoting environmental health and justice.

ZONING AND LAND USE

Cities use their local zoning code to determine how the land can be used and what can be placed where, including commercial, residential, industrial, or agricultural types of land use. **Zoning** codes enable local control over land use and are a powerful regulatory tool that cities can use to implement goals or their vision for a city's future.[16] Cities will create a **comprehensive plan** (master plan, master development plan, or general plan) to create a long-term vision of future **land use** typically for the next 20 years.[17] Local planning commissions, city councils, or another governing body will adopt and implement the comprehensive plan. Though the comprehensive planning process in the United States is evolving to integrate equity, community vision, and community values for example, it has historically been top-down and may prioritize factors such as economic ones.[17] Local authorities can invite industries into their communities to expand their tax base and use the zoning code to determine where they can be placed. There is a strong association between industrial-zoned land in or near communities of color, particularly Black and Hispanic or Latino communities.[6,11,18,19] This siting of industrial and fossil fuel infrastructure not only negatively impacts health for those living nearby, but also worsens the value of nearby land and homes.[20] As discussed in other chapters, discriminatory zoning decisions[21] continue to influence which communities have access to green space and other health-promoting resources and which are zoned in ways that expose them to more pollution from traffic, industry, and other sources.

Redlining, discussed in several other chapters, and zoning are related in complex ways. In many cases, the areas that were redlined and denied financial investment were subsequently subjected to zoning policies that further reinforced segregation. For example, zoning laws could designate certain areas for industrial or commercial development, often leading to the concentration of polluting industries in neighborhoods that had been previously redlined. **Redlining** has been associated with sustained disinvestment in ways that harm physical and mental health.[22-25] Disinvestment worsens neighborhood quality, which affects access to health-promoting resources, such as green space and transportation.[26]

Largely based on race and income, many present-day communities still reflect these patterns and are as segregated as they were 50 years ago.[27] Segregation is associated with chronic diseases and adverse health outcomes and pregnancy outcomes.[28] Though redlining was deemed illegal in 1968 with the passing of the Fair Housing Act, historical and present-day policies and practices continue to reinforce residential racial segregation, such as exclusionary zoning and discriminatory lending practices.[29] For example, applicants of color are more likely to experience a higher mortgage denial rate as compared to White borrowers.[30] Also, exclusionary zoning may set minimum lot sizes or restrictions on multifamily housing, which has been used to maintain racial and economic homogeneity in certain neighborhoods.

TRANSPORTATION PLANNING

Transportation planning practices have major impacts on physical activity, exposure to air pollutants, mental health, and more. To a large extent, communities in the United States have been designed to promote motorized transportation. In cities with a high degree of urban sprawl, workplaces, schools, restaurants, and shopping outlets are located far from urban centers or residential subdivisions. The nation's extensive system of highways, bridges, and roads relies heavily on motorized transportation and has had negative consequences for our health, including decreased physical activity, increased air pollution, and increased traffic collisions.

To enable the car culture further in the United States, the Federal-Aid Highway Act of 1956 authorized the construction of the Interstate Highway System. Highways constructed under this act often cut through communities of color, particularly in urban areas. Highways and other heavily trafficked roadways fragmented communities that had been built over generations in many major cities, dismantling social networks and destroying businesses and cultural institutions throughout the 1950s to 1970s. Examples include the construction of Interstate 95 through Philadelphia's Chinatown and South Philadelphia neighborhoods and Miami's Overtown and Liberty City neighborhoods, Interstate 94 through the Rondo neighborhood in St. Paul, Minnesota, and Interstate 5 through Seattle's Central District, among many, many other instances.

Today, approximately 8% of those living in the United States rely on public transit, and generally, women, Black workers, low-wealth workers, and young adults use public transit more for commuting than other groups.[31,32] Forty-five percent of the United States population does not have access to public transportation, which can disproportionately impact people with disabilities and older adults.[31,33] Lack of or inadequate access to public transit can lead to social isolation, increasing the risk for depression or early death.[31] Research has shown that public transportation reduces vehicle miles traveled, which in turn reduces air pollution and motor vehicle crashes.[31]

There are many benefits from having public transportation options increase alongside dense and compact development, but these benefits are not experienced by all communities. **Gentrification** occurs when new investments in businesses, housing, and infrastructure lead to an influx of wealthier residents and the displacement of low-wealth or working-class residents results,[27,34] often more so affecting communities of color.[27] Gentrification can lead to housing instability or force residents out of accessible areas, resulting in longer commutes with fewer transportation options and job opportunities.[35] Residents who are displaced may have increased stress and depression and decreased economic mobility and power to advocate for change.[34]

INDOOR ENVIRONMENTS

A majority of our time is spent indoors in schools, homes, workplaces, or healthcare facilities, and these indoor environments impact health in many ways:

- Temperature extremes can result in illness and death.
- Indoor air pollutants are connected to asthma, cancer, and development delays and affect the cardiovascular system.
- Housing hazards can result in unintentional injury.
- People may be exposed to higher air-pollutant levels indoors, as much as two to five times higher than outdoor levels.[36]
- Allergens commonly present in schools, such as mold and pests, can trigger asthma symptoms and impact student attendance and performance.[36]
- Exposure to lead, through lead service lines and older buildings and from housing with peeling lead-based paint, disproportionately impacts neighborhoods of low wealth and communities of color.[37]

Beyond the indoor environment, people may be exposed to environmental contaminants, like lead or uranium, through the soils in their yards.

Furthermore, research documents the ways that federally assisted low-wealth housing has been sited on or near contaminated sites like Superfund sites (see Chapter 4, "Environmental Health Policies and Protections: Successes and Failures"). In the United States, residents living in federally assisted housing are primarily people of color, children, older adults, and people with disabilities.[38] Thus, housing programs intended to support those who are marginalized or particularly vulnerable may actually perpetuate environmental health inequities.[38]

Housing affordability can negatively impact mental health and increase the risk of disease.[39] Currently, there is a shortage of affordable homes to purchase or rent across the United States with high home prices and rent. Housing underproduction is linked to restrictive zoning codes, which limits where affordable housing may be developed and prevents development in areas with accessible transportation and employment options.[20,40] Approximately 44 million people rent their homes, and for renters with extremely low incomes, there is a shortage of over seven million affordable and available homes to rent.[13,41] When housing costs are too high, households postpone medical care or the purchase of food.[42] Also, many homes are not designed to accommodate people's functional abilities, which is especially important for older individuals and those with disabilities.[43]

PARKS AND GREEN SPACE

Parks, playgrounds, greenways, trails, and open outdoor spaces can promote health. Parks can encourage physical activity. Studies have shown that when people have access to parks, they exercise more.[44] Exposure to nature in parks or gardens can improve psychological and social health. Parks create opportunities for people of all ages to enjoy themselves and interact with others. In particular, parks provide children with opportunities to play, helping them to develop muscle strength and coordination, language acquisition, and cognitive abilities.[44] Parks can help individuals cope with stress and struggles and have been cited as an important strategy to improve health equity. When designed intentionally and maintained, parks and open spaces also reduce noise, air pollution, and help manage flooding and extreme heat exposure.[45,46]

Despite the importance of parks and other recreational open spaces, many people do not have adequate access to these important resources, showing a lack of distributive justice or inequitable availability of parks and green space. According to a Trust for Public Land analysis, of the 100 most populous cities in the United States, neighborhoods primarily composed of people of color had over 40% less access to park acreage when compared to neighborhoods composed of primarily White populations.[46] It is vital to recognize the historical context in which public parks were created. Public parks were originally created for White families of higher income and led to the displacement of communities of color, with Central Park and Seneca Village, a large community of Black and immigrant property owners, as a prime example.[47] National parks were conceptualized by leaders who believed in creating "untouched" natural spaces for White populations, often in places where Indigenous Peoples had been living on the land for centuries.[48,49] The creation of national parks led to the forced displacement of Indigenous communities in ways that also cut off access to land used for living and cultural practices.[50] Also, Jim Crow laws, which maintained segregation after Reconstruction in the United States, resulted in state parks that were inaccessible to Black people or resulted in parks of lower quality for Black populations.[47] To this day, there are racial disparities in park visitation, and this disparity may be due to a long history of racial exclusion and oppression.[51]

Additional inequities aside from access include park maintenance, size, staffing, and the quality of recreational facilities and amenities.[45] The types of amenities and programming can also influence the use of parks. The enjoyment of parks or open spaces can be influenced by discrimination and by feelings of safety for potential park users. Research has shown that communities of color experience racial profiling, harassment, and criminalization from visitors who are White and park officials.[47] One recent example that gained national attention was of Christian Cooper, a Black man who was birding recreationally in Central Park, and who was threatened by a White woman for requesting that she leash her dog.[52] There are also gender disparities in park use and experience, with many women feeling that they must navigate these public spaces differently because of safety concerns.[53,54] It would help to include diverse voices in the decision-making process involved in codesigning recreational spaces.[55]

> **CASE STUDY 14.1: Elm Playlot, Richmond, California**
>
> Richmond, California, is located in the San Francisco Bay area and is a diverse community that has been home to heavy manufacturing, warehousing, shipyards, and other industrial pollution. Richmond's Iron Triangle neighborhood has experienced many environmental injustices, residential segregation and disinvestment, and residents have poor access to resources such

(continued)

> **CASE STUDY 14.1: Elm Playlot, Richmond, California** (*continued*)
>
> as grocery stores, quality schools, and green spaces.[56,57] The neighborhood, primarily home to Hispanic or Latino and Black populations, is burdened by gun violence, toxic air pollution and poor health outcomes.[57] In 2008, residents formed the Elm Playlot Action Committee (EPAC) to redevelop Elm Playlot, a neighborhood park, into an accessible, safe, and joyful space for the community.
>
> After an unsuccessful city-led attempt at revitalizing the park with playground equipment, EPAC took the lead in planning redevelopment of the park by:
>
> - engaging residents through photovoice, a participatory research or assessment process that invites communities to document and narrate their experiences, perspectives, and priorities using photography;
> - building temporary structures, observing them, and adapting them to residents' interests and needs;
> - facilitating codesign workshops where residents shared ideas for the space; and
> - making plans for daily park maintenance and cleaning.
>
> Through a newly formed community group, Pogo Park, community leaders created a joint-use agreement with the city. *Joint-use agreements* are formal arrangements to share the use of facilities, properties, or resources for mutually beneficial purposes. In partnership with local nonprofits and artists, Pogo Park raised funds to construct, build, and maintain the park by employing residents of the neighborhood. Pogo Park also raised funds to purchase a nearby abandoned house, turning it into a space that housed offices, meeting rooms, a kitchen, and wheelchair-accessible bathrooms for the community. After this, they worked with the city to obtain federal funds to rehabilitate homes nearby without displacing residents.
>
> Through this intentional, community-driven process, the Elm Playlot was redeveloped by 2015, and over 15,000 children visit the park every year. Pogo Park continues to invest in Iron Triangle's community vision of healthier, sustainable places and has gone on to work with the state of California on community development.[55] To learn more about the creation of Elm Playlot and Pogo Park, visit these resources: www.tandfonline.com/doi/full/10.1080/23748834.2023.2230620 and https://pogopark.org.
>
> **REFLECTION QUESTIONS**
>
> *1. How did EPAC's use of the photovoice process and codesign workshops contribute to the redevelopment of Elm Playlot, and what impact did this have on the Iron Triangle community?*
>
> *2. What role did the joint-use agreement and partnerships play in the redevelopment of Elm Playlot, and how might these collaborative efforts impact the Iron Triangle community's health and social outcomes?*

FOOD ENVIRONMENTS

As discussed in depth in Chapter 12, "Food Safety, Security, and Sovereignty," our food environment matters for food security, safety, and sovereignty and greatly impacts human and planetary health. In our communities, our food environment includes the places where we access, grow, purchase, and consume food, including our grocery stores, supermarkets, farmers' markets, food cooperatives, food pantries, food trucks, restaurants, fast-food outlets, and urban farms, for instance. The distribution of these places within our communities significantly affects where, when, and how we eat. For example, in the United States there are many areas with limited access to fresh fruits and vegetables, which leads to disparities in the quality of our diet and health outcomes. Nearly 13% of households were food insecure in 2022, with stark disparities by race and ethnicity and household income.[58] Food insecurity is associated with a higher risk of chronic health conditions such as heart disease, diabetes, and poor mental well-being, which includes stress and depression. Children experience impaired growth and development, behavior problems, and mental health issues.

Zoning and transportation infrastructure influence food accessibility, shaping our diets and health as a result. Various policies can encourage or discourage the development of healthy food environments. Zoning can determine where different types of food retailers are located in a community and what types of agricultural practices are allowable, for instance, whether farms or backyard chickens are permitted in urban areas. Increasingly, there are examples of cities leveraging zoning to promote access to healthy foods. In Philadelphia, Pennsylvania, the Fresh Food Financing Initiative successfully used zoning policies to incentivize the development of grocery stores in areas with relatively high rates of food insecurity and poor access to healthy foods. Similarly, in New York City, decision makers adjusted zoning rules to support the Green Carts Program by allowing mobile produce vendors to sell food in underserved neighborhoods, which led to the expansion of affordable healthy food options.

PATHWAYS BETWEEN THE BUILT ENVIRONMENT AND HEALTH

In the sections that follow, we take a closer look at some of the ways in which policy and planning decisions impact health. Decisions about the built environment can have an effect on air and water quality in communities. The design of transportation, parks, and green space can worsen or reduce rates of injury. Additionally, mental health is influenced by various factors, including commuting time and access to safe green spaces, healthy food environments, and spaces that promote social engagement. In almost all instances, climate change is or will become, a fundamental factor in how the built environment affects community health.

CLIMATE CHANGE

As discussed in Chapter 3, "Confronting the Realities of Climate Change," climate change is a significant threat to health. The negative health impacts of climate change are wide reaching. Extreme heat can lead to increases in heat-related illnesses. Increasing temperatures can reduce air quality, exacerbating chronic conditions such as cardiovascular disease, respiratory disease, and asthma. Rising sea levels and extreme weather events have the potential to cause significant damage to homes and essential services, resulting in flooding and water contamination. These changes in the environment also bring about an increased risk of waterborne diseases. Additionally, there are also potential impacts on vector-borne diseases like Lyme disease and food-related infections such as salmonella.[59]

Urban and suburban areas are high contributors to total greenhouse gas emissions in the United States, and the way areas are developed can exacerbate the impacts of climate change.[60] As demonstrated in the U.S. government's *Fifth National Climate Assessment*, different components of the built environment, such as buildings and roads, city design, and vegetation, affect temperatures in urban areas.[60] Local jurisdictions are using mitigation and adaptation approaches to reduce emissions and climate change impacts. In addition to climate action plans, cities are making changes to the built environment through codes and standards to decrease building emissions, intentionally enhance green spaces, use forward-looking designs, create multi-modal transportation options, and more.

Community-led and grassroots groups are working to ensure that climate actions are equitable. Such efforts may be needed to combat the negative consequences of climate mitigation and adaptation strategies. For instance, many strategies that invest in sustainable spaces and infrastructure may contribute to gentrification, particularly known as climate gentrification. In another example, building retrofits can unintentionally lead to increased indoor air-pollutant exposure.[60] Household strategies for improving energy efficiency, like sealing cracks in the building envelope to reduce air leakage, can also trap volatile organic compounds, radon, or other pollutants inside.

AIR QUALITY

As discussed in Chapter 10, "The Air We Breathe," air pollution greatly affects human health. Over 35% of people living in the United States live in areas with unhealthy ozone or particulate matter pollution. People of color and people of low wealth are more likely to live in areas with poor air quality.[61,62] Climate change impacts the air we breathe, and higher temperatures can lead to an increase in ozone as well as allergens.[63] Exposure to harmful pollutants in the air can reduce life expectancy, exacerbate chronic conditions such as cardiovascular disease and asthma, and contribute to adverse pregnancy and birth outcomes.

For those living near major pollution sources, these impacts are greatest. Power plants, factories, construction sites, equipment, motor vehicles, wood stoves, scrap yards, and more, are all sources of air pollution.[62,64] The transportation sector is another major source of air pollution in the United States. Pollution exposure from cars and trucks is most significant near heavily trafficked roads. Transportation-related air pollution can be reduced through adopting clean-vehicle technology and reducing vehicle miles traveled by, for instance, increasing access to active and public transportation options, creating mixed-use development, and implementing programs that promote ride sharing. Local and state governments can set standards and transition to renewable noncombustible energy, and invest in and increase air-quality monitoring, particularly in communities near polluting sources.[65]

CASE STUDY 14.2: Fighting Pollution in Cancer Alley

Approximately one quarter of petrochemical production in the United States occurs in an 85-mile stretch along the Mississippi River in Louisiana between Baton Rouge and New Orleans. This area is known as "Cancer Alley" due to its high concentration of industry, which began moving to the area during the late 1960s. Rezoning has allowed industries to establish and expand in predominantly Black and low-wealth communities. As recently as 2014, the Fifth District of St. James Parish was rezoned from "residential" to "existing residential/future industrial." Cancer Alley has become a prominent example of environmental racism, as marginalized communities bear a disproportionate burden of environmental hazards. The residents of Cancer Alley are exposed to toxic air and water pollution, leading to elevated cancer rates, respiratory problems, adverse birth outcomes, and other illnesses.

National organizations, such as Human Rights Watch[66] and major news outlets, along with ongoing research like the Louisiana Tumor Registry, have highlighted the disproportionately high cancer rates. In 2021, ProPublica conducted an analysis of cumulative cancer risk from industrial air pollution across the country. Using industry-reported emissions data, the investigative news outlet found that in certain parts of Cancer Alley, the lifetime cancer risk from these chemicals was up to 47 times what the U.S. Environmental Protection Act (EPA) considers acceptable.[67]

Grassroots movements, including organizations like the Louisiana Bucket Brigade, RISE St. James, the Concerned Citizens of St. John Parish, and the Deep South Center for Environmental Justice have been at the forefront of the fight against environmental racism in Cancer Alley for decades. They have organized protests, filed lawsuits against polluting industries, and demanded accountability from government officials. Their efforts gained national attention and support, shining a spotlight on the intersection of environmental degradation and systemic racism in America.

The residents of Cancer Alley have recently collaborated with environmental lawyers at Earthjustice to halt the $9.4 billion Sunshine Project by Formosa Plastics, a Taiwanese petrochemical company. This project would involve the construction of 16 facilities across 2,400 acres, the largest plastics manufacturing complex in the country. The initial state permit in 2019 allowed for the release of 13.6 million metric tons of greenhouse gasses annually and 800 tons of toxic air pollutants, including carcinogens like benzene and ethylene oxide.

Advocates continue to call for policy shifts, improved protections, and corrective actions. These actions could include federal or state moratoriums on new or expanded operations, a transition toward renewable energy, and funding for community-based organizations working on environmental health and justice. Some have called for relocation opportunities for residents as a matter of international human rights. Nationally, there is a push to reassess air-pollution permitting and to develop strategies to hold fossil-fuel companies accountable.

(continued)

> **CASE STUDY 14.2: Fighting Pollution in Cancer Alley** (*continued*)
>
> There are specific demands for the president to develop a Federal Remediation and Relocation Plan, and for the Senate to ratify international human rights conventions. Activists also want the EPA to reject permits for harmful operations and enforce stricter regulations. Similarly, the Louisiana government is encouraged to support a phase-out of fossil fuels and deny permits that disproportionately harm communities. Fossil-fuel companies are urged to comply with environmental laws and take the lead in remediation efforts and corrective actions for residents affected by cumulative impacts.
>
> **REFLECTION QUESTIONS**
>
> 1. How does this case study exemplify environmental racism?
>
> 2. What role do grassroots movements and community organizations play in addressing environmental injustices like those in Cancer Alley?
>
> 3. What are some proposed solutions and policy recommendations for addressing the environmental and public health challenges faced by residents of Cancer Alley?

WATER

As discussed in Chapter 11, "Clean Water for All," water is critical to life and is used for drinking, cooking, bathing, cleaning, and more. Yet over two million people in the United States do not have access to proper sanitation or running water.[68] There are various structural challenges to ensuring that everyone has access to safe water—from dated or inadequate policies and regulations, to aging or lack of infrastructure, to limited funding for water infrastructure, to selective enforcement of drinking water standards.[69,70] Urban sprawl can negatively impact water quality owing to increased surface runoff that carries pollutants into streams and rivers.[71] Extreme weather events associated with climate change stress the existing water infrastructure. This extreme weather is of particular concern for communities that have hazardous facilities, like wastewater treatment plants, that may then contaminate the water supply during flooding events.[69]

Water affordability is another critical factor influencing who has access to water, primarily impacting low-wealth communities and communities of color. Water and sewer costs are increasing for many reasons, such as aging infrastructure and lack of investment, the cost of utility service, and the fragmented ownership and operations of the water sector itself.[72] High water bills can cause household stress and force residents to make difficult choices related to paying bills, and may result in water disconnection, a lien on the property, or eviction. Water-related illnesses include waterborne diseases caused by pathogens; toxins produced by harmful algae and cyanobacteria; and chemicals, like per- and polyfluoroalkyl substances (PFAS), introduced into the environment by human activities. Hygiene and sanitation can also be affected by a lack of access to water or poor wastewater infrastructure.

> **CATHERINE COLEMAN FLOWERS**
>
> "We have to have sustainable solutions for climate change. But we also have to ensure people down here have access to the same infrastructure as wealthy families."
>
> —Catherine Coleman Flowers
>
> In her book *Waste: One Woman's Fight Against America's Dirty Secret,* published in 2020, Catherine Coleman Flowers raises the public's awareness of inadequate infrastructure to support sewage treatment in Lowndes County, Alabama, a majority-Black rural county between Selma and Montgomery with high poverty rates. She uses personal stories, investigative journalism, and other data to expose the profound impact of poor sanitation on human dignity. The county has not provided sewage treatment for the majority of residents, and the private systems are unaffordable for many people. Residents sometimes experience pooling sewage in their yards
>
> *(continued)*

and have sewage coming back through the pipes to their homes. Upon testing the raw sewage, authorities discovered tropical parasites, shocking the public.

Although the problems facing Lowndes County have not been fully solved, Coleman Flowers's book and advocacy have sparked local, state, and national efforts to address these issues. In 2023, the Department of Justice (DOJ) concluded a federal probe that found two areas of concern: the state using fines to punish residents with inadequate home sewage systems and a failure to address the health effects of exposure to raw sewage. The probe resulted in an agreement between the DOJ and the Department of Health and Human Services and state health officials to address long-term wastewater issues. This environmental justice investigation was the department's first under Title VI of the Civil Rights Act of 1964. Today, Flowers continues to lift up community voices and elevate issues facing communities on the front line of similar environmental injustices.[73,74]

INJURY

The ways that communities are designed can influence the risk for injuries, especially those related to transportation. Traffic fatalities have been increasing nationally and are the leading cause of death among children and young adults.[75,76] Pedestrian and cyclist fatalities are increasing at even higher rates. There has been a rising trend of pedestrian deaths since 2010, and 2020 saw over a 4% increase from 2019.[9,77] Individuals living in low-wealth neighborhoods, older adults, and people of color are more likely to be struck and killed than other populations. American Indian and Alaska Native people have over two times the national rate of roadway death than other populations, and Black Americans' fatalities increased by 23% from 2019 to 2020, compared to an overall increase of 7.2%.[75]

The lack of infrastructure, the way our streets and cities are designed, and the policies in place continue to contribute to existing inequities. Arterial roadways, or streets that accommodate a high volume of vehicles, are often placed in low-wealth communities of color and accounted for over 50% of deaths in 2020.[75,78] There is often a lack of or little supportive infrastructure, such as sidewalks, crosswalks, or lights, to allow for other modes of transportation aside from vehicles. Cities have been designed to encourage automobile use, and many streets, especially those outside of a city's urban core, allow for travel at high speeds. Enforcement is a strategy to promote traffic safety and decrease unsafe driving behavior, such as use of seat belts, distracted driving, speeding, and alcohol-impaired driving.[79] High-visibility enforcement campaigns, particularly around seat belt use, have demonstrated effectiveness.[79] However, the use of traffic enforcement to raise revenue for city budgets and the discriminatory traffic stops of people of color have caused a reevaluation and and restructuring of this approach to promote more equitable and safe outcomes.[80,81] People of color, and more specifically Black drivers, are more likely to be pulled over and ticketed or have their car searched for evidence of other crimes, sometimes using low-level traffic violations as a pretextual stop.[82] These interactions with police further exacerbate racial inequities through increased debt, suspension of driver license, loss of employment, and even death.[82,83]

MENTAL HEALTH

The ways our communities are designed can also have profound impacts on our mental health. Our built environment can shape the physical and social contexts in which we live in ways that either facilitate or harm mental health. Access to green spaces, parks, and nature can lead to increased opportunities for coping with stress, engaging in physical activity, and encouraging positive social interactions.[84] Urban greening and tree canopy have been shown to decrease psychological distress and are associated with decreasing firearm violence.[55] The use of parks or green space can be heavily influenced by transportation infrastructure and networks.[85] However, if these spaces are of poor quality or unsafe, they can contribute to feelings of stress, anxiety, and isolation. Also, areas with deteriorating infrastructure, abandoned buildings, and limited economic opportunities may experience higher levels of crime, including gun violence.

Communities with pedestrian-friendly streetscapes, public gathering areas, and diverse amenities can enhance social interactions, build a sense of community, and provide a higher quality of life.[84] Meanwhile, urban sprawl can increase social stratification in communities and the time spent in cars, reducing the time and will to be involved in social activities. Another important community feature to promote social cohesion is creating a mix of housing types that allows individuals with different incomes, ages, and races/ethnicities to live in close proximity. One example of a community designed in ways that promote physical and mental health, as well as equity, is Via Verde in the South Bronx in New York. It serves as a model for how mixed-use developments can improve mental health outcomes without contributing to gentrification. In response to the lack of high-quality affordable housing and high rates of asthma, development in the community was informed by a community-based planning process beginning in the early 1990s that created units for a range of income levels. Among its many amenities, the development supports positive social environments by including an outdoor courtyard accessible for all residents, as well as an intergenerational food-growing space and programs for residents.

WORKING TOWARD ENVIRONMENTAL HEALTH AND JUSTICE

There is a growing understanding of how various sectors must work together with communities to ensure the environmental health, safety, and resiliency for all, but progress is slow. Described at length in Chapter 4, "Environmental Health Policies and Protections: Successes and Failures," the United States has seen unprecedented investments in recent years through the Infrastructure Reduction Act and the Bipartisan Infrastructure Law. For the first time in the nation's history, there is also attention to environmental justice (EJ) through the Justice40 Initiative. These dollars provide an opportunity to do what Jackson and colleagues call "reparative planning practices to address historical injustices and disrupt structural racism in the planning field,"[86(p411)] as well as in related fields. Here we share examples of many strategies, tools, and approaches, as well as examine the ways that we can better integrate environmental health and justice into planning policies and practices. Note that many of the examples we share here are brief and, as described, cannot possibly reflect the messy realities of how conflicts are navigated and decisions are made on the ground within communities and agencies.

IN OTHER WORDS: EQUALITY, EQUITY, AND JUSTICE

Dr. Camara Jones, a renowned public health leader and social epidemiologist, defines health equity as "assurance of the conditions for optimal health for all people. Achieving health equity requires valuing all individuals and populations equally, recognizing and rectifying historical injustices, and providing resources according to need. Health disparities will be eliminated when health equity is achieved."[87(pS74)]

Although equality and equity are often used interchangeably, these terms do not mean the same thing. *Equality* focuses on providing everyone the same opportunities and resources. *Equity* takes into account the needs of specific populations and provides the resources or support needed to thrive. In addition, *justice* entails doing work that eliminates the discrimination, poverty, and other forms of marginalization that lead to these health inequities (Figure 14.1).

(continued)

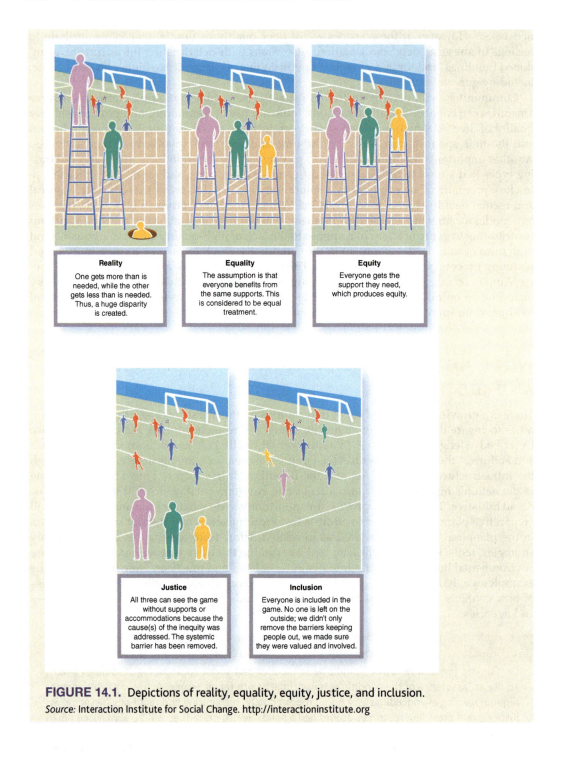

FIGURE 14.1. Depictions of reality, equality, equity, justice, and inclusion.
Source: Interaction Institute for Social Change. http://interactioninstitute.org

CO-GOVERNANCE MODELS, HEALTH IN ALL POLICIES, AND TOOLS FOR EQUITY

Urban and regional planners and transportation engineers and planners undoubtedly have a role to play in achieving environmental health and justice in society. The American Institute of Certified Planners, a professional institute within the American Planning Association, has a Code of Ethics that spells out planners' responsibility to work toward social justice and equity.[88]

Increasingly, these professionals are learning to build trust and form relationships with the communities they serve, as well as changing their traditional practices of community engagement to be more inclusive. Some organizations and academic programs are implementing training specific to cultural humility in recognition of the need for inclusive engagement for our multicultural world.[86] Additionally, some planning agencies offer community-planning academies. These are programs that inform local community leaders and residents about planning and land-use issues in a general way to build relationships between planners and their communities, as well as inform academy participants about the role of planning and how they can be involved.[89]

Of course, many different people must be involved in the design and support of healthy communities. **Co-governance** is a process in which agencies, nonprofit organizations, community groups, and others work together in decision-making. As discussed in several chapters, even with these health equity-minded approaches, it goes without saying that inequities may still persist if underlying factors, like power imbalances and racism, persist.[90] Government and community leaders in all sectors must address the underlying power dynamics and imbalances to promote environmental health and justice in planning policies and practice. In 1969, Sherry Arnstein[91] introduced the conceptual framework known as the "Ladder of Citizen Participation," illustrating a spectrum of engagement ranging from manipulation or tokenism wherein input is solicited merely to legitimize predetermined outcomes to genuine community control over decision-making processes. This framework has been widely referenced and adapted by numerous agencies, organizations, and scholars over time, often with a focus on understanding and addressing underlying power dynamics. More recently, the International Association of Public Participation (IAP2) has proposed a spectrum that spans from informing to consulting, involving, collaborating, and empowering, reflecting the varying degrees of decision-making authority that shift from agency staff or policy makers to the public.[92] In practical terms, this spectrum ranges from simply keeping the public informed about decisions to actively implementing decisions made by the public themselves. Transparency, communication, and accountability about how decisions are made are vital in designing healthy communities.

As discussed in Chapter 2, **Health in All Policies (HiAP)** is an approach that encourages collaboration across all sectors to integrate health considerations into the decision-making process to address the structural determinants of health across sectors.[93] This approach can take many forms, such as:

- housing policies that address issues such as housing insecurity, substandard housing conditions, and neighborhood segregation;
- education policies that address factors influencing student health, such as access to a healthy food environment, outdoor physical activity opportunities, and mental health supports; and
- transportation policies that lead to the creation of walkable and bike-friendly cities.

HiAP can use tools like HIAs to gain an understanding of the health impacts of decisions and work toward health equity.[94] An *HIA* is a systematic process used to evaluate the potential health effects of a policy, program, or project before it is implemented. For instance, imagine that a county government is working to update its comprehensive land-use plan, which includes how officials will move forward with zoning, housing development, and green space preservation. They may conduct an HIA first to evaluate how the plan may influence community safety, mental health, or access to healthcare facilities. Their findings may lead them to alter the plan in meaningful ways to support health.

In the context of new or expanded developments, communities have increasingly begun mobilizing and advocating for **community benefits agreements (CBAs)**. With a CBA, there is a legally-binding contract, usually between developers and coalitions of community-based organizations, in which the developer agrees to specific commitments in response to the priorities and needs of nearby residents.[95] There are many examples of CBAs negotiated in the past few decades. For instance, LA Live, a large entertainment complex in Los Angeles, included a CBA to ensure local hiring, affordable housing, funding for community programming, and support for existing nearby businesses. However, CBAs do not automatically guarantee equity for residents, particularly if negotiations are not inclusive, if there are few or no mechanisms to enforce or ensure that the agreement is upheld, or that it will not lead to further gentrification and displacement. Many large and midsize cities have enacted local ordinances requiring CBAs for developments of a certain size and cost with provisions that consider these issues.

To further address structural racism, some cities, like Asheville, North Carolina, and Evanston, Illinois, are studying and creating reparations initiatives.[86] In 2019, Evanston's city council approved distributing $25,000 to eligible Black households for home repairs, mortgage payments, and down payments or interest rates on property.[96,97] Over a 10-year period, the city committed 10 million dollars, primarily funded by a 3% tax on cannabis sales.[97] As leaders at PolicyLink explain, a reparations and reparative justice framework requires recognizing past harms, reckoning with the systemic causes of these harms, building in accountability moving forward, and making amends through various possible strategies, such as financial compensation, land return, policy reforms, and other forms of redress that rectify past wrongs.[98]

REIMAGINING OUR BUILT ENVIRONMENTS FOR EQUITY: BY DESIGN

As discussed earlier, zoning, the most common way to regulate land use, can have significant impacts on equity. Across the United States, zoning codes are being updated, and localities are using such approaches as up-zoning and inclusionary zoning. *Up-zoning* refers to zoning practices that allow for higher density land uses and may be used to support transit-oriented development and affordable housing. *Inclusionary zoning* is an approach used to increase affordable housing options by requiring or incentivizing developers to include a certain percentage of affordable housing units in new developments. However, these policies must be thought out carefully to avoid abuse by developers driven by profit, creating gentrification and other problems. In general, comprehensive plans are increasingly becoming values driven and include equity, climate change, and health considerations.[17] These plans guide community development and can have lasting impacts on key drivers of environmental health and justice.

Through comprehensive transportation planning and policy, the public's health can be prioritized. Land-use mix, density, connectivity, and design play significant roles in promoting physical activity levels in communities.[99] Policies and strategies can promote active transportation—walking, bicycling, and rolling—as well as the use of public transportation. Dense, compact development is associated with a range of potential benefits, including increased active transportation.[100,101] Infrastructure improvements can support active transportation, for example, by having a highly connected grid or network of streets, dedicated bike lanes, and well-maintained sidewalks. Additionally, community-design features such as improved biking infrastructure, shade, and access to natural amenities can also promote active transportation. Programs like Safe Routes to School can further encourage and facilitate active commuting. The concept of **complete streets** holds that streets should cater to the needs of all users, which include drivers of cars, transit riders, cyclists, and pedestrians. Its main objectives are to prioritize accessibility and safety. There are over 1,700 Complete Streets policies across the nation, and many policies are now prioritizing underinvested and marginalized communities.[102] These efforts are working to make it easier and safer for people to move around using various transportation modes.[103]

Traffic-related injuries and deaths can be prevented by reducing travel demand as well as by redesigning roadways to alter driver behavior. Examples of these strategies include traffic-calming devices such as roundabouts, rumble strips, chicanes or narrowing of roads, speed humps, and street trees.[104] Policies such as speed limits, alcohol-impaired driving enforcement, and teen licensure have also been shown to reduce traffic fatalities.[105] Implementing behavior-change campaigns and enhancing equity and data-driven traffic enforcement are also components of a comprehensive approach to prevent injuries. Creating safer vehicles and using technologies, such as alcohol-detection systems, can improve safety and reduce harm in traffic crashes.[75] By reducing the amount of vehicle miles traveled, such strategies can also positively impact physical activity and benefit the environment. Vision Zero, a multidisciplinary approach to eliminate traffic deaths, brings together traffic planners and engineers, police officers, policy makers, and public health professionals to address the factors that contribute to safe mobility.[106] With the publishing of "The National Roadway Safety Strategy" in January 2022, the Department of Transportation adopted a Safe System Approach to design and engineer a system that is inclusive of all road users.[75] This paradigm shift may help address the inequities experienced by communities of color, particularly around traffic enforcement, because streets will be designed for safety, usage, and human behavior.[107] With the passing of the Bipartisan Infrastructure Law of 2021, increased funds are available to address the inadequate historic transportation policies and practices through such grant opportunities as the Safe Streets and Roads for All Grant Program.[82]

Much work is also being done to advance health and housing equity. Some promising practices and policies include:

- the establishment of community land trusts, whereby a nonprofit organization holds land in trust to preserve the land for the community;
- the adoption of tools like the National Healthy Housing Standard, which complements the International Property Maintenance Code and other housing standards in providing health measures and performance standards to ensure homes are safe and healthy;[108]
- the implementation of proactive housing inspections and informing residents of or applicants for federally assisted housing about environmental contamination and potential health hazards; and
- increasing energy efficiency to reduce energy burden.[27,38,109]

Housing supply can be expanded through land-use reform, as seen in Minneapolis, a city that has been enacting policy changes and land-use reform since 2009. The city created Green Zones by removing minimum parking mandates for new developments, allowing duplex and triplexes rather than only single-family units, and promoting apartment building along commercial corridors.[20,40] Hospitals and health systems are also working upstream to improve health by investing in affordable housing, recognizing that housing instability, affordability, and substandard housing impacts the health of the communities they serve.[110]

Developing and maintaining more accessible and inclusive parks and green space is an approach that governments have employed over the years to make communities healthier. Another strategy involves increasing access to community facilities for people to gather and socialize, such as schools, churches, or community centers. **Shared or joint-use agreements** that outline the terms and conditions for community members to access these resources can help address institutional barriers to their use, such as liability and cost. Increasingly, advocates are calling for a park equity framework, and there are many other promising policies and strategies used throughout the United States. Some antidisplacement strategies for developing and maintaining green and open spaces include:

- first-source hiring, in which employers give priority to long-term residents when hiring;
- maintaining homeownership among low-wealth populations around proposed green or park space through policies such as rent control or restrictions on the demolition of affordable housing;
- establishing community land trusts near new parks;
- engaging community members to share their thoughts and visions for proposed park space at the beginning of the park-planning process, and incorporating community feedback;[40,111] and
- requiring government-funded park-development proposals to include antidisplacement strategies, such as those listed here.

This type of community engagement could employ a co-governance model, which could include shared decision-making authority and participatory budgeting that engages nearby residents in determining how funding will be spent.[112] Additionally, it is vital to engage with all park users, regardless of housing status, and design a park that is an inclusive and welcoming public space that offers a variety of programs and activities appealing to park users.[113]

To improve food environments, there are many possible strategies that support food sovereignty and, consequently, healthy communities. These include:

- providing incentives for grocery store and supermarket development;
- restricting fast-food retail store density;
- increasing fresh produce availability at neighborhood corner stores;
- encouraging community-supported agriculture programs, farmers' markets, community gardens, and mobile produce vendors; and
- improving transportation access to these food environments.[114,115,98]

Zoning codes may also need to be reviewed and adjusted when working toward a regional or local food culture and economy that supports urban agriculture, small businesses, and food ventures. For example, removing restrictions for small-animal husbandry or allowing urban agriculture structures like hoop houses, which are a type of semipermanent greenhouse for growing plants, can enable people to produce an increased variety of foods.[116] Supporting agriculture in communities may also require expanded access to land through land banks and collective land ownership as well as increased protection of Tribal lands. These approaches should be community led, and inequitable food access among communities of color and low-wealth communities should be addressed. Other broader policies and investments might include expanding and strengthening federal assistance programs, such as the Supplemental Nutrition Assistance Program and the Special Supplemental Nutrition Program for Women, Infants, and Children.[117,118]

MAIN TAKEAWAYS

In this chapter, we learned that:

- The built environment affects air quality and water quality, as well as access to spaces that promote or hinder healthy diets, mental health, safety, and physical activity.
- The ways we zone communities, plan transportation infrastructure, site and care for indoor places, and plan and maintain outdoor green spaces all affect community health.
- although there is movement to integrate equity and environmental health and justice more thoroughly into planning practices, implementation and progress are slow.
- Cities are using strategies like zoning reform and CBAs to address health inequities, but attention is needed to ensure that these efforts do not encourage displacement and gentrification.
- With the lasting impacts of historical and ongoing disinvestment through policy and planning, as well as the marginalization of communities of color and low wealth, systemic work is necessary to achieve healthy communities for all.

SUMMARY

The influence of our built environments on environmental health and justice is notably complex. Structural racism and other forms of discrimination have long worsened disparities in accessing safe housing, transportation, and food environments, resulting in inequitable health outcomes for many marginalized communities. Climate change will continue to have major impacts on our communities, and ongoing attention to mitigation and adaptation in our built environments is necessary. Although local, state, and federal policies and planning decisions have contributed to the development of many harmful environments, they also have the potential to transform our communities in equity-minded ways. An HiAP approach and tools such as CBAs and HIAs have been useful to this end. By integrating a consideration of health equity and justice into decision-making and supporting community-led initiatives and community priorities, a transformational shift towards more healthy and just communities is possible.

END-OF-CHAPTER RESOURCES

DISCUSSION QUESTIONS

1. Thinking about your own community, what makes it healthy? What would you change to make it healthier? (Think about land use, infrastructure, zoning, and other policies or programs.)
2. Based on what you have learned in this chapter, think about the role of environmental health practitioners in ensuring a healthy community for all. How would you explain the health impacts of the built environment to a colleague, classmate, or friend who has not read this chapter? What are the different sectors that influence health outcomes?
3. Think of an example of a health disparity in the community where you live or a community you serve. For instance, this example could be disproportionate exposure to air quality for some neighborhoods or disproportionate access to clean, safe parks. What would it look like to address this issue if your goal was equality? What might it look like if your goal was equity?
4. How do zoning practices affect your community? Look up the zoning map for your city. If you live in a rural area or a smaller town, there may not be zoning codes or maps. You can look at a nearby city's map instead. As you look at this map, how does zoning promote health for residents? How might it harm health?
5. Imagine that you are working for a local city or county government and helping to plan new transportation infrastructure. How might you work with community members to ensure that the plan addresses any past harms, reflects their vision, and promotes overall community health?

LEARNING ACTIVITIES

THE TIME IS NOW

Many national environmental organizations work to assess and address issues in our built environment. Search online to identify the people in your community who do this work. Follow them on social media, join their meetings, attend their webinars, and engage. By learning more, you can access training, gain new insights, and explore potential solutions to complex issues. Some examples include the following:

- The Society of Practitioners of Health Impact Assessment (SOPHIA): http://hiasociety.org
- The Urban Land Institute: http://uli.org
- Robert Wood Johnson Foundation: http://rwjf.org
- The Urban Institute: http://urban.org

IN REAL LIFE

Tree equity is the idea that all people deserve trees in their community, regardless of race, color, national origin, or income. Trees are powerful natural resources that can help to manage stormwater, capture pollution, cool urban heat islands, and provide mental health benefits. But who has access to trees in the United States? Take a look at some tree equity scores here: www.treeequityscore.org. Using the group's mapping tool, zoom into a city near you. Open the corresponding Municipal Reports for several Census-block groups. Look at the percentage of children in each Census block group. Look at other demographic and environmental factors. Do you notice any patterns? After looking at and comparing these two reports, what are your thoughts on tree equity?

A robust set of instructor resources designed to supplement this text is located at http://connect.springerpub.com/content/book/978-0-8261-8353-8. Qualifying instructors may request access by emailing textbook@springerpub.com.

REFERENCES

1. Genovese D, Candiloro S, D'Anna A, et al. Urban sprawl and health: a review of the scientific literature. *Environ Res Lett*. 2023;18(8):083004. doi:10.1088/1748-9326/ace986
2. Rutt C, Dannenberg AL, Kochtitzky C. Using policy and built environment interventions to improve public health. *J Public Health Manag Pract*. 2008;14(3):221–223. doi:10.1097/01.phh.0000316479.19394.84
3. The Community Guide. Physical activity: built environment approaches combining transportation system interventions with land use and environmental design. November 1, 2022. https://www.thecommunityguide.org/findings/physical-activity-built-environment-approaches.html
4. Patnaik A, Son J, Feng A, Ade C. Racial disparities and climate change. Princeton Student Climate Initiative. August 15, 2020. https://psci.princeton.edu/tips/2020/8/15/racial-disparities-and-climate-change
5. American Lung Association. Disparities in the impact of air pollution. November 2, 2023. https://www.lung.org/clean-air/outdoors/who-is-at-risk/disparities
6. Ward K Jr. How Black communities become "sacrifice zones" for industrial air pollution. ProPublica. December 21, 2021. https://www.propublica.org/article/how-black-communities-become-sacrifice-zones-for-industrial-air-pollution
7. Meyer MRU, Moore JB, Abildso C, Edwards MB, Gamble A, Baskin ML. Rural active living: a call to action. *J Public Health Manag Pract*. 2016;22(5):E11–E20. doi:10.1097/PHH.0000000000000333
8. Centers for Disease Control and Prevention. Strategies for physical activity through community design. February 8, 2024. https://www.cdc.gov/physicalactivity/community-strategies/activity-friendly-routes-to-everyday-destinations.html
9. Dangerous by design 2022. Smart Growth America. 2022. Accessed June 17, 2024. https://smartgrowthamerica.org/dangerous-by-design/
10. Jacobs DE. Environmental health disparities in housing. *Am J Public Health*. 2011;101 Suppl 1 (suppl 1):S115–S122. doi:10.2105/AJPH.2010.300058
11. Swope CB, Hernández D. Housing as a determinant of health equity: a conceptual model. *Soc Sci Med*. 2019;243:112571. doi:10.1016/j.socscimed.2019.112571
12. Popkin SJ. Disability justice isn't possible without housing justice. Urban Institute. March 1, 2023. https://www.urban.org/urban-wire/disability-justice-isnt-possible-without-housing-justice
13. The Gap. National Low Income Housing Coalition. 2023. Accessed June 17, 2024. https://nlihc.org/gap
14. Taylor L. Housing and health: an overview of the literature. *Health Aff*. Published online June 7, 2018. doi:10.1377/hpb20180313.396577
15. Minkler M, Wakimoto P. *Community Organizing and Community Building for Health and Social Equity*. 4th ed. Rutgers University Press.
16. What are zoning codes? Planopedia. Accessed June 17, 2024. https://www.planetizen.com/definition/zoning-codes
17. Rouse D. Future of the comprehensive plan. *J Comp Urban L Policy*. 2022;5(1):299–326. https://readingroom.law.gsu.edu/cgi/viewcontent.cgi?article=1100&context=jculp
18. NAACP. Fumes across the fence-line: the health impacts of air pollution from oil & gas facilities on African American communities. November 14, 2017. https://naacp.org/resources/fumes-across-fence-line-health-impacts-air-pollution-oil-gas-facilities-african-american

19. American Public Health Association. Addressing environmental justice to achieve health equity. November 5, 2019. https://apha.org/Policies-and-Advocacy/Public-Health-Policy-Statements/Policy-Database/2020/01/14/Addressing-Environmental-Justice-to-Achieve-Health-Equity
20. Velasco G, Cohen O. Three ways zoning can advance housing and climate justice. Housing Matters: An Urban Institute Initiative. March 2, 2022. https://housingmatters.urban.org/articles/three-ways-zoning-can-advance-housing-and-climate-justice
21. American Public Health Association. Separation policy and practice brief. October 2021. https://apha.org/-/media/Files/PDF/topics/equity/Healing_Through_Policy_Separation.ashx
22. Lynch EE, Malcoe LH, Laurent SE, Richardson J, Mitchell BC, Meier HC. The legacy of structural racism: associations between historic redlining, current mortgage lending, and health. *SSM-Popul Health*. 2021;14:100793. doi:10.1016/j.ssmph.2021.100793
23. Krieger N, Van Wye G, Huynh M, et al. Structural racism, historical redlining, and risk of preterm birth in New York City, 2013–2017. *Am J Public Health*. 2020;110(7):1046–1053. doi:10.2105/AJPH.2020.305656
24. Nardone A, Casey JA, Morello-Frosch R, Mujahid M, Balmes JR, Thakur N. Associations between historical residential redlining and current age-adjusted rates of emergency department visits due to asthma across eight cities in California: an ecological study. *Lancet Planet Health*. 2020;4(1):e24–e31. doi:10.1016/s2542-5196(19)30241-4
25. Pappoe YN. Remedying the effects of government-sanctioned segregation in a post-Freddie Gray Baltimore. *U. Md. L.J. Race Relig. Gender & Class*. 2016;16(115). http://digitalcommons.law.umaryland.edu/rrgc/vol16/iss1/6
26. Mendez DD, Hogan VK, Culhane J. Institutional racism and pregnancy health: using Home Mortgage Disclosure Act data to develop an index for mortgage discrimination at the community level. *Public Health Rep*. 2011;126 Suppl 3(suppl 3):102–114. doi:10.1177/00333549111260s315
27. American Public Health Association. Creating the healthiest nation: health and housing equity. May 2020. https://apha.org/-/media/Files/PDF/topics/equity/Health_and_Housing_Equity.ashx
28. Bravo MA, Zephyr D, Kowal D, Ensor K, Miranda ML. Racial residential segregation shapes the relationship between early childhood lead exposure and fourth-grade standardized test scores. *Proc Natl Acad Sci U S A*. 2022;119(34):e2117868119. doi:10.1073/pnas.2117868119
29. Bailey ZD, Krieger N, Agénor M, Graves J, Linos N, Bassett MT. Structural racism and health inequities in the USA: evidence and interventions. *Lancet*. 2017;389(10077):1453–1463. doi:10.1016/S0140-6736(17)30569-X
30. Urban Institute. How local differences in race and place affect mortgage lending. November 15, 2022. https://www.urban.org/urban-wire/how-local-differences-race-and-place-affect-mortgage-lending
31. Health Affairs Health Policy Brief. Public transportation in the US: a driver of health and equity. July 29, 2021. doi:10.1377/hpb20210630.810356
32. Federal Transit Administration. 2022 American Public Transportation Association (APTA) Annual Conference. October 10, 2022. https://www.transit.dot.gov/about/speeches/2022-american-public-transportation-association-apta-annual-conference
33. Public transportation facts. American Public Transportation Association. 2018. Accessed June 16, 2024. https://www.apta.com/news-publications/public-transportation-facts
34. Chapple K, Thomas T, Zuk M. What are gentrification and displacement. Urban Displacement Project. 2021. https://www.urbandisplacement.org/about/what-are-gentrification-and-displacement
35. American Public Health Association. Ensuring equity in transportation and land use decisions to promote health and well-being in metropolitan areas. October 26, 2021. https://www.apha.org/Policies-and-Advocacy/Public-Health-Policy-Statements/Policy-Database/2022/01/10/Ensuring-Equity-in-Transportation
36. Why indoor air quality is important to schools. US EPA. October 27, 2015. Updated November 28, 2023. https://www.epa.gov/iaq-schools/why-indoor-air-quality-important-schools
37. The White House. Fact sheet: the Biden-Harris lead pipe and paint action plan. December 16, 2021. https://www.whitehouse.gov/briefing-room/statements-releases/2021/12/16/fact-sheet-the-biden-harris-lead-pipe-and-paint-action-plan
38. Shriver Center on Poverty Law. Poisonous homes the fight for environmental justice in federally assisted housing. June 2020. https://www.povertylaw.org/wp-content/uploads/2020/06/environmental_justice_report_final-rev2.pdf
39. Housing and homes. Healthy People 2030. Accessed June 16, 2024. https://health.gov/healthypeople/objectives-and-data/browse-objectives/housing-and-homes

40. Pew. Minneapolis land use reforms offer a blueprint for housing affordability. January 4, 2024. https://www.pewtrusts.org/en/research-and-analysis/articles/2024/01/04/minneapolis-land-use-reforms-offer-a-blueprint-for-housing-affordability
41. Harvard Graduate School of Design. America's rental housing. 2022. https://www.jchs.harvard.edu/sites/default/files/reports/files/Harvard_JCHS_Americas_Rental_Housing_2022.pdf
42. Housing burden. National Equity Atlas. Accessed June 15, 2024. https://nationalequityatlas.org/indicators/Housing_burden
43. Scheckler S, Molinsky J, Airgood-Obrycki W. How well does the housing stock meet accessibility needs? An analysis of the 2019 American housing survey. March 2022. https://www.jchs.harvard.edu/sites/default/files/research/files/harvard_jchs_housing_stock_accessibility_scheckler_2022_0.pdf
44. Schipperijn J, Cerin E, Adams MA, et al. Access to parks and physical activity: an eight country comparison. *Urban For Urban Green*. 2017;27:253–263. doi:10.1016/j.ufug.2017.08.010
45. Prevention Institute. Park equity, life expectancy, and power building. Policy Brief. September 2020. https://preventioninstitute.org/sites/default/files/uploads/PI_Park_Equity_Policy_Brief.pdf
46. Trust for Public Land. The power of parks to promote health: a special report. May 2023. https://www.tpl.org/wp-content/uploads/2023/05/The-Power-of-Parks-to-Promote-Health-A-Trust-for-Public-Land-Special-Report.pdf
47. Lee KJ, Fernandez M, Scott D, Floyd M. Slow violence in public parks in the U.S.: can we escape our troubling past? *Soc Cult Geogr*. 2023;24(7):1185–1202. doi:10.1080/14649365.2022.2028182
48. Jacobs JP, Hotakainen R. Racist roots, lack of diversity haunt national parks. E&E News by POLITICO. June 25, 2020. https://www.eenews.net/articles/racist-roots-lack-of-diversity-haunt-national-parks
49. Mock B. The U.S. national park service grapples with its racist origins. Bloomberg. August 26, 2016. https://www.bloomberg.com/news/articles/2016-08-26/at-its-centennial-anniversary-the-u-s-national-park-service-tries-to-diversify-its-visitors-and-workforce
50. Brulliard N. This land is their land. National Parks Conservation Association. October 8, 2020. https://www.npca.org/articles/2742-this-land-is-their-land
51. Hamilton K-A. National parks are travel's next frontier in the movement for racial equality. *Washington Post*. September 17, 2020. https://www.washingtonpost.com/travel/2020/09/17/national-parks-travel-black
52. Hoover FA, Lim TC. Examining privilege and power in US urban parks and open space during the double crises of anti-Black racism and COVID-19. *Socioecol Pract Res*. 2021;3(1):55–70. doi:10.1007/s42532-020-00070-3
53. Wickes R, Kalms N, Ratnam C, Lee M, Matthewson G, Meyer S. Safe spaces: understanding and enhancing safety and inclusion for diverse women. Griffith University. 2023. https://research-repository.griffith.edu.au/bitstream/handle/10072/425309/Wickes8016584.pdf?sequence=1&isAllowed=y
54. Derose KP, Han B, Williamson S, Cohen DA. Gender disparities in park use and physical activity among residents of high-poverty neighborhoods in Los Angeles. *Womens Health Issues*. 2018;28(1):6–13. doi:10.1016/j.whi.2017.11.003
55. Corburn J, Griffin JS, Harris B, Padilla DJ. Co-creating places for urban health & healing: the case of Pogo Park. *Cities & Health*. 2023;7(6):914–925. doi:10.1080/23748834.2023.2230620
56. Mclean J, Wilson L, Kent R. Health in all policies, health data in all decisions. December 2011. https://www.ci.richmond.ca.us/DocumentCenter/View/8663/Health-in-All-Policies-Health-Data-in-all-Decisi?bidId=
57. Pogo Park. Where we work. November 13, 2017. https://pogopark.org/what-we-do/where-we-work/
58. Food security and nutrition Assistance. U.S. Department of Agriculture Economic Research Service. Updated November 29, 2023. https://www.ers.usda.gov/data-products/ag-and-food-statistics-charting-the-essentials/food-security-and-nutrition-assistance
59. Cissé G. Food-borne and water-borne diseases under climate change in low-and middle-income countries: further efforts needed for reducing environmental health exposure risks. *Acta Trop*. 2019;194:181–188. doi:10.1016%2Fj.actatropica.2019.03.012

60. Chu EK, Fry MM, Chakraborty J, et al. Built environment, urban systems, and cities. In: Crimmins AR, Avery CW, Easterling DR, Kunkel KE, Stewart BC, Maycock TK, eds. *Fifth National Climate Assessment*. U.S. Global Change Research Program; 2023. https://nca2023.globalchange.gov/chapter/12/
61. Key findings. American Lung Association. State of the air. 2022. Accessed June 14, 2024. https://www.lung.org/research/sota/key-findings
62. Health impact of pollution. American Lung Association. State of the air. 2022. Accessed June 14, 2024. https://www.lung.org/research/sota/health-risks
63. Centers for Disease Control and Prevention. Climate change decreases the quality of the air we breathe. 2024. https://www.cdc.gov/climate-health/media/pdfs/air-quality-final_508_1.pdf
64. Centers for Disease Control and Prevention. Particle pollution. July 16, 2021. https://www.cdc.gov/air/particulate_matter.html
65. Recommendations for Action. American Lung Association. State of the air. 2022. Accessed June 15, 2024. https://www.lung.org/research/sota/protect-yourself-community
66. Juhasz A. We're dying here. Human Rights Watch. Published online January 25, 2024. https://www.hrw.org/report/2024/01/25/were-dying-here/fight-life-louisiana-fossil-fuel-sacrifice-zone
67. Younes L, Kofman A, Shaw A, Song L. Poison in the air. ProPublica. November 2, 2021. https://www.propublica.org/article/toxmap-poison-in-the-air
68. DigDeep. Draining: the economic impact of America's hidden water crisis. Accessed June 15, 2024. https://www.digdeep.org/draining
69. US Water Alliance. An equitable water future a national briefing paper. 2023. https://uswateralliance.org/wp-content/uploads/2023/09/uswa_waterequity_FINAL.pdf
70. Wilson SM, Heaney CD, Cooper J, Wilson O. Built environment issues in unserved and underserved African-American neighborhoods in North Carolina. *Environ Justice*. 2008;1(2):63–72. doi:10.1089/env.2008.0509
71. Resnik DB. Urban sprawl, smart growth, and deliberative democracy. *Am J Public Health*. 2010;100(10):1852–1856. doi:10.2105/ajph.2009.182501
72. Levine L, Wein O, Lusson K, Haynes B. Water affordability advocacy toolkit. NRDC. June 2022. https://www.nrdc.org/sites/default/files/water-affordability-toolkit-full-report.pdf
73. History. CREEJ. Accessed June 17, 2024. https://www.creej.org/history
74. About. Catherine Coleman Flowers. Accessed June 17, 2024. https://www.catherinecolemanflowers.com/about
75. U.S. Department of Transportation. National roadway safety strategy. January 2022. https://www.transportation.gov/sites/dot.gov/files/2022-02/USDOT-National-Roadway-Safety-Strategy.pdf
76. National Highway Traffic Safety Administration. Children: 2021 data. May 2023. https://crashstats.nhtsa.dot.gov/Api/Public/ViewPublication/813456#:~:text=Child%20traffic%20fatalities%20increased%20by
77. Kim J. U.S. pedestrian deaths reach a 40-year high. NPR. June 26, 2023. https://www.npr.org/2023/06/26/1184034017/us-pedestrian-deaths-high-traffic-car
78. McAndrews C, Pollack KM, Berrigan D, Dannenberg AL, Christopher EJ. Understanding and improving arterial roads to support public health and transportation goals. *Am J Public Health*. 2017;107(8):1278–1282. doi:10.2105/ajph.2017.303898
79. National Highway Traffic Safety Administration. Synthesis of studies that relate amount of enforcement to magnitude of safety outcomes. May 2022. https://www.nhtsa.gov/sites/nhtsa.gov/files/2022-06/NPD-210715-001-15490-Enforcement-to-Magnitude-of-Safety-Outcomes-050522-v5a-tag.pdf
80. McIntire M, Keller MH. The demand for money behind many police traffic stops. *The New York Times*. October 31, 2021. Updated November 2, 2021. https://www.nytimes.com/2021/10/31/us/police-ticket-quotas-money-funding.html?
81. Boddupalli A, Mucciolo L. Following the money on fines and fees the misaligned fiscal incentives in speeding tickets. Urban Institute. January 2022. https://www.urban.org/sites/default/files/publication/105331/following-the-money-on-fines-and-fees_final-pdf.pdf
82. Rau H, Neath J, McDoom M, Resing M. Redesigning public safety: traffic safety. Center for Policing Equity. September 2022. Updated December 2023. https://policingequity.org/traffic-safety/60-cpe-white-paper-traffic-safety/filehave been updated to match the, and publication and updated dates have been addedconfirm

83. Policing Project. NYU School of Law. Why limit pretextual stops? What the data says. 2020. https://static1.squarespace.com/static/58a33e881b631bc60d4f8b31/t/645b9ea85e3f9a7712b2b810/1683725992612/Why+Limit+Pretextual+Stops.pdf
84. Mouratidis K, Poortinga W. Built environment, urban vitality and social cohesion: do vibrant neighborhoods foster strong communities? *Landsc Urban Plan*. 2020;204:103951. doi:10.1016/j.landurbplan.2020.103951
85. Mullenbach LE, Larson LR, Floyd MF, et al. Cultivating social capital in diverse, low-income neighborhoods: the value of parks for parents with young children. *Landsc Urban Plan*. 2022;219:104313. doi:10.1016/j.landurbplan.2021.104313
86. Jackson A, Yerena A, Lee CA, et al. Anti-racist futures: disrupting racist planning practices in workplaces, institutions, and communities. *J Am Plann Assoc*. 2023;89(4):411–422. doi:10.1080/01944363.2023.2244850
87. Jones CP. Systems of power, axes of inequity: parallels, intersections, braiding the strands. *Med. Care*. 2014;52(10 Supp 3):S71–S75. https://www.tfah.org/wp-content/uploads/2020/08/Jones_SystemsofPower.pdf
88. Fierman J, Devastey K, Sveen LW. Equitable community engagement requires learning, self-reflection, and transparency. American Planning Association. March 23, 2023. https://www.planning.org/planning/2023/winter/equitable-community-engagement-requires-learning-self-reflection-and-transparency/
89. Carney DJ. How planners can inspire and empower citizens to get involved. American Planning Association. February 15, 2024. https://www.planning.org/planning/2024/feb/how-planners-can-inspire-and-empower-citizens-to-get-involved/
90. Rogerson B, Lindberg R, Baum F, et al. Recent advances in health impact assessment and Health in All Policies implementation: lessons from an international convening in Barcelona. *Int J Environ Res Public Health*. 2020;17(21):7714. doi:10.3390/ijerph17217714
91. Arnstein SR. A ladder of citizen participation. *J AmInst Plann Assoc*. 1969;35(4):216–224. doi:10.1080/01944366908977225
92. What is public participation. Accessed June 17, 2024. https://www.involve.org.uk/resources/knowledge-base/what/what-public-participation
93. Rudolph L, Caplan J, Ben-Moshe K, Dillon L. *Health in All Policies: A Guide for State and Local Governments*. American Public Health Association and Public Health Institute; 2013.
94. Johnson S, Haney J, Cairone L, Huskey C, Kheirbek I. Assessing air quality and public health benefits of New York City's climate action plans. *Environ Sci Technol*. 2020;54(16):9804–9813. doi:10.1021/acs.est.0c00694
95. Community benefit agreements. Urban Institute. Accessed June 17, 2024. https://www.urban.org/apps/pursuing-housing-justice-interventions-impact/community-benefit-agreements
96. Solman P, Holmes RC.The impact of the nation's first cash reparations program for Black residents. PBS NewsHour. June 22, 2023. https://www.pbs.org/newshour/show/the-impact-of-the-nations-first-cash-reparations-program-for-black-residents
97. Illinois city 1st in US to offer Black residents reparations. AP News. April 20, 2021. https://apnews.com/article/reparations-evanston-illinois-black-residents-752a6fe83c560117523d7f8abba1bfb8
98. Hoang T, Phillips R, Rangel J. Grounding justice: toward reparative spatial futures in land and housing. 2024. https://www.policylink.org/sites/default/files/grounding-justice-010524-d-PL.pdf
99. Wei YD, Xiao W, Wen M, Wei R. Walkability, land use and physical activity. *Sustainability*. 2016;8(1):65. doi:10.3390/su8010065
100. Cong C, Kwak Y, Deal B. Incorporating active transportation modes in large scale urban modeling to inform sustainable urban development. *Comput Environ Urban Syst*. 2022;91(1):101726. doi:10.1016/j.compenvurbsys.2021.101726
101. Transportation Research Board, Institute of Medicine of the National Academies. Does the built environment influence physical activity?: Examining the evidence--special report 282. January 11, 2005. Accessed June 17, 2024. https://www.trb.org/publications/sr/sr282.pdf
102. National Complete Streets Coalition, Smart Growth America. The complete streets policy framework. April 2023. https://smartgrowthamerica.org/resources/elements-complete-streets-policy/
103. American Planning Association. Mobility as a service. January 2, 2024. https://www.planning.org/publications/document/9283316/

104. Speed reduction mechanisms. National Association of City Transportation Officials. Accessed June 17, 2024. https://nacto.org/publication/urban-street-design-guide/design-controls/design-speed/speed-reduction-mechanisms/
105. Notrica DM, Sayrs LW, Krishna N, Rowe D, Jaroszewski DE, McMahon LE. The impact of state laws on motor vehicle fatality rates, 1999–2015. *J Trauma Acute Care Surg*. 2020;88(6):760–769. doi:10.1097/ta.0000000000002686
106. Naumann RB, LaJeunesse S, Keefe E, et al. A novel Vision Zero leadership training model to support collaboration and strategic action planning. *Front Future Transp*. 2023;4:923786. doi:10.3389/ffutr.2023.923786
107. Johns Hopkins Bloomberg School of Public Health. Recommendations of the safe system consortium. 2023. https://publichealth.jhu.edu/sites/default/files/2023-03/recommendations-of-the-safe-system-consortium.pdf
108. National healthy housing standard. National Center for Healthy Housing. Updated January 29, 2020. https://nchh.org/tools-and-data/housing-code-tools/national-healthy-housing-standard/
109. American Public Health Association. Energy justice and climate change: key concepts for public health. 2024. https://apha.org/-/media/Files/PDF/topics/climate/Energy_Justice_Key_Concepts.ashx
110. Reynolds K, Allen E, Fedorowicz M, Ovalle J. Affordable housing investment a guide for nonprofit hospitals and health systems. Urban Institute. August 2019. https://www.urban.org/sites/default/files/publication/100774/affordable_housing_investment_a_guide_for_nonprofit_hospitals_and_health_systems_1.pdf
111. Rigolon A, Christensen J. Greening without gentrification: learning from parks-related anti-displacement strategies nationwide. UCLA Institute of the Environment and Sustainability. 2019. https://www.ioes.ucla.edu/wp-content/uploads/Greening-without-Gentrification-report-2019.pdf
112. Lincoln Institute of Land Policy. Equity in green infrastructure. January 2024. https://go.lincolninst.edu/Mattison_WP24NM1.pdf?_gl=1
113. UCLA Student Reports. Inclusive park design for people of all housing statuses: tools for restoring unhoused individuals' rights in public parks. June 16, 2023. https://escholarship.org/content/qt1f1619sk/qt1f1619sk.pdf?t=rwpccd&v=lg/#_page=2
114. Treuhaft S, Karpyn A. The grocery gap: who has access to healthy food and why it matters. PolicyLink. 2010. https://www.policylink.org/sites/default/files/FINALGroceryGap.pdf
115. American Public Health Association. Creating the healthiest nation: food justice. May 2022. https://apha.org/-/media/Files/PDF/advocacy/CHN_Food_Justice.ashx
116. Healthy Food Policy Project. Zoning for urban agriculture. March 2024. https://healthyfoodpolicyproject.org/key-issues/zoning-for-urban-agriculture
117. Hake M, Engelhard E, Dewey A. Map the meal gap 2023. A report on county and congressional district food insecurity and county food cost in the United States in 2021. Feeding America. 2023. Accessed June 17, 2024. https://www.feedingamerica.org/sites/default/files/2023-05/Map%20the%20Meal%20Gap%202023.pdf
118. The White House. Biden-Harris administration national strategy on hunger, nutrition, and health. 2022. https://www.whitehouse.gov/wp-content/uploads/2022/09/White-House-National-Strategy-on-Hunger-Nutrition-and-Health-FINAL.pdf

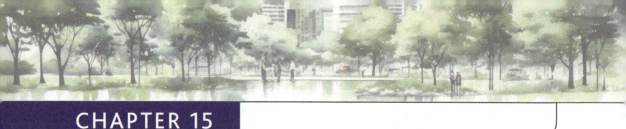

CHAPTER 15

Preparing for and Recovering From Disasters in Our Changing Climate

Mitch Stripling

LEARNING OBJECTIVES

- Understand how existing systems create vulnerability in some communities more than others, resulting in unequal disaster risks and impacts globally.
- Describe how climate change will make disaster risk worse by intensifying impacts and exploiting weaknesses in our physical and social infrastructure.
- Explain how the United States uses disaster frameworks focused on compensation for losses rather than maximization of health outcomes.
- Examine various global-risk reduction frameworks and critically consider their potential to improve the long-term ability of society to address disasters.
- Analyze how disasters make environmental injustice worse, and consider approaches that can lead us toward greater environmental justice.

KEY TERMS

- cascading failure
- collective continuance
- community resilience
- disaster risk
- disaster risk reduction
- disaster swarm
- immediate harm
- mindful muddling
- preparedness cycle
- public health disaster
- social determinants of health (SDOH)
- structural harm
- systems thinking
- vulnerability analysis

OVERVIEW

On September 20, 2017, Hurricane Maria struck Puerto Rico as the strongest storm to hit the island since 1928, with a death toll of nearly 3,000, property damage topping $90 billion, and more than 100,000 islanders displaced from their homes. Flood depths reached 15 feet. Of those fatalities, though, only a handful died directly from the floods. The rest were killed by **cascading failures**, in which the failure of one part of the system led to failures of other connected parts—an annihilated power grid, little clean water, limited medical service—and caused chaos as the infrastructure of modern life was struck down.[1]

In the field of disaster studies, Hurricane Maria is a classic example of a disaster: a devastating impact, to be followed by an immediate response and a long recovery (Case Study 15.1). After the disaster, the island inhabitants readied for the next event through the mitigation of key failures, such as implementing new building codes or a stronger electrical grid, and preparedness activities, such as drafting plans and training residents. These are the four classic phases of emergency management we expand on in this chapter: *response, recovery, mitigation,* and *preparedness*. In emergency plans, they imply a time of disaster (response, recovery) and a time of normality (mitigation, preparedness; Figure 15.1).

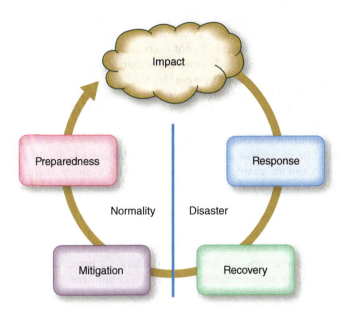

FIGURE 15.1. Emergency management cycle.
In this diagram, the disaster impact sets off a *response* phase, then *recovery*, leading back to normality. During normal periods, *mitigation* and *preparedness* work is done to be ready for the next impact.

This example assumes that Hurricane Maria was the beginning of the story. However, Hurricane Maria was preceded by decades of disinvestment in the territory of Puerto Rico, which still has an ambiguous legal status in the United States. ("A territory is just a nice word for a colony," as Audre Lorde said after she survived the ravages of Hurricane Hugo in 1989 on St. Croix.[2(p53)]) The electrical grid that was decimated during Maria was not up to U.S. mainland standards and had been cobbled together dozens of times after previous storms. Additionally, the island was trapped in an ongoing debt crisis, with high rates of poverty and unemployment, making it more susceptible to ongoing problems in the aftermath.

Hurricane Maria, unfortunately, was not the end of the story either. Afterward, mass protests prompted the resignation of the governor in 2019. Puerto Ricans had reason to hope that the national visibility from the hurricane might change their conditions. But then, in January of 2020, the earthquakes struck. Prompting building collapses and widespread closures of workplaces, schools, healthcare facilities, and government services, more than 250 earthquakes could be felt. In February of 2020, 62% of schools remained closed. Yarimar Bonilla, a Puerto Rican scholar, said that even 6 weeks after one major earthquake, "hundreds of make-shift encampments house the most vulnerable: the young, the elderly, those with special needs, and those with nowhere else to go."[3(p2)] Suicides spiked. Protests were more frequent, less hopeful, and angrier. A month after, in March of 2020, COVID-19 lockdowns began. COVID-19 would eventually kill almost 6,000 Puerto Ricans between 2020 and 2022, a death rate of 1 in 583.[4] This series of events reflects the "repeating disaster" of the Caribbean, according to Bonilla.[3] She explains:

> ... with economic crisis, imperial violence, hurricanes, earthquakes, toxic dumping, climate change, privatization, profiteering, and other forms of structural and systemic violence all acting as a disordered jumble upon a collective body that cannot discern a main event or a discrete set of impacts, only repetitive and enduring trauma.[3(p2)]

Traditional theories of emergency management define disasters as sudden, unexpected events that bring great destruction. As exceptional events, scholars and policy makers have argued, disasters demand exceptional resources and often exceptional ways of handling them. However, the idea of the **disaster swarm** is becoming increasingly familiar as we progress into the 21st century. Since 1980, the United States alone has suffered more than 340 disasters that each resulted in $1 billion or more in damages, toward a total cost of $2.5 trillion. Globally, in 2022 alone, nearly 400 disasters killed 30,000 people at a cost of $270 billion, impacting the lives of more than 185 million people.[5] These numbers do not account for the tens of thousands of small-scale disasters that occur each year, which cause more than 60% of *all* economic loss globally, nor the more than 15 million excess deaths caused by the COVID-19 pandemic, itself a disaster.[6] We are all now, or soon will be, living in the age of the *disaster swarm*, a mass of chronic and acute crises blending ecosystem harm, physical violence, and disparities with rapid impacts that lead to further harm.

Overall, this topic is a difficult and often sad one. **Disaster risk** and disaster impacts are driven by structural disparities based on race, class, and other factors. The impacts of climate change, unsustainable resource usage, and increasing inequity weaken these systems, increasing disaster risk. In turn, as our society is impacted by more and faster disaster events, those events weaken our systems further.

But there is hope in disasters, too. Referenced several times throughout this textbook, the founding principles of the environmental justice (EJ) movement—adopted in 1991 at the National People of Color Environmental Leadership Summit—include interdependence, mutual justice, a right to be free from environmental destruction, universal protection, and self-determination.[7] Taking these principles seriously means making a commitment to work through disasters in ways that enhance environmental and social justice rather than, as often happens, worsening injustices. As Bonilla states, reimagining disaster management requires us to stop focusing on damage repair after disasters and instead to learn from these tragedies and "re-envision the futures we wish to build."[3(p3)] We must adjust, as a planet, to this new era of the disaster swarm and honor these EJ principles in the process.

This chapter explains how we can recalibrate our disaster-management practices to prioritize EJ. We first explore the idea of a *public health disaster* with a consideration of the **social determinants of health (SDOH)**, or the conditions under which one is born and lives that affect a wide range of health outcomes. As we explore this idea with examples, public health disasters can be prompted by underlying inequities, and they can prompt cascading system failures. Then, we discuss how climate change and other factors are driving the swarm of these public health disasters. We examine our current frameworks for addressing these disasters in the United States, as well as the specific roles and responsibilities of environmental health practitioners. None of these frameworks fully embraces the tenets of EJ. So, at the end of this chapter, we explain how these tools should be adjusted to face our new reality.

CASE STUDY 15.1: 2017 Hurricane Maria Impact in Puerto Rico

As the Category 5 Hurricane Maria approached Puerto Rico, 80,000 people were still powerless from Hurricane Irma's strike 14 days before. The island was in a debt crisis, with a fragile power grid, uncertain water treatment, and high levels of both poverty and housing uncertainty. Its cache of emergency supplies was empty, having just been deployed to support storm recovery on other islands.

Maria landed as a strong Category 5 hurricane with a 32-mile-wide eye, giving it a vast area of supercharged wind and rain. Hundreds of thousands of homes were destroyed. Around 95% of cellular networks were down. No aspect of the power grid was spared. Landslides occurred throughout the island. A month later, only 8% of roads had reopened, most hospitals were still on limited backup generators, and half of the sewage treatment plants were not functioning. Helicopters were still required for many supply deliveries. Three months later, nearly half the population (1.5 million people) still had no power. Coffee and other agricultural crops were lost for the year, and growing capacity was impacted for multiple years. By the end of 2021, after impacts from a swarm of earthquakes, political uprisings, and the COVID-19 pandemic, only 1,651 homes had been repaired.[1,3,8–10]

The Puerto Rican government initially reported 64 deaths from Maria. However, the intensity of the damage combined with the ongoing lack of aid and services quickly rendered that

(continued)

> **CASE STUDY 15.1: 2017 Hurricane Maria Impact in Puerto Rico** (*continued*)
>
> number preposterous. Multiple competing analyses were completed, with multiple lawsuits filed. At the behest of the Governor of Puerto Rico, the Milken Institute School of Public Health at George Washington University analyzed the storm's aftermath using a mortality displacement model "in order to predict the expected mortality if Hurricane María had not occurred (predicted mortality) and compare this figure to the actual deaths that occurred (observed mortality)."[11(pi)] Mortality displacement models (also called excess death models) have become the most highly regarded ways of tracking mortality for environmental disasters, which often suffer from poor data collection. For Maria, the researchers estimated a death toll of between 2,658 and 3,290. Only a small number of these deaths were based on initial storm impacts. The rest were driven by lack of public health, basic healthcare, and an environmental health infrastructure in the long months after the storm.
>
> **REFLECTION QUESTION**
>
> 1. Do you agree that mortality displacement is a better way of capturing death rates in an environmental emergency than using death-certificate data? Why or why not?

DEFINING THE PUBLIC HEALTH DISASTER

CLASSIC DEFINITIONS

We can define **public health disasters** in different ways. Disaster research and, to some extent, practice have long focused on the nature of specific hazards. For example, the Integrated Research on Disaster Risk workgroup of the United Nations Office for Disaster Risk Reduction suggests the Sendai Hazard Definitions and Classifications Review, which provides a general overview of the type of hazard that generally initiates disasters (Table 15.1).[12] However, from the perspective of emergency managers, "all hazards" approaches focus less on specific hazards and more on the functions needed to respond to them, many of which are similar, whether dealing with a flood or an earthquake. What matters is the speed with which the disaster occurs, the likelihood of it occurring, and the extent of harm it causes (Table 15.2).[13] Each of the hazards in Table 15.1 (and its associated perils) correspond to different characteristics in Table 15.2. For example, an insect infestation may have a slow speed of onset and a longer time horizon. A wildfire could cover a large expanse of ground and may be over quickly. A pandemic may last for years, but goes through several infectious phases during that time.

Alternately, in their classic book *American Dunkirk*, about the water evacuation of hundreds of thousands from Manhattan after the 9/11 attacks on New York City, James Kendra and Tricia Wachtendorf look at the impacts of the disaster to define it, not its specific characteristics. Instead of using wind speed or earthquake strengths, they say, disasters involve "some notion of a social system being overwhelmed and unable to meet its needs, thus requiring assistance from elsewhere."[14(p22)] This definition is helpful but not sufficient. It implies that there is a distinction between *normality* and *disaster*, which our Puerto Rico example calls into question. Were things "normal" before that one terrible day?

TABLE 15.1. SUGGESTED LIST OF HAZARDS FOR THE PURPOSE OF MEASURING GLOBAL TARGETS OF THE SENDAI FRAMEWORK

BIOLOGICAL	ENVIRONMENTAL	NATURAL	ANTHROPOGENIC (HUMAN-CAUSED)
Animal incident Disease Insect infestation	Environmental degradation	Geophysical Hydrological Meteorological Climatological Extraterrestrial	Technological hazards Chemical and radiological hazards Major transportation accidents Explosions

We can do better in our conception of disaster harms and risks by considering two distinct categories: **immediate harm** and **structural harm,** as well as how these harms cascade through society. Some immediate harms of public health disasters are listed in Table 15.3.[15-19] These harms are likely familiar from the news media reports, and they show up frequently in disaster movies (e.g., *The Day After Tomorrow, Greenland,* and *San Andreas,* among countless others). Various hazards catalyze specific immediate harms. For instance, storms cause evacuations that can lead to an immediate or long-term lack of housing. Disasters also cause or worsen structural harms. For example, they can cause economic breakdowns that lead to economic

TABLE 15.2. DISASTER TYPOLOGY

CLASSIFICATION SYSTEM	DESCRIPTION
Speed of onset	How fast or slowly a disaster occurs (e.g., wildfires are rapid; hurricanes are comparatively slow)
Time horizon	How finite or more permanent a disaster is (e.g., earthquakes are time limited; pandemics have more sustained impacts)
Spatial concentration	How large or small the harm distribution (e.g., tornados have a narrow focus, while food contamination can spread widely)
Affected population needs	How similar or complex the disaster is (e.g., flooding is common and has well-documented impacts; a radiation incident creates complicated monitoring roles for humans and their environment)
Perceived probability of occurrence	Assumed to be less or more likely to happen (creates bias toward making the system less or more prepared; e.g., weather events are known and cyclical, human-caused events like bio-terrorism are harder to predict)
Perceived magnitude of occurrence	Anticipated amount of harm (affects how pre-event systems are prepared (e.g., heat waves are often perceived as minor events, while nuclear incidents can cause major infrastructure damage)

TABLE 15.3. SPECIFIC DISASTER HARMS

IMMEDIATE HARMS	BROADER SOCIAL DETERMINANTS OF HEALTH IMPACTS
• Death • Illness and injuries • Loss of clean water • Loss of shelter • Loss of personal and household goods • Loss of sanitation and routine hygiene • Disruption of solid waste management • Public concern for safety • Increased pests and vectors • Loss or damage to the healthcare system • Worsening of chronic illness • Food scarcity • Standing surface water • Toxic exposures • Secondary environmental damage • Psychological or behavioral damage • Spontaneous population movement (i.e., displacement)	• Economic infrastructure breakdown • Wage earner loss • Loss of power • Loss of communication infrastructure • Contamination of agriculture • Social cohesion impacts • Reduction in livelihood • Loss of meaning and purpose • Sustained educational impacts

depression, or they can contaminate agricultural areas to hinder long-term food production. They can produce anxiety or other mental health effects. Even when the harms are far reaching, they may be delayed, be seemingly unrelated to the disaster, and be overlooked by the media or government agency reports.

CASCADING DISASTERS

A little-understood feature of disasters is that they tend to cascade, typically making harms worse and inequitable. A disaster cascades either through:

1. setting off one or more secondary crises, often based on human systems being overwhelmed, or
2. when multiple hazards impact the same area within a short duration, causing interrelated harms.[20]

The 2011 Tohoku earthquake in Japan, which led to the Fukushima nuclear power plant failure, was an example of the first type of cascade.[21] Puerto Rico's disaster swarm of Hurricane Maria, earthquakes, and COVID-19 highlights what happens when communities experience multiple hazards in a short time. As Thomas makes clear, in these instances the suffering compounds.[20]

One disaster in one location can also ripple outward with harms that help us to see other disasters. As the Flint Water Crisis unfolded in 2014 and in the years that followed (Case Study 15.2), many reports concerning levels of lead contamination in other cities emerged. Largely related to aging infrastructure, paint in old homes, and contaminated soil from current or legacy industries, the lead contamination was ongoing but underreported. In another example of ripple effects, the U.S. response to COVID-19 caused structural harm. As healthcare systems redirected resources and routine care slowed, deaths by chronic diseases spiked. We also saw a 35% increase in gun deaths from both murders and suicides early in the pandemic.[22] In children, these issues corresponded to an estimated 733 additional deaths, nearly identical to the 752 children who died from COVID-19 in the same period.[23] The number of lives saved through public-health interventions was many times greater than these cascades of harm from COVID-19. Still, the equivalence of harm for children emphasizes that cascades matter, and again we see that suffering is often compounded.

CASE STUDY 15.2: 2014–2018 Flint, Michigan, Water Crisis

The city of Flint, Michigan, mandated that the city's water mains be laid with lead pipe in 1897, with water sourced from the nearby Flint River. In 1967, flush with cash from the postwar boom brought on by the auto industry, Flint switched to purchasing treated water from the Detroit Water and Sewage Department. By 2013, however, Flint was reeling from the fallout of the 2008 financial crisis and a sharp decline in local manufacturing. To save money, the city joined a consortium of cities in building a pipeline to bring down water from Lake Huron. So the city did not renew its long-term contract with Detroit; however, the pipeline was not built yet, and Detroit would not agree to a short-term contract with Flint. During this time, in 2011, Governor Rick Snyder stripped power from elected officials and installed an Emergency Manager, which led to the prioritization of cost savings over resident health. Flint brought its aged equipment back online and started doing something it had not done in almost 50 years: treating water from the Flint River and distributing it to residents, the majority of whom were of people of color and with low wealth.

Multiple officials shared their concerns, and the switch was never formally authorized, presumably because it was viewed as temporary. However, in May 2014, Flint switched the source water and the crisis began. Red water and discoloration suffused the system. Children were experiencing raised red welts on their skin. Water mains began to break. General Motors complained that the water was corroding its engines (never a good sign) and switched their water source, but the residents, already facing high levels of unemployment, could not.

(continued)

> **CASE STUDY 15.2: 2014–2018 Flint, Michigan, Water Crisis** (*continued*)
>
> *Escherichia coli* caused three boil-water alerts in 3 weeks that summer. Trihalomethane (more commonly known as TTHM)—a cancer-causing by-product of imbalanced water chlorination concentrations—broke regulatory limits too, which the state flagged as a violation of the Safe Drinking Water Act (SDWA). Blood lead levels in children shot up by a factor of 2.5; lead samples in the water were elevated for months, sometimes up to eight times the legal limit. Unbeknownst to officials at the time, people were also dying of *Legionella*, with 91 cases and 12 deaths from 2014 to 2015. Before the switch, in 2013, Flint had seen about nine cases. Residents took to the streets, demanding action, until officials consented to investigate.
>
> The water had not been treated correctly and it was corrosive, causing lead to leech from the pipes. Flint did not switch back to buying water from Detroit until October of 2015. Neither the city nor the state declared a state of emergency until after the water source had been switched back. In 2016, based on federal funding received as a result of these emergency declarations, the state of Michigan committed to replacing all lead pipes in Flint with upgraded copper pipes, a process that was still unfinished in mid-2023. During this long recovery period, bottled water was distributed to residents, support was given to health centers, and different types of water analysis were attempted. Multiple state officials were charged with crimes for their negligence, including involuntary manslaughter, though nearly all the charges were dismissed.
>
> However, there were cascading impacts beyond the water crisis. The disaster drove a crash in the Flint housing market and sharpened its economic downturn. The state of Michigan spent nearly $1 billion to contain the crisis, between funding infrastructure and a settlement for victims, on top of a $100 million investment by the U.S. Environmental Protection Agency. Moreover, the perceived likelihood of the issue of lead levels in water increased throughout the country, causing other cities to search for, and often find, contaminated water.
>
> The Flint experience shows how neglected infrastructure, in combination with environmental racism, can generate environmental emergencies. Almost a decade later, the infrastructure may have been repaired but, for many, the trust in city leadership and environmental agencies has not.[24–27]
>
> **REFLECTION QUESTION**
>
> 1. When did the emergency in Flint really begin? What was the root cause?

DISASTER RISKS

The concept of disaster risk also needs reconsideration. **Disaster risk** is the likelihood and scale of harm caused by a disaster's impacts. Structural disparities based on race, class, and other factors can worsen risk. Disaster sociologist Kathleen Tierney makes the point that, "the root causes of disasters are to be found in the social order itself—that is, in social arrangements that contribute to the buildup of risk and vulnerability."[28(p12)] In looking at a tsunami, for example, the commonsense thinking might be that the disaster is inherent in the force of rushing water. However, the risk is embedded within society's structures itself; that is, in how we have allowed buildings to be constructed, where we have allowed them to be placed, and the robustness of the medical systems we provide—structures and systems that were designed before the water ever strikes.

In this model, the causal agent of the disaster shifts. The disaster in a tsunami is caused by society's failure to protect certain people from a known hazard, allowing them to live in risky areas, and to establish systems to provide the immediate care they need. Absent the risks and vulnerabilities society has allowed, a tsunami is just a wave. In this sense, disasters are not—or are not *merely*—acute events. They are chronic failures built into societal structures waiting to emerge when prodded by an external force, whether natural, human caused, or pathogenic.[29]

REDEFINING A PUBLIC HEALTH DISASTER

Structural harm to our SDOH leads to disasters, which then inflicts more harm against the underlying SDOH.[30] For our purposes then, a *public health disaster* is an impact that overwhelms a social system, whatever the cause, and causes harm to the underlying structure that supports human health and flourishing. Crucially, it encompasses all those current public health issues in the present with the potential to allow or provoke those consequences when triggered by an external hazard.

This definition is nonlinear. It assumes that the disasters of the future are with us now—in the inequities we allow today—that future incidents will weaponize against us.

IMPACTS OF CLIMATE CHANGE

Unfortunately, part of the reason we need to reestablish the definition of a public health disaster at this moment, is that climate change is moving us further into the world of Bonilla's disaster swarm. As discussed in Chapter 3, "Confronting the Realities of Climate Change," climate change will increase both the frequency and intensity of these disasters. Hurricanes in the Atlantic Ocean, for example, are likely to be both more intense and likely to make landfall. For example, recent studies have shown that tropical cyclone precipitation rates are likely to increase by 7% per degree Celsius of warming. Climate change helped to supercharge the intense 2020 hurricane season, increasing the amount of rain that extreme hurricanes dumped in three hours by 11% on people who live in communities at risk. That is the equivalent of another heavy storm and enough to lead to regional flooding.[31] Furthermore, vector-borne and zoonotic diseases like malaria, dengue, and Lyme disease could see increased spread. Cases of foodborne illnesses like *Salmonella* are on the rise as temperatures increase. Increased ozone concentrations in the air, which we often see with heat, drive mortality events too, as discussed in more detail in Chapter 10, "The Air We Breathe."[32] Yet, this intensification is not the whole story.

First, *these increases are differential*, meaning that they vary substantially around the world and between populations. Even with just 1.5 degree Celsius of warming, for example, the Intergovernmental Panel on Climate Change (IPCC) predicts that "twice-per-century" heat events could happen every 6 years. These events will hit some areas harder than others. Residents of the Pacific Northwest, never threatened by extreme heat, saw their thermometers hit 116 degrees Fahrenheit in 2021, a "once-in-a-millennium" event that they could now experience every 10 years if current climate trajectories continue (Case Study 15.3).[33] It is not just geographic impacts that are different, though. The IPCC has found that disasters related to climate change make existing inequalities worse. Women and children, for example, are 14 times more likely to die or be injured in a disaster than men. These harms too cascade. For example, 71% of Bangladeshi women have experienced violence during disaster recovery.[34] In the United States, a systematic review showed the intense physical and mental toll these climate-driven disasters take on marginalized populations including older adults, individuals of lower wealth, and institutionalized people—a toll that lingers, often prevents full recovery, and mounts over time with various impacts.[18]

Second, *climate change will lead to more cascading failures*. For example, in 2020 the World Bank estimated that climate change could pull 100 million people into poverty by 2030, based on impacts to agricultural productivity, food prices, lowering of labor productivity, increases in childhood and chronic diseases, and other increased losses from natural disasters.[35] Climate change lowers agricultural productivity, for example, and prompts additional droughts and floods, which lower that productivity still further. Because we know that more communities who are already at increased risk from structural inequalities do worse in natural disasters, a vicious cycle occurs.

CASE STUDY 15.3: 2021 Northwest Heat Wave

Mondays are always busy at the Harborview Emergency Medical Center in downtown Seattle. The Monday of June 28, 2021, started off much worse: Beds were short, staff were burned out from more than a year of battling COVID-19, and the last two days had been the hottest in the city's history, topping out at 104°F. Area hospitals were struggling. One had lost power. Another's lab had gone down. That Monday would be the hottest day in Seattle's history, hitting 108°F.

Heat injuries are cumulative. Day by day they compound if the temperature does not break, and that Monday Harborview saw a hundredfold increase in heat injury patients. Many died prior to arrival; one paramedic showed the burns on his knees from intubating heat stroke patients for hours on end. The region saw 3,500 emergency department visits for heat injury, with 400 known deaths in a four-state region and a thousand more in Canada. Until this event, no one had ever seen a temperature record broken by 10 full degrees.

Heat waves produce significant direct mortality, but their other environmental impacts can be overlooked. The air quality index (AQI) in Los Angeles during this heat wave reached 760 on a scale only designed to reach 500, meaning that air pollution was literally off the charts. Chronic care patients were hit hard, as ambulance wait time skyrocketed, and the heat contributed to strange medication interactions. Electrical consumption soared as residents rushed to buy air conditioners, prompting rolling power outages in Spokane. Sidewalks buckled, and melting roads had to be closed. Workers without air conditioning walked off their jobs. Cherry, blackberry, and other crops were lost. More than a billion seashore animals were essentially boiled to death.

The heat contributed to substantial fires as well, burning hundreds of thousands of acres, leading to evacuations and more service closures. The First Nation's settlement of Lytton in British Columbia was burned to the ground. Floods came too. There was rapid glacier melt, closing roads and flooding towns throughout British Columbia. Diseases spiked as well, as *Vibrio* bacteria levels in oysters rose and the people eating them were sickened.

These downstream impacts, which produced healthcare effects for months, show how environmental disasters cause cascading failures that impact every aspect of society. Over and over again, health officials emphasize how preventable heat wave deaths are. Regionwide emergency plans continue to improve. They have evolved to include better warning systems, more effective ambulance routing, and stronger communications and social services, including ensuring that vulnerable residents can be checked on and supported outside of medical centers. Many jurisdictions also provide free or discounted air conditioners to those without them. This air conditioner program is important for human health but ironic, considering that the units contribute to climate change and make these events worse.[33,36–39]

REFLECTION QUESTION

1. Can you think of ways to halt or slow some of the cascading impacts from an event like this 2021 heat wave?

MANAGING PUBLIC HEALTH DISASTERS

In the face of this vicious cycle of disaster swarm, what is it that we should attempt to do? How is true recovery possible in these conditions? As noted, disasters produce both immediate and structural harms. These harms disrupt a community's ability to function in various ways. The goal of any kind of public-health disaster readiness is to limit these disruptions and ensure that communities recover their strength *or even build back better* after a disaster.

Disaster readiness, response, and recovery can be effectively understood and managed through a systems-thinking model. **Systems thinking** is a holistic approach that views problems and solutions as interconnected pieces of a larger system. When applied to disaster management, the approach helps in understanding the complexity of disasters, their causes, and the various factors involved in preparedness and recovery. The first step in systems thinking in disasters is to identify the key components within the system, which may include vulnerabilities and available resources, as well as the root causes of the components, like structural inequalities that lead to vulnerability. The next step is to understand how these pieces of the system are interconnected and what feedback loops exist that can be both positive (like education training) and negative (like limited resources). Collaborating with partners like affected communities, healthcare providers, and emergency responders, among others, to understand how systems work leads to continuous learning and improvement.

Globally, there are many approaches for public-health disaster management. It is a complex field, and those leading the work must continue to critically evaluate large-scale management decisions in our new era of crisis. They must return to these two questions: How effective will their approach be in the era of the disaster swarm? Do they manage disasters in ways that improve EJ?

THE PUBLIC HEALTH AND ENVIRONMENTAL HEALTH ROLE

To understand better what public health does regarding emergency preparedness before, during, and after an event, it is helpful to look at both the areas that the Public Health Emergency Preparedness Program at the U.S. Centers for Disease Control and Prevention (CDC) focuses on (Figure 15.2) and the 15 capabilities that they developed. The capabilities are a framework for state, local, Tribal, and territorial preparedness programs to evaluate their ability to plan for, respond to, and recover from emergencies (Table 15.4).

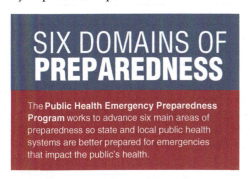

Community resilience: Preparing for and recovering from emergencies

Incident management: Coordinating an effective response

Information management: Making sure people have information to take action

Countermeasures and mitigation: Getting medicines and supplies where they are needed

Surge management: Expanding medical services to handle large events

Biosurveillance: Investigating and identifying health threats

www.cdc.gov/cpr/readiness

FIGURE 15.2. Six domains of preparedness.

Source: Six domains of preparedness. Centers for Disease Control and Prevention. Updated October 6, 2020. https://www.cdc.gov/orr/readiness/sixdomains.htm

TABLE 15.4. DOMAINS AND ASSOCIATED CAPABILITIES FOR PUBLIC HEALTH EMERGENCY PREPAREDNESS AND RESPONSE

DOMAIN	CAPABILITY
Community resilience	Community preparedness
	Community recovery
Incident management	Emergency operations coordination
Information management	Emergency public information
	Information sharing
Countermeasures and mitigation	Medical countermeasure dispensing and administration
	Medical material management and distribution
	Nonpharmaceutical interventions
	Responder safety and health
Surge management	Fatality management
	Mass care
	Medical surge
	Volunteer management
Biosurveillance	Public health laboratory testing
	Public health surveillance and epidemiologic investigation

Source: Adapted from *Public health emergency preparedness and response capabilities*. Centers for Disease Control and Prevention. 2018. Updated April 23, 2024. https://www.cdc.gov/readiness/php/capabilities/index.html

In general, these domains and capabilities rely on the environmental health activities discussed throughout this book, for example, surveillance, information management, and mitigation techniques like nonpharmaceutical interventions (e.g., masking, distancing guidance).

There is a common refrain among practitioners that public environmental health work during disaster response is just "public health on steroids." Many tasks are much like the daily work of practitioners. The CDC's *Environmental Health Training in Emergency Response* (EHTER) courses, for example, cover many standard issues like water safety; food safety; wastewater; building assessments; vectors and pests; and solid waste and debris.[40] There are some specific tasks in these areas, though, that require new or adjusted skills worth describing in more detail.

Considering Social Determinants of Health

As we have seen, SDOH are quite broad and are broadly impacted after public health disasters. The CDC has rightly asked for public health responders to consider SDOH during disaster phases by, for example, incorporating them into community **vulnerability analyses** and connecting them to the 10 Essential Public Health Services. This important task is complicated, though. Response goals like minimizing social disruption or accelerating recovery likely mean different choices than another essential response goal of ensuring equity. The first two goals require a quicker return to normalcy; the third requires different operations, resources, and perspectives because it is a goal to improve SDOH. The SDOH mission is tricky for pragmatic reasons too, because many areas influencing SDOH are managed by other people involved in the the disaster-management enterprise who have vastly different expertise from environmental health practitioners, such as economists or representatives from law enforcement.

In addition, we know that public health disasters overwhelmingly make underlying inequities worse, and governmental responses tend to reinforce those inequities, not improve them.[29] During the COVID-19 pandemic, jurisdictions across the country were quick to realize that if they focused only on the medical impacts of COVID-19 without addressing the SDOH, it would create substantial harm. Instead, public health authorities used an SDOH framework to push for changes in areas such as home evictions, child tax credits, and unemployment benefits. These changes allowed jurisdictions to respond to impacts across the social determinants, both those caused directly by COVID-19 and those made worse by stay-at-home orders. However, in New York City, the enforcement of efforts like social distancing was still heavily racialized, with only 7% of those arrested being White, even as people of color were disproportionately contracting and dying of the virus.[41] In data from the Kaiser Family Foundation, as of mid-2022 age-standardized death rates showed that American Indian and Alaska Native (AIAN), Hispanic, Asian, Native Hawaiian and Other Pacific Islander (NHOPI), and Black people were about twice as likely to die from COVID-19 as their White counterparts.[42] A study on these disparities in Black populations found that the relationship between race and COVID-19 disappeared when key SDOH were accounted for.[43] These disparities are preventable, as the study illustrates.[43]

EQUITY AND JUSTICE IN DISASTER MANAGEMENT

Over time, the United States has adopted various ways to manage what we call **public health disasters,** and it is important to understand underlying the implications of disaster management for equity and justice. In *The Sympathetic State*, legal scholar Michele Dauber reviewed the history of U.S. disaster relief and concluded that the underlying ethic for domestic-disaster response was not justice or even "relief," but restitution. That means that disaster relief did not evolve to provide aid, but only to restore verified losses back to the status quo. As she writes:

> [T]here is a direct relationship in the American context between the ability to represent a loss as blameless and the amount of aid that can be claimed. It is far better when requesting federal funds to be standing hip deep in water than to be standing in an unemployment line. That is not because we have two different logics for resolving claims on public resources, an openhanded one for disaster victims and a skeptical one for the needy. We have one logic that sorts claimants into more or less generous systems depending on their ability to demonstrate that their deprivation is not their own fault.[44(p162)]

Another way to say it: Many frameworks discuss disaster aid as a way to bring justice or, at least, humanitarian aid that leads to improved welfare for recipients. However, even though many heroic responders strive to make life better for disaster victims, in this country our management approach has been based on the idea of making things exactly the way they were before.

As one example, a 2022 study by ProPublica and the Times-Picayune showed that federal authorities calculated the housing rebuilding costs after Hurricane Katrina in 2005 partially based on the prestorm value of the house, not just on how much it would cost to rebuild that house.[45] This meant that victims in higher poverty areas often did not get sufficient funds to rebuild their properties. Though this policy is no longer used, it speaks to the underlying model of federal disaster assistance. Victims do not receive what they need to achieve a just recovery, but rather (in theory) only enough to regain their prestorm status quo. This generally means that wealthy or middle-class homeowners receive significantly more in aid than poor households, which are generally households of color in more at-risk areas. Federal and state governments often put in place many other supplementary grants or aid mechanisms to offset this logic, but they rarely change the underlying calculus.

Disaster-management practice is slowly evolving to consider issues of equity and justice. We look briefly at these frameworks to understand opportunities for EJ: crisis response, the disaster preparedness cycle, community resilience, and disaster risk reduction. All of them are currently in use in various ways. They often overlap, even within the same location or for the same incident. We discuss how they function, their relevant policy aspects, and how they do or do not align with the EJ principles discussed earlier in this chapter.

CRISIS RESPONSE

Domestically, the oldest known disaster aid was given by Congress to Portsmouth, New Hampshire, after a fire in 1802. The aid provided relief from bond payments to city residents. This amount of aid was small. Yet it highlights how U.S. disaster response was based on a federalist system, with state governments taking primary responsibility for emergencies and disasters. Impacted towns request assistance from counties (generally) that, in turn, request assistance from the states. States then can request various forms of assistance from the federal government.

Actions taken directly in response to a public health disaster are part of a *crisis response framework*. Most U.S. crisis-response efforts are governed by the Robert T. Stafford Disaster Relief and Emergency Assistance Act (The Stafford Act) passed in 1989 and last amended in 2021. The Stafford Act is used, on average, each week within the United States and covers two types of incidents: minor emergencies and major disasters. It provides both public assistance and individual assistance during disasters. President Trump engaged Section 501b clause of the Stafford Act to declare the COVID-19 pandemic a "nationwide emergency" in 2020. This was the first time that the Stafford Act had been used to declare a nationwide emergency; the declaration invited governors and territorial leaders to request major disaster declarations, which they all subsequently did. It also marked the first time the "major disaster" clause had been used for any infectious disease agent.[46]

Separately, Section 319 of the Public Health Service Act gives the federal Secretary of Health the authority to declare a public health emergency (PHE) when:

- a disease or disorder presents a PHE; or
- a PHE, including significant outbreaks of infectious disease or bioterrorist attacks, otherwise exists.[47]

The federal government has declared PHEs for hurricanes like Katrina, Sandy, and Maria; infectious diseases like H1N1, Zika, and SARS-CoV-2 (the virus that causes COVID-19); and broader health concerns such as the national opioid crisis.[48]

Declared disasters and PHEs prompt substantial coordinated action, generally managed by versions of the Incident Command System (ICS), a paramilitary management model developed to combat California wildfires in the 1970s. Through coordinative structures called Emergency Operations Centers (EOCs), government leaders gather to make decisions. During the COVID-19 pandemic, for example, the PHE designation helped to ensure insurance coverage for COVID-19 services and testing, telehealth usage, and billions of dollars in aid to states and localities for their public health efforts.

Alignment With Environmental Justice

These crisis response actions are important because disaster and PHE declarations provide meaningful help and support to victims. However, the disasters are generally treated as unprecedented, urgent, and somehow disconnected from "normal" reality. They rely on what we explained earlier as outmoded "natural" ideas of public health disasters, rather than on the idea that their impacts are constructed by societal risk. Philosopher Kyle Whyte describes this as *crisis epistemology*, a way of "knowing the world in such a way that a certain present is experienced as new."[49(p52)] This way of viewing disasters also rarely accounts for, focuses on, or changes the underlying discriminatory structures that drive disasters—exactly those structures that must change to achieve EJ. Addressing public health disasters only within crisis-response frameworks often leads to unjust outcomes.

> **IN OTHER WORDS: CRISIS EPISTEMOLOGY**
>
> Did you know that during emergencies the brain's processing capacity drops substantially? It is hard to see the past or the future because the focus is on staying alive or minimizing the damage in your community or home. That is what *crisis epistemology* can be like—decisions are made in the moment in reaction to events without considering the past. These decisions may help you to avoid immediate danger, but not to think and plan long term.

DISASTER PREPAREDNESS CYCLE

During the Civil Defense period in the 1950s, when the United States prepared for potential nuclear war with the Union of Soviet Socialist Republics, the idea of the **preparedness cycle** took shape. It advanced the idea of crisis response. This cycle attempts a set of activities to make communities ready for public health disasters in advance and to connect those activities to a better crisis response. The classic preparedness cycle moves a given system through a version of these phases (defined according to the Federal Emergency Management Agency [FEMA] curriculum)[50]:

- **Mitigation:** Includes any activities that prevent an emergency, reduce the chance of an emergency happening, or reduce the damaging effects of unavoidable emergencies.
- **Preparedness:** Includes plans or preparations made to save lives and to help response-and-rescue operations.
- **Response:** Includes actions taken to save lives and prevent further property damage in an emergency.
- **Recovery:** Includes actions taken to return to a normal or, possibly, a safer situation following an emergency.

The Stafford Act also provides for FEMA to have a coordinating role in these disaster-preparedness activities around the country under its Titles 2 and 6. One recent study shows the value of these preparedness efforts, estimating, in particular, that FEMA's Emergency Management Performance Grant (EMPG) program (which provides money for all-hazards efforts such as planning and training) "generates economic returns, in the form of avoided damage, with a range of 3–5 dollars on average [per dollar spent] and even higher in coastal counties, of 14–27 dollars."[51(p16)]

Similarly, multiple enhancements have been made to public health statutes to emphasize preparedness, though, if anything, this field has been in greater flux. The graphic from Jennifer Horney (Figure 15.3) describes the relationship between public health incidents from the turn of the 21st century until today. Measuring the success of these systemic-preparedness efforts has proved difficult. One high-profile effort, the Global Health Security Index (which assessed factors like preparedness planning, training, and capacity), failed rather spectacularly. A higher score on this index (indicating a country was more prepared) actually correlated with higher numbers of COVID-19

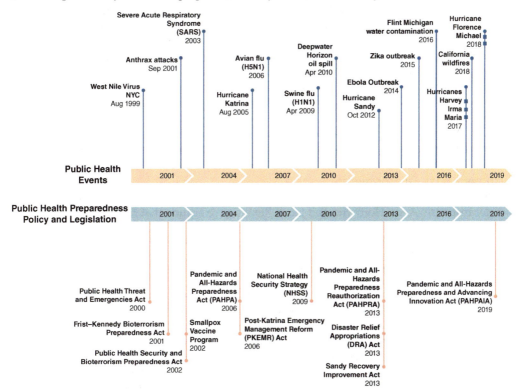

FIGURE 15.3. Public health events and corresponding policy and legislation.

Source: Adapted from Horney J. The public health emergency preparedness and response system: a comprehensive review. Paper commissioned by the Committee on Evidence-Based Practices for Public Health Emergency Preparedness and Response. Unpublished. 2019.

cases and deaths in multiple studies.[52] Partly, this is an artifact of the fact that the United Nation's Human Development Index (HDI)—which measures factors like life expectancy and education—also correlated with higher COVID-19 deaths. Still, the situation seems a bit backwards.

Alignment With Environmental Justice

making plans and providing training and exercises can improve a systemic response to disasters, but they do not make the underlying systems more functional. Activities categorized as "mitigation" within the preparedness cycle framework (e.g., building seawalls, installing backup generators) can be helpful, but they still do not address the community-function elements or the structural discrimination that drives EJ issues. It may be better than crisis response, but it is still just working around the edges.

Ethicist Naomi Zack emphasizes the moral duty society owes to prepare *before* a disaster. She warns against crisis thinking in which leaders prioritize "saving the greatest number" over "saving all who can be saved." For example, planning elements like Crisis Standards of Care were adopted in some hospitals during COVID-19 that anticipated having to make hard choices based on scarce resources or staff, such as how to allocate ventilators. Planning ahead can support more ethical decision-making.

COMMUNITY-RESILIENCE FRAMEWORKS

In the last few years, and particularly as we wrestle with complex events like Hurricane Maria and COVID-19, more officials have advocated for use of a **community resilience** framework. Preparedness approaches attempt to make systems more prepared for public health disasters through activities like training or mitigation projects, hardening systems against disaster impacts from the outside. Community-resilience approaches attempt to better center and support existing community systems.

Community resilience is defined in the CDC's 2008 *Ethical Guidance for Public Health Emergency Preparedness and Response* as "the capacity of a (natural or social) system to absorb external disturbances without losing its essential continuity and coherence."[x(p40)] If a community is resilient, it aims to support hyperlocal social services and private sector enterprises so that it can continue operating in the face of public health disasters, lessening the need for an outside crisis response. Both the federal Department of Health and Human Services and the CDC promote programs that seek to support local social services in public health disasters.

Connections both within a community and between that community and its political power structures have real impact.[17,18] Daniel Aldrich and his colleagues studied resilience early in the COVID-19 pandemic. His team found, persuasively, that bridging social capital (i.e., creating strong links between different groups) could reduce the spread of COVID-19.[17,32,35]

Alignment With Environmental Justice

EJ calls for us to remove discriminatory structures, not strive to bounce back to them as part of disaster response. Andy Horowitz and Jacob Remes have argued that resilience is:

> *A thoroughly political concept: it asserts the goals of a community's response to a disaster—conservative goals, to be sure, as "resilient" means a durable status quo—and also creates the conditions in which the community attempts to reach those goals.*[53(p3)]

In their emphasis on returning to a preexisting status, resilience frameworks implicitly serve those who are better off, not those who were already struggling.

Also, resilience is not designed as a "positive-sum game," and the same policies and practices that increase resilience in some components of a system may decrease resilience in others.[54] That is, by focusing on recovering the "essential continuity and coherence" of any given community, resilience will enrich or protect some communities at the expense of others. Again, COVID-19 provides an example. Lower-income workers were forced to travel from their own "less resilient" communities to work in service jobs so that wealthier people could successfully stay home in their own "more resilient" communities.[55] This discrepancy between communities led to higher rates of mortality for the travelling workers. The resilience of some communities can be sacrificed to improve the resilience of others in a phenomenon called *parasitic resilience*.[a]

DISASTER RISK-REDUCTION FRAMEWORKS

Globally, the last decades have seen a notable shift from disaster management toward disaster risk reduction. According to the United Nations Office for Disaster Risk Reduction, applying a **disaster risk reduction (DRR)** framework means focusing on prevention of new disasters, decrease of current risks, and management of any remaining risks.[56] The underlying goals are to strengthen resilience and achieve sustainability. DRR frameworks improve upon community resilience frameworks in two ways.

First, DRR is explicitly connected to sustainable development goals, which call for ongoing community improvements. DRR does not accept the status quo. The connection between DRR and sustainable development is not accidental. Many countries and international organizations, in particular the United Nations and the Organisation for Economic Co-operation and Development, advocate for policies that consider sustainable development, climate change adaptation, and DRR in an integrated approach.[57] DRR was officially first called for in the Hyogo Framework for Action in 2005 and is currently governed by the United Nations' Sendai Framework for Disaster Risk Reduction, which is in effect through 2030.

Second, the DRR framework more fully considers SDOH. Its explicit goal is to "prevent new and reduce existing disaster risk through the implementation of integrated and inclusive economic, structural, legal, social, health, cultural, educational, environmental, technological, political and institutional measures."[58(p12)] FEMA and the CDC might analyze community measures holistically, but their interventions will generally be focused on specific disaster readiness, such as hospital preparation or flood mitigation. By contrast, the global DRR framework has realized that the most powerful interventions to reduce disaster risk are not "disaster specific" at all but are aimed at core human issues like poverty alleviation, stable infrastructure, and good governance. Global DRR frameworks have been able to connect these baseline interventions to disaster risk in a way not yet accomplished in the United States.

Alignment With Environmental Justice

Although the DRR framework addresses some of the problematic aspects of community resilience, such as returning to a (possibly unjust) status quo, it still does not fully account for the drivers of injustice. DRR still considers community resilience. However, it shows that vulnerability and resilience are created by policy choices grounded in interdependence between communities. In short, disaster vulnerability is produced by society, but DRR is only focused on the effects, not the cause. DRR frameworks might argue that a community should alleviate flood risk, for example. However, it would not focus on changing the flow of money that generated the poverty that required the community to be located in a flood-prone area in the first place. Even DRR cannot likely achieve EJ in the age of the disaster swarm without additional systems' change.

HOW DO WE DO BETTER IN THE ERA OF THE DISASTER SWARM?

There are many definitions of EJ, for many purposes, by many people. Here is a simple one from the philosophers Kristie Dotson and Kyle Whyte:

> Environmental justice seeks fairness in how environmental burdens and risks are visited on poor people, women, communities of color, Indigenous Peoples, minorities, and citizens of developing countries. It also concerns whether members of these same groups have fair access to environmental goods such as urban green spaces, forested areas, and clean water.[59(p1)]

---

[a] Parasitic resilience is defined and expanded on in the article "Parasitic Resilience: The Next Phase of Public Health Preparedness Must Address Disparities Between Communities" in the *Journal of Health Security* by Mitch Stripling and Jordan Pascoe, December, 2023.

None of the public health disaster-management strategies we have reviewed so far can achieve this ideal. None of them work to undo the deep societal structures that prevent us from creating and sustaining fairness. Undoing these structures requires fundamental changes in how we approach public-health disaster risk.[b]

STRIVING FOR COLLECTIVE CONTINUANCE

First, the underlying focus would need to shift from "recovery" or "resilience" to what the philosopher Whyte calls **collective continuance.** In his work on Indigenous climate adaptation, Whyte defines this idea as "a community's aptitude for being adaptive in ways sufficient for the livelihoods of its members to flourish into the future."[60(p602)] Note that collective continuance is not a phase of preparedness, like recovery, nor a hard-and-fast status quo, like resilience. For Whyte, collective continuance is a marker of the health of an interdependent system made from "relationships and responsibilities" between humans as well as between humans and the environment.

To achieve collective continuance, public-health disaster work could no longer treat vulnerability as a characteristic of specific communities but, instead, as a result of ongoing structural discrimination. Just as modern disaster management works to improve a failing disaster grid so that it will survive the next storm, emergency practitioners would unpack and address the structural roadblocks that create disparities that end up making public health disasters so much worse. The revised goal is now not to return a community to its precrisis state, but to recognize interdependence between communities and make sure everyone affected can flourish after a disaster. This new goal is forward looking, not backward looking like current restitution-based recovery frameworks.

IN OTHER WORDS: COLLECTIVE CONTINUANCE

Unlike crisis epistemology, *collective continuance* always keeps the endgame in mind, even if that endgame is a human civilization flourishing a thousand years in the future. It means that decisions made in the moment must serve the future too.

As an example, most disaster responses bring in huge numbers of federal contractors and military personnel, who work quickly but are extremely expensive. Communities have found that they are sometimes unfamiliar with local values, are unfriendly, and are inflexible in letting local neighborhoods use resources to manage their own recoveries the way they want to, ultimately making these communities weaker. However, collective continuance does not mean giving up immediate, lifesaving responses. Instead, it guides the response in a way that sets up affected communities for a more hopeful future, not one that is just living from emergency to emergency.

THE ROLE OF MUTUAL AID IN DISASTERS

Mutual aid entails communities uniting to confront a common issue through both resource sharing and advocacy for systems change. Mutual aid is *not* charity but an approach wherein everyone plays their part in collective care. In the spirit of *mindful muddling*, mutual aid networks often mobilize during disasters to fill gaps where government systems have fallen short or failed, particularly in ways that have harmed historically marginalized communities.

Mutual aid has existed for centuries but became more well known early in the COVID-19 pandemic with the emergence of countless local mutual-aid response groups across the United States. During a time of deep uncertainty and disconnect, communities rallied to ensure that their neighbors' basic needs could be met through community-initiated interventions for child care, transportation, and food delivery, for instance.

(continued)

---

[b] Jordan Pascoe and Mitch Stripling expand on these arguments in their book *The Epistemology of Disasters and Social Change: Pandemics, Protests, and Possibilities* (2024) from Rowman & Littlefield.

A quick search of "mutual aid" on social media will yield hundreds of such networks. In New Orleans, for instance, powerful examples include Mutual Aid New Orleans and Imagine Water Works' Mutual Aid Response Network.

To learn more, read Dean Spade's *Mutual Aid: Building Solidarity During this Crisis (and the Next)*. Verso Books; 2020.

MINDFUL MUDDLING: SUPPORTING SELF-MANAGED RESPONSE

The underlying structure of our disaster frameworks must shift from their current top-down approach. Even disaster risk reduction, our current best model, generally functions by imposing the external beliefs of external command structures onto disaster communities. Whyte argues that, although this thinking is well intentioned, it emerges from a settler-colonialist mindset, which erases the real needs and strengths of impacted communities.[61]

Disaster scholarship shows how impractical top-down approaches actually are in disaster response. In *American Dunkirk*, Kendra and Watchtendorf showed how crisis response frameworks like ICS can easily fail to accomplish coordinated centralization during emergencies. In their extensive research on New York City's response to the terrorist attacks on 9/11, for example, they documented "thousands" of responding organizations, orders of magnitude more than the dozen that appeared in official reports.[62] They recommend **mindful muddling,** which is a much more decentralized system that may be realistically fragmented but allows for self-managed response toward an aligned set of goals.[14] Note that this system does not take away the responsibility of larger governmental structures—it just obliges them to provide resources to impacted communities in more trusting, decentralized ways. Everybody helps and everyone responds.

HOPEFUL PESSIMISM: RETHINKING "NORMAL TIME" AND "DISASTER TIME"

Disaster management must abandon its core division between "normal time" and "disaster time"—this idea from the preparedness cycle that there is a long era in which we get ready and a focused period of response. Accepting the interdependency of human populations and their environments means that we are all one complex social-ecological system. In the disaster swarm, some aspect of that system will always be facing an impact or recovering from one, learning to adapt to one or predicting another. All parts of the cycle will be happening, all at once. This picture is not a hopeful one. To Bonilla, in writing about Puerto Rico, it has meant giving up the "modernist assumptions of a better future"[63(p156)] that are part of the idea of a linear progression from response to recovery.

At the same time, understanding that disasters are always with us means accepting the responsibility for reducing future disaster risk even while we are responding to a current disaster. This idea helps ground the decisions we make during disaster impacts in collective continuance. In other words, even in the heat of a disaster impact, we cannot make decisions just for the moment, but always with our interdependent future in mind. Figure 15.4 shows the logic model developed by the global health experts at ICAP at Columbia University and adopted by the New York City Pandemic Response Institute. This model is not meant to be linear, in the manner of the four emergency management phases; rather it shows interlocking cycles of learning, with the idea that communities and populations may be preparing for, responding to, or working to prevent future impacts all the time, all at once.

This change means that during a crisis, there is no more "but it's an emergency" excuse for making some workers suffer more than others (as in COVID-19) or to address short-term issues at the expense of sustainable infrastructure (as in Hurricane Maria) or valuing property based on preexisting socioeconomic structures (as in Hurricane Katrina). A response cannot involve quickly bringing in outside contractors that destroy local economies (as in Alaska) or cutting

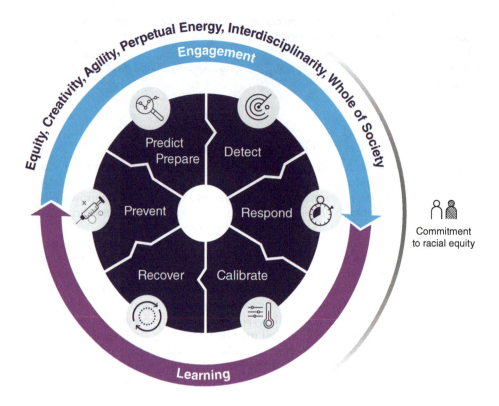

FIGURE 15.4. A nonlinear public-health disaster readiness model.

In this figure, the various phases are likely happening simultaneously in different parts of the world, creating nonlinear responses that should be oriented toward the future.

Source: ICAP @ Columbia University, 2022 NY, NY.

corners on safe, long-term infrastructure (as in Flint) based on the excuse of short-term urgency. This change does not mean that the impacts will stop coming, whether they are weather events or chemical spills. These hazards are unfortunately baked into both the reality of climate change and the nature of our high-risk approach to environmental extraction. However, in this nonlinear model, we understand that these horrors have occurred before; they will happen again. Disasters are neither unusual nor unprecedented. Our responsibility is not to make things the way they were before, but to responsibly support human flourishing in each moment by strengthening relationships, rebuilding sustainably, and ensuring communities that are able to adapt and grow continuously throughout periods of turmoil.

In the climate-change-driven era of Bonilla's disaster swarm, environmental health practitioners must reframe public health disaster work toward collective continuance, decentralized coordination, and an ongoing, nonlinear approach that never rests or assumes things should be put back the way they were before. It is an approach that always works to create communities based on environmental sustainability not environmental dominance, and that consistently focuses on the holistic experience of being human. Bonilla calls this approach *hopeful pessimism*, in that it has given up on the dream that there is some kind of perfect future, but, at the same time, gives all of us an "engine for worldmaking."[63(p161)] To give the last word to Bonilla, "this kind of hopeful pessimism forces us to recognize the hard tasks that must be taken on in order to transform the here and now to hopefully make our world anew."[63(p162)]

> **IN OTHER WORDS: HOPEFUL PESSIMISM**
>
> What is *hopeful pessimism*, and is it really so sad? It is really about giving up a story of one dominant rise to glory of civilization always becoming more modern. In other words, it allows a new kind of creativity; the idea that a new kind of future for the planet can be built. In one of Bonilla's examples, performance artist Macha Colón, said it this way, "[Hurricane Maria] allowed people to explore things that they couldn't do, now they realize that they can do it, and who the heck is going to tell them no? . . . it was sort of like we could do things without having to ask permission."[63(p160)] This part of disaster-management work is to keep this freedom safe and use it as the ground for a future that improves well-being, even without the idea of heading to some perfect, modern utopia.

MAIN TAKEAWAYS

In this chapter, we learned that:

- Our risk for disasters is not natural or external to our day-to-day lives but embedded in the inequitable systems and structures of society. Climate change is driving both more intense and more frequent disasters. The related risks are not borne equally around the world, and they primarily impact populations already living in conditions of environmental injustice.
- Responding to these public health disasters as discrete events that disrupt an underlying normality is not sufficient under these conditions. Public health disasters are a continuum that require a nonlinear approach.
- Environmental health practitioners have three kinds of roles in public health disasters:
  1. performing their everyday functions in extraordinary conditions (for issues like water safety),
  2. ensuring they can address specific environmental health issues brought on by the disaster (e.g., radiation monitoring or ventilation assessment), and
  3. evaluating and addressing broader impacts across the SDOH.
- Disaster management has used multiple frameworks over time:
  - **Crisis response:** Reactively addressing disasters after they happen
  - **Preparedness:** Focusing on disaster readiness work (e.g., training, mitigation) to help existing systems respond more effectively to disasters.
  - **Community resilience:** Focusing on supporting existing community systems themselves so that they recover more quickly from disasters.
  - **Disaster risk reduction:** Looking holistically at disaster risk in terms of progressive, sustainable development. This framework has shown itself to be the most effective.
- To achieve both a more successful and more environmentally just disaster response, risk frameworks would need to address the underlying drivers of vulnerability, not just the current outcomes of those drivers.
- Disaster frameworks based on EJ need to focus on collective continuance, mindful muddling, and hopeful pessimism.

SUMMARY

Climate change is driving us toward an era of persistent, ongoing disasters. These disasters will cause immediate harms, like death and destruction, but also structural harms, like economic collapse and social disruption. Public health disasters are the impacts, harms, and risks resulting largely from the choices society makes. Environmental health practitioners have a major role to play within the context of these public health disasters. We must analyze the various types of disaster management frameworks used in the United States and globally.

Then we can adjust to better address the climate change-driven reality of the next decades. Ultimately, an EJ-driven approach can help us achieve what Yarimar Bonilla describes as *hopeful pessimism*.

> **ENVIRONMENTAL HEALTH IN PRACTICE**
> **Resources**
>
> - **For sheltering operations**, environmental health practitioners often need to calculate health and safety requirements for sheltering populations using the Centers for Disease Control and Prevention (CDC's) tools for shelter assessment (https://emergency.cdc.gov/shelterassessment/index.asp).
> - **Chemical and bacterial water-supply contamination** often accompany disaster situations. As one example, after the February 2023 train derailment in East Palestine, Ohio, which released toxic chemicals including vinyl chloride, multiple teams were deployed to the scene for environmental health assessments and the state of Ohio situated a toxicologist on site for several weeks.[64]
> - **Mass feeding sites** present specific issues after disasters because they are often operated by noncertified volunteers. Taking an educational, rather than regulatory stance, can help support the community's engagement and solidarity while keeping the public safe.
> - **Nonstructural building-related safety and health hazards** are often part of the environmental health disaster portfolio. These are similar to standard indoor air assessments but may involve much broader types of contamination. In COVID-19, for example, many environmental health offices assessed filtration systems in accordance with the CDC's guidance on ventilation and transmission. Assessments to find and remove mold are common after hurricanes, as well, to prevent issues such as invasive mold infections.
> - **Radiation assessments** during small emergencies such as radiation source leakage or larger disasters such as dirty bombs (i.e., explosives laced with radioactive material) are often coordinated by environmental health offices, even though many local health departments no longer have this expertise. The CDC has standby teams and resources for this eventuality. Local health departments may also deploy *Community Reception Centers* (CRCs) during radiation events. CRCs are monitoring facilities that measure population radiation levels and provide decontamination services that require environmental health expertise.[65]
> - **Communicating to nontechnical audiences** is often required of environmental health practitioners in multiple disasters, likely because environmental health work is often so site specific. As one example, when a patient in New York City was determined to have Ebola during 2014, public health officials retraced his steps, and found that a bowling alley he visited needed cleaning. Environmental health officials then needed to both determine an appropriate cleaning protocol and justify that cleaning protocol publicly within a brief period.

END-OF-CHAPTER RESOURCES

DISCUSSION QUESTIONS

1. How are SDOH, EJ, and disaster-related risk related? Use examples to discuss the relationship.
2. This chapter discusses fundamental changes needed in how we approach public-health disaster risk. Select one of the case studies in this chapter. In the context of that example, how would disaster response look different if there were a shift from *recovery* or *resilience* to *collective continuance*?
3. How would you explain Bonila's concept of *hopeful pessimism* to someone unfamiliar with disaster preparedness?

LEARNING ACTIVITIES

THE TIME IS NOW

Environmental health practitioners are particularly well suited to communicate the idea that disaster risk is embedded in society. Building healthy communities is what we are all about. Think about the communities you are part of and examine how they approach disaster risk reduction.

- What information is available from your city, university, or workplace about emergency management or disaster response?
- What frameworks from this chapter do your campus or community appear to use? What language is used? What resources exist?

After reading this chapter, what would you ask of the people leading this work? Have a conversation to share your thoughts and questions. That is disaster risk reduction in action!

IN REAL LIFE

Oftentimes, public health disasters seem abstract until you are in one. As discussed in this chapter, one of the most important aspects in responding to a disaster is *social cohesion*. So one thing you can do is have a party!

- Gather friends who live near you and look up your risks, vulnerability, and relative community resilience on FEMA's National Risk Index Map: https://hazards.fema.gov/nri.
- Choose a hazard you are most at risk for and imagine it was happening.
- Discuss what you think makes your area more susceptible or resilient. Think about these issues based on their root causes, not just current characteristics.
- Talk through what you would do when a disaster occurred, and then afterward, to help the community recover. Remember to consider your community's needs and assets. You cannot simply provide everyone with go-kits (i.e., kits with batteries, water, and first aid).

By having this discussion at a potluck or small gathering, you are halfway to having a team you can trust to support each other if a public health disaster should occur.

A robust set of instructor resources designed to supplement this text is located at http://connect.springerpub.com/content/book/978-0-8261-8353-8. Qualifying instructors may request access by emailing textbook@springerpub.com.

REFERENCES

1. Cruz-Cano R, Mead EL. Causes of excess deaths in Puerto Rico after hurricane Maria: a time-series estimation. *Am J Public Health*. 2019;109(7):1050–1052. doi:10.2105/AJPH.2019.305015
2. Rowell CH, Lorde A. Above the wind: An interview with Audre Lorde. *Callaloo*. 2000 Jan 1;23(1):52–63. https://www.jstor.org/stable/3299518?mag=how-audre-lorde-weathered-the-storm&seq=2
3. Bonilla Y. The swarm of disaster. *Polit Geogr*. 2020;78:102182. https://yarimarbonilla.com/wp-content/uploads/2020/04/swarm-of-disaster.pdf
4. COVID data tracker. Centers for Disease Control and Prevention. March 28, 2020. Updated May 10, 2024. https://covid.cdc.gov/covid-data-tracker
5. Disaster losses & statistics. PreventionWeb. Accessed June 20, 2024. https://www.preventionweb.net/understanding-disaster-risk/disaster-losses-and-statistics
6. The Invisible Toll of Disasters in 2022. United Nations Office for Disaster Risk Reduction. Accessed June 20, 2024. https://www.undrr.org/explainer/the-invisible-toll-of-disasters-2022

7. The principles of Environmental Justice (EJ). Community Commons. Accessed June 20, 2024. https://www.communitycommons.org/entities/f5511283-eaa3-4c01-9c63-31ba3a4a6ad9
8. Andrade EL, Barrett ND, Edberg MC, Seeger MW, Santos-Burgoa C. Resilience of communities in Puerto Rico following hurricane Maria: community-based preparedness and communication strategies. *Disaster Med Public Health Prep.* 2023;17:e53. doi:10.1017/dmp.2021.306
9. Borges-Méndez R, Caron C. Decolonizing resilience: the case of reconstructing the coffee region of Puerto Rico after hurricanes Irma and Maria. *J Extreme Events.* 2019;6(1):1940001. doi:10.1142/S2345737619400013
10. admin. Best practices and lessons learned from community engagement and data collection strategies in Post-Hurricane Maria Puerto Rico. GSTDTAP. Published online April 27, 2021. http://119.78.100.173/C666//handle/2XK7JSWQ/325103
11. Milken Institute School of Public Health. Ascertainment of the Estimated Excess Mortality from Hurricane María in Puerto Rico. https://publichealth.gwu.edu/sites/g/files/zaxdzs4586/files/2023-06/acertainment-of-the-estimated-excess-mortality-from-hurricane-maria-in-puerto-rico.pdf
12. Hazard definition and classification review: technical report. United Nations Office for Disaster Risk Reduction. Accessed June 15, 2024. https://www.undrr.org/publication/hazard-definition-and-classification-review-technical-report
13. Mackay J, Munoz A, Pepper M. A disaster typology towards informing humanitarian relief supply chain design. *J Humanit Logist Supply Chain Manag.* 2019;9(1):22–46. doi:10.1108/JHLSCM-06-2018-0049
14. Kendra JM, Wachtendorf T. *American Dunkirk: The Waterborne Evacuation of Manhattan on 9/11.* Temple University Press; 2016.
15. Keim M, Giannone P. Disaster preparedness. *Disaster Med.* 2006:164–173. doi:10.1016/B978-0-323-03253-7.50032-7
16. Noji EK. Public health issues in disasters. *Crit Care Med.* 2005;33(1):S29–S33. doi:10.1097/01.ccm.0000151064.98207.9c
17. Horney JA. Introduction: mental health impacts of disasters and emergencies. In: Horney JA. *COVID-19, Frontline Responders and Mental Health: A Playbook for Delivering Resilient Public Health Systems Post-Pandemic.* Emerald Publishing Limited; 2023:1–8.
18. Benevolenza MA, DeRigne L. The impact of climate change and natural disasters on vulnerable populations: a systematic review of literature. *J Hum Behav Soc Environ.* 2019;29(2):266–281. doi:10.1080/10911359.2018.1527739
19. Burström B, Tao W. Social determinants of health and inequalities in COVID-19. *Eur J Public Health.* 2020;30(4):617–618. doi:10.1093/eurpub/ckaa095
20. Thomas DS, Jang S, Scandlyn J. The CHASMS conceptual model of cascading disasters and social vulnerability: the COVID-19 case example. *Int J Disaster Risk Reduct.* 2020;51:101828. doi:10.1016/j.ijdrr.2020.101828
21. Pescaroli G, Alexander D. Critical infrastructure, panarchies and the vulnerability paths of cascading disasters. *Nat Hazards.* 2016;82:175–192. doi:10.1007/s11069-016-2186-3
22. Tanne JH. US gun deaths increased by 35% during the early covid-19 pandemic. *BMJ.* 2022;379. doi:10.1136/bmj.o2430
23. Peña PA, Jena A. Child deaths by gun violence in the US during the COVID-19 pandemic. *JAMA Netw Open.* 2022;5(8):e2225339. doi:10.1001/jamanetworkopen.2022.25339
24. Buckley P, Fahrenkrug E. The Flint, Michigan water crisis as a case study to introduce concepts of equity and power into an analytical chemistry curriculum. *J Chem Educ.* 2020;97(5):1327–1335. doi:10.1021/acs.jchemed.9b00669
25. Butler LJ, Scammell MK, Benson EB. The Flint, Michigan, water crisis: a case study in regulatory failure and environmental injustice. *Environ Justice.* 2016;9(4):93–97. doi:10.1089/env.2016.0014
26. DeWitt RD. Pediatric lead exposure and the water crisis in Flint, Michigan. *Jaapa.* 2017;30(2):43–46. doi:10.1097/01.jaa.0000511794.60054.eb
27. Ezell JM, Griswold D, Chase EC, Carver E. The blueprint of disaster: COVID-19, the Flint water crisis, and unequal ecological impacts. *Lancet Planet Health.* 2021;5(5):e309–e315. doi:10.1016/s2542-5196(21)00076-0
28. Tierney K. *Disasters: A Sociological Approach.* John Wiley & Sons; 2019.
29. Tierney K. *The Social Roots of Risk: Producing Disasters, Promoting Resilience.* Stanford University Press; 2014.

30. Yearby R. Structural racism and health disparities: reconfiguring the social determinants of health framework to include the root cause. *J Law Med Ethics*. 2020;48(3):518–526. doi:10.1177/1073110520958876
31. Reed KA, Wehner MF, Zarzycki CM. Attribution of 2020 hurricane season extreme rainfall to human-induced climate change. *Nat Commun*. 2022;13(1):1905. doi:10.1038/s41467-022-29379-1
32. Ebi KL, Vanos J, Baldwin JW, et al. Extreme weather and climate change: population health and health system implications. *Annu Rev Public Health*. 2021;42(1):293–315. doi:10.1146/annurev-publhealth-012420-105026
33. Patel L, Conlon KC, Sorensen C, et al. Climate change and extreme heat events: how health systems should prepare. *NEJM Catal Innov Care Deliv*. 2022;3(7):CAT-21. doi:10.1056/CAT.21.0454
34. Reggers A. Climate change is not gender neutral: gender inequality, rights and vulnerabilities in Bangladesh. In: Huq S, Chow J, Fenton A, Stott C, Taub J, Wright H, eds. *Confronting Climate Change in Bangladesh: Policy Strategies for Adaptation and Resilience*. Springer; 2019:103–118.
35. Jafino BA, Walsh B, Rozenberg J, Hallegatte S. Revised estimates of the impact of climate change on extreme poverty by 2030. The World Bank. Published online 2020. https://documents.worldbank.org/en/publication/documents-reports/documentdetail/706751601388457990/revised-estimates-of-the-impact-of-climate-change-on-extreme-poverty-by-2030
36. Hasan F, Marsia S, Patel K, Agrawal P, Razzak JA. Effective community-based interventions for the prevention and management of heat-related illnesses: a scoping review. *Int J Environ Res Public Health*. 2021;18(16):8362. doi:10.3390/ijerph18168362
37. Henderson SB, McLean KE, Lee MJ, Kosatsky T. Analysis of community deaths during the catastrophic 2021 heat dome: early evidence to inform the public health response during subsequent events in greater Vancouver, Canada. *Environ Epidemiol*. 2022;6(1):e189. doi:10.1097/ee9.0000000000000189
38. Hess JJ, Errett NA, McGregor G, et al. Public health preparedness for extreme heat events. *Annu Rev Public Health*. 2023;44:301–327. doi:10.1146/annurev-publhealth-071421-025508
39. White RH, Anderson S, Booth JF, et al. The unprecedented Pacific Northwest heatwave of June 2021. *Nat Commun*. 2023;14(1):727. doi:10.1038/s41467-023-36289-3
40. EHS, CDC. Environmental Health Training in Emergency Response (EHTER). March 20, 2023. https://www.cdc.gov/nceh/ehs/elearn/ehter.htm
41. Kajeepeta S, Bruzelius E, Ho JZ, Prins SJ. Policing the pandemic: estimating spatial and racialized inequities in New York City police enforcement of COVID-19 mandates. *Crit Public Health*. 2022;32(1):56–67. doi:10.1080/09581596.2021.1987387
42. Ndugga N, Hill L, Artiga S. COVID-19 cases and deaths, vaccinations, and treatments by race/ethnicity as of fall 2022. KFF. November 17, 2022. https://www.kff.org/coronavirus-covid-19/issue-brief/covid-19-cases-and-deaths-by-race-ethnicity-current-data-and-changes-over-time/
43. Dalsania AK, Fastiggi MJ, Kahlam A, et al. The relationship between social determinants of health and racial disparities in COVID-19 mortality. *J Racial Ethn Health Disparities*. 2022;9(1):288–295. doi:10.1007/s40615-020-00952-y
44. Dauber ML. *The Sympathetic State: Disaster Relief and the Origins of the American Welfare State*. University of Chicago Press; 2013.
45. Webster RA, Adelson J, Hammer D, Chou S. The federal program to rebuild after hurricane Katrina shortchanged the poor. New data proves it. ProPublica. December 11, 2022. https://www.propublica.org/article/how-louisiana-road-home-program-shortchanged-poor-residents
46. Goitein E. Emergency powers, real and imagined: how president Trump used and failed to use presidential authority in the COVID-19 crisis. *J Natl Sec Pol*. 2020;11:27.
47. A public health emergency declaration. Administration for Strategic Preparedness & Response. Accessed June 15, 2024. https://aspr.hhs.gov:443/legal/PHE/Pages/Public-Health-Emergency-Declaration.aspx
48. Declarations of a public health emergency. Administration for Strategic Preparedness & Response. Accessed June 15, 2024. https://aspr.hhs.gov:443/legal/PHE/Pages/default.aspx
49. Whyte K. *Against Crisis Epistemology*. Routledge. Published online 2021:52–64. https://papers.ssrn.com/sol3/papers.cfm?abstract_id=3891125
50. IS-10.A: animals in disasters: awareness and preparedness. FEMA—Emergency Management Institute (EMI) Course. April 3, 2023. https://training.fema.gov/is/courseoverview.aspx?code=IS-10.a&lang=en

51. Miao Q, Davlasheridze M. Estimating the loss reduction effects of disaster preparedness: an empirical study of U.S. coastal states. Coastal Response Research Center. Published online 2021. Accessed June 15, 2024. https://scholars.unh.edu/crrc/30/
52. Kumru S, Yiğit P, Hayran O. Demography, inequalities and global health security index as correlates of COVID-19 morbidity and mortality. *Int J Health Plann Manage*. 2022;37(2):944–962. doi:10.1002/hpm.3384
53. Remes JA, Horowitz A. *Critical Disaster Studies*. University of Pennsylvania Press; 2021.
54. Matyas D, Pelling M. Positioning resilience for 2015: the role of resistance, incremental adjustment and transformation in disaster risk management policy. *Disasters*. 2015;39(s1):s1–s18. doi:10.1111/disa.12107
55. Boz HA, Bahrami M, Balcisoy S, et al. One city, two tales: using mobility networks to understand neighborhood resilience and fragility during the COVID-19 pandemic. ArXiv Prepr ArXiv221004641. Cornell University. October 2, 2022. https://arxiv.org/abs/2210.04641
56. Disaster risk reduction. United Nations Office for Disaster Risk Reduction. Accessed June 15, 2024. https://www.undrr.org/terminology/disaster-risk-reduction
57. Mena R, Brown S, Peters LE, Kelman I, Ji H. Connecting disasters and climate change to the humanitarian-development-peace nexus. *J Peacebuilding Dev*. 2022;17(3):324–340. doi:10.1177/15423166221129633
58. Sendai framework for disaster risk reduction 2015–2030. UN Office for Disaster Risk Reduction. 2015. Accessed June 15, 2024. http://www.undrr.org/publication/sendai-framework-disaster-risk-reduction-2015-2030
59. Dotson K, Whyte K. Environmental justice, unknowability and unqualified affectability. *Ethics Environ*. 2013;18(2):55–79. doi:10.2979/ethicsenviro.18.2.55
60. Whyte KP. Indigenous women, climate change impacts, and collective action. *Hypatia*. 2014 Jul;29(3):599–616. doi:10.1111/hypa.12089
61. Whyte K. Settler colonialism, ecology, and environmental injustice. *Environ Soc*. 2018;9(1):125–144. doi:10.3167/ares.2018.090109
62. Wachtendorf T. *Improvising 9/11: Organizational Improvisation Following the World Trade Center Disaster*. Ph.D Dissertation. University of Delaware; 2004. https://www.proquest.com/docview/305206641/abstract/AB41B20EF89A4760PQ/1
63. Bonilla Y. Postdisaster futures: hopeful pessimism, imperial ruination, and la futura cuir. *Small Axe Caribb J Crit*. 2020;24(2 (62)):147–162. doi:10.1215/07990537-8604562
64. Ohio Department of Health. Ohio Department of Health to open East Palestine Health Assessment Clinic. February 21, 2023. https://odh.ohio.gov/media-center/feature-stories/odh-to-open-east-palestine-health-assessment-clinic
65. Choudhary E, Agnihotri S, Nitschke D. Population monitoring after a radiological emergency: the Community Reception Center Electronic Data Collection Tool (CRC eTool). 2018 CSTE Annual Conference, West Palm Beach, Florida. CSTE; 2018.

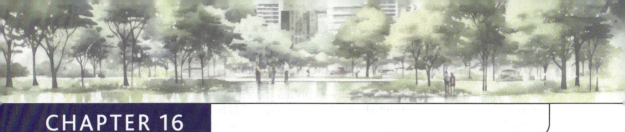

CHAPTER 16

Ensuring Occupational Health

Eric Persaud and Devan Hawkins

LEARNING OBJECTIVES

- Share a brief history of occupational health.
- Describe the relationship between occupational health and environmental health and justice.
- Describe the agencies and policies responsible for protecting occupational health.
- Identify health inequities within occupational settings in the United States and globally.
- List the solutions that may protect the health of workers and promote health equity.

KEY TERMS

- ergonomics
- industrial hygiene
- occupational epidemiology
- occupational hazards
- occupational health and safety

OVERVIEW

As a field, **occupational health and safety** seeks to understand and control hazards within the workplace to safeguard workers. In the 18th and 19th centuries, the field primarily emerged to address hazards following a rapid shift from agricultural-based economies to industrialized ones. The need for occupational health became more apparent as workers faced dangers like exposure to chemicals, unsafe machinery, long working hours, and poor ventilation. In response, labor laws and regulations were established, occupational medicine as a specialized field emerged, and labor unions advocating for worker safety were formed. Despite much progress toward protecting workers over the last century, many workers still face dangerous or exploitative work environments in the United States and beyond.

In recent years, society has also changed in notable ways. In our fissured economy, we are seeing fewer long-term commitments to specific employers with more contract-based work.[1] What does occupational health mean in a "gig economy" where there may be uncertain work arrangements, more autonomy and isolation, flexible hours, and decreased access to employer-sponsored healthcare? And, of course, workplaces must now also consider climate change.[2] For instance, do policies and practices exist to protect outdoor workers from extreme heat or poor air quality as a wildfire rages nearby? Are workplaces and the healthcare sector accounting for shifts in allergies, respiratory illnesses, and vector-borne diseases that may impact workers? Society must confront these questions as the nature of work continues to change.

In this chapter, readers are introduced to the basics of occupational health as it relates to environmental health and justice. Readers will learn about the history of the field and the policies and practices that shape occupational health today. We must also recognize the strong connections between occupational health and environmental justice (EJ), as some communities are harmed by hazardous working conditions and environmental pollutants more than others. This chapter introduces solutions for achieving occupational health for all.

A BRIEF HISTORY OF OCCUPATIONAL HEALTH

The American Civil War was essentially a conflict rooted in the moral justice of labor, albeit forced labor, or slavery.[3] For nearly the first 100 years of U.S. history, the ability to own and enslave humans was governed by law and permitted by the United States Constitution. Slavery was "justified" based on racism. Enslaved people were exploited for free labor and were regarded as property, with little to no rights, forced into unsanitary, inadequate, and often violent conditions.

Following the Civil War, the U.S. economy transitioned from being predominantly agriculturally based and rural to increasingly industrialized and urban.[4] This changeover led to the increased employment of workers in factories, mills, and other new types of jobs. In the 1820s, one of the earliest of America's industrial cities was Lowell, Massachusetts. Many young women (also known as "Mill Girls" at the time) were attracted to the wages offered by the Lowell textile mills (Figure 16.1). However, when textile prices plummeted, wages were cut. The mill workers went on strike. At first, they failed. Years later, in 1854 during a market boom, they launched another strike and formed the first union of working women in American history. Employers eventually met their demands for a fair wage. Their lessons paved the way for the U.S. labor movement—a movement that has evolved and continues today.

Throughout U.S. history, there are many landmark examples of workers facing difficult working conditions, sometimes resulting in tragic injuries or death. One of the deadliest in history was the 1911 Triangle Shirtwaist Factory fire in New York City.[5] Because the doors of the factory were locked to prevent theft, the mostly Italian and Jewish immigrant female workers could not escape when a fire broke out on the 8th-to-10th floors. The 146 workers,

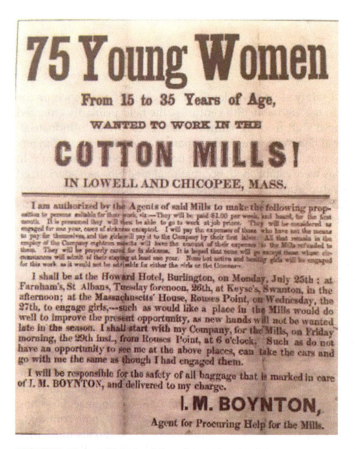

FIGURE 16.1. Mill Girls of Lowell recruitment poster.

Source: The Mill Girls of Lowell. National Park Service. Updated April 8, 2024. https://www.nps.gov/lowe/learn/historyculture/the-mill-girls-of-lowell.htm

including 123 women, were killed. The fire spurred action to create fire safety standards and contributed to the growth of the International Ladies Garment Workers Union that had been recently established in 1900.

During the 1930 Hawks Nest Tunnel disaster in West Virginia, an estimated 764 workers, the majority of whom were Black, died owing to silica dust exposure while excavating to build the tunnel. The workers performing this excavation were tasked with digging a tunnel through stone without masks. Managers stood nearby wearing protective masks, suggesting that they knew that silica exposure is particularly hazardous to the lungs.[6] The workers' exposure to silica dust in a difficult, contained work environment led to the largest death toll due to silicosis in U.S. history. The long-term health effects of silica dust exposure likely resulted in additional delayed but premature deaths for many more workers (Figure 16.2). With the country dealing with the Great Depression, workers often had to migrate for job opportunities, which were sparse. The tunnel workers were unprotected at the time without laws to enforce a safer environment, address harms, or provide compensation. The disaster eventually led to the recognition of silicosis as an occupational disease, as well as to legislation for workers' compensation.

In response to the Great Depression and high unemployment, President Franklin D. Roosevelt enacted a series of social reforms, referred to as the New Deal, which included some safeguards for workers.[7] In 1935, the National Labor Relations Act (NLRA) safeguarded labor organizing by legally protecting the ability of employees of private-sector workplaces to collectively bargain, or form a union. Unfortunately, some of those reforms excluded Black workers, and the NLRA permitted Black workers to segregate into separate unions. It was through President Roosevelt's Secretary of Labor, Frances Perkins, the first woman to serve in a presidential cabinet, that the New Deal emphasized national labor issues (Figure 16.3).

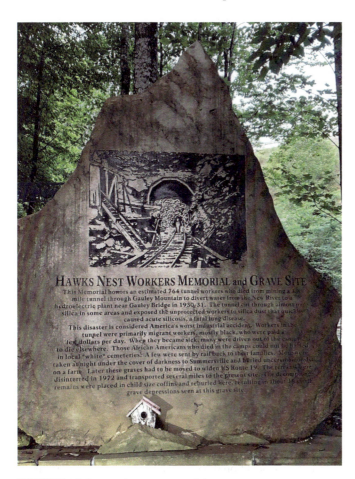

FIGURE 16.2. Hawks Nest tunnel disaster.

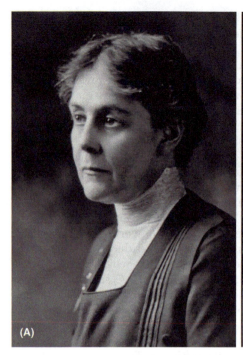 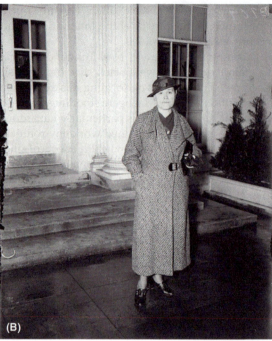

FIGURE 16.3. Early leaders in occupational health.

Dr. Alice Hamilton (A) helped to pioneer the field of industrial medicine through on-site industrial worksite investigations in the early-20th century. Frances Perkins (B) was President Roosevelt's Secretary of Labor, and the first woman to serve in a presidential cabinet. Some of Perkins's major contributions included federal laws regulating child labor and the creation of unemployment insurance and social security.

Source: (A) Photograph courtesy of the Department of Health and Human Services, National Institutes of Health; (B) Photograph courtesy of the Library of Congress.

Later in 1970, during a time of increased social awareness and activism related to environmental issues, the U.S. Congress passed the Occupational Safety and Health (OSH) Act, which led to the creation of the Occupational Safety and Health Administration (OSHA) and the National Institute for Occupational Safety and Health (NIOSH).[8] NIOSH is a research agency dedicated to workplace health and safety and provides OSHA with recommendations based on scientific findings. See Chapter 4, "Environmental Health Policies and Protections: Successes and Failures," and Chapter 7, "Understanding the Environment and How It Relates to Health Using Toxicology and Epidemiology Research Methods," for discussion of regulatory science.

Much of this awareness was inspired by Dr. Alice Hamilton and other leaders who pioneered the field of industrial medicine through on-site industrial worksite investigations in the early 20th century (see Figure 16.3).[9] The Governor of Illinois had commissioned Dr. Hamilton's "shoe-leather" epidemiologic investigations (i.e., wearing out shoes by going door-to-door to track and control disease). The goal was to better understand the dangerous industrial and occupational exposures. This led to state legislators in Illinois passing safety standards for chemicals in 1911. Shortly after Dr. Hamilton's death in 1970, the OSH Act gave the federal government authority to create and enforce standards of safety and health in most workplaces for the first time.[10] In 1970, on average, there were 38 workplace deaths per day; by 2020 the number of workplace deaths has been reduced to 13 deaths per day.

OCCUPATIONAL HAZARDS

Broadly speaking, **occupational hazards** can be divided according to the threats negatively impacting workers' health. Major categories for hazards in the workplace include safety, chemical, biological, and psychosocial hazards. Some additional hazards include ergonomic hazards, radiation, noise, and temperature levels, as well as how work is organized, as described with

SAFETY HAZARDS

Safety hazards can cause injuries or death when owners and managers do not take the proper steps to prevent physical harm to workers. Safety hazards at the workplace are responsible for many injuries. According to the Bureau of Labor Statistics' (BLS) Survey of Occupational Injuries and Illnesses, there were 2.2 million occupational injuries in the United States in 2022.[11] Due to underreporting of occupational injuries and illnesses, these numbers are likely an undercount. According to the BLS's Census of Fatal Occupational Injuries, in 2021 there were 4,764 work-related fatalities.[12]

The Occupational Injury and Illness Classification System (OIICS) coding system is used to define occupational injury and illnesses characteristics in a consistent way.[13] Table 16.1 provides details about different factors used to define injuries using this system.

Injuries and illnesses at the workplace can also be characterized by the occupation and industry of the impacted worker. Occupation refers to the actual job performed by the worker (sometimes called "job title"), and industry refers to where the worker works. For example, *janitor* is an example of an occupation. A janitor could be employed in different *industries* such as healthcare (e.g., hospitals, private clinics) or education (e.g., middle school, college). Different standard coding systems are used for coding occupation and industry (the BLS Standard Occupational Classification [SOC]; North American Industry Classification System; and Census Industry and Occupation Codes). The International Labor Organization (ILO) uses the International Standard Classification of Occupation system for coding occupation.[15]

Information about occupation and industry can be useful for identifying high-risk industries and occupations, and this information can inform protective policies and programs. According to industry data from the Department of Labor, in 2021 healthcare and social assistance had the highest number of injuries, while agriculture, forestry, fishing, and hunting had the highest rate of injuries.[11] In healthcare, workers may face hazards such as injuries from lifting, violence, stress, and exposure to infectious diseases. In agriculture, workers may face hazards associated with frequent pesticide exposures or injuries from repetitive activities or tragic accidents.

In addition to using data about injuries and safety hazards at work to identify the common types of injuries and the occupations and industries most impacted, these data can also be used to identify trends in incidents at work. For example, a 2021 BLS report about nonfatal injuries and illnesses in 2021 reported that retail trade and transportation and warehousing industries had the biggest increase in incidents. Trend analyses may also look at different types of injuries. One report using the BLS Survey of Occupational Injuries and Illnesses data highlighted increasing rates of violence in the healthcare and social assistance industry (Figure 16.4).[16]

TABLE 16.1. FACTORS FOR CLASSIFYING OCCUPATIONAL INJURIES AND ILLNESSES

FACTOR	DEFINITION	EXAMPLES
Nature	Characteristic(s) of the injury	Sprain, strains, or tears; fractures; and cuts, lacerations, or punctures[14]
Body part affected	The primary part of the body that was harmed	Upper extremities and lower extremities; head
Source	The primary physical factor(s) that caused the injury	People (either the workers themselves or someone else); floors, walkways, and ground surfaces; and containers
Event	How the injury occurred[13]	Overexertion and bodily reaction; falls, slips, and trips; and contact with objects or equipment

Source: Adapted from Occupational Injury and Illness Classification System. Centers for Disease Control and Prevention. Updated December 9, 2023. https://wwwn.cdc.gov/wisards/oiics; Injuries, illnesses, and fatalities. U.S. Bureau of Labor Statistics. 2023. https://www.bls.gov/iif

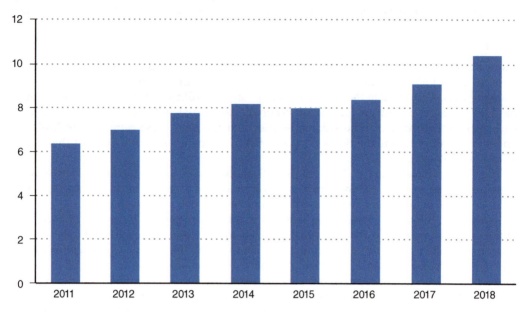

FIGURE 16.4. Incidence rate of nonfatal workplace violence to healthcare workers, 2011–2018.
Source: Injuries, illnesses, and fatalities: Workplace violence in healthcare, 2018. U.S. Bureau of Labor Statistics. April 2020. https://www.bls.gov/iif/factsheets/workplace-violence-healthcare-2018.htm

CHEMICAL HAZARDS

Chemical hazards in the workplace are toxic substances that have the potential to damage health when workers are exposed to unsafe concentrations. Broadly speaking, the hazards presented by chemicals in the workplace can be divided by whether they cause acute or chronic health effects, as well as the types of physical damage they may cause.

If exposure to toxic chemicals leads to health impacts over a short timeframe (on the scale of minutes to hours), these are considered acute effects. For example, exposure to high levels of carbon monoxide in a workplace could lead to acute health effects. Exposure to carbon monoxide is a concern especially for workers in industries that involve combustion, such as work involving automobiles in enclosed spaces.[17] Carbon monoxide is a particular concern because it is odorless and colorless, requiring carbon monoxide detectors to alert workers when the levels of exposure are dangerously high. When concentrations of carbon monoxide are high enough and inhaled, it can combine with hemoglobin and negatively impact oxygen delivery throughout the body. This can cause loss of consciousness, suffocation, and death. Because of concerns about the acute effects of carbon monoxide, OSHA requires that all employees be evacuated from workplaces if carbon monoxide concentrations exceed defined safe limits.

In addition to acute effects, chemicals can also have chronic effects caused by long-term exposure. With chronic health effects, workers are often exposed at low doses that may not produce any acute health effects. One example of a chemical with a chronic toxic health effect is benzene. Benzene is used in a wide variety of industrial processes as a solvent, and it is also found in fossil fuels and by-products derived from fossil fuels. Exposure to benzene from rapid inhalation or skin exposure can also cause acute effects like dizziness, headache, vomiting, rapid heart rate, unconsciousness, and even death. Long-term exposure to benzene has been linked with leukemia, a type of blood cancer.[18] Because of chronic and acute effects of benzene exposure, OSHA has many regulations regarding the use of benzene in occupational settings such as general industry, maritime work, and construction.

For both acute and chronic health effects, chemicals can be classified in terms of how they enter the body while performing work activities. The routes of entry for chemical hazards include:

- inhalation,
- ingestion,
- injection, and
- contact with the skin and eyes.[19]

Additionally, chemicals can also be classified according to the organs that they affect. For example, the chemical arsenic can enter the body through a variety of routes including inhalation, skin contact, and ingestion.

Once in the body, there are different target organs (or organs on which the chemical has a toxic effect) including the kidneys and the central nervous system. Some chemicals are classified as *sensitizers*, which are chemical types that create an allergic reaction among those exposed. Formaldehyde, which is a commonly used industrial chemical, is one example of a sensitizer that can trigger asthma.[20]

Workplace chemical regulations regulate exposure levels based on (a) concentrations of the chemical (how much of the actual chemical is in the work environment), and (b) time of exposure to the chemical (the amount of time the worker is exposed to the chemical). OSHA sets limits on the amount of chemical hazards workers can be exposed to, which are referred to as permissible exposure limits (PELs). These PELs are often expressed as time-weighted averages (TWAs), which are calculated by summing the total concentration a worker is exposed to over specific time periods (such as 15-minute intervals) throughout the workday and dividing that number by 8 to get an average level of exposure during an 8-hour workday. Workers' exposures are said to exceed the PEL if the TWA of their exposure is higher than that listed by OSHA. Concentrations will usually be listed as parts per million and/or milligrams per cubic meter. For example, the PEL for aluminum dust is a TWA of exposure to 15 milligrams per cubic meter (Table 16.2). OSHA acknowledges that "many of its [PELs] are outdated and inadequate for ensuring protection of worker health. Most of OSHA's PELs were issued shortly after adoption of the [OSH] Act in 1970, and have not been updated since that time."[21(para1)] NIOSH has its own recommended exposure limits (RELs), which are not enforceable by OSHA, but are often lower than those issued by OSHA. Most NIOSH RELs are listed as 10-hour TWAs. Additionally, California's OSHA (CalOSHA) has their own PELs.

TABLE 16.2. EXAMPLE OF DIFFERENT EXPOSURE LIMITS FOR ALUMINUM DUST

ORGANIZATION	EXPOSURE LIMIT NAME	EXPOSURE LIMIT
OSHA	Permissible exposure limits (PELs)	15 mg/m^3 (total dust), 5 mg/m^3 (respirable fraction)
NIOSH	Recommended exposure limits (RELs)	10 mg/m^3 (total dust), 5 mg/m^3 (respirable fraction)
CalOSHA	Permissible exposure limits (PELs)	10 mg/m^3 (total dust), 5 mg/m^3 (respirable fraction)

CalOSHA, California Division of Occupational Safety and Health; NIOSH, National Institute for Occupational Safety and Health; OSHA, Occupational Safety and Health Administration

Source: Aluminum, metal (as Al). U.S. Department of Labor, Occupational Safety and Health Administration. Updated March 27, 2024. https://www.osha.gov/chemicaldata/496

BIOLOGICAL HAZARDS

Biological hazards at work refer to exposure to infectious agents, including bacteria, viruses, parasites, and fungi. Workers in a variety of industries face the risk of exposure to biological hazards at work. For example, healthcare workers and other workers in the industry are at risk because of their frequent contact with sick patients and medical waste. During the COVID-19 pandemic, studies showed that healthcare workers were at an elevated risk for contracting COVID-19 and dying from it.[22-24] Agriculture workers, because of their contact with animals, risk becoming infected with animal-acquired infections.[25] In a similar way, laboratory workers who work with infectious agents face the risk of infection.[26]

When trying to control exposure to biological hazards in the workforce, one of the first steps is identifying the source of the exposure. For example, in the healthcare setting one source of dangerous infections is blood-borne pathogens. *Blood-borne pathogens* are infectious diseases that are primarily spread through contact with blood or other bodily fluids and include hepatitis B and C and HIV. One method by which healthcare workers can be exposed to blood-borne pathogens is by being stuck with needles and other sharp devices that are contaminated with blood. OSHA currently has a blood-borne pathogen standard, which was implemented with the goal of preventing these types of dangerous exposures to healthcare workers. The standard requires healthcare facilities to implement exposure control plans, engineering controls, safe work practices, hepatitis B vaccination, and education plans, among other protocols.[26]

PSYCHOSOCIAL HAZARDS

Occupational psychosocial hazards refer to workplace exposures that negatively impact workers' mental, social, and emotional health. These hazards can have downstream impacts on workers' health behaviors, physical health, and overall quality of life. There are a wide variety of specific psychosocial hazards, such as high job demands, low job control, and low social support. These hazards are less understood and may be more difficult to measure and characterize than physical, chemical, and biological hazards at the workplace.

Occupational stress is a category of psychosocial hazard associated with both mental and physical health.[27] Different models have been used to conceptualize occupational stress:

- *The Demand–Control Model* classifies jobs according to two axes: (1) job demands and (2) decision latitude (i.e., control over tasks; Figure 16.5). Jobs with high demands and low decision latitude are considered "high-strain" jobs and are generally linked to worse health outcomes. High-strain jobs contribute to elevated rates of coronary heart disease and depression for workers, among other health outcomes. The model has also been revised to include a third dimension—social support—which may offer some health protection in high-strain jobs.
- *The Effort–Reward Imbalance Model* hypothesizes that there will be negative health consequences when there is an imbalance between the amount of effort someone perceives that they put into their work versus the rewards and benefits that they receive from it. Effort–reward imbalance has been found to be associated with a variety of health outcomes, including depressive symptoms and poor cardiovascular health.

Researchers have also investigated how job precarity and job insecurity impact health. *Precarious employment* has been defined in different ways and entails different dimensions of work, including stability of employment, rights at work, and pay and benefits.[28] *Job insecurity* is a potential consequence of job precarity and refers to concerns about losing employment. Increasingly, researchers are looking to assess both the physical and mental health consequences of both job precarity and job insecurity, which have major implications for quality of life for much of society.

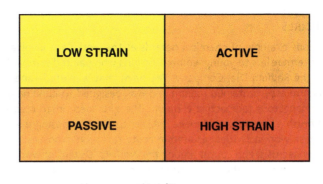

FIGURE 16.5. Demand–Control Model by Robert Karasek.

Jobs with high demands and low decision latitude are considered "high-strain" jobs and are generally linked to worse health outcomes. High-strain jobs contribute to elevated rates of coronary heart disease and depression for workers, among other health outcomes.

Source: Karasek RA. Job demands, job decision latitude, and mental strain: implications for job redesign. *Adm Sci Q.* 1979;24(2):285–308. doi:10.2307/2392498.

ERGONOMIC HAZARDS

Ergonomic hazards at the workplace refers to hazards that cause wear and tear on the body through exposure to lifting, uncomfortable postures, repetitive motion, and other types of physically demanding activities. Workers can develop musculoskeletal disorders, which entail harm to different organs in the body, especially muscles, bones, and nerves, brought about by these ergonomic hazards.[29] Different interventions can be applied to protect workers from these workplace hazards, including:

- engineering controls, such as patient-lifting devices to prevent healthcare workers from injuring themselves when moving and repositioning patients;
- administrative controls, such as modified work routines with more microbreaks or different shifts; and
- personal protective equipment, such as knee pads, for those whose daily work often entails kneeling (e.g., plumbers, tilers, roofers).

RADIATION HAZARDS

Workers in industries that use radioactive materials face the risk of radiation exposure and its serious health effects.[30] Radiation is a health concern because of its potential to damage cells. There can be acute impacts, particularly acute radiation syndrome (also called radiation sickness) from a high dose of radiation in a short time span. There can also be chronic health effects, such as certain cancers.

OSHA has standards for both ionizing and nonionizing radiation. Medical workers who perform imaging (such as x-rays and computed tomography [CT] scans) and workers at nuclear power plants and weapons facilities may experience exposure to ionizing radiation. These workplaces are sources of ionizing radiation, which has enough energy to knock off electrons from atoms. Potential occupational exposure to nonionizing radiation occurs in a wide range of industries from healthcare to construction, as it is used in radio waves, lasers, and ultraviolet light. Nonionizing radiation does not have enough energy to knock off electrons from atoms.

> **RADIUM GIRLS**
>
> One infamous example of chemical hazards at the workplace involved the so-called "Radium Girls." The term refers to young women and girls who painted watch dials in the late 1910s and 1920s for the Radium Dial Company. The paint that was used—and which the workers were told was harmless—contained radium and was designed to illuminate the dials. Radium is an extremely dangerous radioactive element. The girls were instructed to use their lips to give the paint brush a fine point and make it easier to paint, exposing them to radium around their mouth. These work activities resulted in acute radiation exposure and related symptoms like anemia, jaw necrosis, and cancer among the workers. Dozens of workers fell ill, and many died. There were years of litigation for surviving workers before any compensation was received. The case of the Radium Girls is another important inspiration for the labor movement's fight to protect workers' health and safety.

NOISE HAZARDS

Exposure to loud noises at work is an occupational health concern because these noises can cause temporary or permanent damage to workers' hearing.[31] Short term exposure to loud noises may cause temporary loss of hearing, while long term exposure may contribute to tinnitus and permanent hearing loss. NIOSH recently estimated that 22 million workers in the United States are exposed to dangerous levels of noise at work.[32] Industries with a high prevalence of occupational noise exposure include mining, construction, manufacturing, and airport mechanics and ramp work. Noise exposure at the workplace may also have impacts beyond just hearing itself. Research suggests that exposure to loud noises at work may also be associated with a higher risk for cardiovascular disease and poor mental health.

TEMPERATURE HAZARDS

Exposure to extremes of hot and cold is another occupational health concern.[33] Workers can experience extreme high temperatures when working in outdoor environments (e.g., in agriculture, construction, landscaping, mail delivery) or in indoor environments with heat sources or poor ventilation (e.g., in food preparation, manufacturing, warehouses). The physical demands of the job and personal risk factors may increase the likelihood of suffering from occupational heat-related illnesses. Heat-related illnesses include heat stress and stroke, which may only be further exacerbated with increasing temperatures due to climate change. Few protections, such as access to water, rest, and shade, exist for outdoor workers and none exist at the federal level and only five states with heat regulations as of 2023.

Workers can also be exposed to extreme cold temperatures, which poses health risks. Jobs that are at an increased risk from cold exposure include outdoor labor during winter weather and indoor work in cold and damp environments. Workplace controls, such as not scheduling work on extremely cold days, and personal protection, such as insulating clothing, may protect workers from injuries and illnesses caused by exposure to environmental cold. Working in the cold may also exacerbate other health problems such as pain, respiratory difficulties, and cardiovascular health.[34]

WORK-ORGANIZATION HAZARDS

Work organization is a broad term referring to how work processes are carried out and the relationship between workers and their employers.[35] The impact of different aspects of work organization is a growing area of research in occupational health. Some aspects of work organization that have received particular attention include long work hours, irregular shifts (evening, night, rotating), telecommuting, and technological monitoring of employees. For example, irregular shifts may lead to increased risk of psychological, gastrointestinal, and cardiovascular disorders.[36]

OCCUPATIONAL HEALTH FIELDS

Occupational Medicine

One of the first fields to specifically concern itself with occupational exposures was occupational medicine. Although different individuals within the medical and scientific fields had previously described how work-related factors could impact health, the Italian physician Bernardino Ramazzini, born in 1633, is often considered one of the most significant figures in the field of occupational medicine. His book *De Morbis Artificum Diatriba* (Dissertation on Workers' Diseases) describes various diseases and health outcomes associated with different occupations and ways to treat those diseases. Since the time of Ramazzini, occupational medicine physicians have continued to diagnose and study diseases, injuries, and illnesses among workers and sought to identify methods to control these health outcomes.

Occupational Epidemiology

Occupational epidemiology is concerned with assessing the distribution and determinants of work-related injuries, illnesses, and fatalities. It applies the methodology of epidemiology to studying these problems. Because of the nature of occupational health issues, occupational epidemiology is primarily an observational field using observational study designs (e.g., cohort, case-control, cross-sectional) to make inferences about etiologic factors contributing to occupational health concerns. In most instances, it would be unethical to conduct an experimental occupational epidemiologic study. For instance, it would be inappropriate to conduct a randomized controlled trial to study a harmful chemical like benzene, because by design it would entail intentionally exposing some workers to benzene.

Occupational health surveillance uses different data sources to continuously track occupational injuries, illnesses, and fatalities, with the goal of understanding the extent of these health problems, the factors associated with them, and the industries and occupations at a high risk. These findings are then communicated to the relevant interested parties, for example, community leaders, healthcare professionals, and researchers, and government and labor representatives. The data sources used for occupational health surveillance include surveys, medical records, OSHA and other injury logs, workers' compensation data, and death certificates.

Industrial Hygiene

Industrial hygienists seek to identify, measure, and control harmful exposures in the workplace. Ideally industrial hygienists will be able to practice primary prevention by monitoring and evaluating workplaces before workers are harmed by dangerous exposures. Industrial hygienists will frequently use exposure-monitoring tools to both identify harmful exposures and to measure potential exposures. They will then seek to identify the sources of exposures with the goal of eventually controlling them. Industrial hygienists will also often engage in hazard communication (discussed later in the chapter) to inform workers about any risks associated with their work.

Ergonomics

Ergonomics (sometimes referred to as human factors and ergonomics) is a field concerned with engineering products to meet humans' physical and psychological needs.[29] With respect to occupational health, ergonomics is relevant because it can be applied to understanding how workplace design and work processes might contribute to physical health concerns (e.g., injuries, pain) and how to redesign the workplace to make work less harmful. The application of ergonomics to work is often referred to as "fitting the job to the person." For instance, in office settings, ergonomics has led to options such as wrist rests, curved keyboards, adjustable monitors, and stand-up desks.

Industrial and Organizational Psychology

Industrial and organizational psychology (sometimes referred to as occupational psychology) is a field of psychology concerned with how the organization of work and stressors in the workplace have an impact on psychological health and well-being. The field conducts assessments of these factors, with the goal of organizing work in such a way as to make it less harmful and more productive.

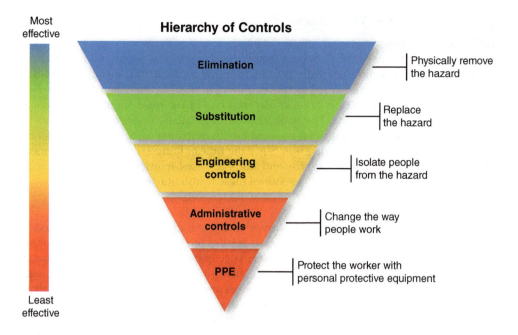

FIGURE 16.6. Hierarchy of Controls by the National Institute for Occupational Safety and Health.
PPE, personal protective equipment.
Source: The National Institute for Occupational Safety and Health. Hierarchy of Controls. Centers for Disease Control and Prevention. Updated January 17, 2023. https://www.cdc.gov/niosh/topics/hierarchy/default.html

Toxicology

Toxicology is a scientific field that studies how chemicals are absorbed, metabolized, and excreted from the body and how chemicals may be hazardous for different target organs in the body. The principles of toxicology are also applied in studying different chemical hazards in the workplace (see the "Chemical Hazards" section earlier and Chapter 7, "Understanding the Environment and How It Relates to Health Using Toxicology and Epidemiology Research Methods").

Safety Engineering

Safety engineering is a subfield of engineering that uses design principles to increase safety, and it frequently applies the Hierarchy of Controls to identify worker protections.[37] The *Hierarchy of Controls* is often visualized as an upside-down triangle (Figure 16.6). Generally, the most effective methods of control are listed at the top of the triangle and less effective methods are listed at the bottom. For example, elimination (completely removing the hazard) is at the top, while personal protective equipment is listed at the bottom. In between the least and most effective methods are substitution, engineering controls, and administrative controls.

REGULATING OCCUPATIONAL HEALTH

There are various levels of policies and regulations that govern occupational health in the United States at the federal, state, county, and Tribal levels. Although some policies have been effective, others have been inadequate. Politics, industry, and public awareness are among the many factors that play a role in the regulatory science of occupational health. In this section, some major occupational health-related policies, challenges facing occupational health policies, and potential solutions are discussed.

As mentioned earlier in this chapter, the 1970s were a landmark era in the federal regulation of occupational health and safety. The U.S. Congress passed new federal laws related to occupational and environmental health, and President Richard Nixon signed the OSH Act in

1970. He had authority to regulate occupational health under the Interstate Commerce Clause in the Constitution. This clause is frequently invoked for environmental laws because it allows the federal government to regulate any activity that affects interstate commerce. Indeed, the economic burdens of worker injuries, illnesses, and deaths have this ability to affect interstate commerce.

With the passage of the OSH Act, workers in the United States had the right to a safe and healthy workplace for the first time. The General Duty Clause of the OSH Act required that workplaces provide "employment and a place of employment which are free from recognized hazards that are causing or are likely to cause death or serious physical harm."[38(Sec5)] The OSH Act led to the adoption of OSHA standards that were enforced through awareness and assistance. Researchers have repeatedly found that these policies are effective in protecting workers from injuries and illnesses.[39]

However, there are political and legal barriers to OSHA's effectiveness. Through inspections, OSHA reviews worksites to ensure proper healthy working conditions. Unfortunately, there are a total of 2,000 OSHA federal and state plan inspectors, or 5.6 inspectors for every one million covered workers. It would take over 150 years for OSHA to visit each worksite at least once.[40] Even when OSHA reviews a worksite, the fines imposed for violations are often minimal and do not deter companies that profit significantly from unhealthy practices. Also, industry lobby groups often fight implementation of these protections, because occupational health protections are seen as being too costly.

Not all workers are fully covered under OSHA. For instance, there are millions of unprotected public employees and workers on small farms. Additionally, many workers today are part of the gig economy, taking on temporary roles, working as contractors, and providing short-term staffing support. This shift has resulted in a fissured economy in which employers in these settings can potentially avoid some or all OSHA requirements, leaving their workers with less protection. Although all workers have the right to file complaints, unstable conditions often discourage them from doing so, leading to underreporting. For instance, undocumented Americans may choose not to report workplace hazards owing to concerns about employer retaliation and the risk of deportation.

WORKPLACE STANDARDS

OSHA standards have changed workplaces for the better by creating protections against hazards like asbestos, lead, falls, and countless others.[8] However, because it takes significant periods of time to pass legislation that updates the standards, and because doing so is not a priority of elected leaders, OSHA standards are rarely improved. Most of the standards for safe and permissible exposure to chemicals, for example, were enacted in the 1960s and are woefully outdated. Some of today's most pressing workplace safety issues have not been addressed by any standard, such as:

- protections to address the health effects of extreme heat, which is exacerbated by climate change;[41]
- assurance of ergonomic interventions (though there was a quickly repealed federal standard in effect from January 2000 to March 2000 requiring workplaces to assess ergonomic risks);[42] and
- workplace violence, which thousands of workers experience every year.[43]

ASBESTOS IN LIBBY, MONTANA

Beginning in 1919, vermiculite mining was common in the small town of Libby, Montana. From 1963 to 1990, W. R. Grace and Company operated the vermiculite mine in the region. Vermiculite is a mineral used in various construction and industrial applications, and it was particularly prized for its fire-resistant and insulating properties.

(continued)

> The vermiculite ore in Libby was contaminated with a highly toxic form of asbestos called tremolite asbestos. Asbestos is a group of naturally occurring minerals that, when disturbed, can release tiny, airborne fibers; when these fibers are inhaled, they can cause serious health problems, including lung cancer, asbestosis, and mesothelioma. There was widespread exposure of miners, their families, and the community for many years. Although the dangers of asbestos were known by 1930, its use and exposure continued in Libby and the United States for decades.
>
> In this small town of under 3,000 people, approximately 700 exposed adults and children have died, with numbers still rising owing to the long latency period between exposure to asbestos and development of asbestosis and mesothelioma. In 2002, the U.S. Environmental Protection Agency (EPA) designated Libby as a Superfund site, recognizing the extensive asbestos contamination, and in 2009 the situation was officially declared an environmental public health emergency. W. R. Grace agreed in a 2008 settlement to pay the EPA $250 million for cleanup work. Cleanup was officially completed in Libby in 2019.
>
> Zonolite (a brand of a specific type of vermiculite insulation) was used across the United States in millions of homes, and it remains in the walls and floors of many. Therefore, ongoing efforts are essential for outreach and education, screening, ongoing medical care, and financial compensation. In 2024, the EPA finally put legislation into place to ban asbestos.[44]

RIGHT TO WORK

The U.S. Congress passed the Taft–Hartley Act in 1947, which amended sections of the NLRA of 1935. The NLRA had secured the rights of employees to join or form unions and engage in organizing activities to address working conditions. The Taft–Hartley Act restricted the power of labor unions, however, and allowed "right-to-work" laws in the private sector. These laws make it optional for employees to join a union or pay union dues,[45] and they were passed in many states. In 1977, the Supreme Court had ruled in favor of public workplaces maintaining collective bargaining fees in *Abood v. Detroit Board of Education*. However, in 2018, the Supreme Court case *Janus v. AFSCME*, ruled that public employees could not be required to pay union fees as a condition of employment, effectively making all states right-to-work states.

Right-to-work laws remain heavily debated. Many argue that workers should have the freedom to associate with a union or not. Many others argue that having fewer members weakens a union's ability to bargain collectively, and nonmembers still benefit from the union. The long-term impacts of the Janus decision could result in the erosion of union power in the United States. Considering the success that labor unions have had historically in providing better working conditions, this outcome may be troubling for the overall well-being of workers.

WORKERS' COMPENSATION

Workers injured at work or who have developed a disease from exposures at their workplace may need wage replacement, medical treatment, and rehabilitation. In 1970, injured workers were not entitled to such compensation by their employers in 19 states, while other states only covered some limited worker benefits.[46] Now, workers injured on the job have the right to receive compensation by law in all states.

Evidence suggests that many workers who need compensation and are entitled to such benefits do not receive them. This is in part because many state governments have created limitations to reduce employer costs, such as requiring clear and convincing evidence from workers. These requirements create challenges for workers, as it may be difficult to find medical evidence to *prove* that the injury or illness was caused by workplace conditions. For example, a worker may be denied workers' compensation if they have common injuries (e.g., leg pain) or diseases that may manifest long after the worker is at the company where the exposure occurred (e.g., cancer).

MINE SAFETY

In 1969, the U.S. Congress passed the Coal Mine Safety and Health Act. It created a federal-compensation system for victims of black lung disease. *Black lung disease* is scarring in the lungs caused by continued inhalation of coal dust. In 1977, Congress passed the Federal Mine Safety and Health Act, or the Mine Act, following a mine disaster that killed several miners. The Mine Act expanded the rights of miners to request inspections, and it enabled the Mine Safety and Health Administration to impose strict penalties for violators of mine regulations.

PAID SICK AND PARENTAL LEAVE

As of 2023, there are no federal legal requirements for paid sick leave in the United States. With no guaranteed paid sick leave, many workers who feel unwell may still report to work rather than risk the loss of pay or, potentially, their employment. Without paid sick leave employers risk their workers' health as well as the health of their greater community. For example, during the COVID-19 pandemic, workers who felt unwell may have had to continue working because they did not have paid sick leave, putting other workers at risk of exposure.

Paid parental leave is crucial for the physical and mental well-being and stability of families. However, it is alarming to note that the United States is the only high-income nation that lacks a national paid-maternity-leave program. This lack of support is not unrelated to the fact that the United States has the highest maternal mortality rate of any industrialized nation, with significant disparities by race.[47] Additionally, the overturning of *Roe v. Wade* by the Supreme Court in 2022 has far-reaching implications for the health of pregnant people and their families. Abortion care is often seen as a personal issue, with professional consequences for parents. However, in a nation lacking universal healthcare, government-subsidized child care, or paid parental leave, personal and professional considerations often cannot be separated.

For nearly 50 years, the right to an abortion was guaranteed under constitutional law by *Roe v. Wade*. However, since its overturning by the Court in 2022, several states have enacted abortion bans or are expected to ban abortions with varying degrees of circumstances. These recent changes make protecting the health and safety of mothers and infants even more critical.

OCCUPATIONAL HEALTH INEQUITIES

Just like most health issues, the burden of workplace exposure to health hazards and the probability of working in the most hazardous industries and occupations are not borne equally across society. Although all workers face hazards at work, some workers are more at risk than others. In particular, the risk of these hazards differs according to industry and occupation. Workers in the most hazardous jobs tend to be disproportionately people of color and people from lower wealth backgrounds. Thus, intervening to prevent exposure to workplace hazards can be an effective means for reducing health inequities.[48]

WORK AS A SOCIAL DETERMINANT OF HEALTH

Work relates to most social determinants of health (SDOH), as we look at the "causes of the causes" of health inequities. The U.S. Department of Health and Human Services divides the SDOH into five categories:

- economic stability,
- education access and quality,
- healthcare access and quality,
- neighborhood and built environment, and
- social and community context.

For example, a living wage and secure and consistent work can contribute to economic stability. Additionally, work is an important determinant of health insurance coverage. In 2021, over 54% of people in the United States had an employer-based health insurance plan, greater than any other insurance source, including Medicare and Medicaid combined.[49]

Work is also an important element of access to other benefits. Although the most common type of retirement income is social security, 57% of retirees get income from a pension.[50] Over time there has been a decline in the number of workers with access to defined-benefit pension plans, in which retirees are entitled to a set amount of money upon retirement, and an increase in defined-contribution plans, in which the amount of money that workers receive on retirement is based on the money that they put into retirement accounts and how well those investments perform in the market. Such defined-contribution systems are more precarious because money can be lost when the value of the investments decline. Other types of benefits available to some workers include leave benefits, such as sick leave, parental leave, and vacation leave. Unlike almost all high-income countries, the United States is unique in not providing guaranteed access to these types of leave benefits.

UNDERSTANDING WORK, SOCIOECONOMIC STATUS, AND HEALTH

Public health research has frequently characterized the differences in health according to socioeconomic status. *Socioeconomic status (SES)*, also called socioeconomic position, refers to someone's relative position in society with respect to income and wealth, as well as other factors like education and occupation. Many studies have examined the relationship between SES and health by using occupation as an indicator of SES. For example, the Whitehall Study, an influential longitudinal study of British civil servants, used "employment grade" as a measure of SES. Employment grade classifies workers according to whether their jobs fit into one of these categories: (1) administrative, (2) professional/executive, (3) clerical, and (4) other. The initial Whitehall study documented a clear gradient in coronary heart disease mortality, with the highest risk among the lowest SES workers.[51] Some theorize that this SES gradient in health outcomes is due to work-related psychosocial hazards, including high demands and low decision latitude among lower SES workers.

Educational attainment is strongly associated with occupation.[52] According to data from the 2019 U.S. Census, the five most-common occupations for people with less than a high school education were: (1) driver/sales workers and truck drivers; (2) first-line supervisors of retail sales workers; (3) managers, all others (meaning managers that could not be assigned a more specific type of management job); (4) janitors and building cleaners; and (5) customer service representatives. For those with a graduate degree, the five most-common job titles were: (1) elementary and middle school teachers; (2) lawyers; (3) managers, all others; (4) postsecondary teachers; and (5) other physicians.[53] In comparing the occupations in these two lists, it is more likely that people who have less than a high school education will be exposed to a range of workplace hazards than people who have graduate degrees.

WORK-RELATED HEALTH INEQUITIES

In the United States, there are large, well-documented racial and ethnic health disparities, and work is a key contributor to this health inequity. In 2021, the life expectancy at birth (in years) was 76.4 for White, non-Hispanic individuals; 70.8 for Black, non-Hispanic individuals; and 65.2 for American Indian/Alaskan Native non-Hispanic individuals.[54] Work contributes to these health disparities in a variety of ways. Across various occupational health outcomes, workers of color tend to face higher risks when compared to their White counterparts. For example, Hispanic workers have been found to have a higher rate of occupational fatalities compared to non-Hispanic workers.[55] The share of occupational fatalities among Hispanic or Latino workers has been consistently increasing. Previous research has established Black and

Hispanic or Latino workers to have the highest risk for nonfatal occupational injuries.[56] Additionally, evidence indicates that workers of color are more likely to be exposed to hazardous chemicals in the workplace and are at a greater risk of occupational disease.[57]

Different factors may account for these racial and ethnic disparities in occupational health outcomes. For example, some of the disparities may be due to occupational segregation, in that workers of color are more likely to be employed in hazardous jobs. During the COVID-19 pandemic, workers of color were more likely to be employed in high-risk jobs interacting with the public, which may have contributed to racial and ethnic disparities in COVID-19 mortality by occupation.[58]

Additionally—even within the same occupation—workers of color may face worse exposures than White workers. One study examining the prevalence of occupational psychosocial and work organization exposures found that differences in employment patterns by occupation accounted for only some of the higher risk of exposure to job insecurity among Hispanic and Asian workers, shift work among Black workers, and employment in alternative work arrangements among Hispanic workers. These results indicate that some of these differences in exposure are not related solely to employment patterns by race and ethnicity, but may also be due to racism and discrimination at the workplace.[59]

Immigrant and migrant workers are more likely to experience harmful exposures in the workplace.[60] Migrant workers are more likely to be employed in dangerous and harmful industries and occupations. They also face exploitation in the labor force. This exploitation includes high rates of child labor among migrant children.[61] Additionally, some migrant workers may not be aware of the legal protections that they have at the workplace or fear retaliation, including deportation, if they report unsafe conditions.[62]

The impacts of work on health also differ according to gender. Research finds that men are more likely to be exposed to physical hazards than women. In contrast, women have been identified as facing a higher risk of psychosocial hazards related to bullying, harassment, and discrimination. These differences are not solely due to gender differences in employment patterns by industry and occupation. Also there is minimal research that sheds light on the experiences of transgender and nonbinary workers. It important to be inclusive and to recognize gender as a construct that affects occupational health in complex ways.[63]

The issue of aging and how it is related to the health and safety of workers are an increasingly important topic. The median age of workers in the United States has been consistently rising and is projected to continue for a variety of reasons, including increases in the median age population in the United States and retirement age.[64] Workers over the age of 65 are one of the fastest-growing segments of the U.S. workforce. Their greater numbers are a concern because fatal occupational injuries, along with other health concerns, are more common among older workers.

Occupational segregation, referring to different patterns of employment according to demographic factors, such as sex, gender, and race/ethnicity, and discrimination at work, may lead to some workers facing hazardous exposures at greater rates than other groups. For example, poultry workers tend to work in southern states where labor unions are rare. Poultry workers also tend to be people of color, immigrants, and women, in an industry filled with health and safety hazardous exposures (Figure 16.7).

Work-related factors are also likely to contribute to global disparities in health. Article 23 of the Universal Declaration of Human Rights affirms several rights related to work, including the right "to work, to free choice of employment, to just and favorable conditions of work and to protection against unemployment . . . equal pay for equal work."[65(Article23)] Despite these affirmations, throughout the world workers suffer from unsafe and unjust working conditions. With globalization, many manufacturing jobs have been exported to low- or middle-income countries. While this movement of labor has created economic opportunities for many people in these countries, the work is often done in unsafe conditions. The collapse of Rana Plaza garment factory in 2013 in Bangladesh, which resulted in over 1,000 deaths, unfortunately highlighted these unsafe conditions. The movement of these manufacturing jobs may make such disasters and other occupational health concerns a greater concern in these countries in the future.

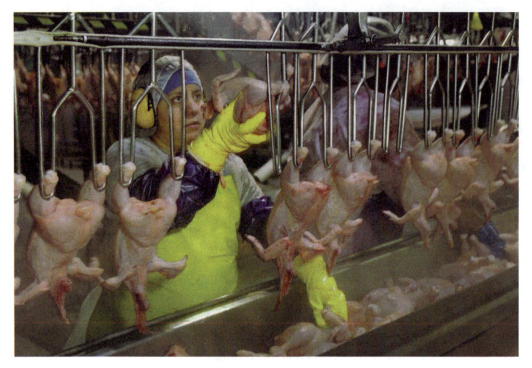

FIGURE 16.7. Hispanic poultry worker on chicken-processing line, Montgomery, Alabama.
Source: Photograph courtesy of Earl Dotter © www.earldotter.com

WORKING TOWARD ENVIRONMENTAL HEALTH AND JUSTICE

Decades ago, occupational safety and public health research viewed health inside and outside of the workplace as separate issues. However, we now know, as it has been validated by a significant amount of data and research, that worker health affects general health, and vice versa. In other words, conditions that impact an individual in the workplace can have an impact on life outside of work, and their life outside of work can affect their health outcomes at work. This concept is known as *Total Worker Health*® (TWH), a valuable framework to lean on as we continue to improve occupational health (Figure 16.8).

Advocacy is needed to bring about policy changes and improve efforts in occupational health toward EJ.[8] Workplace injustices and discrimination persist and are associated with adverse mental, physical, and emotional health outcomes. Discrimination based on one's race, age, sex, gender, and documentation status, and often a combination of these factors, takes place within the workforce daily. Having described the inequities facing workers in the previous section, we focus in this next section on how these inequities can be addressed for all workers, regardless of their race, sex, income, political party, or documentation status.

ADVANCING OCCUPATIONAL HEALTH AND SAFETY PROTECTIONS

There are many ways in which OSHA could be strengthened, for instance:

- **A more timely and effective process in setting standards:** To do so can help address existing and emerging threats to health, for example, the constant creation and introduction of new chemicals and new technologies. A solution may be to allow OSHA to easily adopt recommendations by experts.
- **Increased penalties for employers who violate OSHA policies:** As of 2022, the penalty for violations is approximately $12,000 at maximum (adjusted annually for inflation), which is not a meaningful deterrent for large corporations. Raising the financial penalties may incentivize more industries to comply with rules and regulations.

FIGURE 16.8. Issues relevant to advancing worker well-being using *Total Worker Health*® Approaches.
Source: Lee MP, Hudson H, Richards R, Chang CC, Chosewood LC, Schill AL. *Fundamentals of* Total Worker Health® *Approaches: Essential Elements for Advancing Worker Safety, Health, and Well-Being*. Department of Health and Human Services. Publication No. 2017-112. December 2016. https://www.cdc.gov/niosh/docs/2017-112/default.html

- **Assurances for workers that they can alert OSHA and other agencies to unsafe workplace practices:** *Whistleblowing* occurs in the workplace when an employee reports their employer for breaking the law or covering up criminal activities. Strengthening whistleblower protections can prevent employer retaliation and underreporting of harmful work spaces.
- **Expansion of OSHA coverage to public employees, workers on small farms, and gig workers:** This expansion is particularly important in light of the growth of the gig economy. There is also a need for a federal standard to require states to ensure that worker compensation systems cover all workers who may be injured or sickened on the job.

Also, while some states require that employers provide workers with paid sick leave and other types of leave, there is no national law. Such policies mean that many workers lack access to paid sick and parental leave, which are key components of protecting health, including reproductive and maternal health. Globally, the United States can learn from a variety of models in other countries where different types of paid leave are supported with notable benefits to public health.

TRAINING AND EDUCATION

Workers may face a variety of dangerous and precarious situations that can lead to injury, illness, and death. Effectively delivered training, regardless of job classification and across occupations and industries, may contribute to preventing such harm.[66] Training may raise the awareness of the worker, supervisor, and employer so that they become more aware of hazards in the workplace and identify actions that can reduce those hazards and promote well-being. By raising awareness and teaching skills, workers can take back the lessons learned to their workplaces and communities, which may empower them to take actions against such injustices. Training and education can help workers prevent and recognize the links between injustices and poor working conditions, such as a lack of protective equipment and engineering controls that can lead to increases in workplace injuries. The long-term impacts of worker training may improve safety, reduce injuries, illness, and disparities in the workplace, and increase community protection from environmental injustices. Moreover seeking out the input of workers with lived experiences can help ensure accuracy when developing training curricula and other materials and resources.

> ### IN OTHER WORDS: RIGHT-TO-KNOW
>
> Learn, understand, and share information about the laws affecting workers' rights. These laws, often referred to as "Right-to-Know" laws or "Hazard Communication" laws, are regulations designed to ensure that employees have access to information about the potential hazards associated with the chemicals and substances they may come into contact with in the workplace. See these related OSHA cards available in over 20 languages.
>
> **AS A WORKER you have the right to:**
> - a safe and healthful workplace
> - tools and equipment needed to do your job safely
> - training in a language you understand
> - and more...
>
> If you think your job is unsafe and you have questions, call OSHA.
>
> **It's confidential. We can help!**
>
> 1-800-321-OSHA (6742)
> TTY 1-877-889-5627
> osha.gov/workers
>
>
>
> **No one should have to be injured or killed for a paycheck.**
>
> If you think your job is unsafe and you have questions, call OSHA.
>
> **It's confidential. We can help!**
>
>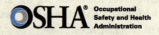
>
> 1-800-321-OSHA (6742)
> TTY 1-877-889-5627
> osha.gov/workers
>
>
>
> OSHA 3392-07R 2023
>
> *Source:* Occupational Safety and Health Administration.

> ### CASE STUDY 16.1: Superfund Training
>
> In the 1970s, the public became alarmed about the risks hazardous waste sites posed following a series of national stories about hazardous waste sites, including Love Canal and the Valley of the Drums. In 1980, the U.S. Congress responded to the discovery of thousands of such hazardous waste sites by passing the Comprehensive Environmental Response, Compensation and Liability Act (CERCLA), commonly called the Superfund. This act gave the U.S. Environmental Protection Agency (EPA) authority to clean up thousands of untreated contaminated sites throughout the United States. CERCLA requires the responsible parties to remove the contamination or pay back the government for the cleanup. If a responsible party is unavailable, then the Superfund provides funds to clean up the hazardous waste site.[67]

(continued)

CASE STUDY 16.1: Superfund Training (continued)

With the Superfund, there was a need to create green jobs to prepare workers, especially from impacted communities, for cleaning up contaminated sites and gain economically from the work. Multiple job-training programs have been developed nationwide, including the National Institute of Environmental Health Sciences (NIEHS) Worker Training Program (WTP) for training workers in these clean-up activities.[68] The WTP focused on providing safety and health training for hazardous-waste and emergency-response workers. One of the main program areas of the WTP is the Environmental Careers Worker Training Program (ECWTP).[69] For over 25 years, the ECWTP has focused on training and job placement for over 14,000 disadvantaged and underrepresented workers. The trainees included many workers who were struggling in life, from being unemployed and underemployed, homeless, formerly incarcerated, and more. ECWTP graduates have reported a high rate of job placements and higher wages, but also stability, self-confidence, and empowerment to give back to their communities. The ECWTP's innovative workforce development model aims to not just provide occupational safety and health and technical training, but also basic skills, life skills, and other preemployment training to prepare trainees to deal with everyday life challenges. There are ECWTP programs throughout the country through organizations such as the Atlantic Center for Occupational Health and Safety Training, the Center for Construction Research and Training, the Deep South Center for Environmental Justice and Texas Southern University, OAI, Sustainable Workplace Alliance, and Western Region Universities Consortium (Figure 16.9).

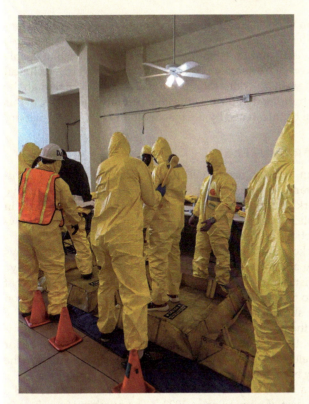

FIGURE 16.9. Training at the Los Angeles Black Worker Center, a partner organization of the UCLA Labor Occupational Safety and Health Program, part of the Western Region Universities Consortium.

REFLECTION QUESTION

1. Can you think of any other programs that support occupational safety and health and jobs in the community?

TECHNOLOGY EQUITY

As online methods are increasingly used to reach wider audiences for training and educational sessions, bear in mind that not all people have equitable access, fluency, and comfort using such platforms. Workplaces can provide training in technology use, either in computers or digital applications, but also in the latest devices. Preparing workers for using and communicating on such platforms and ensuring access to those resources are an important step toward technological justice.

Technological justice refers to inequity in access to and use of technologies needed to participate in society, such as cell phones, internet access, and adaptive technologies for people with disabilities. Technological injustice can contribute to workers being less able to enter the workforce because they do not know how to find and apply for jobs and struggle when they do enter the workforce because they lack adequate technological skills required for many jobs. For example, during the COVID-19 pandemic, some Native American workers on Tribal lands lacked internet access and were unable to receive online training, as opposed to other workers who did have access.[67]

LANGUAGE JUSTICE

Although English is the primary language used in the United States, it is far from the only language spoken. To reach a wider audience, it is necessary to ensure that multiple languages are used in workplaces and in training and education.[71] Too often English is the only language provided, excluding many workers from properly understanding the risks associated with their job duties.

Also, simply providing information in one's language is not enough. The use of plain language (as covered in depth in Chapter 5, "Environmental Health Science for the People") ensures information can be accessed, used, and understood by everyone in ways that enable them to take action. For example, a workplace's safety protocol may be written in a technical or legal language that does not have clear instructions for reporting concerns. Even though the information is written in English or is translated into workers' other primary languages, in this scenario, occupational health may still be threatened by the inaccessibility of the information.

LABOR UNIONS AND WORKER CENTERS

As this chapter illustrates, there is an ongoing need to address worker rights across occupations and industries. In some instances, workers and employers can have a productive dialogue to ensure safe, healthy work environments for all. Workers can educate those in leadership positions to implement policies and programs that ensure their rights. Often, however, leadership does not take such actions without the call to act from workers.

Of course, dialogue between workers and employers and supervisors does not always result in meaningful change. Forming a union and collectively bargaining are other effective ways to ensure that legal language exists for a just and equitable workplace. The first step that workers can take to form a union is to get together with other coworkers to discuss common interests and needs. Next the group should talk with a union organizer to strategize. The employer may voluntarily recognize the union if a majority of coworkers sign union authorization cards. If the employer does not, then a petition should be filed with the National Labor Relations Board (NLRB) to hold an election. If more than 50% of the workers vote for the union, the employer must collectively bargain with the union over working conditions.

Even though forming and joining a union may be ideal for some populations, only 11.3% of workers in the United States were part of a union as of 2022.[72] The number of workers in unions has steadily declined over the past several decades. When a worker is unable to join a collective bargaining organization or is legally excluded from U.S. labor laws, nonprofit worker centers offer an alternative.[73] Beginning in the late 1990s and early 2000s, worker centers began serving as bases for workers to mobilize, particularly low-wage workers, workers of color, and undocumented workers. Worker centers have had successes with initiatives such as raising minimum wages, securing immigrant worker protections, and stopping wage theft. They serve as a mechanism for workers to build social capital by coming together and positioning themselves to face fundamental occupational injustices.

CASE STUDY 16.2: International Labor Organization and India

While this chapter focused on the United States, it is important to keep in mind the occupational hazards to health that exist globally. These issues are prevalent in so-called developing countries or low- and middle-income countries. Globally, of the billions of people who work, 2.3 million workers die annually from occupational injury and illness. Work-related accidents that result in disability and the need to take time off from work account for over 300 million workers per year.[74] Surveillance systems vary by country, and the figures gathered may underrepresent injuries and deaths attributed to work-related causes.

Workers in places without stringent safety standards may work in precarious situations (Figure 16.10). From 2012–2016, this included 1.5 billion workers globally, including 134 million child laborers.[75]

Organizations throughout the world work to achieve global occupational justice, including the International Labour Organization (ILO). The ILO works to achieve labor rights and social justice by setting labor standards and policies for decent work among their 187 member states. The ILO was awarded the Nobel Peace Prize in 1969 for fostering dialogue on equitable work conditions.

In India, the ILO has been working to prevent forced labor, promote gender equality in the workplace, and strengthen national and state capacity, among other initiatives.[76] Successes of the ILO in India include the ratification of ILO's core conventions on child-labor minimum age, the training of over 370,000 women migrant workers to reduce their risk of becoming trafficked into forced labor, and supporting over 10,000 young persons in rural communities to set up their own businesses. The important work of international organizations such as the ILO and others can help workers in India and throughout the world continue towards occupational and social justice.

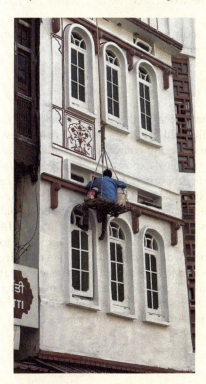

FIGURE 16.10. Worker painting a wall in Amritsar, India.
Source: Photograph courtesy of Eric Persaud.

REFLECTION QUESTIONS

1. Can you think of occupational and environmental issues that persist in other countries?
2. What steps are being taken by the ILO or other international organizations to address those issues? If you cannot find any activism publicly taking place, what do you recommend needs to be done?

MAIN TAKEAWAYS

In this chapter, we learned that:

- There are a variety of hazards facing workers, including physical, chemical, and psychosocial hazards. These hazards contribute to the risk for injuries, acute health effects, chronic health effects, mental health disorders, and fatalities.
- Much of the work of occupational health and safety involves characterizing the health impacts of specific hazards and identifying and implementing methods to control these hazards.
- Occupational health practitioners often make use of the Hierarchy of Controls for addressing occupational health concerns. The Hierarchy of Controls encourages addressing hazards in more fundamental ways—first, when possible, eliminate the hazard, before focusing on more downstream methods to control the hazard, such as personal protective equipment or education.
- Exposure to these hazards and their associated health outcomes vary across occupation and industry and demographics. In many instances, the worst impact of these hazards is felt among already marginalized communities, such as people of color, recent immigrants, women, and disabled people.
- Policies such as workplace inspections, fines, and worker's compensation have contributed to healthier workplaces, while inadequate financial penalties and enforcement barriers remain an issue.
- By supporting policies to address inequities in the workplace, we can improve conditions for all.
- Labor unions and worker centers are powerful tools for addressing shortcomings in existing occupational health policies and protecting workers.

SUMMARY

For decades, the field of occupational health and safety has successfully addressed many occupational health hazards, but millions of workers globally still face occupational risks. New hazards are emerging with new forms of work and the changing context of climate change. Traditional hazards, such as unsafe working conditions, chemical exposures, and psychosocial hazards, remain a concern. Many of these hazards fall disproportionately on communities of color. With globalization, much of the most dangerous types of work, especially in the manufacturing sector, have been exported to low-income countries. There are many policies that exist to protect workers, including inspections and fines from government bodies like OSHA and workers' compensation, to ensure that the cost of medical care and lost wages due to work-related injuries and illnesses are covered, but much work is needed to achieve equity and justice in accessing these protections. Work is still needed to improve access to benefits that protect workers further, such as paid sick and parental leave. Regulations, labor unions, worker centers, and general support for labor, as well as a progressive and expanded understanding of what worker well-being means may help accomplish safer and healthier workplaces.

END-OF-CHAPTER RESOURCES

DISCUSSION QUESTIONS

1. The mission of OSHA is "to assure America's workers have safe and healthful working conditions… by setting and enforcing standards… [and by] providing and supporting training, outreach, education, and assistance."[77(para1)] Refer back to the themes of the chapter to explore the barriers that prevent OSHA from achieving its mission. Is there anything that you would change or update in the mission statement?

2. Read the article "California Workers Who Cut Countertops Are Dying of an Incurable Disease," published by the *Los Angeles Times*: www.latimes.com/california/story/2023-09-24/silicosis-countertop-workers-engineered-stone. What are some themes from the chapter that are highlighted here? Who is affected? How do we promote equity in the workplace with safety communication? What are some barriers to prevention and treatment? Using this example, what are some ways (as described in the chapter) that we can advance occupational safety protections and EJ?
3. Refer back to the OSHA cards that specify worker Right-to-Know laws: www.osha.gov/workers. Have you ever had a safety walk-through for a particular place of employment? What was included on the tour? Are these laws something you were made aware of?
4. NIOSH began utilizing the TWH model in 2011. Its intention is to integrate occupational health with health promotion. Discuss a few issues under each header and what they mean to you in the context of TWH and the broader ideas of environmental health and EJ (refer back to Figure 16.8).

LEARNING ACTIVITIES

THE TIME IS NOW

If you are interested in engaging with other advocates, researchers, and students around the United States, consider joining a local or national trusted organization. One such organization is the American Public Health Association's (APHA) Occupational Health and Safety Section. The APHA Occupational Health and Safety Section aims to address workplace-related barriers to equity for all workers through policy proposals and collaborations throughout the year and during an annual meeting. The annual meeting is an ideal place for students and researchers to share their work and learn about ongoing efforts to advance worker health and safety. The APHA has many other sections, including the Environmental Health Section, focused on advancing policies and programs to protect people and communities through healthier environments. One thing an APHA section member can become involved in is working to propose specific policies. Such policies are created within and across sections to address some of the most pressing matters in public health and, if passed, become the official policies of the APHA and are often used in legislative arguments.

IN REAL LIFE

Think of the type of work environment you have experienced or hope to have in the future. Examples include working outside, in office settings, in laboratories, or in healthcare facilities. Research common occupational hazards, safety measures, and relevant regulations from your work environment, drawing information from sources like OSHA (www.osha.gov), NIOSH (www.cdc.gov/niosh), and the World Health Organization (WHO) (www.who.int/teams/environment-climate-change-and-health/occupational-health). Answer the following questions as part of your investigation:

1. What new information did you learn about occupational health in your work environment?
2. How can the safety measures you researched be applied in real-life scenarios?
3. Were there any surprises or unexpected findings in your research?
4. How do you think awareness of occupational health issues can affect your future workplace behavior or choices?
5. Discuss any personal experiences you or your friends and family may have experienced and how they relate to the broader concepts of occupational health.

A robust set of instructor resources designed to supplement this text is located at http://connect.springerpub.com/content/book/978-0-8261-8353-8. Qualifying instructors may request access by emailing textbook@springerpub.com.

REFERENCES

1. Weil D. The future of occupational safety and health protection in a fissured economy. *Am J Public Health*. 2020;110(5):640–641. doi:10.2105/ajph.2019.305550
2. Ferrari GN, Leal GCL, Thom de Souza RC, Galdamez EVC. Impact of climate change on occupational health and safety: a review of methodological approaches. *Work*. 2023;74(2):485–499. doi:10.3233/wor-211303
3. Oakes J. Capitalism and slavery and the civil war. *Int Labor Work Class Hist*. 2016;89:195–220.
4. Dray, P. *There Is Power in a Union: The Epic Story of Labor in America*. Anchor Books; 2011.
5. Stein L. *The Triangle Fire*. ILR Press; 2011.
6. Crandall WR, Crandall RE. Revisiting the Hawks Nest Tunnel incident: lessons learned from an American tragedy. *J Appalachian Stud*. 2002;8(2):261–283.
7. Rosner D, Markowitz G. A short history of occupational safety and health in the United States. *Am J Public Health*. 2020;110(5):622–628. doi:10.2105/ajph.2020.305581
8. Michaels D, Barab J. The occupational safety and health administration at 50: protecting workers in a changing economy. *Am J Public Health*. 2020;110(5):631–635. doi:10.2105/ajph.2020.305597
9. Baron SL, Brown TM. Alice Hamilton (1869–1970): mother of US occupational medicine. *Am J Public Health*. 2009;99(suppl 3):S547–S549. doi:10.2105%2FAJPH.2009.177394
10. OSH Act of 1970. Occupational Safety and Health Administration. Accessed June 17, 2024. https://www.osha.gov/laws-regs/oshact/completeoshact
11. Employer-reported workplace injuries and llnesses, 2021–2022. United States Department of Labor. Updated November 9, 2023. https://www.bls.gov/news.release/osh.nr0.htm
12. Bureau of Labor Statistics. National census of fatal occupational injuries in 2021. December 19, 2023. https://www.bls.gov/news.release/pdf/cfoi.pdf
13. Occupational injury and illness classification system. Centers for Disease Control and Prevention. Updated December 9, 2023. https://wwwn.cdc.gov/wisards/oiics/
14. Injuries, illnesses, and fatalities. United States Department of Labor. 2023. Accessed June 17, 2024. https://www.bls.gov/iif/
15. International Labour Organization. International standard classification of occupations. Accessed June 17, 2024. https://ilostat.ilo.org/methods/concepts-and-definitions/classification-occupation/
16. United States Department of Labor. Workplace violence in healthcare, 2018. April 2020. https://www.bls.gov/iif/factsheets/workplace-violence-healthcare-2018.htm
17. Occupational Safety and Health Adminstration. Carbon monoxide poisoning. 2012. https://www.osha.gov/sites/default/files/publications/carbonmonoxide-factsheet.pdf
18. Khalade A, Jaakkola MS, Pukkala E, Jaakkola JJK. Exposure to benzene at work and the risk of leukemia: a systematic review and meta-analysis. *Environ Health*. 2010;9(1):31. doi:10.1186/1476-069x-9-31
19. Occupational Safety and Health Administration. Understanding chemical hazards. Accessed June 16, 2024. https://www.osha.gov/chemical-hazards
20. Medical management guidelines for Formaldehyde. Agency for Toxic Substances and Disease Registry. Updated October 21, 2014. https://wwwn.cdc.gov/TSP/MMG/MMGDetails.aspx?mmgid=216&toxid=39#
21. Permissible exposure limits-annotated tables. United States Department of Labor. Accessed June 16, 2024. https://www.osha.gov/annotated-pels
22. Gaffney A, Himmelstein DU, McCormick D, Woolhandler S. COVID-19 risk by workers' occupation and industry in the United States, 2020–2021. *Am J Public Health*. 2023;113(6):647–656. doi:10.2105/ajph.2023.307249.
23. Billock RM, Steege AL, Miniño A. COVID-19 mortality by usual occupation and industry:46 states and New York City, United States, 2020. *Natl Vital Stat Rep*. 2020;71(6):1–33.
24. Hawkins D, Davis L, Kriebel D. COVID-19 deaths by occupation, Massachusetts, March 1–July 31, 2020. *Am J Ind Med*. 2020;64(4):238–244. doi:10.1002/ajim.23227
25. Agricultural operations. United States Department of Labor. Accessed June 16, 2024. https://www.osha.gov/agricultural-operations/hazards
26. Bloodborne pathogens and needlestick prevention. United States Department of Labor. Accessed June 16, 2024. https://www.osha.gov/bloodborne-pathogens/standards
27. Sohail M, Rehman CA. Stress and health at the workplace—a review of the literature. *J Bus Stud Q*. 2015;6:94–121.

28. Bodin T, Çağlayan Ç, Garde AH, et al. Precarious employment in occupational health—an OMEGA-NET working group position paper. *Scand J Work Environ Health*. 2020;46(3):321–329. doi:10.5271/sjweh.3860
29. Ergonomics. United States Department of Labor. Accessed June 16, 2024. https://www.osha.gov/ergonomics
30. Radiation. Occupational Safety and Health Adminstration. Accessed June 16, 2024. https://www.osha.gov/radiation
31. Occupational noise exposure. Occupational Safety and Health Adminstration. Accessed June 16, 2024. https://www.osha.gov/noise/health-effects
32. Noise and hearing loss. Centers for Disease Control and Prevention. Accessed June 16, 2024. https://www.cdc.gov/niosh/noise/?CDC_AAref_Val=https://www.cdc.gov/niosh/topics/noise/default.html
33. Heat. Occupational Safety and Health Adminstration. Accessed June 16, 2024. https://www.osha.gov/heat-exposure
34. Kinen TM, Hassi J. Health problems in cold work. *Ind Health*. 2009;47(3):207–220. doi:10.2486/indhealth.47.207
35. Centers for Disease Control and Prevention. The changing organization of work and the safety and health of working people 2002. Accessed June 16, 2024. https://www.cdc.gov/niosh/docs/2002-116/pdfs/2002-116.pdf
36. Costa G. Shift work and health: current problems and preventive actions. *Saf Health Work*. 2010;1(2):112–123. doi:10.5491/SHAW.2010.1.2.112
37. About hierarchy of controls. Centers for Disease Control and Prevention. Updated April 10, 2024. https://www.cdc.gov/niosh/topics/hierarchy/default.html
38. OSH Act of 1970. Occupational Safety and Health Adminstration. Accessed June 16, 2024. https://www.osha.gov/laws-regs/oshact/section5-duties
39. Tompa E, Kalcevich C, Foley M, et al. A systematic literature review of the effectiveness of occupational health and safety regulatory enforcement. *Am J Ind Med*. 2016;59(11):919–933. doi:10.1002/ajim.22605
40. AFL-CIO Organizations. Death on the job: the toll of neglect, 2011. April 28, 2011. https://aflcio.org/reports/death-job-2011
41. Hawkins D, Ibrahim M. Characteristics of occupational environmental heat injuries/illnesses, survey of occupational injuries and illnesses, 2011 to 2019. *J Occup Environ Med*. 2023;65(5):401–406. doi:10.1097/jom.0000000000002794
42. Delp L, Mojtahedi Z, Sheikh H, Lemus J. A legacy of struggle: the OSHA ergonomics standard and beyond, Part I. *New Solut*. 2014;24(3):365–389. doi:10.2190/ns.24.3.i
43. Hawkins D, Ghaziri ME. Violence in health care: trends and disparities, Bureau of Labor Statistics survey data of occupational injuries and illnesses, 2011–2017. *Workplace Health Saf*. 2022;70(3):136–147. doi:10.1177/21650799221079045
44. U.S. Environmental Protection Agency. Biden-Harris Administration finalizes ban on ongoing uses of asbestos to protect people from cancer. March 18, 2024. https://www.epa.gov/newsreleases/biden-harris-administration-finalizes-ban-ongoing-uses-asbestos-protect-people-cancer
45. Eisenberg-Guyot J, Hagopian A. Right-to-work-for-less: how *Janus v. AFSCME* threatens public health. *New Solut*. 2018;28(3):392–399. doi:10.1177/1048291118784713
46. Boden LI. The occupational safety and health administration at 50-the failure to improve workers' compensation. *Am J Public Health*. 2020;110(5):638–639. doi:10.2105/ajph.2019.305549
47. Worrell FC. Denying abortions endangers women's mental and physical health. *Am J Public Health*. 2023;113(4):382–383. doi:10.2105/ajph.2023.307241
48. Centers for Disease Control and Prevention. *Community Health and Program Services (CHAPS): Health Disparities among Racial/Ethnic Populations*. Department of Health and Human Services; 2008.
49. United States Census Bureau. Health insurance coverage in the United States. 2022. Accessed June 16, 2024. https://www.census.gov/library/publications/2022/demo/p60-278.html
50. Board of Governors of the Federal Reserve System. Economic well-being of US households 2023. Accessed June 16, 2024. https://www.federalreserve.gov/publications/files/2023-report-economic-well-being-us-households-202405.pdf
51. Marmot MG, Rose G, Shipley M, Hamilton PJ. Employment grade and coronary heart disease in British civil servants. *J Epidemiol Community Health*. 1978;32(4):244–249. doi:10.1136/jech.32.4.244
52. Employment projections. United States epartment of Labor. Updated September 6, 2023. https://www.bls.gov/emp/tables/educational-attainment.htm
53. Detailed cccupation by sex education age earnings: ACS 2019. United States Census Bureau. May 2022. Updated June 1, 2022. https://www.census.gov/data/tables/2022/demo/acs-2019.html

54. Arias E, Tejada-Vera, B, Kochanek KD, Ahmad FB. Provisional life expectancy estimates for 2021. National Center for Health Statistics. August 31, 2022. doi:10.15620/cdc:118999
55. Centers for Disease Control and Prevention. Occupational fatal injuries and rates, by industry, sex, age, race, and Hispanic origin: United States selected years 1995–2011. Accessed June 16, 2024. https://www.cdc.gov/nchs/data/hus/2013/038.pdf
56. Seabury SA, Terp S, Boden LI. Racial and ethnic differences in the frequency of workplace injuries and prevalence of work-related disability. *Health Aff*. 2017;36(2):266–273. doi:10.1377/hlthaff.2016.1185
57. Stanbury M, Rosenman KD. Occupational health disparities: a state public health-based approach. *Am J Ind Med*. 2014;57(5):596–604. doi:10.1002/ajim.22292
58. Faghri PD, Dobson M, Landsbergis P, Schnall PL. COVID-19 pandemic: what has work got to do with it? *J Occup Environ Med*. 2021;63(4):e245–e249. doi:10.1097/jom.0000000000002154
59. Hawkins D, Alenó Hernández KM. Racial and ethnic differences in the prevalence of work organization and occupational psychosocial exposures. *Am J Indl Med*. 2022;65(7):567–575. doi:10.1002/ajim.23368
60. Moyce SC, Schenker M. Migrant workers and their occupational health and safety. *Annu Rev Public Health*. 2018;39:351–365. doi:10.1146/annurev-publhealth-040617-013714
61. Rascoe A. Hundreds of migrant children work long hours in jobs that violate child labor laws. *NPR*. 2023. Accessed June 16, 2024. https://www.npr.org/2023/03/05/1161192379/hundreds-of-migrant-children-work-long-hours-in-jobs-that-violate-child-labor-laws.
62. O'Connor T, Flynn M, Weinstock D, Zanoni J. Occupational safety and health education and training for underserved populations. New Solut. 2014;24(1):83-106. doi:10.2190/NS.24.1.d
63. Messing K, Punnett L, Bond M, et al. Be the fairest of them all: challenges and recommendations for the treatment of gender in occupational health research. *Am J Ind Med*. 2003;43(6):618–629. doi:10.1002/ajim.10225
64. Bentley T, Onnis L-a, Vassiley A, et al. A systematic review of literature on occupational health and safety interventions for older workers. *Ergonomics*. 2023;66(12):1968–1983. doi:10.1080/00140139.2023.2176550
65. Universal declaration of human rights. General Assembly resolution 217 A. United Nations. December 10, 1948. https://www.un.org/en/about-us/universal-declaration-of-human-rights
66. The National Institute for Occupational Safety and Health. Assessing occupational safety and health training: a literature review 1998. Accessed June 16, 2024. https://stacks.cdc.gov/view/cdc/11254
67. Superfund history. U.S. Environmental Protection Agency. Updated October 30, 2023. https://www.epa.gov/superfund/superfund-history
68. About the Worker Training Program (WTP). National Institute of Environmental Health Sciences. Updated October 26, 2023. https://www.niehs.nih.gov/careers/hazmat/about_wetp/index.cfm
69. Beard S, Freeman K, Richards D, Lee Pearson J. Government program celebrates 25 years of commitment to environmental justice movement. *New Solut* 2023;32(4):277–287. doi:10.1177/10482911221150832
70. National Institute of Environmental Health Sciences. Worker training program. COVID-19 biosafety training and infectious disease response evaluation report 2021. Accessed June 16, 2024. https://tools.niehs.nih.gov/wetp/public/hasl_get_blob.cfm?ID=13641
71. Persaud E. Undocumented Americans need equitable language in worker training. *Health Equity*. 2022;6(1):638–639. doi:10.1089/heq.2022.0006
72. U.S. Department of Labor, Bureau of Labor Statistics. Union members. January 23, 2024. https://www.bls.gov/news.release/pdf/union2.pdf
73. Monforton C, Von Bergen JM. *On the Job: The Untold Story of Worker Centers and the New Fight for Wages, Dignity, and Health*. The New Press; 2021.
74. International Labour Organization. Safety and health at work: a vision for sustainable prevention. 2014. Accessed June 16, 2024. https://www.ilo.org/publications/safety-and-health-work-vision-sustainable-prevention
75. International Labour Organization. Global estimates of child labour results and trends, 2012–2016. 2017. Accessed June 16, 2024. https://www.ilo.org/publications/global-estimates-child-labour-results-and-trends-2012-2016
76. International Labour Organization. The ILO in India. Accessed June 16, 2024. https://www.ilo.org/publications/ilo-india-1
77. OSHA. U.S Department of Labor, Occupational Safety and Health Administration. https://www.osha.gov/aboutosha

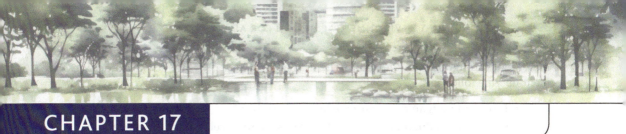

CHAPTER 17

Ensuring Children's Environmental Health and Justice

Nsedu Obot Witherspoon and Leyla Erk McCurdy

LEARNING OBJECTIVES

- Describe the field of children's environmental health.
- Demonstrate children's vulnerabilities to chemical, biological, and built environment hazards.
- Identify how children from marginalized communities are at a higher risk of negative physical and mental health outcomes due to toxic chemical exposures and climate change.
- Identify examples of community and national programs and efforts that work to protect children from harm.
- Define the mental and physical health benefits of healthy natural environments for children.

KEY TERMS

- child-protective policies
- children's environmental health
- climate change
- cumulative exposures
- mental health
- social determinants of health (SDOH)
- windows of susceptibility

OVERVIEW

Children today live in an environment that is vastly different from that of previous generations. Advances in technology, increased access to information, a growing population, and the rapid production of material goods at the end of the 20th century have greatly impacted society. These changes impact not only the environment around us, but also our health and the health of our children for generations to come. Environmental health challenges can result from the built, natural, biological, and chemical environments to which we and our children are exposed.

Children's environmental health, which includes exposures and outcomes across the preconception,[1] prenatal, infant, toddler, adolescent, and young adult life stages, has been identified by the American Public Health Association (APHA), the National Institute of Environmental Health Sciences (NIEHS), the Environmental Protection Agency (EPA), and the World Health Organization (WHO) as a critical focus area for the study of environmental health.[2] The elegance and delicacy of the development of a human being from conception through adolescence affords particular windows of vulnerability to environmental hazards. Preconception is also a critical exposure window, as described in Chapter 7, "Understanding the Environment and How It Relates to Health Using Toxicology and Epidemiology Research Methods." Exposure at those moments of vulnerability can lead to damage that is often permanent.

All children are affected by environmental hazards. Extensive scientific evidence shows how and why environmental stressors, toxicant exposures, and certain settings specifically affect children and how early-life exposures can affect the health and development of an individual throughout the life span.[3] The available science over the last three decades has identified the following:

- Lead and inorganic mercury are linked to autism.[4]
- Certain air pollutants are linked to the onset and development of asthma.[5]
- Air pollution from vehicles, pesticides, paints, and solvents are linked to childhood cancer.[6]
- Lead, organophosphate pesticides, manganese, and phthalates,[7] a group of chemicals used to make plastics more durable, are linked to attention deficit hyperactivity disorder (ADHD).

We in the United States are living among the first generation of children predicted to be less healthy than their ancestors before them.[8] Pollution and environmental degradation are found at the neighborhood, county, state, regional, national, and global levels. Contaminants are transported through many media including air, water, soil, food, the built environment, and products throughout the world. The environments of our homes, child-care facilities, K–12 schools, and colleges and universities, as well as community and work settings, are all important to consider in the efforts to protect children from harm. The places where children spend much of their time, both indoors and outdoors, are critical to their health and well-being.

Protecting the children of today and tomorrow is vital for human survival. The implications from institutional and structural racism have and continue to create barriers to achieving health equity for all communities.[9] Children are uniquely vulnerable in our changing climate as well.[10] This chapter provides an overview of the field of children's environmental health; describes how all children—especially the most marginalized—experience risks to their health, safety, and well-being; and offers examples of equitable solutions for doing better by our youngest members of society.

STATE OF CHILDREN'S ENVIRONMENTAL HEALTH

The prevalence of childhood chronic diseases and developmental disorders have risen dramatically, and environmental exposures are significant contributors. Air pollutants such as ozone and particulate matter (PM) increase the risk of lung and heart disease, along with other health concerns. Poor water quality resulting from industrial waste and pollution, as well as a lack of proper water treatment can cause gastrointestinal illness, developmental effects like learning disorders, endocrine disruption, and cancer. Additionally, exposure to contaminated food, harmful chemicals in everyday household items, and materials and furnishings found in homes, child-care centers, schools, and workplaces are all linked to poor indoor air quality.

These exposures contribute to a number of diseases in children. About 14% of the U.S. population, or over 10 million children younger than 18 years, are estimated to have asthma.[9] An estimated one in six children aged 3 to 17 years old have one or more developmental disabilities.[11] Conditions range from mild disabilities, such as speech and language impairments, to serious developmental disabilities, such as intellectual disabilities and autism.[12] Autism rates have been increasing, impacting approximately 1 in 44 children.[11,12] As of 2022, approximately 6.4 million children ages 4 to 17 years had been diagnosed with ADHD.[13] The prevalence of obesity has increased as well; the percentage of U.S. children ages 6 to 11 years with obesity increased from 7% in 1980 to nearly 21% in 2020. These trends continue, with the percentage of adolescents ages 12 to 19 years with obesity increasing from 5% to 22% over the same period.[14] Simultaneously, we are witnessing rising trends in comorbidities such as type 2 diabetes, which has increased approximately 33% from 2001 to 2017 in children between 10 and 19 years of age.[15] Childhood cancer incidence has increased steadily since 1975,[6] with trends showing that the demographics have been shifting to disproportionately affect people of color, especially Black populations. Moreover, the types of pediatric cancer are shifting, with a growing prevalence of renal and thyroid cancer among children.[16]

These health issues bring a host of complications for children and their families. For example, poor air quality can create or exacerbate asthma symptoms, which can lead to missed school days and result in diminished academic performance.[17] Childhood cancer survivors are at a higher risk for infertility, sleeping disorders, anxiety, and other forms of cancer.[6]

When society makes greater investments to safeguard children's overall health, we benefit by having better educated adolescents and adults who can thrive.[18] Table 17.1 identifies the extremely small amount of U.S. investment in children's environmental health between 2017 and 2023. Children born into low-wealth families tend to have poorer health in childhood, receive fewer investments in their future, and have a higher potential for lower wages as adults, adding to a generational cycle of disinvestment for their children.[18] Beyond economic factors,[19] racial disparities are critical to understanding the full picture of children's environmental health and related risks. This concept is explored more throughout the chapter.

REASONS FOR CHILD VULNERABILITY

Children, beginning at the fetal stage and continuing through adolescence, are physiologically very different from adults. As identified by the EPA, these differences include less effective filtration in nasal passages, highly permeable skin, a more permeable blood–brain barrier, lower levels of circulation of plasma proteins, and the continuous development of the digestive system, metabolic pathways, renal clearances, and vital organs.[20] Science and human experience have demonstrated that the timing and dose of environmental exposures play a critical role in determining health outcomes, especially during the development of an organ or organ system, pathway, or behavior. The terms **windows of susceptibility** or *critical windows of exposure* refer to specific periods of time when children are most susceptible to the effects of environmental agents.[21] Each stage of a child's development influences their susceptibility to various environmental exposures.[22]

Children are in a dynamic state of growth, with cells multiplying and organ systems developing at a rapid rate.[23] They also have higher metabolic rates and a higher proportionate intake of food and liquid than do adults.[24] At birth, their nervous, respiratory, musculoskeletal, reproductive, and immune systems are not yet completely developed.[23] In the first 4 months of life, an infant more than doubles its weight. Young children take in more air and breathe more rapidly in proportion to their body weight than do adults.

The rate at which children absorb nutrients likewise increased, potentially impacting their exposure to naturally produced toxins, as well as toxicants that are produced by, or are by-products of, human activities. For example, children have a greater need for calcium to support bone development than do adults and will absorb more calcium when it is present in the gastrointestinal tract. However, when lead has been ingested into the gut, the body will absorb it in place of calcium. As a result, an adult will absorb 10% of ingested lead, while a toddler will absorb 50% of ingested lead.[25] Because metabolic systems are still developing in the fetus and in children, they are not able to detoxify and excrete toxicants as well as adults, and thus are more vulnerable to them.[3]

Child behaviors, especially in early childhood, also affect a child's exposure to toxicants. In the first year of life a young child spends hours close to the ground where they may be exposed to toxicants in dust, soil, and carpets as well as to pesticide vapors in low-lying layers of air. Before a child can walk, crawling occurs on ground surfaces like floors,[26] increasing exposures. As part of the natural curiosity and developmental stages that children—especially toddlers—exhibit, hand-to-mouth and hand-to-object behaviors are common.[26] This normal development in early childhood may increase exposure to such toxicants as lead in paint dust or chips and to pesticide residues. Children also spend more time outdoors than do most adults, often engaged in

TABLE 17.1. TOTAL SPENDING ON CHILDREN'S ENVIRONMENTAL HEALTH—FIRST FOCUS ON CHILDREN: CHILDREN'S BUDGET 2017–2023

	2017	2018	2019	2020	2021	2022	2023
Spending level	$0.42B	$0.53B	$0.58B	$0.64B	$0.72B	$0.78B	$0.97B
Real change from prior year	15.78%	21.80%	7.97%	9.13%	9.53%	0.36%	20.68%
Share of total spending	0.011%	0.013%	0.013%	0.010%	0.011%	0.013%	0.017%

Source: Children's budget. First Focus on Children; 2023. https://firstfocus.org/childrens-budget

vigorous play. Because children breathe more air per pound of body weight than adults and because their respiratory systems are still developing, they are prone to greater exposure to and adverse effects of air particulates, ground-level ozone, and other chemicals that pollute outdoor air.[27]

A child's environment and diet also differs from that of an adult. In the first environment, the mother's womb, the fetus may be permanently damaged by exposure to a wide variety of chemicals that can cross the placenta. These chemicals include lead,[28] human-made chemicals called polychlorinated biphenyls (PCBs),[29] methylmercury,[30] ethanol and nicotine from environmental tobacco smoke,[31] arsenic,[32] and endocrine disrupting chemicals.[33] Because children eat more fruits and vegetables and drink more liquids in proportion to their body weight, their potential exposure to ingested toxicants such as lead, pesticides, and nitrates is greater.

Owing to exposures to toxicants at an early age, children have more time to develop environmentally triggered diseases with long latency periods, such as cancer[6] and Parkinson disease.[34] Additionally, multiple and cumulative exposures to toxicants and their potential coactions are not well known and demand further research.

> **IN OTHER WORDS: GROWING BODIES AND ENVIRONMENTAL EXPOSURES**
>
> Children, from when they are babies, are very different from adults when it comes to how their bodies deal with the world around them and the exposures they encounter. Their noses are not as good at filtering, their skin lets exposures in more easily, and their organs are still developing because they are always growing. They also eat, drink, and breathe more in comparison to their size, and generally they act differently, crawling around and playing on the floor, putting things in their mouth, and playing outside. All of these factors mean that exposures are different for them, and their bodies handle the exposures in a unique way. *When* they are exposed and the *amount* to which they are exposed can also make a big difference in their health. We need to put children first and consider these differences when looking at exposures in our environment.

CRITICAL EXPOSURES

SETTINGS AND SURROUNDINGS

The indoor and outdoor built environment, including human-made or modified structures, connects with all aspects of our lives. Indoor furnishings, such as carpets, curtains, mattresses, wall decorations, and some furniture, may be treated with chemicals and are potentially dangerous.[35] For a few days after installation, new carpets emit volatile organic compounds (VOCs),[36] which are chemicals associated with carpet manufacturing that can be harmful to humans and the environment. Pesticides are one of the most common reported substances in poison control centers, with poisoning in children being a major concern.[37] Gas stoves, wood-burning fireplaces and stoves, and kerosene heaters may also release dangerous chemicals. Building materials such as particle board, insulation, asbestos, and treated wood (used for decks and outdoor furniture) can also pose health threats. Lead in indoor environments can be found in paint (if the building was built before the late 1970s) and as a result of dust from remodeling or destruction projects. Other indoor sources of lead can include toys, cosmetics, jewelry, and lead-glazed pottery.[38] Some play sets and toys, as well as outdoor swing sets and playgrounds, may also be treated with toxic chemicals, be made from toxic plastics, or include hazardous materials.[39] The more time that children spend playing in such an environment, the higher their exposure to toxic chemicals and the greater the risk to their health.

Considering where children spend the most time, homes, child-care centers, and K–12 schools are critical environments in which to prioritize protective actions, in addition to actions to provide healthy outdoor environments. The first few years of children's lives are critical for shaping their future health and development. Increasing evidence shows that early-life exposures and the environments in which children grow up contribute to mental health and cognitive developmental challenges.[40] Children who experience cumulative exposures from climate change, air pollution, and water and food contamination within their homes and learning facilities face higher risks for negative health outcomes. Research also shows that childhood stress increases the risk of poor physical and mental health later in life.[41]

Early-care and education programs play an important role in helping children reach their full potential in school and throughout their lives. An estimated 30% of children under the age of 5 years in the United States are in some form of child care.[42] Exposure to environmental hazards in child care and schools can have short- and long-term impacts on the health of children and staff.[43] Some of the impacts from unhealthy school environments include negative influences on attendance, concentration, and performance.[43] According to the U.S. Centers for Disease Control and Prevention (CDC), an estimated 1 in 6 U.S. children have a learning or developmental disability.[44] The National Academy of Sciences estimates that environmental factors, including toxic chemicals, cause or contribute to at least a quarter of learning and developmental disabilities in American children.[45] In addition, schools that do not work to address environmental exposure concerns can inevitably encounter expensive remediation needs in the future. Childcare providers and schools that work to reduce exposures to harmful chemicals can help prevent illnesses and conditions like asthma, developmental disorders, and even some forms of cancer.

CASE STUDY 17.1: The Children & Nature Network

The Children & Nature Network works to create healthy environments for all children in addition to removing harmful exposures. The Children & Nature Network supports communities and schools in creating nature-based play scapes and advocating for equitable access to green space, which is shown to improve general well-being. Here are a few examples of such efforts supported by the Network:

- Fairfax County Public Schools in Virginia launched the Get2Green program in 2010 to engage PreK–12 students in environmental stewardship and to incorporate sustainability in the classroom. They now have 150 schools participating, 90 edible gardens, and more than 100 wildlife habitats.
- For over 30 years, leaders in Harris County, Texas, have run the Spark School Park Program, which has led to the establishment of over 200 parks across 17 school districts. Community members, students, teachers, parents, and others all participate in the design process, and the program specifically addresses gaps in park access.
- Santa Cruz City Schools in California run the Life Lab program at four elementary schools. Life Lab lessons incorporate California Science standards, environmental awareness, and nutrition education in engaging students to actively learn in their nature-based outdoors.

Communities developing such interventions must stay keenly aware of threats to environmental health (e.g., checking outdoor air quality when children are playing outdoors, testing the soil when developing school or community gardens to ensure the produce is safe to eat).

REFLECTION QUESTIONS

1. How does the Spark School Park Program in Harris County, Texas, address gaps in park access, and what community-driven aspects contribute to the success of this program in creating equitable green space?

2. How does the Life Lab program at Santa Cruz City Schools integrate different aspects of learning to enhance students' experiences?

CHEMICALS IN OUR DAILY ENVIRONMENT

During the last 50 years, hundreds of thousands of chemicals have been developed.[46] Since the 1950s, synthetic chemical production has increased 50-fold, and by 2050 that number is predicted to triple again.[47] Chemicals are ubiquitous in environments worldwide, and trace toxicants are found in all humans and animals.[48] Common environmental chemicals or substances to which children are exposed include lead, arsenic, pesticides, mercury, bisphenol A (BPA), bisphenol S (BPS), phthalates, combustion-related air pollutants, and flame retardants like polybrominated diphenyl ethers (PBDEs) and organophosphate ester flame retardants (OPFRs), which are classes of chemicals that are added to certain manufactured products, such as children's pajamas, in order to reduce the chances that the products will catch on fire. A University of California–San Francisco study of the blood of pregnant individuals and their children detected 109 chemicals, including 55 chemicals not previously reported in people and 42 "mystery chemicals," whose sources and uses are unknown,[49] but which most likely come from consumer products or other industrial sources.[50]

Currently, use of more than 86,000 chemicals is allowed in the United States as part of the EPA's list of substances that are included in the Toxic Substances Control Act.[51] Children are uniquely vulnerable to exposure and harm from environmental agents where they live, learn, and play.[2] Little is known about the health effects of the majority of these chemicals on children.[3] We know that chemicals are ubiquitous in built and natural environments because in the past several decades, health effects due to chemical exposures have been noted in wildlife. Exposures to some environmental toxicants, such as lead, are now known to cause permanent damage to a child's nervous system.[52] Other toxicants are implicated in causing adverse health effects in children.[3] Cumulative risks, even at low doses, from other sources can compound the adverse effects of exposure to harmful chemicals or biological agents and require concerted, intentional efforts to protect the youngest and most vulnerable. Moreover, the social determinants of health (SDOH) interact with these exposures to create an increasing risk for further disparities among children.[2]

Household products such as detergent, floor and furniture polish, paints, and various cleaners for glass, wood, metal, ovens, toilets, and drains may contain hazardous chemicals such as ammonia, sulfuric and phosphoric acids, lye, chlorine, formaldehyde, and phenols.[53] Air fresheners can also contain chemicals, like VOCs and phthalates, that are harmful to health. Art supplies (e.g., markers, paint, glue), toys, personal care products, and other children's products may also contain toxic materials. If not properly handled, these products can make homes, child-care centers, or work environments dangerous places. When considering equity, families who frequently shop at discount retailers have a high potential of bringing home products that contain hazardous chemicals. In a 2022 study, the Campaign for Healthier Solutions found that 50% of the products screened in these stores contained one or more chemicals of concern.[54]

CASE STUDY 17.2: Flame Retardants

In the mid-1900s, cigarette companies faced much scrutiny because cigarettes posed a fire hazard and could ignite furniture and other materials. In response, tobacco companies began developing fire-safe cigarettes. Next, they strategized to shift the blame away from cigarettes as the primary cause of household fires. Working with chemical and furniture manufacturers, they lobbied for flame-retardant regulations and standards. In 1975, a California law (TB 117) began mandating the treatment of all upholstered furniture on the market with flame-retardant chemicals like polybrominated diphenyl ethers (PBDEs). Around this time, Congress mandated that children's sleepwear be flame resistant too, so manufacturers started adding flame-retardant chemicals to children's sleepwear.

Many advocates have called for an end to the use of flame retardants because, despite industry claims, these chemicals can cause neurological damage, hormone disruption, and cancer. Flame retardants bioaccumulate in humans—their levels increase in the body—and pose long-term health risks. In response to decades of advocacy by a California-based coalition that included environmental groups and firefighters, California updated TB 117 in 2013 to reduce the need for flame-retardant chemicals. In 2018, California banned the use of flame retardants in furniture, mattresses, and children's products. Firefighters played a crucial role in these efforts, as exposure to flame retardants and other chemicals in their line of duty significantly contributes to their leading cause of death: cancer. While some states have taken similar actions, there are currently no federal laws that regulate flame retardants.

Today, consumers may be confused by labeling information on products as it relates to fire safety. For instance, anyone who has bought children's pajamas may have seen a yellow tag or label that reads "For child's safety, garment should fit snugly. This garment is not flame resistant. Loose-fitting garment is more likely to catch fire." These labels do nothing to explain the benefits of not having flame retardant chemicals in pajamas, and very few other products containing these chemicals are well labeled. Consumers are left to educate themselves on the dangers of flame retardants and weigh the risks of exposure to them against the safety of products in the case of a fire.

(continued)

> **CASE STUDY 17.2: Flame Retardants** *(continued)*
>
> **REFLECTION QUESTIONS**
> *1. Why did the cigarette companies lobby for flame-retardant regulations and standards in the 1970s?*
> *2. How did the collaboration between concerned groups and the California-based coalition contribute to the update of TB 117 in 2013 and the subsequent ban on flame retardants?*

AIR, WATER, AND FOOD

As discussed in Chapter 10, "The Air We Breathe," air pollution has significant impacts on health. It affects children more severely due to their still developing lungs and higher rates of air intake compared to adults. Exposure to pollution can result in reduced lung size and function, respiratory conditions like asthma and bronchitis, and some forms of cancer.[55] Among the most prevalent health outcomes, outdoor air pollution is associated with cognitive impairments, asthma attacks, bronchitis, hospital and emergency room visits, missed school and work days, respiratory symptoms, and premature mortality.[56] Poor indoor air quality can cause or contribute to infections, lung cancer, and chronic lung diseases.[57] With the U.S. population spending 90% of their time indoors, an increasing body of scientific evidence has indicated that indoor air in homes, schools, and other buildings can be more seriously polluted than outdoor air.[58]

Clean water and sanitation are a human right and essential to the health and development of all people, especially children. However, despite the importance of clean water, it remains out of reach for some of the most vulnerable children in the United States and the communities where they live, including Black, Hispanic or Latino, and Indigenous communities and communities in areas of low wealth. Children are especially vulnerable to the adverse impacts of pollutants in drinking water because children drink more water per pound of body weight when compared to adults, which can result in higher exposures because their bodies, immune systems, and brains are still developing.[59] Maternal exposure to harmful pollutants is also a concern to the developing fetus.[60] Contaminants of concern in drinking water in the United States include lead, pesticides, arsenic, nitrates, and per- and polyfluoroalkyl substances (PFAS), a class of millions of chemicals that are found in most everyday products. PFAS and other chemicals are also known to pass from mother to child through breastfeeding. However, the benefits of breastfeeding outweigh the potential risk of exposure to chemicals through breast milk for most infants.

Several chemicals that can be found in foods have been associated with adverse health outcomes, including developmental, reproductive, and neurological outcomes.[61] For example, organophosphate pesticides used in agricultural practices can expose workers (including pregnant individuals) who can then expose their children. Recent research suggests that even low levels of pesticide exposure can affect young children's neurological and behavioral development.[62] The health risks from chemicals in food are dependent on both the actual level of a chemical in the food as well as the amount of the food consumed. In addition to pesticides, chemicals of concern for children's health in the food system include methylmercury, PCBs, PBDEs, BPA, phthalates, PFAS, and perchlorate.[63] There are several challenges to consider regarding community access to healthy and safer food choices. As discussed in earlier chapters, food apartheid and the availability of organic foods can vary depending on the region and community. On average, organic foods can cost 50% more than nonorganic options.[64] Additionally, finding organic foods can be difficult in lower income communities.

CLIMATE CHANGE

Climate change is arguably the greatest public health threat that society is facing.[65] Urgent action is needed to protect children from the mental and physical health impacts of climate change upon children in all phases of their lives.[66] Decreased air quality and rising temperatures affect children by increasing asthma and upper respiratory attacks, allergies, negative pregnancy outcomes, food insecurity, mental health challenges, developmental delays, and epigenetic changes.[67] Health effects from climate change also include increased vector-borne diseases such as malaria; increased exposures to toxic chemicals; worsened poverty; increased physical insecurity and the need for migration; and increased morbidity and mortality from extreme weather.[68] In particular,

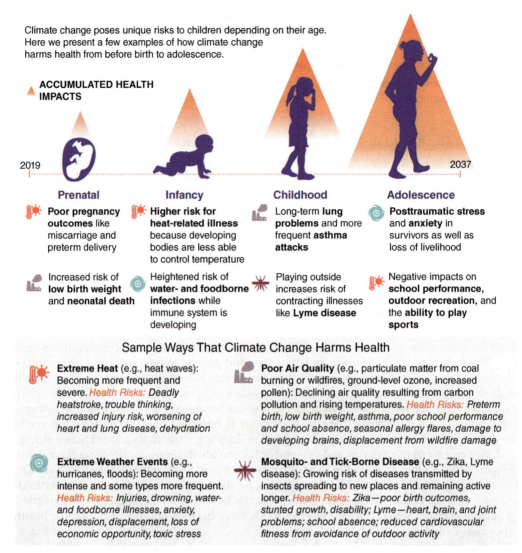

FIGURE 17.1. Climate change harms the health of children.
Source: Clayton S, Manning CM, Hill AN, Speiser M. *Mental Health and Our Changing Climate: Children and Youth Report 2023.* American Psychological Association, ecoAmerica; 2023. https://www.apa.org/news/press/releases/2023/10/mental-health-youth-report-2023.pdf

a rising heat index—the measure of how hot it really feels when relative humidity is factored in with the actual air temperature—is connected to diminished school performance and exacerbation of health disparities.[68] With about half of the world's child population living in areas at risk of the impacts of climate change, their exposure to multiple climate and environmental insults, combined with inadequate essential services, such as water and sanitation, healthcare, and education, is serious.[69,70] Figure 17.1 depicts the impacts on children from climate change at various stages of their critical growth. Climate change has the likely potential to reverse the advancements made in child health survival and well-being over the last several decades.[71]

> **MENTAL, PHYSICAL, AND COMMUNITY WELL-BEING: LINKS TO INEQUITY**
>
> Physical health, mental health, and community well-being have an interconnected relationship. The following graphic highlights how climate change and inequities affect these aspects of well-being and how family and household health play a role in the health outcomes of children. This graphic was adapted from the 2021 report *Mental Health and Our Changing Climate*.[72]

(continued)

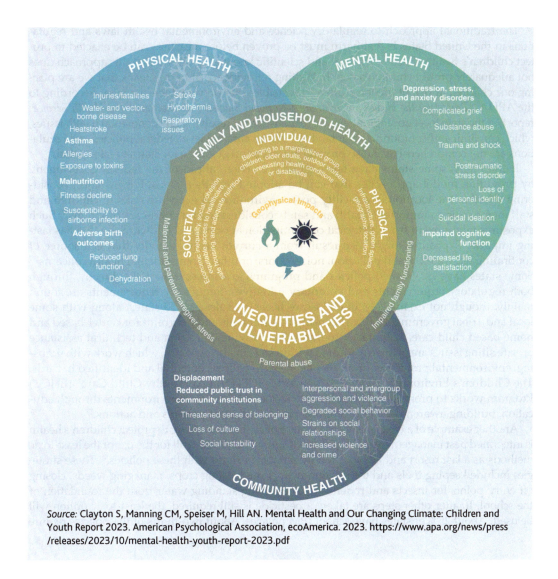

Source: Clayton S, Manning CM, Speiser M, Hill AN. Mental Health and Our Changing Climate: Children and Youth Report 2023. American Psychological Association, ecoAmerica. 2023. https://www.apa.org/news/press/releases/2023/10/mental-health-youth-report-2023.pdf

RELATED POLICIES

In 1997, President Clinton signed Executive Order 13045, which established the Task Force on Environmental Health Risks and Safety Risks to Children.[73] This task force remains in effect today to accomplish the goals outlined in the executive order.[73] The group encourages various government agencies to participate in and fulfill federal strategies for children's environmental health and safety. Goals also include targeted annual priorities to guide the federal approach, and recommendations for appropriate partnerships among federal, state, local, and Tribal governments, and the private, academic, and nonprofit sectors.[73] Many research agencies, committees, and organizations were created as a result of the premise of Executive Order 13045 to mitigate environmental health risks to children, especially the most marginalized. Specifically, the EPA established the Children's Health Protection Advisory Committee in 1997 to advise the agency on regulations, research, and communications related to children's health; the NIEHS, along with the EPA, established the Children's Environmental Health and Disease Prevention Research Centers in 1998; and the regional Pediatric Environmental Health Specialty Units (PEHSUs; also discussed in Chapter 18, "Integrating Environmental Health and Justice Into Healthcare") were created to provide consultation to public agencies, support communities in protecting children from environmental hazards, and educate health professionals on protecting children from environmental exposures.[74]

The traditional approach to regulatory science and environmental health laws and regulations in the United States is that harm must be proven before measures can be enacted to protect children's health. Current medical and scientific knowledge shows that this approach does not adequately protect children's health. Waiting for evidence of harm means that we are placing our children at risk of life-long, often irreversible—yet preventable—damage. According to the APHA's *Protecting the Health of Children: A National Snapshot of Environmental Health Services* report, at the state level no single agency is responsible for resolving environmental health issues, which can limit and confound accountability.[75] At the national level, federal policies and regulations are not comprehensive and so provide limited or no guidance for states to take action.

Increasingly, some states have taken proactive action, ahead of the federal government, by providing model approaches that can be adopted by other states. For instance, considering whether the location of a facility poses environmental exposure risks to children and staff members is an important health and safety consideration for child-care programs.[76] Such exposures might result from historical contamination at or near a child-care site that has lasting impacts. Exposures might also result from a current nearby activity that is a source of continuing air, water, or soil pollution; noise; odors; or other environmental health concerns.[77] Some states have established policies and programs to address these risks directly, through both regulatory requirements and voluntary initiatives. Regulatory requirements are found mainly, though not exclusively, in child-care licensing rules. All 50 states, along with some local and Tribal governments, have licensing requirements and programs for center-based and home-based child care. Voluntary programs that provide education and technical assistance on safe siting issues are primarily located within state health agencies, which work with licensing, environmental protection, and other agencies to address potential and identified hazards. The Children's Environmental Health Network's (CEHN) Eco-Healthy Child Care® (EHCC) Program works to promote safe and healthy indoor and outdoor environments through education, building awareness, and promoting **child-protective policies** and actions.[78]

Another example of a type of environmental policy that is working to protect children's health is integrated pest management (IPM) policies (Figure 17.2), which call for the use of the least-toxic methods as a last resort and are adopted by schools in states with these policies.[79] These strategies include keeping tools and the environment clean, rotating crops, managing weeds, closing off entry points for insects and rodents, and removing standing water from the foundation of the school. If, after other steps are taken, a pesticide is still required, the least-toxic option will be used. About 25% of states have school IPM policies. About two-thirds of the policies require

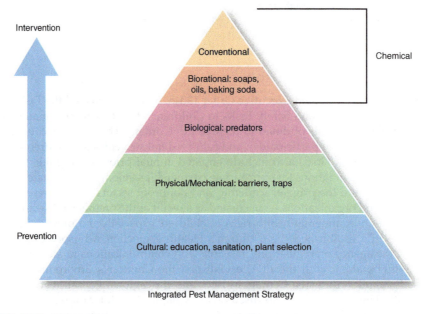

FIGURE 17.2. IPM strategy.
IPM, integrated pest management.

schools to develop an IPM plan or program, though these laws vary in the extent to which they establish minimum elements of an IPM plan.[80] These IPM policies are a step in the right direction toward using available science and community experience to take action in school environments where children spend the majority of their time between kindergarten and 12th grade. Child-care facilities could also use such state-driven policies since children from 6 weeks to 5 years in age use various forms of child care in the United States. The irony here, however, is that a state such as Louisiana, home to "Cancer Alley"—the area between New Orleans and Baton Rouge with some of the highest rates of cancer and asthma in the country—is one of the states that has IPM school policies, but also does not effectively protect its fenceline communities from industrial pollution.[81]

ENVIRONMENTAL HEALTH INEQUITIES

Children living in poverty and children in racial or ethnic communities are at a disproportionate risk for exposure to environmental hazards, including the potential for premature death.[82] One in six children in the United States lives in poverty, and 73% of them are children of color.[83] Although we have already pointed out several environmental health inequities affecting these children, they cannot be overstated.

White neighborhoods have an average of four times as many supermarkets as predominantly Black communities.[84] As a result, *food apartheid*—the system of segregation that divides those with access to an abundance of nutritious food and those who have been denied that access due to systemic injustice—impacts an estimated 24 million U.S. individuals, of which 5 million are children.[85] Access is limited in lower wealth communities where residents do not have safe and convenient access to supermarkets or other food retailers that carry affordable and nutritious food. Communities with limited or no transportation options rely more on smaller neighborhood stores that may not carry healthy foods or may offer them only at higher prices.

Lack of housing, poor housing conditions, limited access to recreational outlets and nature, and inadequate child-care and school conditions are not experienced equally. Middle-class Black Americans (making $50,000–60,000 a year) are more likely to live in polluted areas than White Americans with low income (those making less than $10,000 a year), and Black children are five times more likely to develop health problems due to their proximity to waste.[63] An estimated 76% of residents living within a 3-mile radius of the 12-worst polluting facilities are Indigenous, Black, and Brown individuals.[9,50] This exposed population includes children in these communities who experience higher levels of pollution from all sources. Low-wealth communities; Black, Indigenous, and Hispanic or Latino individuals; and families with children are also most likely to have significantly less access to natural spaces, limiting their ability to benefit from the physical and mental health values of being outdoors in nature.[86]

The poorest and most marginalized students often attend schools in the worst condition, placing them at an increased risk for adverse health outcomes as well as diminished learning.[87] Research shows that when compared to middle- and upper-class White children, Black children, those with less wealth, and those in other marginalized communities exhibit poorer school performance.[88] Environmental exposures are also connected to the achievement gap, with lead poisoning serving as one of the well-known pathways impacting cognitive abilities. Research on the discrepancies in exposures to air pollution, especially related to proximity to industrial areas and high-traffic areas, is well documented. Schools with higher populations of lower wealth or ethnically diverse students tend to have higher concentrations of two air pollutants: fine particulate matter ($PM_{2.5}$), which can increase the risk for asthma and heart disease, and nitrogen dioxide, which can also increase respiratory conditions.[89,90] To control the spread of airborne viruses in schools (e.g., COVID-19), it is important to have high-functioning ventilation and air conditioning systems to reduce the potential for airborne transmission of viruses and pollutants, particularly in schools located in marginalized communities.[91]

Children from low-wealth communities and children of color are most often exposed to adverse environmental factors and have fewer protective resources available to them. This combination results in negative health outcomes for children who fall into this cycle, impacting their current and future physical and mental health, wellness, and safety.[92] This scenario can be viewed as an intergenerational cycle of health disparities, since economic and epigenetic impacts persist across generations.[92]

Considering the range of environmental stressors and exposure pathways endured by our most marginalized children for decades, the negative health outcomes that are found in these communities are a direct result of those realities. Children from low-wealth communities and communities of color often have a greater risk of exposures to pollution, higher levels of contaminants in their bodies, and more illness or disability such as asthma and learning disabilities.[93] More than twice the number of Black children have elevated blood lead levels as compared to White children of the same age.[94] Hispanic or Latino, Black, and Indigenous children suffer from asthma the most, while Black children are five times more likely to be hospitalized for asthma, and three times more likely to die of asthma than White children.[95,96]

Children from underserved communities and communities of color are more susceptible to the adverse effects of climate change. Many are forced to live near hazardous waste sites, coal-fired power plants, or polluting industries that often present significant exposure crises during natural disasters and flooding. Community members often also lack the social and economic resources necessary to either relocate or to purchase the necessary materials or services to adapt to climate change where they live. As a result, low-wealth and Black, Brown, and Indigenous children are at a higher risk of suffering during extreme weather events as a result of direct harm from natural disasters; through potential increased air or water pollution, food contamination, or rising temperatures; or from displacement, among other effects.[97]

Communities of color are more likely to reside in inadequate and unsafe housing, attend schools and child-care facilities, and live in neighborhoods that tend to be closer in proximity to polluting industrial facilities and high-traffic roads.[98] Racist policies and practices—including redlining, the placement of hazardous waste facilities, intentional disinvestment in affordable housing and rental assistance programs, and systemic exclusion from shared resources—have allowed these statistics, patterns, and stories to proliferate and recreate generational patterns that have existed for far too long.[99]

WORKING TOWARD ENVIRONMENTAL HEALTH AND JUSTICE

While federal spending on children's environmental health more than doubled from 2017 to 2023 (Table 17.1), the overall share of budget spending was 0.017% of federal spending.[19] This level of investment does not keep up with the fact that almost every child in the world is exposed to at least one major climate or environmental hazard, shock, or stress, resulting in a variety of mental and physical health implications.[100] There is a proven return on investment in children and on the prevention of disease.[101] Preventing illness costs much less than treating negative health outcomes. The steps taken in Executive Order 13045 to place children first in decision-making and to provide capacity support for communities to protect children were important. However, the overall intent of the executive order has yet to be fulfilled. Federal agencies, academic research centers, and nonprofit organizations often take the lead on preventive research for children's environmental health, and yet funding for this work does not come close to meeting the various needs of preventing illness and supporting the growing number of children with negative health outcomes.

ADDRESSING INEQUITIES IN CHILDREN'S ENVIRONMENTAL HEALTH

Well-intentioned programs and policies may improve public health for some but perpetuate or miss opportunities to reduce inequities. Deeply rooted systemic inequities require transformational and bold shifts. Most efforts to address environmental health issues, in general, would benefit children's environmental health—across all sectors; with community, academic, government, and private partners; and at local, state, and national levels.

A recent report, *Racism That Upends the Cradle*, examines how Black children are differentially vulnerable to impacts from the syndemics of the economic crisis, the COVID-19 pandemic, and climate change.[102] (See Chapter 5, "Environmental Health Science for the People," for further discussion of syndemics.) To address environmental health inequities, the report explains how food, energy, water, and transportation systems must prioritize people over profits, including a transition away from a dependency on synthetic chemical production to fuel our economy. For these efforts to be sustained, they must include stringent standards and adequate investment in the monitoring and enforcement of all major routes of environmental exposures (e.g., clean water, clean air, uncontaminated soil, toxic-free building materials, toxic-free household products, toxic-free homes, and safe child-care centers and schools).

The authors also describe a large range of cross-sector strategies needed to address these deeply rooted inequities, beginning with the integration of anti-racism principles and accountability measures using tools such as the Government Alliance on Race and Equity Racial Equity Toolkit. The report calls for more equitable education systems that ensure quality, regardless of residence, race, gender, immigration status, disability, or any other factors. Early learning facilities and K–12 schools must be publicly financed instead of relying on property taxes—a system that deepens and exacerbates inequities. As the report explains, these changes all require transparent, participatory processes at community water and air boards and environmental agencies, school boards, zoning boards, housing associations, and community advisory boards, as well as participatory budgeting that engages residents in decision-making for city or state budgets.

Long-standing environmental justice (EJ) organizations, such as West Harlem Environmental Action for Environmental Justice (WE ACT), have called out and fought against various injustice challenges for the protection of the communities they are a part of and serve. EJ advocates help provide education and guidance on working toward community-driven solutions. WE ACT and the APHA's *Addressing Environmental Justice to Achieve Health Equity* policy statement offer many essential steps to improving health outcomes and mitigating injustices.[102,103] For instance, we can support communities with information, resources, scientific collaborations, funding, and additional capacity and spaces for networking and sharing to document and address health inequities through a child-protective lens with attention to health equity. We can also use child health indicators, such as physical health and safety, mental health, education, and learning, to help in the beginning of community decision-making, standard-setting, and policy making.[104] Over time, the tracking and sharing of such indicators will help us to understand where more work is needed in the United States and perhaps which programs or policies may be working to improve children's environmental health.

CRITICAL COMPETENCIES IN CHILDREN'S ENVIRONMENTAL HEALTH

The Community Preventive Services Task Force has identified education as the social determinant of health with the best evidence of effective interventions that lead to improved health status.[105] The Critical Competencies table (Table 17.2) identifies key areas in which to educate and motivate students, healthcare professionals, community and public health leaders, and child health advocates trained in children's environmental health at various educational levels.[106] Community leaders have an opportunity to learn about and promote these competencies as advocates for children. Similarly, the Break the Cycle of Health Disparities program works to mentor university and college students in the field of children's environmental health while they complete a community project in which they implement these competencies. Also bringing attention to children's environmental health is the CEHN's Children's Environmental Health Day, which is a day of action in October for and with youth to place children's health first through a variety of activities. The National Center for Healthy Housing (NCHH) works to utilize the competencies critical to children's environmental health through efforts to incentivize healthy housing practices (see Table 17.2). The CEHN incorporates these competencies in the larger children's environmental health movement in its efforts to educate healthcare professionals, environmental leaders, policy makers, and early child-care professionals.

EVERYONE HAS A ROLE IN PROTECTING THE HEALTH OF OUR MOST VULNERABLE

The CEHN's *Blueprint for Protecting Children's Environmental Health: An Urgent Call to Action* is a resource that can be used to frame action steps and guide priority setting.[107] The blueprint was developed with a broad base of input and consensus from key federal officials; pediatric and public health professionals; leaders in sustainable businesses, agriculture, transportation, and urban planning; child health and EJ advocates; and other traditional and nontraditional

TABLE 17.2. CRITICAL COMPETENCIES IN CHILDREN'S ENVIRONMENTAL HEALTH

COMPETENCY NUMBER	DESCRIPTION
1	Assess a children's environmental health concern, risk, or potential exposure in a community and develop a briefing paper.
2	Present information to stakeholders about children's environmental health threats and prevention methods.
3	Develop, implement, and evaluate a community-based intervention to mitigate a children's environmental health threat.
4	Increase children's exposure to healthy natural environments.
5	Monitor and report child health indicators to the state or local public health department.
6	Communicate to the media promoting children's environmental health through traditional and nontraditional outlets (e.g., social media).
7	Identify how climate change and environmental exposures (e.g., pesticides) affect children's short- and long-term health.
8	Be able to recognize or assess structural and systemic harms (e.g., built environment, climate change, risks associated with exposure) on children's health.
9	Identify federal, state, and local regulations as they relate to children's health and the environment.
10	Prepare and present testimony about children's health and the environment before local and state legislators.
11	Identify actions and evaluate yearly progress toward the reduction of greenhouse gas emissions and the carbon footprint of an organization (i.e., state or local health department).
12	Design environmental health guidelines that account for children's unique vulnerabilities and long-term susceptibility to health effects.

Source: Del Rio M, Lasley P, Tallon L, et al. Critical competencies in children's environmental health. *J Environ Health.* 2023;85(6):26–29. https://www.cmhnetwork.org/wp-content/uploads/2023/01/JEH1-2.23-Spec-Report-Critical-Competencies-Childrens-EH.pdf

partners.[107] Coordinated, comprehensive, and intentional efforts to reduce or eliminate environmental risks to all children are a valuable investment in children's health and long-term development and in the well-being of future generations.

Government agencies, public health practitioners, policy makers, community-based and EJ organizations, health economists, communication leaders, business leaders, and researchers must work together to advance policy and planning activities that incorporate or address the following objectives in relevant legislation or public health priority-setting regulations. The following calls to action are an adapted subset of those proposed in APHA's Protecting Children's Environmental Health Policy Statement[2]:

1. **Public health agencies, national and community organizations, and research and science institutions** need to create clear and accessible information to support effective action on children's environmental health. These groups should continue to identify gaps in research and information, strengthen the understanding about the connection between children and their environment, create a credible source of information, and develop a robust national research-translation agenda to build on existing research efforts.

2. **Federal and state agencies, sometimes with private institutions,** can support local health departments and community partners in promoting healthy neighborhoods, activities, and play environments for children, including access to parks and green

spaces, safe routes for biking and walking, public transportation, and access to universal playgrounds designed to be accessible to all children, including those with disabilities. Also, the development of new integrated county, city, and state systems could respond to, evaluate on site, and track and report the children who are at risk for suspected exposures. Each system should include an increased presence for pediatric environmental health experts, new healthcare provider protocols for uncovering or assessing environmental exposures and potential health risks, and specialized services for families with at-risk children.

3. **Other sectors** have important roles to play. Housing industry leaders and advocates need to adopt the evidence-based Healthy Housing Standard, a tool developed by APHA and the NCHH, for property owners, advocates, elected officials, code agency staff, public health leaders, and all who recognize the impact that housing has on community health. Also, public housing agencies and private management companies should ensure compliance. Leaders in creating and maintaining the built environment, such as engineers, design professionals, transportation officials, and urban planners need to create and maintain buildings, streets, neighborhoods, parks, and other elements of the built environment in ways that prioritize children's health and well-being.

4. **Educators and educational affiliates at all levels, such as boards of education, school administrators, teachers, and parent–teacher associations** are urged to recognize the environmental hazards that may be present in child-care facilities, K–12 schools, and colleges or universities; to monitor schools for the presence of these hazards; to remediate them when they are present; and to proactively establish protective environments moving forward. State and local child-care licensing officials are called on to adopt the environmental health standards included in the third edition of *Caring for Our Children*[108] as required regulations for licensing. They can encourage no idling for vehicles and adopting healthy cleaning policies at child-care facilities, the regular testing of water, and the implementation of IPM strategies. Environmental health improvements might also entail classroom clean-up days, outdoor beautification days, and community and school gardens. Schools are also encouraged to implement IPM strategies, healthy cleaning, and maintenance policies. Many schools have tried clubs to help keep momentum going each year and to support the school in child and environmental health protective practices.

5. **Scientists and advocates** with expertise in regulatory science, chemistry, and healthcare can inform policy reforms in chemicals use. They can advocate for bans or standards that reduce children's exposure to toxic chemicals found in many consumer products, for instance.

MAIN TAKEAWAYS

In this chapter, we learned that:

- Children are exposed to environmental exposures as early as the preconception and prenatal stages of development.
- Due to their unique vulnerabilities, children are more susceptible to environmental-hazard exposures and related negative health outcomes that can impact the entirety of their lives.
- As a result of structural and environmental racism, children of color and those living in low-wealth communities are frequently at risk for increased and cumulative amounts of environmental hazard exposures.
- Disinvestment in children's environmental health overall has resulted in a range of negative physical, mental, and overall quality-of-life indicators that can have current and life-long implications.
- Climate change is one of the most critical influences in the field of children's environmental health. Intentional community-based solutions that place children first need to be a top priority.

- Community advocates and nonprofit organizations need to work together at the national, state, and local levels to increase diverse partnerships and leverage capacity toward comprehensive and greater child health protections.
- the places where children spend the most time, such as homes, child-care centers, and schools, require focused attention to ensure that they are as safe and healthy as possible.
- Focused attention on reducing dependency on fossil fuels, plastics, and synthetic fabrics requires dedicated advocacy to ensure that children are not harmed owing to industry practices, their resulting products, and the legacy of increased waste in the environment.
- There are a range of actions that individuals, as well as community, national, and government organizations, can take to promote better protections for children.

SUMMARY

Children generally lack awareness and control over their environmental exposures, and they depend on adults for protection. While some exposures to environmental hazards have decreased because of new regulations and standards, children continue to be exposed to harmful toxicants in the air, water, food, products, and built environment. Overall, prenatal and preconception care are especially viewed as critical to risk reduction and healthy child development, especially with respect to the developmental origins of health and disease. Ensuring the well-being of all children, especially those who are repeatedly marginalized, requires proactive measures to break the cycle of health disparities exacerbated by environmental injustice and climate change. Comprehensive community responses are needed, focusing on proactive actions to safeguard children in their surroundings, including their homes, schools, child-care centers, and play spaces. Coordinated and comprehensive child-centered solutions are needed to prevent environmental risks for all children, to protect their health and well-being. Government agencies, public health practitioners, community-based and EJ organizations, youth leaders, child health advocates, policy makers, health economists, engineers, community planners, social service leaders, and researchers must all partner to advance policy and planning priorities to improve child health protections.

ACKNOWLEDGMENT

The authors wish to acknowledge the valuable time and feedback provided by Kristie Trousdale, MPH, Deputy Director, CEHN, in reviewing the material presented in this chapter.

END-OF-CHAPTER RESOURCES

DISCUSSION QUESTIONS

1. Thinking about your own city or hometown, in what ways are children's environmental health supported? In what ways could protections be improved? Think about the places where children are likely to spend most of their time.
2. Families with children have a lot of responsibility as they care for newborns and small children. Considering environmental exposures in the built environment, various chemical exposures in our daily life, and the threats of climate change, how can we prepare families for navigating these many risks? In your opinion, how can this be done in ways that educate, support, and empower families without overwhelming them further?
3. Throughout this text, there is much discussion about how chemicals in the United States are mostly "innocent until proven guilty." This chapter explains that the traditional approach to environmental health laws and regulations is that harm must be

proven before we can enact measures to protect children's health. In your opinion, what changes are needed in regulatory science to better protect children from environmental health issues?
4. Review the CEHN's *Blueprint for Protecting Children's Environmental Health: An Urgent Call to Action*. If you were an elected official, which of these actions would you prioritize? Can you think of other ways to promote children's environmental health equity that are not included?

LEARNING ACTIVITIES

THE TIME IS NOW

How Can We Prepare the Next Generation for Climate Change?

The APHA's Children's Environmental Health Committee recently developed the Climate and Health Lesson Plan for Grades 9–12 Toolkit. This toolkit, designed for public health and healthcare professionals and students, aims to educate and inspire young people about climate solutions. Additionally, the Committee has partnered with the APHA Center for Climate, Health and Equity to launch the Climate and Youth Education Toolkit, which is available on their website at: https://apha.org/Topics-and-Issues/Climate-Change/Education. With this resource, you can volunteer to teach a Climate and Health Lesson Plan at high schools in your community.

IN REAL LIFE

UNICEF is a United Nations agency that works to provide humanitarian and developmental assistance to children and mothers in low- and middle-income countries. UNICEF focuses on promoting children's rights; providing healthcare and immunizations; ensuring access to clean water and nutrition; and offering education and protection from violence, exploitation, and discrimination. Its mission is to advocate for the protection and well-being of children globally, particularly those who are most vulnerable or marginalized.

As such, the agency has developed a Climate Risk Index to examine how climate change is impacting children globally. (Similar to tools discussed in Chapter 8, "Mapping Environmental Health and Justice Issues," this is an interactive GISc tool.) As explained on the UNICEF website, the index ranks countries based on children's exposure and vulnerability to climate and environmental events like cyclones and heat waves.[109]

Go to the Children's Climate Risk Index: https://data.unicef.org/resources/childrens-climate-risk-index-report. Which countries can anticipate the greatest climate and environmental shocks? Which are the most vulnerable? Based on what you see, how might you prioritize action for those most at risk?

A robust set of instructor resources designed to supplement this text is located at http://connect.springerpub.com/content/book/978-0-8261-8353-8. Qualifying instructors may request access by emailing textbook@springerpub.com.

REFERENCES

1. Wesselink A, Wellenius GA. Impacts of climate change on reproductive, perinatal, and paediatric health. *Paediatr Perinat Epidemiol*. 2022;36(1):1–3. doi:10.1111/ppe.12839
2. American Public Health Association Policy Statements. Protecting children's environmental health: a comprehensive framework. November 7, 2017. https://www.apha.org/policies-and-advocacy/public-health-policy-statements/policy-database/2018/01/23/protecting-childrens-environmental-health
3. Carroquino MJ, Posada M, Landrigan PJ. Environmental toxicology: children at risk. *Environ Toxicol*. 2012;239–291. doi:10.1007/978-1-4614-5764-0_11

4. Yassa HA. Autism: a form of lead and mercury toxicity. *Environ Toxicol Pharmacol*. 2014;38(3): 1016–1024. doi:10.1016/j.etap.2014.10.005
5. Tiotiu A, Novakova P, Nedeva D. Impact of air pollution on asthma outcomes. *Int J Environ Res Public Health*. 2020;17(17):6212. doi:10.3390/ijerph17176212
6. Childhood Cancer Prevention Initiative and Cancer Free Economy Network. Childhood cancer: cross-sector strategies for prevention. 2020. https://www.cancerfreeeconomy.org/wp-content/uploads/2020/09/CFE_ChildhoodCancerPrevention_Report_F2.pdf
7. Zota AR, Calafat AM, Woodruff TJ. Temporal trends in phthalate exposures: findings from the national health and nutrition examination survey, 2001–2010. *Environ Health Perspect*. 2014;122:235–241. doi:10.1289/ehp.1306681
8. Grabmeier J. Health declining in Gen X and Gen Y, national study shows. Ohio State News. March 19, 2021. https://news.osu.edu/health-declining-in-gen-x-and-gen-y-national-study-shows/
9. Hoover E, Cook K, Plain R, et al. Indigenous peoples of north America: environmental exposures and reproductive justice. *Environ Health Perspect*. 2012;120(12):1645–1649. doi:10.1289/ehp.1205422
10. Climate change and children's health and well-being in the United States. U.S. Environmental Protection Agency. April 2023. Updated May 30, 2023. https://www.epa.gov/cira/climate-change-and-childrens-health-and-well-being-united-states-report
11. CDC's work on developmental disabilities. Centers for Disease Control and Prevention. Accessed June 17, 2024. https://www.cdc.gov/ncbddd/about/index.html
12. Data and statistics on autism spectrum disorder. Centers for Disease Control and Prevention. https://www.cdc.gov/autism/data-research/index.html
13. Centers for Disease Control and Prevention. Attention-deficit/hyperactivity disorder (ADHD). May 15, 2024. http://www.cdc.gov/ncbddd/adhd/data.html
14. Centers for Disease Control and Prevention. Childhood Obesity Facts. April 2, 2024. https://www.cdc.gov/obesity/data/childhood.html#:~:text=Obesity%20prevalence%20was%2012.7%25%20among,more%20common%20among%20certain%20populations
15. Lawrence JM, Divers J, Isom S, et al. Trends in prevalence of type 1 and type 2 diabetes in children and adolescents in the US, 2001–2017. *JAMA*. 2021;326(8):717–727. doi:10.1001/jama.2021.11165
16. Siegel DA, King J, Tai E, Buchanan N, Ajani UA, Li J. Cancer incidence rates and trends among children and adolescents in the United States, 2001–2009. *Pediatrics*. 2014;134:e945–e955. doi:10.1542/peds.2013-3926
17. U.S. Environmental Protection Agency. *America's Children and the Environment*. 3rd ed. CreateSpace Independent Publishing; 2013. https://cfpub.epa.gov/si/si_public_record_report.cfm?Lab=NCEE&dirEntryID=217843
18. Belli P, Bustreo F, Preker A. Investing in children's health: what are the economic benefits? *Bull World Health Organ*. 2005;83(10):777–784.
19. Dallafior M, Troe J, Kayal M, Sasner C, Gomez O, eds. *Children's Budget 2022*. First Focus on Children; 2022. https://firstfocus.org/wp-content/uploads/2022/10/ChildrensBudget2022.pdf
20. Firestone M, Berger M, Foos B, Etzel R. Two decades of enhancing children's environmental health protection at the U.S. Environmental Protection Agency. *Environ Health Perspect*. 2016;124(12):A214–A218. doi:10.1289/EHP1040
21. Perlroth NH, Castelo Branco CW. Current knowledge of environmental exposure in children during the sensitive developmental periods. *J Pediatr*. 2017;93(1):17–27. doi:10.1016/j.jped.2016.07.002
22. Agency for Toxic Substances and Disease Registry. Principles of pediatric environmental health: why are children often especially susceptible to the adverse effects of environmental toxicants? Updated May 25, 2023. https://www.atsdr.cdc.gov/csem/pediatric-environmental-health/why_children.html
23. An introduction to children's environmental health. Children's Environmental Health Collaborative. 2009. Accessed June 16, 2024. https://ceh.unicef.org/resources/introduction-childrens-environmental-health-course
24. Susceptible populations. Agency for Toxic Substances and Disease Registry. Choose safe places for early care and education. Updated October 30, 2018. https://www.atsdr.cdc.gov/safeplacesforECE/cspece_guidance/susceptible.html
25. Bearer CF. Environmental health hazards: how children are different from adults. *Future Child*. 1995;5(2):11–26.

26. Protecting children's environmental health. U.S. Environmental Protection Agency. October 2016. Updated April 12, 2024. https://www.epa.gov/children
27. Bates DV. The effects of air pollution on children. *Environ Health Perspect*.1995;103(6):49–53. doi:10.1289/ehp.95103s649
28. Wani AL, Ara A, Usmani JA. Lead toxicity: a review. *Interdiscip Toxicol*. 2015;8(2):55–64. doi:10.1515/intox-2015-0009
29. Nakajima S, Saijo Y, Kato S, et al. Effects of prenatal exposure to polychlorinated biphenyls and dioxins on mental and motor development in Japanese children at 6 months of age. *Environ Health Perspect*. 2006;114(5):773–778. doi:10.1289/ehp.8614
30. Sakamoto M, Tatsuta N, Izumo K, et al. Health impacts and biomarkers of prenatal exposure to methylmercury: lessons from Minamata, Japan. *Toxics*. 2018;6(3):45. doi:10.3390/toxics6030045
31. Bruin JE, Gerstein HC, Holloway AC. Long-term consequences of fetal and neonatal nicotine exposure: a critical review. *Toxicol Sci*. 2010;116(2):364–374. doi:10.1093/toxsci/kfq103
32. Tofail F, Vahter M, Hamadani JD, et al. Effect of arsenic exposure during pregnancy on infant development at 7 months in rural matlab, Bangladesh. *Environ Health Perspect*. 2009;117(2):288–293. doi:10.1289/ehp.11670
33. Tanner EM, Hallerback MU, Wikstrom S, et al. Early prenatal exposure to suspected endocrine disruptor mixtures is associated with lower IQ at age seven. *Environ Int*. 2020;134:105185. doi:10.1016/j.envint.2019.105185
34. Chen H, Ritz B. The search for environmental causes of parkinson's disease moving forward. *J Parkinsons Dis*. 2018;8(suppl 1):S9–S17. doi:10.3233/JPD-181493
35. Loftness V, Hakkinen B, Adan O, Nevalainen A. Elements that contribute to healthy building design. *Environ Health Perspect*. 2007;115(6):965–970. doi:10.1289/ehp.8988
36. Hodgson AT, Wooley JD, Daisey JM. Emissions of volatile organic compounds from new carpets measured in a larger-scale environmental chamber. *Air Waste*. 1993;43(3):316–24. doi:10.1080/1073161x.1993.10467136
37. Roberts RR, Karr CJ; Council on Environmental Health. Pesticides exposure in children. *Pediatrics*. 2012;130(6):e1765–1788. doi:10.1542/peds.2012-2758
38. U.S. Health and Human Services, Centers for Disease Control and Prevention. Prevent children's exposure to lead. Accessed June 17, 2024. https://www.cdc.gov/lead-prevention/about/index.html
39. Children's Environmental Health Network. Eco-Healthy Child Care® plastics & plastic toys factsheet. 2016. https://cehn.org/wp-content/uploads/2017/07/Plastics_Plastic_Toys_6_16.pdf
40. Kamp IV, Persson W, Kerstin, et al. Early environmental quality and life-course mental health effects: the equal-Life project. *Environ Epidem*. 2022;6(1):e183. doi:10.1097/EE9.0000000000000183
41. Bjorkenstam E, Burstrom B, Brannstrom L Vinnerljung B, Björkenstam C, Pebley AR. Cumulative exposure to childhood stressors and subsequent psychological distress. An analysis of U.S. panel data. *Soc Sci Med*. 2015;142:109–117. doi:10.1016/j.socscimed.2015.08.006
42. Environmental Law Institute and Children's Environmental Health Network. Reducing environmental exposures in child care facilities. January 2015. https://www.eli.org/research-report/reducing-environmental-exposures-child-care-facilities-review-state-policy
43. About the state school environmental health guidelines. U.S. Environmental Protection Agency. Updated April 5, 2024. https://www.epa.gov/schools/about-state-school-environmental-health-guidelines
44. CDC's work on developmental disabilities. U.S. Health and Human Services, Centers for Disease Control and Prevention. Accessed June 17, 2024. https://www.cdc.gov/ncbddd/about/helping-children.html
45. About LDA's healthy children project. Learning Disabilities Association of America. Accessed June 17, 2024. https://healthychildrenproject.org/about-ldas-healthy-children-project/
46. Naidu R, Biswas B, Willett IR, et al. Chemical pollution: a growing peril and potential catastrophic risk to humanity. *Environ Int*. 2021;156:106616. doi:10.1016/j.envint.2021.106616
47. Persson L, Almroth BMC, Collins CD, et al. Outside the safe operating space of the planetary boundary for novel entities. *Environ Sci Technol*. 2022;56(3):1510–1521. doi:10.1021/acs.est.1c04158
48. Colborn T, Dumanoski D, Myers JP. *Our Stolen Future: Are We Threatening Our Fertility, Intelligence, and Survival?* Penguin; 1997.
49. Wang A, Abrahamsson DP, Jiang T, et al. Suspect screening, prioritization, and confirmation of environmental chemicals in maternal-newborn Pairs from San Francisco. *Environ Sci Technol*. 2021;55(8):5037–5049. doi:10.1021/acs.est.0c05984

50. Fleischman L, Franklin M. *Fumes Across the Fence-Line: The Health Impacts of Air Pollution from Oil and Gas Facilities on African American Communities*. National Association for the Advancement of Colored People, Clean Air Task Force; 2017.
51. About the TSCA chemical substance inventory. U.S. Environmental Protection Agency. Updated June 9, 2023. https://www.epa.gov/tsca-inventory/about-tsca-chemical-substance-inventory
52. Sanders T, Liu Y, Buchner V, Tchounwou PB. Neurotoxic effects and biomarkers of lead exposure: a review. *Rev Environ Health*. 2009;24(1):15–45. doi:10.1515/reveh.2009.24.1.15
53. Children's Environmental Health Network. Eco-Healthy Child Care® household chemicals factsheet. January 2022. Accessed June 17, 2024. https://cehn.org/download/household-chemicals-fact-sheet/
54. Campaign for Healthier Solutions. Toxic chemicals in dollar store products: 2022 report. 2022. https://www.ecocenter.org/sites/default/files/2022-04/Toxic%20Chemicals%20in%20Dollar%20Store%20Products-%202022%20Report.pdf
55. Children's Environmental Health Network. Air quality fact sheet. October 2020. Accessed June 17, 2024. https://cehn.org/download/air-quality-fact-sheet/
56. Outdoor air quality. 2022. U.S. Environmental Protection Agency. Updated July 4, 2023. www.epa.gov/report-environment/outdoor-air-quality
57. American Lung Association. What Makes Indoor Air Unhealthy? Accessed June 17, 2024. https://www.lung.org/clean-air/at-home/indoor-air-pollutants
58. The inside story. A guide to indoor air quality. U.S. Environmental Protection Agency. Updated June 22, 2023. https://www.epa.gov/indoor-air-quality-iaq/inside-story-guide-indoor-air-quality#:~:text=In%20the%20last%20several%20years,percent%20of%20their%20time%20indoors
59. Landrigan PJ, Kimmel CA, Correa A, Eskenazi B. Children's health and the environment: public health issues and challenges for risk assessment. *Environ Health Perspect*. 2004;112(2):257–265. doi:10.1289/ehp.6115
60. U.S. Health and Human Services, Centers for Disease Control and Prevention. Childhood lead poisoning prevention: pregnant women. April 2, 2024. https://www.cdc.gov/nceh/lead/prevention/pregnant.htm
61. Environments and contaminants—chemicals in food. U.S. Environmental Protection Agency. Updated October 9, 2023. www.epa.gov/americaschildrenenvironment/environments-and-contaminants-chemicals-food#:~:text=Chemicals%20of%20concern%20for%20children"s,%2C%20perchlorate%2C%20and%20organophosphate%20pesticides
62. Liu J, Schelar E. Pesticide exposure and child neurodevelopment. *Workplace Health Saf*. 2012;60(5):235–243. doi:10.3928/21650799-20120426-73
63. Bullard RD, Mohai P, Saha R, Wright B. *Toxic Wastes and Race at Twenty, 1987–2007: A Report Prepared for the United Church of Christ Justice & Witness Ministries*. United Church of Christ; March 2007. https://www.ucc.org/wp-content/uploads/2021/03/toxic-wastes-and-race-at-twenty-1987-2007.pdf
64. West Virginia University. Organic vs. locally grown food. February 23, 2022. https://diningservices.wvu.edu/allergy-and-dietary-resources/the-dietitian-dish/blog/2022/02/23/organic-vs-locally-grown-food-february-2022#:~:text=Data%20has%20shown%20that%20on,as%20much%20as%20conventional%20foods.&text=Another%20issue%20is%20that%20organic,have%20a%20shorter%20shelf%2Dlife
65. World Health Organization. Climate change and health. https://www.who.int/news-room/fact-sheets/detail/climate-change-and-health
66. Watts N, Amann M, Arnell N, et al. The 2019 report of The *Lancet* Countdown on health and climate change: ensuring that the health of a child born today is not defined by a changing climate. *Lancet*. 2019;394(10211):1836–1878. doi:10.1016/s0140-6736(19)32596-6
67. Rider CF, Carlsten C. Air pollution and DNA methylation: effects of exposure in humans. *Clin Epigenet*. 2019;11(1):131. doi:10.1186/s13148-019-0713-2
68. Sheffield PE, Landrigan PJ. Global climate change and children's health: threats and strategies for prevention. *Environ Health Perspect*. 2011;119(3):291–298. doi:10.1289/ehp.1002233
69. American Public Health Association Policy Statement. Addressing the impacts of climate change on mental health and well-being. November 5, 2019. https://www.apha.org/Policies-and-Advocacy/Public-Health-Policy-Statements/Policy-Database/2020/01/13/Addressing-the-Impacts-of-Climate-Change-on-Mental-Health-and-Well-Being
70. Climate change. UNICEF USA. Accessed June 16, 2024. https://www.unicefusa.org/what-unicef-does/emergency-response/climate-change

71. World Health Organization and United Nations Environment Programme. *Healthy Environments for Healthy Children: Key Messages for Action.* World Health Organization; 2010.
72. Clayton S, Manning CM, Speiser M, Hill AN. *Mental Health and Our Changing Climate: Children and Youth Report 2023.* American Psychological Association and ecoAmerica; 2023.
73. U.S. Environmental Protection Agency. President's task force on environmental health and safety risks to children presidential executive order 13045: protection of children from environmental health risks and safety risks. https://www.gpo.gov/fdsys/pkg/FR-1997-04-23/pdf/97-10695.pdf
74. Paulson JA, Karr CJ, Seltzer JM, et al. Development of the pediatric environmental health specialty unit network in north America. *Am J Public Health.* 2009;99:S511–S516. doi:10.2105/AJPH.2008.154641
75. American Public Health Association. *Protecting the Health of Children: A National Snapshot of Environmental Health Services.* American Public Health Association; 2019. https://www.apha.org/-/media/Files/PDF/topics/environment/Protecting_the_Health_of_Children.ashx
76. Agency for Toxic Substances and Disease Registry. Choose safe places for early care and education. March 2020. https://www.rdhrs.org/wp-content/uploads/2020/07/Choose-Safe-Places-for-Early-Care-and-Education-Disaster-Recovery-Supplement-ATSDR-March-2020.pdf
77. Environmental Law Institute. Selected state policy and program strategies for integrating safe siting considerations into the child care licensing process. September 2022. https://www.eli.org/sites/default/files/files-pdf/ELI%20Safe%20Siting%20Policy%20Actions%20Sept.%202022.pdf
78. Eco-Healthy Child Care®. Children's Environmental Health Network. Accessed June 17, 2024. https://cehn.org/our-work/eco-healthy-child-care/
79. McIntyre T, Gutner R, Cohen H, Silvasy T, Momol E. A florida-friendly landscaping (TM) approach to pest management in your edible landscape. ENH1365/EP629. University of Florida. January 9, 2023. https://edis.ifas.ufl.edu/publication/EP629
80. Environmental Law Institute. Integrated pest management in schools: overview of state laws. Accessed June 17, 2024. https://www.eli.org/sites/default/files/files-pdf/ipm_tseh_6.pdf
81. Baurick T, Younes L, Meiners J. Welcome to "Cancer Alley," where toxic air is about to get worse. October 30, 2019. Accessed June 17, 2024. https://www.propublica.org/article/welcome-to-cancer-alley-where-toxic-air-is-about-to-get-worse
82. Princeton University. Racial disparities and climate change. August 15, 2020. https://psci.princeton.edu/tips/2020/8/15/racial-disparities-and-climate-change
83. The state of America's children 2021. Children's Defense Fund. 2021. https://www.myflfamilies.com/sites/default/files/2023-05/The-State-of-Americas-Children-2021.pdf
84. Food Empowerment Project. Food deserts. Accessed June 17, 2024. https://foodispower.org/access-health/food-deserts/
85. Key statistics and graphics. U.S Department of Agriculture. Updated October 25, 2023. https://www.ers.usda.gov/topics/food-nutrition-assistance/food-security-in-the-u-s/key-statistics-graphics/
86. Perry MJ, Arrington M, Freisthler MS, et al. Pervasive structural racism in environmental epidemiology. *Environ Health.* 2021;20:119. doi:10.1186/s12940-021-00801-3
87. American Public Health Association Policy Statement. Establishing environmental public health systems for children at risk or with environmental exposures in schools. November 7, 2017. https://www.apha.org/policies-and-advocacy/public-health-policy-statements/policy-database/2018/01/18/establishing-environmental-public-health-systems-for-children
88. Walters PB. The limits of growth: school expansion and school reform in historical perspective. In: Hallinan MT, ed. *Handbook of the Sociology of Education.* Kluwer Academic/Plenum Publishers; 2000:241–261.
89. American Geophysical Union. Air pollution high at US public schools with kids from marginalized groups. 2022. Accessed June 17, 2024. https://www.sciencedaily.com/releases/2022/11/221117135603.htm
90. University of North Carolina Gillings School of Global Public Health. New UNC study quantifies disparity among marginalized communities exposed to traffic-related air pollution across the US. June 1, 2023. https://sph.unc.edu/sph-news/new-unc-study-quantifies-disparity-among-marginalized-communities-exposed-to-traffic-related-air-pollution-across-the-u-s/
91. Indoor air and coronavirus (COVID-19). U.S. Environmental Protection Agency. Updated May 6, 2024. https://www.epa.gov/coronavirus/indoor-air-and-coronavirus-covid-19

92. Rubin IL, Witherspoon NO. Climate change, environmental justice and children's health: break the cycle of climate change by cultivating future leaders. *J Appl Res Children*. 2021;12(1). doi:10.58464/2155-5834.1466
93. Children's Environmental Health Network. Children and health disparities. February 2018.
94. Yeter D, Banks EC, Aschner M. Disparity in risk factor severity for early childhood blood lead among predominately African-American Black children: the 1999 to 2010 US NHANES. *Int J Environ Res Public Health*. 2020;17(5):1552. doi:10.3390/ijerph17051552
95. Castleden H, Watson R, Tui'kn Partnership, et al. Asthma prevention and management for Aboriginal people: lessons from Mi'kmaq communities, Unama'ki, Canada, 2012. *Prev Chronic Dis*. 2016;13:150244. doi:10.5888/pcd13.150244external icon
96. U.S. Department of Health and Human Services, Office of Minority Health. Asthma and African Americans. Accessed June 17, 2024. https://minorityhealth.hhs.gov/omh/browse.aspx?lvl=4&lvlid=15
97. Morello-Frosch R, Pastor M, Sadd J, Shonkoff SB. The Climate Gap: Inequalities in How Climate Change Hurts Americans & How to Close the Gap. University of Southern California Equity Research Institute. May 2009. https://dornsife.usc.edu/eri/publications/the-climate-gap-inequalities-in-how-climate-change-hurts-americans-how-to-close-the-gap/
98. Park YM, Kwan MP. Multi-contextual segregation and environmental justice: toward fine scale spatiotemporal approaches. *Int J Environ Res Public Health*. 2017;14(10):1205. doi:10.3390/ijerph14101205
99. Patterson J, Witherspoon NO. Racism that upends the cradle: how Black children are differentially vulnerable to impacts of the syndemic—the economic crisis, COVID 19 pandemic, and climate change, 2022.
100. Congressional Budget Justification Department of State, foreign operations, and related programs fiscal year 2023. 2022. https://www.state.gov/wp-content/uploads/2022/06/FY-2023-Congressional-Budget-Justification_Final_508comp.pdf
101. Trasande L. Economics of children's environmental health. *Mt Sinai J Med*. 2011;78(1):98–106. doi:10.1002/msj.20234
102. American Public Health Association Policy Statement. Addressing environmental justice to achieve health equity. November 5, 2019. https://www.apha.org/policies-and-advocacy/public-health-policy-statements/policy-database/2020/01/14/addressing-environmental-justice-to-achieve-health-equity
103. Equitable and Just National Climate Platform. A vision for an equitable and just climate future. Accessed June 17, 2024. https://ajustclimate.org/
104. Children's Environmental Health Network. Children's environmental health indicators: a summary and assessment. January 25, 2018. https://cehn.org/wp-content/uploads/2018/02/CEH-Indicators-report-FINAL.1.pdf
105. Community Preventive Services Task Force. Task force findings for health equity. Accessed June 17, 2024. https://www.thecommunityguide.org/content/task-force-findings-health-equity#education-programs-policies
106. Del Rio M, Lasley P, Tallon LA, et al. Critical competencies in children's environmental health. *J Environ Health*. 2023;85(6):26–29.
107. Blueprint for protecting children's environmental health: an urgent call to action. Children's Environmental Health Network. 2015. Accessed June 17, 2024. https://cehn.org/resources/blueprint-for-protecting-childrens-health/
108. American Academy of Pediatrics. *Caring for Our Children, National Health and Safety Performance Standards*. 4th ed. American Academy of Pediatrics; 2019. doi:10.1542/9781610022989
109. United Nations Children's Fund. The climate crisis is a child rights crisis: Introducing the Children's Climate Risk Index. August 19, 2021. https://data.unicef.org/resources/childrens-climate-risk-index-report

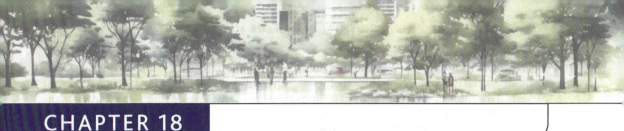

CHAPTER 18

Integrating Environmental Health and Justice Into Healthcare

Maida P. Galvez, Emma N. Chang, Perry E. Sheffield, Hannah M. Thompson, Blair J. Wylie, and Tatiana C. Height

LEARNING OBJECTIVES

- Describe priority environmental health concerns for adults, children, and pregnant individuals.
- Integrate environmental health screening for priority environmental health concerns into clinical practice.
- Apply a key messages (risk-communication) framework to screen, counsel, and refer patients to environmental interventions.
- Discuss evidence-based resources for environmental health information.

KEY TERMS

- environmental medicine
- exposome
- occupational health
- pediatric environmental health
- reproductive environmental health
- risk communication

OVERVIEW

Over the past century, research has significantly advanced our understanding of the key role that physical and social environments play in shaping human health throughout the life span. The life span refers to the course of one's life from preconception to pregnancy, infancy to childhood, and from adolescence to adulthood. We now recognize that environmental exposures during critical windows of development contribute to diseases across the life span and impact future generations. As has been discussed throughout this book, we know that environmental health exposures—broadly defined to include chemical (e.g., lead) and nonchemical (e.g., stress) factors—can drive health disparities. Another notable advancement in environmental health research is the shift from the traditional *one-exposure* approaches to an examination of the **exposome**—the totality of all external and internal exposures (e.g., chemical, social, genetic, metabolomic, and microbial) across the life span, using novel laboratory and geospatial statistical approaches.[1–7] We can measure over 265 chemicals in humans through cutting-edge biomonitoring and environmental-exposure assessment methods that continue to evolve. All these advancements have propelled the practice of environmental medicine forward and made these techniques possible today.[8]

The field of environmental health has grown by cultivating clinical and public health leaders.[9,10] With the recent increased integration of environmental health into medical education, the clinical practice of environmental occupational medicine, environmental pediatrics, and reproductive environmental health has expanded.[11–14] **Environmental medicine** is rooted in the intersection of diverse fields, including toxicology, genetics, epidemiology, primary care medicine, behavioral health, sociology, and public health.[15] While occupational medicine is firmly established and environmental pediatrics is growing, **reproductive environmental health** remains in the early stages of integration into clinical practice.

Clinicians, including nurses, nurse practitioners, physicians, physician assistants, medical assistants, social workers, respiratory therapists, community health workers, patient navigators, patient advocates, and others in clinical settings refer to evidence-based guidelines for the management of environment-related conditions. Clinical evaluations are rooted in taking an environmental history as part of the patient assessment, and then counseling the patient on ways to prevent and reduce exposure. The Occupational Safety and Health Administration (OSHA),[16] The American College of Occupational and Environmental Medicine (ACOEM),[17] The American Academy of Pediatrics,[18] The American College of Obstetricians and Gynecologists (ACOG),[19] the United States Preventive Services Task Force (USPSTF),[20] and the U.S. Centers for Disease Control and Prevention (CDC)[21,22] are credible sources for these practice guidelines.

the integration of environmental health into primary care remains limited largely due to time constraints and a general lack of training of primary care clinicians in environmental health.[23] Still, significant gains have been made in select areas. For example, many decades after the harmful effects of childhood lead poisoning were established, we now finally see a national shift toward the primary prevention of lead exposure, beginning with screening homes for lead rather than waiting for children to be exposed before remediation.[24] For these reasons, it is imperative that environmental health research be translated into changes at the clinical, educational, program, and policy levels in direct benefit to families and communities.[25-36]

OCCUPATIONAL HEALTH AND HEALTHCARE

Occupational health and safety are discussed at length in Chapter 16, "Ensuring Occupational Health," and they are relevant in the context of clinical environmental health. According to the U.S. Census Bureau, over 166 million individuals worked in some capacity in 2021, with 70% working full time throughout the year.[37] Given that this number represents a significant portion of the population, it is important for clinicians to understand the unique hazards faced by workers. Although there are overarching safety standards, every workplace needs to tailor safety programs and protocols to its unique environment. Additionally, our world is changing, and we need to be aware of and learn about new hazards that present themselves in order to continue to protect workers.

As introduced in Chapter 16, "Ensuring Occupational Health," there are multiple types of work hazards, and a worker may face several hazards within the same workplace.[38] A workplace hazard can be defined as a possible source of damage or adverse effect.[39] Although a hazard may not always lead to harm, it is important to recognize hazards, understand the risk for harm, and identify potential methods of controlling the exposure of workers to hazards.[39] Safety hazards can exist for workers using machinery or electrical equipment, or even in the form of cluttered floors that create slip and trip hazards. Other hazards can include biological exposures, such as infectious agents encountered when working with humans or animals; chemical exposures; and ergonomic issues, such as awkward postures needed to perform certain tasks and lifting.[38] The workplace itself can become a hazard depending on the stress experienced by the worker related to workplace tasks, pace, and structure, and even the social environment. Another important hazard to understand is the physical environment within which the worker is performing their job tasks. Noise, radiation, and even the indoor and outdoor climate, including temperature, humidity, and weather conditions, can contribute to a dangerous physical work environment.

For a worker who becomes injured or ill on the job, the Workers' Compensation program provides wage replacement in addition to covering medical costs for these workers. Physicians are central to this program since workers are generally required to get an official medical diagnosis to qualify for compensation. This system is largely state based, with the Office of Workers' Compensation Programs, under the United States Department of Labor, providing coverage for specific workers under several programs: the Federal Employees' Compensation Program, the Longshore and Harbor Workers' Compensation Program, the Federal Black Lung Program, and the Energy Employees Occupational Illness Compensation Program.[40] Workers' compensation is a no-fault legal system in which the determination of the work-relatedness of an injury is decided by the states.[41]

TAKING AN OCCUPATIONAL HEALTH HISTORY

Taking an occupational health history is a crucial part of assessing an individual's health and well-being, especially when their work environment may expose them to health risks. A detailed occupational history is typically conducted by healthcare professionals, and the primary goals are to identify potential work-related health hazards, provide appropriate guidance, and prevent work-related illnesses or injuries. The occupational history includes the following information:

- work history, including the years worked and previous jobs and industries;
- job tasks and the exposures or hazards encountered;
- work environment, including physical conditions, social aspects of work, and the use of personal protective equipment (PPE);
- outside hobbies and lifestyle factors; and
- medical history that includes preexisting conditions and those that may be aggravated by occupational factors.[42]

The key pieces of an occupational history are an individual's occupation and industry. An occupation is defined by the National Institute for Occupational Safety and Health (NIOSH) as an individual's job, such as a registered nurse, waitress, construction worker, or teacher.[43] An industry refers to the type of business. For example, a registered nurse (occupation) could work in a hospital (industry), in a school (industry), or in an outpatient clinic (industry). While the difference may be subtle, it is important to collect both types of information given that the hazards and job tasks may vary. It may also be important to ask an individual's employment status, in other words, if they are currently employed, unemployed, retired, not able to work, enrolled as a student, or other employment status.[44]

Additional details of an individual's occupational history can be asked on the basis of the clinical scenario and should be combined with the other parts of a medical and environmental history. For example, a primary care physician seeing a patient who has an elevated blood lead level may need to understand all their occupational sources of lead exposure (from both current and past occupations and industries), along with possible environmental exposures. An occupational medicine clinician seeing a patient with a work-related hand laceration may only need information on the patient's current occupation and industry.

An occupational history may be an overlooked and potentially complex part of a patient's medical history, but the information obtained may be imperative for a patient's diagnosis. It also can be easily tailored to fit many clinical scenarios. Employers should routinely implement needed environmental safety measures in the workplace, as well as train and enforce the use of personal protective measures that can prevent and reduce environmental exposures. It is important that employees be aware of possible exposures in the workplace and any associated symptoms. Should an exposure happen in the workplace, they also need to understand that early and coordinated communication is vital.

ENVIRONMENTAL PEDIATRICS

Approximately 74 million children under the age of 18 years live in the United States, making up approximately 20% of the total U.S. population.[45] Globally, there are approximately 2.4 billion children in this same age group. Children represent a sizable proportion of the population, and because they do, as discussed in Chapter 17, "Ensuring Children's Environmental Health and Justice," we now have a critical opportunity to influence their health trajectory for life, their overall life expectancy, and the health of subsequent generations via epigenetic mechanisms. A consideration of the environmental influences on child health has long been unaddressed by clinicians, starting with a lack of training and manifesting itself in a lack of integration into pediatric clinical care. While incredible gains have been made in terms of addressing the infectious disease threats to children over the past half century, children face a new pediatric morbidity driven by lifestyle and dietary changes, our pervasive chemical exposures, and the changing global climate. With the increasing integration of environmental health into medical education, clinicians can now gain the needed knowledge base and skills to address common environmental concerns during every clinical encounter with a child.

Since most children, particularly in the United States, do not work, the concepts of occupational health do not specifically apply; however, many of the same key concepts are applicable for the clinician to consider. Instead of a workplace, the environments of interest for children are the places where they spend their time—their homes, schools, child-care centers, and play spaces in the community—understanding that the time spent in each environment changes as children age. Their "work" is that of learning and development. As such, their activities include developmentally appropriate behaviors; school-based activities; and the hobbies, sports, or jobs they have as they get older. One concept that sets environmental pediatrics apart is the importance of considering children's unique developmental and physiological vulnerabilities specific to their still-growing and developing bodies, organ systems, and brains.[46] Children possess distinct attributes, such as higher respiratory rates, breathing zones closer to the ground, a higher consumption of food and drink relative to their body weight, age-appropriate hand-to-mouth behaviors, and unique dietary preferences. These factors all make children uniquely vulnerable to environmental exposures as compared to adults in the very same environments.[46] As they enter the workforce in adolescence, these special considerations should be taken into account.

TAKING AN ENVIRONMENTAL HEALTH HISTORY FOR A CHILD

A child's environmental health history has significant overlap with an adult environmental health history, replacing the concept of the work setting with a child-care setting or school and introducing particular attention to unique child behaviors that influence their exposure. The go-to resource for pediatric clinicians on environmental health is *Pediatric Environmental Health*, Fourth Edition, published by the American Academy of Pediatrics and also known as "The Green Book."[47] In the book, the recommended environmental health questions are grouped into five categories: surroundings (home, school, child care, community); tobacco smoke or other nicotine exposure; water sources; dietary exposures; and sun or other ultraviolet radiation. Each category has guidance on specific questions to ask children's caregivers, such as "Do you have carbon monoxide (CO) detectors in your home?" and "Do you use tap water, and does it come from a well?" This resource also offers guidance on additional or alternative targeted questions to ask when a child presents with symptoms that are unusual or persistent or when symptoms affect multiple people in an area where a child is spending time. These questions are meant to complement existing environmental health standards of care such as blood-lead-level tests for children at 12 and 24 months and annual screening questions about potential lead exposures until age 6.

Within a particular child-serving clinical setting, targeted screening linked to both local needs and available resources helps motivate clinicians to continue to incorporate this content and strengthens relationships with families who appreciate actionable questions. National **pediatric environmental health** experts created the Prescriptions (Rx) for Prevention program to support the inclusion of such locally relevant, actionable topics.[48] If, for example, a family reports insect problems in their home, they will be given guidance about options for safer pest control to minimize their toxic exposures. Addressing the insect issue can both reduce a potential asthma or allergy trigger from the insects, while also avoiding a second respiratory irritant from unnecessary spraying of pesticides.

In pediatrics, screening for lead and environmental asthma triggers is the area in which the greatest gains have been made with respect to integration of environmental health into clinical practice. This screening for lead and asthma triggers parallels the growth in screening for the social determinants of health (SDOH). Federal and state mandates specifically for lead have driven clinical action. At the federal level, Medicaid requires that all children entitled to this benefit receive childhood lead testing.[49] At the state level, certain states have expanded the program to require health providers to test all children for lead,[50-53] while other states simply include children receiving Special Supplemental Nutrition Program for Women, Infants, and Children (WIC) or Medicaid.[54] In this example, all of these policies refer back to the CDC reference values (set in 2021 at a blood lead level of 3.5 mcg/dL),[55] which are based on data from the National Health and Nutrition Examination Surveys (NHANES),[22] and these values are updated every 4 years. For asthma, screening for environmental triggers has become more routine, although the accessibility and availability of healthy home interventions remain limited, and costs can be a barrier in the absence of insurance reimbursement for needed interventions. Value-based payment pilot programs are underway to build a case for insurance reimbursement for interventions that prevent and reduce morbidity and mortality from asthma. For emerging topics of concern, such as per- and polyfluoroalkyl substances (PFAS) and wildfire smoke, where there has been additional concern, safety messaging, and regulatory guidance since the last edition of "The Green Book," the Pediatric Environmental Health Specialty Units (pehsu.net)[56] offer both national and regional specific information online.

> ### CASE STUDY 18.1: Environmental Health and Cancer in the United States
>
> The occurrence of childhood cancer is closely tied to a country's level of wealth, with a higher incidence in high-income nations but higher mortality rates in low-income countries. The most common cancers in childhood include leukemia and lymphoma. According to the American Cancer Society, about 9,900 children are diagnosed with cancer each year. However, survival has improved substantially from 58% in the 1970s to about 85% today.[57]
>
> There are several factors that contribute to the relatively higher rates of childhood cancer in the United States. The United States has powerful diagnostic tools to detect cancer and a large (but largely imperfect) healthcare system. Diets and physical activity levels may also be factors. However, potential environmental factors, which likely play a role in these disparities, are less often discussed. More research is needed to understand the many contributing factors to childhood cancer rates in the United States.
>
> Recognizing this knowledge gap, the Pediatric Environmental Health Specialty Units are "a national network of experts in the prevention, diagnosis, management, and treatment of health issues that arise from environmental exposures from preconception through adolescence."[58(para1)] They are supported by the Centers for Disease Control and Prevention/Agency for Toxic Substances and Disease Registry (CDC/ATSDR), the U.S. Environmental Protection Agency (EPA), and the American Academy of Pediatrics.
>
> As one of the 10 regional federally-funded clinical and educational centers, the Western States Pediatric Environmental Health Specialty Unit has developed materials that consider environmental factors in childhood cancer (see https://wspehsu.ucsf.edu/main-resources/videos/community-outreach-tools).
>
> #### REFLECTION QUESTIONS
> 1. Rates of childhood leukemia have increased in the past few decades, and increasing evidence suggests that the environment may play a role. Name some of the environmental exposures known to be associated with leukemia or other cancers.
> 2. Since preconception or prenatal exposure to some pesticides are associated with an increased risk of certain childhood cancers, describe some strategies to reduce exposures.

ENVIRONMENTAL HEALTH AND PRENATAL HEALTHCARE

Although no area of health is immune to the potential for adverse impact from environmental exposures, the prenatal period is a particularly critical time for clinicians to screen for environmental exposures and provide counseling about reducing exposure because periconceptual and prenatal exposures can adversely impact the pregnancy, negatively affect the health of the pregnant individual, and have lasting lifelong consequences for the developing fetus. Physiologic changes during pregnancy may change exposure concentrations in the bloodstream that pass through the placenta; as an example, delayed gastric emptying may increase the absorption of toxicants in the diet. Likewise, elevated minute ventilation and higher tidal volumes may increase respiratory toxin absorption. Fetuses, even to a greater extent than young children, are particularly susceptible to the effects of environmental toxicants as their exposures are greater per body weight compared to adults and older children and their metabolic pathways are immature. Development is rapid across gestation, and certain periods may be susceptible to unique problems from toxicant exposures. During organogenesis, congenital anomalies may result, whereas during the latter half of pregnancy, the same exposures may negatively impact connections in the developing brain or alter fetal growth. The *epigenome*, or the expression of genes (see Chapter 7, "Understanding the Environment and How It Relates to Health Using Toxicology and Epidemiology Research Methods," for more information), is reprogrammed during embryonic and fetal life. Epigenetic effects can echo across the life span and additionally carry the potential for transgenerational harm.

Antenatal care before a child is born, with repeated and frequent interactions between patients and the healthcare teams, affords an opportunity to improve the environmental health of both the pregnant individual and the growing family. Counseling can be provided on specific actions that may minimize exposure to hazards and outside resources can be accessed if necessary (see "Environmental Health in Practice" at the end of the chapter). Increased awareness of behavioral actions that can reduce exposures may prevent future childhood environmental health problems such as elevated lead before harm has occurred. That said, there are numerous challenges to the practicing clinician that may limit what is being routinely offered currently in reproductive environmental health counseling. Environmental health screening must compete with other antenatal care priorities. A tension also exists between education about potential harms and increasing undue anxiety, especially concerning ubiquitous exposures that may be challenging to eliminate in modern life. Moreover, a vast number (more than 80,000) of potentially harmful chemicals exist in consumer products with little regulatory oversight.[59] While there has been an exponential increase in epidemiologic literature linking some of these chemicals with adverse pregnancy outcomes, it may be challenging for the clinician to stay up to date and translate this emerging information into meaningful recommendations for individual patients. Nonetheless, there are several key priority environmental health concerns that clinicians caring for pregnant individuals should have knowledge of and be able to screen and provide basic counseling about to their patients. Many of these concerns are similar to those detailed in the "Environmental Pediatrics" section and are summarized briefly in the following.

Heavy metals, such as mercury and lead, have been known for quite some time to harm the developing fetus. Both are potent neurotoxicants but also have other wide-ranging effects in pregnancy, including miscarriage, impaired fetal growth, and preterm birth. For mercury, neurodevelopmental toxicity was established following several industrial disasters leading to severe methylmercury poisoning from the ingestion of contaminated fish in Minamata, Japan, and at other locations and from contaminated grain in Iraq.[60,61] The association of lower exposure levels with impaired neurodevelopment was documented in a birth cohort in the Faroe Islands in a population reliant on seafood in their diet.[62,63] Prenatal exposure largely results from consuming contaminated fish because mercury, released into the atmosphere from industrial pollution that contaminates the water, bioaccumulates, with the highest concentrations occurring among large predatory fish. Professional organizations, such as the ACOG, have provided recommendations for limiting the consumption of fish likely to contain higher mercury levels for pregnant and lactating individuals.[64] The challenge in risk communication has been how to avoid messaging that results in the elimination of fish altogether from diets, as fish low in mercury contains other dietary benefits, like omega-3 fatty acids, which provide benefits to fetal neurodevelopment. Perhaps unsurprisingly, researchers from Massachusetts documented a reduction in all fish consumption among pregnant participants following the release of the initial federal advisory in 2001 to limit consumption of higher-mercury-containing fish.[65]

Lead has been a historical focus for years for its potential to impair cognitive development, reduce IQ, and a myriad of other health effects. The recognition that prenatal exposure alone may affect neurocognition in offspring has increased the awareness among obstetric clinicians of lead as an important toxicant of concern.[66] Elevated lead levels in the maternal blood have also been associated with gestational hypertension and, as such, carry negative consequences for the health of the pregnant person as well as the developing fetus. The ACOG recommends that prenatal providers adopt a risk-factor-based approach to lead screening in pregnancy rather than universal screening, reserving laboratory evaluation of blood lead levels for pregnant individuals with risk factors such as recent immigration from areas of ambient lead contamination, behaviors like pica (an eating disorder in which a person eats nonfood items), use of imported cosmetics, high-risk occupations or hobbies, known water contamination, or renovations of pre-1978 homes, which is the year lead paint was banned in the United States.[67] In an evaluation of lead screening in a Massachusetts cohort of pregnant individuals, 78% had at least one risk factor for elevated lead, yet none had a venous blood lead level sent by their clinical team.[68] This study underscores that the recommended current approach is both too cumbersome (too many risk factors) and too nonspecific to be easily put into practice by prenatal care providers and highlights the challenges of incorporating environmental health into routine prenatal care.

There is a growing recognition that several chemicals in consumer products can function as endocrine disruptors with wide-ranging effects on reproduction and during pregnancy, including early pregnancy loss, preterm delivery, impaired fetal growth, gestational hypertension, gestational diabetes, and stillbirth. Exposure classes include pesticides, plastics (e.g., phenols, phthalates), PFAS used for their nonstick repellent qualities, and parabens. Exposure to endocrine-disrupting chemicals can occur from the dietary ingestion of food and water, cooking practices, use of personal care products, consumer goods from furniture to toys, inhalation of fumes, and many other sources in the modern world. Teasing out association from causation and estimating the effect size of exposures in isolation and in mixtures with other chemicals are emerging areas of focus. A priority among practicing prenatal providers is to be able to provide actionable information, acknowledging the emerging, yet incomplete, scientific information while also discussing methods to reduce personal exposure. Some chemicals with short half-lives, like phenols or phthalates, may be more amenable to personal behavioral changes to reduce exposures. Others with long half-lives that persist in both the environment and in the body, like PFAS, which are also known as "forever chemicals," may be more resistant to reduction through personal behavior changes, requiring policy changes such as restrictions around commercial and residential use before body burdens diminish. Counseling requires careful nuance to empower individuals to reduce their own exposures, when possible, without unduly placing blame.

Finally, climate-change-related factors are emerging among obstetric providers as high-priority environmental health exposures. Heat waves and poor air quality—from wildfire smoke or traffic—are increasingly raised by pregnant and lactating patients as concerns for their potential to adversely impact their reproductive health. Providing clear messaging about potential risks and strategies to minimize exposure to hazards like heat and air pollution will be increasingly necessary in this time of a warming climate.

TAKING AN ENVIRONMENTAL HEALTH HISTORY

The principles that underlie conducting an environmental health history in pregnancy are similar to those detailed earlier in the sections focused on workers and children. Ideally, a structured environmental health history would be incorporated into routine prenatal care as part of the social history and positive responses to specific exposures would be followed with targeted counseling about reduction of exposures. In a U.S. national online survey among ACOG fellows ($n = 2514$), the majority (78%) agreed about the importance of reducing patient exposures to potential environmental health hazards through screening and counseling; however, fewer than 20% of them routinely asked their pregnant patients about environmental exposures during the course of prenatal care.[69] Cited barriers to taking a routine environmental health history included concerns about their own lack of training on the topic and therefore uncertainty about how to respond, as well as concerns about sparking anxiety among patients.

Efforts are underway to create web-based or mobile applications to walk a patient through a series of questions related to the environment from housing to diet, to the use of consumer products, to lifestyle. on the basis of a patient's responses, targeted advice is provided about potential risks with identified exposures and suggested ways to reduce exposure. Innovation that engages the patient, provides curated and relevant messaging, and identifies resources where both the patient and clinician can seek more detailed information is likely to help close the gap between the intent to screen and counsel pregnant patients on environmental hazards and the reality of practice.

> **CASE STUDY 18.2: Integrating Environmental Health Into Clinical Case Studies**
>
> In clinical care, case studies are powerful tools that can be used to document stories of patient interactions and treatment and discuss both the common and rare situations that clinicians might face. Clinicians document specific cases to inform clinical studies, to inspire new perspectives, to advance medicine and healthcare practices, and to prepare future clinicians.[70] They do not tell other clinicians exactly what to do for every case, but they show how clinicians have worked with patients before. Here is one clinical case example that integrates environmental health issues:
>
> ### AN INDIVIDUAL WITH WORKPLACE-RELATED CARPAL TUNNEL SYNDROME
>
> *A 45-year-old right-hand-dominant female presented to the occupational medicine clinic with right wrist and hand pain on the palm side. The pain is associated with tingling in her thumb and second and third fingers, especially in the evening. She reports that she will sometimes wake up and need to shake her hands to improve the tingling. She also notes her symptoms are worse after a full day of work but improve on the weekends. Her past medical history includes hypertension. She has not had any surgeries and does not have any significant family history. She is an accountant and works on the computer for the majority of her 8-hour workday. On physical examination, her body mass index is 37. She has a full range of motion and strength in her wrists bilaterally. She has decreased sensation to light touch over her thumb and second and third digits with normal sensation over her fourth and fifth digits. The carpal-compression test was positive.*
>
> Taking an occupational history can provide the clinician and treatment team with vital information and help with treatment planning. In this patient's case, the work she does is more likely than not contributing to her symptoms. By identifying this cause early in her treatment course, the treatment team can provide her with referrals to an ergonomist for any needed accommodations for work and an occupational medicine specialist for possible worker's compensation. This holistic approach that encompasses the patient's work environment can be helpful in the recovery process, in returning to work sooner, and in limiting future injury.
>
> ### REFLECTION QUESTIONS
>
> 1. What aspects of her case make it possible that her occupation contributed to the development of her symptoms?
> 2. What other tests may need to be done to evaluate other contributing factors to this diagnosis?

HEALTHCARE POLICY AND ENVIRONMENTAL HEALTH

Healthcare does not start and end in the hospital. Many policies are relevant to the integration of environmental health into healthcare. In general, healthcare can be inaccessible to those who do not have sufficient health insurance, transportation, or time off from work.[71,72] Passed in 2010, the Affordable Care Act was the most recent major expansion of healthcare access via health insurance for millions—many, of course, whose health is harmed by environmental exposures.[73]

The role of hospitals can also be reimagined, expanding beyond direct patient care to comprehensively addressing community health, including environmental factors. In order to retain their tax-exempt status, private nonprofit hospitals have a legal obligation under the Affordable Care Act to conduct community-health needs assessments, to adopt an implementation strategy every 3 years, and to give back to their communities.[74] These actions can include nutrition and housing initiatives, as well as grants to community coalitions doing this work.[75] This law obliges clinical institutions to get more involved in preventive and environmental interventions.

States may also propose policies that integrate environmental health into healthcare. One example of proposed legislation was a bundled payment program for high-risk pediatric asthma cases under the Medicaid program in Massachusetts.[77] This program would have paid for regular monitoring and testing, home environmental assessments, care coordination, and even air filters and pest-management supplies. Community health workers would have played a big role in this program and could even assist with advocacy with landlords to address environmental issues. Although the program was ultimately not implemented, it offers one possible vision for a better integration of environmental health promotion, clinical practice, and reimbursement. Pilot programs including insurance plans that provide insurance reimbursement for healthy homes interventions for children with asthma are underway (e.g., in New York City and New York State). In these ways, hospitals could expand health promotion by partnering with community-based organizations to better address the environmental health needs of the communities they serve.

As another relevant policy, and as referenced earlier, employees who believe they are ill due to an environmental exposure from work may seek workers' compensation as covered under the Federal Employee's Compensation Act (FECA).[77] However, receiving compensation can be difficult because OSHA Standard 1904.5(b)(2) states that employers are not required to report an illness if it results solely from a nonwork-related exposure.[78] This standard puts the onus on the worker and their primary care provider to prove that their ailment is caused by their work environment. OSHA has also publicly acknowledged that their permissible exposure limits (PELs) are often out-of-date,[79] reflecting a mismatch between policy and regulatory science (see Chapter 16, "Ensuring Occupational Health").

> **IN OTHER WORDS: RISK COMMUNICATION**
>
> A core component of environmental medicine is counseling on environmental risks. **Risk communication** is rooted in providing patients with evidence-based information that they can use to make informed decisions about what is best for themselves or their families.[80,81] Often the public first hears about concerns related to environmental exposures from headlines in the news. These headlines, designed to grab the public's attention, can be very alarming. Common questions from families in response to these headlines are: Why did we not know about this exposure, what does it mean for our health, and what can we do about it? To effectively respond, root clinical counseling by answering the following three questions: What? Define the exposures. So what? Explain why we care and outline the health effects. Now what? Walk through the simple steps families can take to prevent and reduce exposures. This highly effective three-key-messages framework was developed by risk-communication experts and can be used for a variety of messaging needs, including counseling patients and communities, speaking to the media, and informing decision makers.[82,83] Each key message can have three additional supporting facts to be completed and shared as is helpful or needed. Each supporting fact can have additional supporting facts as needed. The key messages risk communication template is shown in Figure 18.1, along with a sample message map on mercury in fish (Figure 18.2).
>
> Individuals experience mental noise when under high stress, making it challenging for messages to be heard.[80–82] To address this issue, keep messages short and use plain language. This approach increases the likelihood that messages are heard, understood, and can lead to actions that protect health. Placing environmental exposures into context requires careful consider-

(continued)

IN OTHER WORDS: RISK COMMUNICATION (continued)

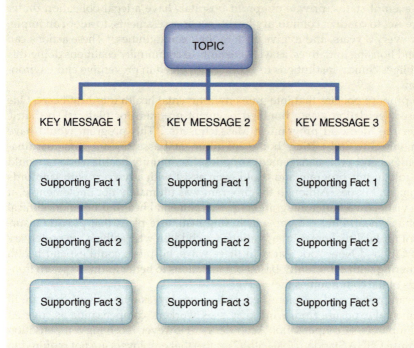

FIGURE 18.1. Template message map for risk communication.

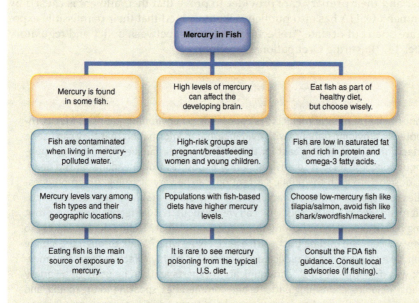

FIGURE 18.2. Message map on mercury in fish.
Source: Region 2. Pediatric Environmental Health Specialty Units. Accessed June 18, 2024. https://www.pehsu.net/region2.html

ation with respect to what is an appropriate comparison. The lessons learned after 9/11 included use of historical background levels for comparison when available (e.g., comparing lead levels in the air post-9/11 at Ground Zero with lead levels in the air in the 1970s).[82]

(continued)

> **IN OTHER WORDS: RISK COMMUNICATION (*continued*)**
>
> Once appropriate messages are developed, ensure clarity and consistent messaging by having diverse experts, including families, target community members, and partners from various disciplines, review the messages prior to disseminating. Finally, consider trust determination with respect to who is the best messenger to convey the messages, especially in high-stress scenarios (e.g., community-level environmental exposure cases).[83] Clinicians are often considered trusted messengers. Appropriately match the message to the messenger to ensure a high level of confidence when communicating complex environmental information. Clinical environmental health counseling tools have been developed (e.g., New York State Children's Environmental Health Centers [NYSCHECK] Prescription [Rx] for Prevention)[48] so that key messages on common environmental concerns are at the ready for use by busy clinicians.[84] Consider the need for translation into different languages as well as closed captioning and American Sign Language to meet the needs of diverse communities. Disseminating messages through local, city, state, and national partners and especially community partners can be a highly effective way to ensure that messages reach diverse communities.

ENVIRONMENTAL HEALTH INEQUITIES IN CLINICAL PRACTICE

Access barriers create clinical inequities, which in turn create environmental health inequities. Employment can impact healthcare access both through time-off restrictions and employer control over health insurance options.[85] Contracted employees may not be provided safety training, access to occupational health and safety services, and awareness of worker rights.[86] The Personal Responsibility and Work Opportunity Act (PRWORA) of 1996 gives states discretion to bar legally documented noncitizens from receiving Medicaid during the 5 years after they secure qualified immigrant status.[86]

Geographic location in either rural or underserved areas, and transportation accessibility can also move healthcare out of reach. Individuals at risk for access difficulties include those with low income, and those who are elderly, disabled, incarcerated, and documented or undocumented immigrants.[87] Anyone with limited healthcare access will have decreased chances for screening and treatment for environmental-related health issues. Clinicians must consider the intersections of race, socioeconomic and political status, disability, culture, language, and geography to seek out patients who may not be receiving adequate care for many reasons. An example of this lack of access is the fact that Black patients who have cancer are often diagnosed at later stages and consequently experience worse outcomes.[88]

Healthcare institutions have also abused the trust that is required for an effective clinical relationship with communities of color. Due to the historical and current instances of discrimination that these communities have experienced while seeking healthcare, many patients decline to seek care or follow prescribed treatments.[89,90] Trust will have to be rebuilt both on an interpersonal level with more respect, fairness, and honesty between clinicians and patients, as well as on an institutional level.[89]

This is not to say that clinical access and trust are the only complications in the diagnosis and treatment of environment-related illnesses, although they can often perpetuate inequities. Environmental health-related diseases can be hard to diagnose. The EPA recognizes that biomonitoring is not source specific, is difficult to interpret regarding health risks, and can be costly.[91] There is also often a long latency period from exposure to disease for many environmental exposures. The barriers mentioned previously in this chapter include the difficulty of proving the source of disease among many potential causes, limited research examining multiple cumulative exposures throughout the life span, and a flawed regulatory framework not yet rooted in prevention or the precautionary principle, as well as clinician workload and familiarity with these issues.

MEDICAL RACISM

Risk characterization (discussed in Chapter 6, "Understanding (Unequal and Cumulative) Risks in Our Daily Environment") includes determining the likelihood of adverse human health outcomes based on the hazard, dose-response, and exposure assessment. In addition, it was noted that risk assessment must account for the complexity among the various human and nonhuman components of the world to enhance responses to risks. We also described how various forms of racism act as root causes for health disparities. When many people think of racism, they imagine explicit and overt discrimination, at the interpersonal level, based on race. While this is not an untrue depiction of how racism can operate, racism is often much more sinister and covert. Further, many people continue to believe that racism is a problem within individuals that can be solved simply by removing some "bad apples" from the bunch. However, this thinking ignores the all-too-prevalent reality that racism is baked into our very systems and will continue to function with or without bad apples. One of the many systems that has been founded on racism is healthcare.

Racism has been ingrained into the structuring and financing of the healthcare system since the Jim Crow era, with examples like underfunded federal programs disproportionately affecting Black Americans and racially discriminatory provisions to build separate and unequal healthcare facilities in the Hill–Burton Act of 1946.[92] According to Braveman and colleagues, "Systemic and structural racism are forms of racism that are pervasively and deeply embedded in systems, laws, written or unwritten policies, and entrenched practices and beliefs that produce, condone, and perpetuate widespread unfair treatment and oppression of people of color, with adverse health consequences."[93(p171)] Included in this dynamic, *medical racism* is defined as "the systematic and widespread racism against people of color within the medical system."[94(para1)] Bronson goes on to share that Black people are more likely to develop respiratory illnesses such as asthma because of the prevalence of polluting facilities in their communities, a fact that was likely compounded during the COVID-19 pandemic, as Black people were 3.57 times as likely to die from the virus than White people.[95] Washington describes the disproportionate lead exposure that low-income and racially minoritized people face in urban communities.[96] Taylor details the birth defects that newborn infants in environmental justice (EJ) communities have because of toxic exposures their mothers experienced during pregnancy.[97] This is particularly startling given the fact that Black, Indigenous, and People of Color (BIPOC) mothers in the United States are three times more likely to die of pregnancy-related causes than White women, thus compounding the potential threat to mothers in EJ communities. In addition to mothers, Black people in the United States in general face higher rates of morbidity and mortality than their White counterparts.

Twenty years ago, the Institute of Medicine Committee on Understanding and Eliminating Racial and Ethnic Disparities in Health Care published a report that indicated that racism is the primary driving factor of healthcare disparities.[98] Those disparities continue today.[99] Black people's perceptions of healthcare in the United States have been hampered by a history of medical malpractice and carelessness by White doctors toward Black patients.[100] For example, some White doctors have a perception that Black patients have a higher pain tolerance, are less medically cooperative, and fake chronic pain for the purposes of securing prescription pain medicine.[100,101] In addition to experiencing racial microaggressions from White doctors, Black and Hispanic or Latino communities in the United States face barriers to accessing health insurance and are less likely to have paid sick days from work, while predominantly Black communities are 67% more likely to lack enough primary care physicians.[102,103] These facts have undoubtedly contributed to the CDC's declaration that racism is a threat to public health.[104] The purpose of this segment of the chapter is to explain medical racism in the United States, frame medical racism in the context of environmental racism, and describe how these two problems compound one another in EJ communities.

The history of placing environmentally hazardous facilities in low-wealth or BIPOC communities has been well documented.[97] Communities that have repeatedly borne the burden of these siting patterns are known as EJ communities. The ease with which corporations have been able to place such facilities within or adjacent to marginalized communities has been advanced as a result of segregation caused by housing discrimination, restrictive covenants, exclusionary zoning, redlining, predatory lending, and other factors.[97,105] The presence of a polluting facility often triggered a systematic disinvestment in the community by businesses and residents with the means to relocate, which further stripped the community of resources such as job opportunities or medical facilities. Moreover, the placement of these facilities has had documented negative health impacts.[93] While these negative health impacts are sometimes noticed rather quickly by community members, in other cases it takes years of rigorous research to substantiate the claims of EJ community residents. Additionally, there are sometimes long latency periods, or long periods of time, between exposure and health deterioration, making it more difficult to prove harm.[93] Not only do BIPOC people in EJ communities risk negative health outcomes as a result of exposure patterns, but these outcomes are exacerbated by a lack of access to health-promoting resources, substandard school environments, and a troubling history that has led to distrust for medical providers.[93,96]

For example, in the 1930s, a young Black man was admitted into a St. Louis hospital, where he would ultimately die of pneumonia. Rather than respect his body, his remains were used for medical research for decades to come.[106] According to the CDC, "The data show that racial and ethnic minority groups, throughout the United States, experience higher rates of illness and death across a wide range of health conditions, including diabetes, hypertension, obesity, asthma, and heart disease, when compared to their White counterparts. Additionally, the life expectancy of non-Hispanic/Black Americans is four years lower than that of White Americans."[104(para4)]

Even BIPOC people within the healthcare system are not shielded from racism. One study found that physicians of color reported regularly experiencing their services being denied based upon race, in addition to other microaggressions from patients.[107] In a related instance, the Kaiser Permanente health system's medical school is facing legal action for allegedly promoting anti-Blackness.[108]

Personal actions that can be taken against medical racism may begin with the following:

- Spread awareness about medical racism and vote for politicians who support anti-racist healthcare policies.
- Visit your neighborhood bookstore or local library to find books on the topic, such as *Medical Bondage* by Deirdre Cooper Owens.
- Use social media to learn more about Black Maternal Health week—visit Blackmamasmatter.org or @BlkMamasMatter on Twitter to learn more about Black Maternal Health Week.

WORKING TOWARD ENVIRONMENTAL HEALTH AND JUSTICE

This chapter provides an overview of environmental health in clinical settings, with a focus on pregnant people, children, and workers. Focused environmental health screening and counseling on priority areas of concern can be employed within the time limitations of a clinic visit. There is increasing recognition of the importance of incorporating environmental health considerations into medical practice, particularly as some healthcare training includes lessons on SDOH. Efforts to enhance clinical education must be continued by integrating more robust environmental health components and providing resources to support healthcare professionals in addressing environmental exposures in patient care effectively.

TACKLING CLIMATE CHANGE WITHIN HEALTHCARE

More work is needed to integrate environmental health and healthcare systems, especially in our changing climate. Healthcare is increasingly recognizing climate change's impact on public health. There are two aspects to this recognition: (1) healthcare providers recognizing and reducing their carbon footprint; and (2) healthcare providers preparing for the reality of climate change as a physical and mental health crisis. This crisis will continue to worsen existing health disparities without significant efforts across many sectors, including healthcare. In partnership with the Alliance of Nurses for Healthy Environments, the American Psychological Association, Kaiser Permanente, the National League for Nursing, and the National Environmental Health Association, ClimateRx is a particularly useful resource that provides peer-reviewed and vetted education, training, guidance, and opportunities for action to assist healthcare professionals and their patients to care for their health and the climate.

Healthcare providers must engage in efforts to prevent and manage health-related risks. These efforts may entail patient education on heat-related illnesses, air quality, vector-borne diseases, and other climate-related health risks. For instance, imagine a patient undergoing a serious heart surgery in the summer during an extreme heat event. Healthcare providers should consider whether the patient has a safe, cool place to recover without suffering heat stroke after their release from the healthcare facility, since extreme heat can be particularly dangerous for patients with underlying health issues and patients taking multiple medications.

Healthcare providers can advocate for improved and more sustainable workplaces. The Practice Greenhealth[109] network offers a program called Health Care Without Harm,[110] which works with healthcare organizations to increase sustainability in healthcare and gives awards to hospitals that achieve green milestones. See Chapter 13, "Waste and Sustainability," for more information about healthcare waste.

CLIMATE CHANGE IN MEDICAL EDUCATION

In recent years, medical school curricula have started including climate change topics, largely in response to pressure from advocates and the next generation of clinicians. In 2019, medical students at the University of California San Francisco School of Medicine launched the Planetary Health Alliance and started working with various organizations and student leaders to grade medical schools globally. They rate programs on the basis of their climate-related curriculum, research, advocacy, community outreach, support for student-led initiatives, and sustainability efforts. Some of their many criteria, which can be asked of other healthcare programs, include:

- Does your curriculum address the impacts of extreme weather events on individual health and/or on healthcare systems?
- Does your curriculum address the impact of climate change on the changing patterns of infectious diseases?
- Does your curriculum address the mental health and neuropsychological effects of environmental degradation and climate change?
- In training for patient encounters, does your curriculum introduce strategies to have conversations with patients about the health effects of climate change?
- Does your school employ a faculty member to specifically oversee and take responsibility for the incorporation of planetary health and sustainable healthcare as themes throughout the course?
- Does your school and/or institution have an Office of Sustainability?

ANTI-RACIST HEALTHCARE AND ENVIRONMENTAL HEALTH

In Chapter 5, "Environmental Health Science for the People," we learned about anti-racist approaches to environmental health research. Similarly, many clinicians, particularly in the current generation, are calling for anti-racist approaches to healthcare and clinical education. Medicine has long adhered to biomedical models, heavily focusing on the genetic, biological, and behavioral factors contributing to health outcomes, while overlooking structural factors, including racism. A consideration of environmental factors in healthcare aligns well with these calls for a more equitable and anti-racist healthcare system. We can move toward a more equitable system by identifying and correcting institutional harms and patterns that perpetuate racism and updating clinical curricula to foster awareness of structural drivers of health (e.g., environmental injustice), while not overtaxing Black, Hispanic or Latino, and other healthcare providers of color to lead this work.[111]

INTERPROFESSIONAL EDUCATION TO ADDRESS ENVIRONMENTAL HEALTH AND JUSTICE

Van Diggele and colleagues describe interprofessional education (IPE) as

a critical approach for preparing students to enter the health workforce, where teamwork and collaboration are important competencies. IPE has been promoted by a number of international health organisations, as part of a redesign of healthcare systems to promote interprofessional teamwork, to enhance the quality of patient care, and improve health outcomes.[112(p1)]

Increasingly, universities are creating opportunities for IPE. For instance, the University of Michigan's Center for Interprofessional Education (Center for IPE) brings students together from different schools and programs, including students studying dentistry, kinesiology, medicine, nursing, pharmacy, social work, public health, health sciences, and health and human services. The Center for IPE facilitates modules and events that use a team approach to to navigate real and hypothetical case studies that benefit from multiple perspectives and skill sets. The Center also offers courses in topics such as "Breaking Bad News," "Health and Disabilities," "Interprofessional Team-Based Care," and "Current Issues and Interprofessional Perspectives in Occupational and Environmental Health and Safety." IPE may be one more tool to support integration of environmental health into healthcare.

COMMUNITY HEALTH WORKERS AND ENVIRONMENTAL HEALTH

Community health workers play a crucial role in healthcare by serving as a bridge between healthcare providers and the communities they serve. They often come from the communities they serve, speaking the local language and understanding cultural nuance. In some Hispanic or Latino communities, community health workers are referred to as *promotoras*. They may take on a wide range of roles, including informal counseling, social support, and health education. They might assist in scheduling appointments, arranging transportation, supporting individuals with chronic illnesses, or helping during crises or emergencies, among many other roles. They are on the ground in communities and households, making them uniquely situated to understand and help to address patients' environmental exposures. Community health workers play a vital role in our healthcare system and are critical to the integration of environmental health into clinical practice.

ENVIRONMENTAL PRECISION MEDICINE

As we call for integration of environmental health into clinical care, we must also judiciously approach the growing field of precision medicine. *Precision medicine*, also known as personalized medicine, is an approach to healthcare that considers individual differences in genetics, environment, and lifestyle when tailoring medical care and treatment plans for patients. Instead of the traditional one-size-fits-all approach, precision medicine aims to deliver the right intervention to the right patient at the right time. The field uses advanced technologies to analyze an individual's genetic makeup, including variations in genes, proteins, and other molecular markers. Specifically, work in the field of environmental epigenetics (discussed in Chapter 7, "Understanding the Environment and How It Relates to Health Using Toxicology and Epidemiology Research Methods"), may be useful for understanding how various environmental exposures alter how our genes are expressed. A precision medicine approach may involve tailored plans to prevent or treat cancer, cardiovascular disease, and various chronic conditions.

Environmental precision medicine, as a relatively new field, raises many concerns about privacy and equity that must be addressed: Who owns this genetic data? Who will have access to effective services informed by environmental precision medicine, and who will not? Will insurance cover such tailored services for everyone? Could increased personalized information lead to discrimination in employment, insurance, or in other areas? Healthcare professionals, policy makers, patients, and the public may need to consider the ethical aspects of this medical approach when integrating environmental health into healthcare.

HEALTHCARE PROFESSIONALS AS ADVOCATES

Outside of work, clinicians can use their trusted voices by becoming active in local politics, writing op-eds, and signing petitions, as well as educating decision makers.[113] Of course, this political activism requires a time commitment and policy or media advocacy skills. Organizations such as the Alliance of Nurses for Healthy Environments engage healthcare professionals through education and news updates about possible courses of action.[114] In the American Medical Association's *Journal of Ethics*, Macphereson and Wynia discuss the criteria for when a healthcare professional might consider stepping into advocacy.[115] The criteria include relevant expertise, proximity to the community or issue at hand, likelihood of effectiveness, severity of the issue, and public trust, as the public generally trusts clinicians as messengers. They also discuss risk and note that risk and cost of stepping into advocacy varies depending on a variety of individual and societal factors. There are many avenues for healthcare professionals to become more active on environmental health issues within and outside of the healthcare system. Several physician advocates are introduced in Box 18.1.

BOX 18.1. PHYSICIAN ADVOCATES

Learn more about physicians who have used their expertise, power, and privilege to advocate on climate change:

Dr. Jay Lemery is an emergency physician and codirector of the Climate and Health Program at the University of Colorado. Dr. Lemery is actively engaged in research and advocacy regarding climate change and health. He coedited the book *Enviromedics: The Impact of Climate Change on Human Health* and frequently speaks about the health implications of environmental changes.

Dr. Harleen Marwah is the Founding Chair of Medical Students for a Sustainable Future. Dr. Marwah earned the 2020 Health Care Without Harm Emerging Physician Leader Award in recognition of her work in founding and leading Medical Students for a Sustainable Future. She collaborated with the United Nations on the Paris Climate Agreement, attending the COP20 in Lima, Peru, and the COP21 in Paris, France.

Dr. Lisa Patel is the Executive Director of the Medical Society Consortium on Climate and Health and a member of the American Academy of Pediatrics Council on Environmental Health and Climate Change. She is a practicing pediatric hospitalist, is Clinical Associate Professor of Pediatrics at Stanford University, and works on projects related to climate-resilient schools, environmental justice (EJ), sustainable healthcare, and medical education curriculum reform.

Dr. Mona Sarfaty is the director of the Program on Climate and Health at George Mason University's Center for Climate Change Communication. She is also a family physician and has been involved in advocating for policies addressing climate change's health impacts. She emphasizes the importance of healthcare professionals' role in raising awareness and addressing climate-related health challenges.

MAIN TAKEAWAYS

In this chapter, we learned that:

- Pregnant individuals, infants, and children have physiological changes that increase their likelihood of environmental harms. Exposures during critical windows of human development have impacts throughout the life span and can also impact future generations.
- Further research and regulation are necessary in the face of the multitude of available chemicals and products. Preventive policies and the elimination of hazards are the best treatment. Prevention is the cure.
- Many barriers remain in the integration of environmental health into clinical care. Many resources are available for healthcare professionals seeking guidance. Innovations that automate screening and reduce the workload on clinicians can be beneficial.
- The field of clinical environmental health must consider the exposome, or totality of exposures in an individual's environment. This means considering the patient's regular behaviors and frequently occupied spaces when taking a health history, conducting patient assessment, and counseling via the "What–So What–Now What" framework.
- Healthcare providers need to address climate change's impact on health by reducing their carbon footprint, educating patients on climate-related health risks, and engaging in advocacy.
- Important aspects of environmental health in clinical care include anti-racist approaches to environmental health research, IPE as an essential component, the critical role of community health workers, and environmental precision medicine.

SUMMARY

Within clinical practice, this chapter provides a brief introduction to and helpful resources for some of the top concerns in environmental health. Challenges to the clinical visit include time limits, clinician confidence, and the balance of not overwhelming the patient, but instead giving them actionable messages that address their priority concerns. As healthcare providers take a patient's history, they must consider the various exposures their patients may incur at work, at school, at early learning facilities, or at home. Everyday culprits include lead, mercury, mold, pesticides, plastics, PFAS, parabens, and air pollutants, among many others. Workplace hazards are often more varied than those at home, including biological, chemical, ergonomic, stress, noise, or radiation exposures. As a clinician, you may not be sure how to counsel patients, and as a patient you might not be sure what to advocate for when talking to clinicians. Some of the go-to resources in this chapter may help.

Although this chapter focuses on the clinical evaluation and treatment of environmental health hazards, we know that prevention is always better than cure. The number of new chemicals and exposures continues to grow, outpacing research, regulation, and clinical understanding. Communities already overburdened with environmental hazards often face barriers to accessing healthcare, high-quality early learning opportunities, healthier foods, and safer products. Climate change will disproportionately impact these same communities and present multiple threats, from extreme weather to infectious diseases. For these reasons, there must be a shift from medical management, or tertiary prevention and care after people are already exposed and sick, to a focus on prevention. The ultimate goal is to improve the SDOH and advocate for healthier environments for all.

ENVIRONMENTAL HEALTH IN PRACTICE

Occupational

Websites

- **Agency for Toxic Substances and Disease Registry (ATSDR):** An agency under the United States Department of Health and Human Services that provides information on specific toxic substances. It also has an informative guide for more information on taking an exposure history. (atsdr.cdc.gov)
- **American College of Occupational and Environmental Medicine (ACOEM):** A physician-led organization focused on occupational health and safety. Their website includes information on the specialty of occupational and environmental medicine, educational resources, publications, guidance, and position statements. (acoem.org)
- **American Industrial Hygiene Association (AIHA):** Agency focused on occupational and environmental health and safety largely consisting of certified industrial hygienists; it has a number of resources including guidelines for occupational exposures. (aiha.org)
- **National Institute for Occupational Safety and Health (NIOSH):** Provides a wealth of information regarding their programs and research, including links to data sets that include work-related variables and their publications. They also have easy-to-understand information on various hazards, chemicals, industries and occupations, and work-related diseases and injuries. Through its website, one can access their *NIOSH Pocket Guide to Chemical Hazards*, which includes the Relative Exposure Limits, discussed in Chapter 16. (cdc.gov/niosh/data/default.html)
- **Occupational Safety and Health Administration (OSHA):** Through the OSHA website, one can access the OSHA standards as well as important information on filing a complaint. The website also provides resources and education. (osha.gov)
- **Office of Workers' Compensation Programs (OWCP):** Provides key information on their specific programs. For state-specific workers' compensation information, including benefits, impairment guidelines, drug formularies, and medical-treatment guidelines, there are also lists to state websites. (dol.gov/agencies/owcp/wc)

Pediatric

Websites

- **American Academy of Pediatrics (AAP):** An organization focused on pediatric care. It has a number of landing pages on various environmental health topics with key messages and links to additional resources. (aap.org/en/patient-care/environmental-health/promoting-healthy-environments-for-children)
- **Children's Environmental Health Network (CEHN):** The preeminent national nonprofit organization focused on children's environmental health. It has long-standing programs focused on reducing toxic exposures in child-care settings (Eco-Healthy Child Care®), EJ, climate change, childhood cancer, and other policy-focused efforts. (CEHN.org)
- **HealthyChildren.Org:** This resource, also maintained by the American Academy of Pediatrics, is intended to be a go-to resource for families on a variety of topics, including a growing number of environmental-health-related ones. (healthychildren.org)
- **NYS Centers of Excellence in Children's Environmental Health (NYSCHECK):** The NYSCHECK website houses the Prescriptions for Prevention clinical tools that provide evidence-based actionable guidance for educating clinicians and provide a way to connect families to environmental health resources. (nyscheck.org)[48]
- **Pediatric Environmental Health Specialty Units (PEHSU):** The PEHSUs are a national network of experts in the prevention, diagnosis, management, and treatment of health issues that arise from environmental exposures from preconception through adolescence. Educational material for both clinicians and patients is available at the website for free, along with access to regional PEHSU experts. (pehsu.net)[57]

(continued)

- **Promoting Healthy Environments for Children:** The American Academy of Pediatrics has a number of landing pages on various environmental health topics, with key messages and links to additional resources. (aap.org/en/patient-care/environmental-health/promoting-healthy-environments-for-children)

OB/GYN

Websites
- **MotherToBaby:** A service of the nonprofit Organization of Teratology Information Specialists, which is dedicated to providing information to mothers and healthcare providers on medications and other exposures during pregnancy and breastfeeding. Also provides a hotline to call or email for additional advice (866-626-6847). Many patient-facing fact sheets available online for free on a variety of environmental exposures (carbon monoxide, lead, insect repellants, methylmercury, hair treatments, etc.) in addition to medication exposures. (mothertobaby.org)
- **REPROTOX:** An information system developed by the Reproductive Toxicology Center. It contains commentaries on the potentially harmful effects of chemicals and physical agents on human pregnancy, reproduction, and development. It is available for a fee online (reprotox.org).

Books
- **American Academy of Pediatrics,** *Pediatric Environmental Health* **("The Green Book").**[47] A textbook on environmental health for clinicians, it provides sources of exposure and potential developmental susceptibility. It also contains relevant prenatal and early childhood information throughout. Available online for purchase at www.aap.org.

Articles
- Environmental exposures: how to counsel preconception and prenatal patients in the clinical setting.[116] Sathyanarayana S, Focareta J, Dailey T, Buchanan S.
- International Federation of Gynecology and Obstetrics Opinion on Reproductive Health Impacts of Exposure to Toxic Environmental Chemicals.[117] Di Renzo GC, Conry JA, Blake J, et al.
- Exposure to toxic environmental agents.[118] ACOG Committee Opinion Number 575.
- Lead screening during pregnancy and lactation.[67] ACOG Committee Opinion Number 533.
- Update on Seafood Consumption during pregnancy.[64] ACOG Practice Advisory.
- Occupational and environmental risks to reproduction in females: Specific exposures and impact.[119] UpToDate, 2023, updated and reviewed yearly. Goldman RH, Wylie BJ.
- Overview of occupational and environmental risks to reproduction in females.[120] UpToDate, 2023, updated and reviewed yearly. Goldman RH, Wylie BJ.

END-OF-CHAPTER RESOURCES

DISCUSSION QUESTIONS

1. From what you read in this chapter (and from your own experience), what are some ways we can reimagine the U.S. healthcare system to better integrate environmental health issues into patient care?
2. Throughout this book, you have read about a variety of environmental health exposures—from lead to PFAS, from polychlorinated biphenyls (PCBs) to cumulative impacts. Think of a chemical exposure that concerns you. How might healthcare professionals advocate for protections or programs to reduce exposure?
3. The realities of our healthcare system are that many clinicians experience burnout at some point in their career. This is more common for women and health workers of color. Surgeon General Vivek Murthy has prioritized this issue and examines underlying causes—from excessive workloads to administrative burdens, from

extended hours to workforce shortages. As we work to integrate environmental health into healthcare, how do we support the healthcare workforce in taking on one more heavy issue—climate change?

4. In your own words, what is interprofessional education, and how might it support efforts to integrate environmental health into healthcare? Use examples for what this might look like.

LEARNING ACTIVITIES

THE TIME IS NOW

Clinicians have a lot to keep track of, including emerging technologies, new pharmaceuticals and treatments, and ever-changing evidence-based guidelines. They may not have training on climate change and health. Next time you go to a primary care provider for a check-up, engage them in a discussion about climate change and health. Some may be well prepared to discuss the health effects of extreme weather events, changing patterns in infectious disease, or other climate-related concerns you may have. If not, share what you know about various organizations doing this work with opportunities for continuing education:

- Medical Students for a Sustainable Future
- The Global Consortium on Climate and Health Education
- Climate for Health Ambassador Training
- The Climate Health Alliance
- Practice Greenhealth
- Health Care Without Harm
- Physicians for Social Responsibility

IN REAL LIFE

Most everyone has completed a health-history form or answered a set of health history questions given by a healthcare provider. For instance, we are often asked to report on our family's health history or our own dietary, exercise, substance use, and sexual behaviors. Do you recall ever being asked about potential environmental factors in your workplace, home, or community? If you are comfortable with this issue, reflect on it or discuss it with others. What do you think would be helpful for your clinical team to know?

A robust set of instructor resources designed to supplement this text is located at http://connect.springerpub.com/content/book/978-0-8261-8353-8. Qualifying instructors may request access by emailing textbook@springerpub.com.

REFERENCES

1. Bello GA, Arora M, Austin C, Horton MK, Wright RO, Gennings C. Extending the distributed lag model framework to handle chemical mixtures. *Environ Res*. 2017;156:253–264. doi:10.1016/j.envres.2017.03.031
2. Cote I, Andersen ME, Ankley GT, et al. The next generation of risk assessment multi-year study-highlights of findings, applications to risk assessment, and future directions. *Environ Health Perspect*. 2016;124(11):1671–1682. doi:10.1289/EHP233
3. Cui Y, Balshaw DM, Kwok RK, Thompson CL, Collman GW, Birnbaum LS. The exposome: embracing the complexity for discovery in environmental health. *Environ Health Perspect*. 2016;124(8):A137–A140. doi:10.1289/EHP412
4. Gennings C, Curtin P, Bello G, Wright R, Arora M, Austin C. Lagged WQS regression for mixtures with many components. *Environ Res*. 2020;186:109529. doi:10.1016/j.envres.2020.109529

5. Payne-Sturges DC, Scammell MK, Levy JI, et al. Methods for evaluating the combined effects of chemical and nonchemical exposures for cumulative environmental health risk assessment. *Int J Environ Res Public Health*. 2018;15(12):2797. doi:10.3390/ijerph15122797
6. Stingone JA, Buck Louis GM, Nakayama SF, et al. Toward greater implementation of the exposome research paradigm within environmental epidemiology. *Annu Rev Public Health*. 2017;38:315–327. doi:10.1146/annurev-publhealth-082516-012750
7. Wright RO. Environment, susceptibility windows, development, and child health. *Curr Opin Pediatr*. 2017;29(2):211–217. doi:10.1097/MOP.0000000000000465
8. Centers for Disease Control and Prevention. Fourth national report on human exposure to environmental chemicals. 2015. Accessed date June 18, 2024. doi:10.15620/cdc:105345
9. Landrigan PJ, Braun JM, Crain EF, et al. Building capacity in pediatric environmental health: the academic pediatric association's professional development program. *Acad Pediatr*. 2019;19(4):421–427. doi:10.1016/j.acap.2019.01.001
10. Landrigan PJ, Woolf AD, Gitterman B, et al. The ambulatory pediatric association fellowship in pediatric environmental health: a 5-Year assessment. *Environ Health Perspect*. 2007;115(10):1383–1387. doi:10.1289/ehp.10015
11. Anderson ME, Zajac L, Thanik E, Galvez M. Home visits for pediatric asthma—a strategy for comprehensive asthma management through prevention and reduction of environmental asthma triggers in the home. *Curr Probl Pediatr Adolesc Health Care*. 2020;50(2):100753. doi:10.1016/j.cppeds.2020.100753
12. Galvez M, Collins G, Amler RW, et al. Building New York State Centers of Excellence in children's environmental health: a replicable model in a time of uncertainty. *Am J Public Health*. 2019;109(1):108–112. doi:10.2105/AJPH.2018.304742
13. Galvez MP, Balk SJ. Environmental risks to children: prioritizing health messages in pediatric practice. *Pediatr Rev*. 2017;38(6):263–279. doi:10.1542/pir.2015-0165
14. Wellbery C, Sheffield P, Timmireddy K, Sarfaty M, Teherani A, Fallar R. It's time for medical schools to introduce climate change into their curricula. *Acad Med*. 2018;93(12):1774–1777. doi:10.1097/ACM.0000000000002368
15. Landrigan PJ. Children's Environmental health: a brief history. *Acad Pediatr*. 2016;16(1):1–9. doi:10.1016/j.acap.2015.10.002
16. Medical screening and surveillance requirements in OSHA standards: a guide. U.S. Department of Labor Occupational Safety and Health Administration. 2014. https://www.osha.gov/sites/default/files/publications/osha3162.pdf
17. Practice resources. American College of Occupational and Environmental Medicine. Accessed June 18, 2024. https://acoem.org/Practice-Resources/Practice-Guidelines-Center
18. Key points about taking an environmental history. American Academy of Pediatrics. February 14, 2023. Updated October 1, 2024. https://www.aap.org/en/patient-care/environmental-health/promoting-healthy-environments-for-children/taking-an-environmental-history/
19. Reducing prenatal exposure to toxic environmental agents. ACOG committee opinion No. 832. American College of Obstetricians and Gynecologists. *Obstet Gynecol*. 2021;138:e40–e54. https://www.acog.org/clinical/clinical-guidance/committee-opinion/articles/2021/07/reducing-prenatal-exposure-to-toxic-environmental-agents
20. Screening for Breast Cancer. U.S. Preventive Service Task Force. Accessed June 18, 2024. https://www.uspreventiveservicestaskforce.org/uspstf/
21. Guidelines for the identification and management of lead exposure in pregnant and lactating women. Accessed June 18, 2024. 2021. https://stacks.cdc.gov/view/cdc/147837
22. Centers for Disease Control and Prevention. Blood lead reference value. April 17, 2024. https://www.cdc.gov/lead-prevention/php/data/blood-lead-surveillance.html?CDC_AAref_Val=https://www.cdc.gov/nceh/lead/data/blood-lead-reference-value.htm
23. U.S. Environmental Protection Agency. NIEHS/EPA Children's Environmental Health and Disease Prevention Research Centers impact report: protecting children's health where they live, learn, and play. EPA Publication No. EPA/600/R-17/407. 2017. https://www.epa.gov/sites/production/files/2017-10/documents/niehs_epa_childrens_centers_impact_report_2017_0.pdf?pdf=chidrens-center-report
24. Garcia K, Grybauskas N, Colarusso A, et al. A roadmap to eliminating childhood lead exposure. LeadFreeNYC. 2019. https://www.nyc.gov/assets/leadfree/downloads/pdf/Lead_Report_2019_Full.pdf

25. Andra SS, Austin C, Arora M. The tooth exposome in children's health research. *Curr Opin Pediatr.* 2016;28(2):221–227. doi:10.1097/MOP.0000000000000327
26. Arora M, Austin C, Sarrafpour B, et al. Determining prenatal, early childhood and cumulative long-term lead exposure using micro-spatial deciduous dentine levels. *PLoS One.* 2014;9(5):e97805. doi:10.1371/journal.pone.0097805
27. Bose S, Ross KR, Rosa MJ, et al. Prenatal particulate air pollution exposure and sleep disruption in preschoolers: windows of susceptibility. *Environ Int.* 2019;124:329–335. doi:10.1016/j.envint.2019.01.012
28. Evans SF, Raymond S, Sethuram S, et al. Associations between prenatal phthalate exposure and sex-typed play behavior in preschool age boys and girls. *Environ Res.* 2021;192:110264. doi:10.1016/j.envres.2020.110264
29. Petrick LM, Arora M, Niedzwiecki MM. Minimally invasive biospecimen collection for exposome research in children's health. *Curr Environ Health Rep.* 2020;7(3):198–210. doi:10.1007/s40572-020-00277-2
30. Sathyanarayana S, Grady R, Redmon JB, et al. Anogenital distance and penile width measurements in The Infant Development and the Environment Study (TIDES): methods and predictors. *J Pediatr Urol.* 2015;11(2):76.e1–76.e6. doi:10.1016/j.jpurol.2014.11.018
31. Sheffield PE, Herrera MT, Kinnee EJ, Clougherty JE. Not so little differences: variation in hot weather risk to young children in New York City. *Public Health.* 2018;161:119–126. doi:10.1016/j.puhe.2018.06.004
32. Sheffield PE, Shmool JLC, Kinnee EJ, Clougherty JE. Violent crime and socioeconomic deprivation in shaping asthma-related pollution susceptibility: a case-crossover design. *J Epidemiol Community Health.* 2019;73(9):846–853. doi:10.1136/jech-2018-211816
33. Sorek-Hamer M, Just AC, Kloog I. Satellite remote sensing in epidemiological studies. *Curr Opin Pediatr.* 2016;28(2):228–234. doi:10.1097/MOP.0000000000000326
34. Wolff MS, Pajak A, Pinney SM, et al. Associations of urinary phthalate and phenol biomarkers with menarche in a multiethnic cohort of young girls. *Reprod Toxicol.* 2017;67:56–64. doi:10.1016/j.reprotox.2016.11.009
35. Wu S, Gennings C, Wright RJ, et al. Prenatal stress, methylation in inflammation-related genes, and adiposity measures in early childhood: the programming research in obesity, growth environment and social stress cohort study. *Psychosom Med.* 2018;80(1):34–41. doi:10.1097/PSY.0000000000000517
36. Zajac L, Kobrosly RW, Ericson B, Caravanos J, Landrigan PJ, Riederer AM. Probabilistic estimates of prenatal lead exposure at 195 toxic hotspots in low- and middle-income countries. *Environ Res.* 2020;183:109251. doi:10.1016/j.envres.2020.109251
37. Bureau of Labor Statistics. Work experience of the population—2022. News Release, U.S. Department of Labor. December 8, 2022. https://www.bls.gov/news.release/pdf/work.pdf
38. Hazard identification and assessment. Occupational Safety and Health Administration. Accessed June 18, 2024. https://www.osha.gov/safety-management/hazard-Identification
39. Canadian Centre for Occupational Health and Safety. Hazard and risk. June 13, 2023. https://www.ccohs.ca/oshanswers/hsprograms/hazard/hazard_risk.html
40. Workers' compensation. U.S. Department of Labor. Accessed June 18, 2024. https://www.dol.gov/general/topic/workcomp
41. Knoblauch DK, Cassaro S. Workers compensation. In: *StatPearls.* StatPearls Publishing; 2023. http://www.ncbi.nlm.nih.gov/books/NBK448106/
42. Taking the occupational history. *Ann Intern Med.* 1983;99(5):641–651. doi:10.7326/0003-4819-99-5-641
43. National Institute for Occupational Safety and Health. Collecting and using industry and occupation data. Centers for Disease Control and Prevention. Updated June 29, 2022. https://www.cdc.gov/niosh/topics/coding/collect.html
44. National Institute for Occupational Safety and Health. Chart the 2013–2015 BRFSS data. Centers for Disease Control and Prevention. Accessed June 18, 2024. https://wwwn.cdc.gov/NIOSH-WHC/
45. Child population: number of children (in millions) ages 0–17 in the United States by age, 1950–2022 and projected 2023–2050. Childstats Forum on Child and Family Statistics. Accessed June 18, 2024. https://www.childstats.gov/americaschildren/tables/pop1.asp

46. Landrigan PJ, Etzel RA, eds. *Textbook of Children's Environmental Health*. 2013; (online ed., Oxford Academic, May 1, 2014). doi:10.1093/med/9780199929573.001.0001
47. American Academy of Pediatrics Council on Environmental Health. Taking an environmental history and giving anticipatory guidance. In: Etzel RA, Balk SJ, eds. *Pediatric Environmental Health*, 4th ed. American Academy of Pediatrics; 2019:47–68.
48. New York State prescriptions for prevention—English. New York State Children's Environmental Health Centers. Accessed June 18, 2024. https://nyscheck.org/rx/
49. Lead screening. Medicaid. Accessed June 18, 2024. https://www.medicaid.gov/medicaid/benefits/early-and-periodic-screening-diagnostic-and-treatment/lead-screening/index.html
50. Relates to prevention and screening for elevated lead levels in children, S 5024-D, New York State Senate, 2021–2022 legislative session. Signed August 17, 2022. Accessed June 18, 2024 https://www.nysenate.gov/legislation/bills/2021/S5024
51. Childhood Blood Lead Test Act, S 522, Pennsylvania State Senate, 2021–2022 Legislative Session. Passed November 3, 2022. https://legiscan.com/PA/text/SB522/id/2611503
52. Relating to childhood lead poisoning prevention, H 222, Delaware State House. Passed June 30, 2021. https://legiscan.com/DE/text/HB222/2021
53. Learn about lead screening and reporting requirements. Mass.Gov. Accessed June 18, 2024. www.mass.gov/service-details/learn-about-lead-screening-and-reporting-requirements#:~:text=The%20Lead%20Law%20and%20screening,and%20again%20at%20age%203
54. Swinburne M. State lead testing policies for children not enrolled in medicaid. The Network for Public Health Law. May 9, 2018. https://www.networkforphl.org/wp-content/uploads/2019/12/50-State-Survey-Lead-Screening-for-Children-Not-Enrolled-in-Medicaid.pdf
55. Recommended actions based on blood lead levels. Centers for Disease Control and Prevention. December 2, 2022. https://www.cdc.gov/nceh/lead/advisory/acclpp/actions-blls.htm
56. Pediatric Environmental Health Specialty Units. Home. Accessed June 18, 2024. https://www.pehsu.net/index.html
57. American Cancer Society. Key statistics for childhood cancers. January 12, 2023. Accessed June 18, 2024 https://www.cancer.org/cancer/types/cancer-in-children/key-statistics.html
58. About the PEHSU program. Pediatric Environmental Health Specialty Units. Accessed June 18, 2024. https://www.pehsu.net/About_PEHSU.html
59. Sutton P, Woodruff TJ, Perron J, et al. Toxic environmental chemicals: the role of reproductive health professionals in preventing harmful exposures. *Am J Obstet Gynecol*. 2012;207(3):164–173. doi:10.1016/j.ajog.2012.01.034
60. Amin-Zaki L, Elhassani S, Majeed MA, Clarkson TW, Doherty RA, Greenwood M. Intra-uterine methylmercury poisoning in Iraq. *Pediatrics*. 1974;54(5):587–595.
61. Harada M. Congenital Minamata disease: intrauterine methylmercury poisoning. *Teratology*. 1978;18(2):285–288. doi:10.1002/tera.1420180216
62. Grandjean P, Weihe P, White RF, et al. Cognitive deficit in 7-year-old children with prenatal exposure to methylmercury. *Neurotoxicol Teratol*. 1997;19(6):417–428. doi:10.1016/s0892-0362(97)00097-4
63. Debes F, Budtz-Jørgensen E, Weihe P, White RF, Grandjean P. Impact of prenatal methylmercury exposure on neurobehavioral function at age 14 years. *Neurotoxicol Teratol*. 2006;28(3):363–375. doi:10.1016/j.ntt.2006.02.004
64. Toxic chemicals: Steps to stay safer before and during pregnancy. The American College of Obstetricians and Gynecologists. October 2022. Accessed June 18, 2024. https://www.acog.org/womens-health/faqs/toxic-chemicals-steps-to-stay-safer-before-and-during-pregnancy
65. Oken E, Kleinman KP, Berland WE, Simon SR, Rich-Edwards JW, Gillman MW. Decline in fish consumption among pregnant women after a national mercury advisory. *Obstet Gynecol*. 2003;102(2):346–351. doi:10.1016/s0029-7844(03)00484-8
66. Bellinger D, Leviton A, Waternaux C, Needleman H, Rabinowitz M. Longitudinal analyses of prenatal and postnatal lead exposure and early cognitive development. *N Engl J Med*. 1987;316(17):1037–1043. doi:10.1056/NEJM198704233161701
67. Committee on Obstetric Practice. Committee opinion No. 533: lead screening during pregnancy and lactation. *Obstet Gynecol*. 2012;120(2 Pt 1):416–420. doi:10.1097/AOG.0b013e31826804e8
68. Johnson KM, Specht AJ, Hart JM, et al. Risk-factor based lead screening and correlation with blood lead levels in pregnancy. *Matern Child Health J*. 2022;26(1):185–192. doi:10.1007/s10995-021-03325-x

69. Stotland NE, Sutton P, Trowbridge J, et al. Counseling patients on preventing prenatal environmental exposures—a mixed-methods study of obstetricians. *PLoS One*. 2014;9(6):e98771. doi:10.1371/journal.pone.0098771
70. Budgell B. Guidelines to the writing of case studies. *J Can Chiropr Assoc*. 2008;52(4):199–204. https://www.ncbi.nlm.nih.gov/pmc/articles/PMC2597880/
71. Smith LB, Karpman M, Gonzalez D, Morriss S. More than one in five adults with limited public transit access forgo health care because of transportation barriers. Robert Wood Johnson Foundation. April 26, 2023. https://www.rwjf.org/en/insights/our-research/2023/04/more-than-one-in-five-adults-with-limited-public-transit-access-forgo-healthcare-because-of-transportation-barriers.html
72. Five key barriers to healthcare access in the United States. Wolters Kluwer. July 27, 2022. Accessed June 18, 202.4 https://www.wolterskluwer.com/en/expert-insights/five-key-barriers-to-health-care-access-in-the-united-states
73. Affordable Care Act (ACA). HealthCare.Gov. www.healthcare.gov/glossary/affordable-care-act/
74. Charitable hospitals—general requirements for tax-exemption under section 501(c)(3). Internal Revenue Service. July 13, 2023. https://www.irs.gov/charities-non-profits/charitable-hospitals-general-requirements-for-tax-exemption-under-section-501c3
75. Hostetter M, Klein S. In focus: hospitals invest in building stronger, healthier communities. The Commonwealth Fund: Improving Health Care Quality. September 23, 2016. https://www.commonwealthfund.org/publications/2016/sep/focus-hospitals-invest-building-stronger-healthier-communities?redirect_source=/publications/newsletters/transforming-care/2016/september/in-focus
76. Spencer A, Lloyd J, McGinnis T. Using medicaid resources to pay for healthrelated supportive services: early lessons. Center for Health Care Strategies, Inc. December 2015. http://www.chcs.org/media/Supportive-Services-Brief-Final-120315.pdf
77. Federal Employees' Compensation Act (FECA) claims administration. US Department of Labor. Accessed June 18, 2024. www.dol.gov/agencies/owcp/FECA/about#:~:text=The%20Federal%20Employees%27%20Compensation%20Act%20gives%20injured%20workers%20the%20right,and%2C%20if%20necessary%2C%20beyond
78. Occupational safety and health standards: determination of work-relatedness (Standard No. 1904.5). Occupational Safety and Health Administration. 2001. Accessed June 18, 2024. https://www.osha.gov/laws-regs/regulations/standardnumber/1904/1904.5
79. Permissible exposure limits—annotated tables. Occupational Safety and Health Administration. Accessed June 18, 2024. https://www.osha.gov/annotated-pels
80. National Research Council. *Improving Risk Communication*. National Academies Press; 1989:1189. doi:10.17226/1189
81. Covello VT. Best practices in public health risk and crisis communication. *J Health Commun*. 2003;8 (suppl 1):5–8; discussion 148–151. doi:10.1080/713851971
82. Galvez MP, Peters R, Graber N, Forman J. Effective risk communication in children's environmental health: lessons learned from 9/11. *Pediatr Clin North Am*. 2007;54(1):33–46, viii. doi:10.1016/j.pcl.2006.11.003
83. Peters RG, Covello VT, McCallum DB. The determinants of trust and credibility in environmental risk communication: an empirical study. *Risk Anal*. 1997;17(1):43–54. doi:10.1111/j.1539-6924.1997.tb00842.x
84. Galvez MP, Herlache A, Anderko L, et al. Speaking with one voice: lessons learned on effective communication of environmental health risk. *Environ Justice*. 2021;14(4):235–242. doi:10.1089/env.2020.0074
85. Hojat LS. Breaking down the barriers to health equity. *Ther Adv Infect Dis*. 2022;9:20499361221079453. doi:10.1177/20499361221079453
86. McCauley LA. Immigrant workers in the united states : recent trends, vulnerable populations, and challenges for occupational health. *AAOHN J*. 2005;53(7):313–319. doi:10.1177/216507990505300706
87. Mechanic D, Tanner J. Vulnerable people, groups, and populations: societal view. *Health Aff*. 2007;26(5):1220–1230. doi:10.1377/hlthaff.26.5.1220
88. Woods LM, Rachet B, Coleman MP. Origins of socio-economic inequalities in cancer survival: a review. *Ann Oncol*. 2006;17(1):5–19. doi:10.1093/annonc/mdj007
89. Hostetter M, Klein S. Understanding and ameliorating medical mistrust among Black Americans. The commonwealth fund: advancing health equity. January 14, 2021.

https://www.commonwealthfund.org/publications/newsletter-article/2021/jan/medical-mistrust-among-black-americans

90. Williams DR, Rucker TD. Understanding and addressing racial disparities in health care. *Health Care Financ Rev*. 2000;21(4):75–90.
91. Exposure assessment tools by approaches—exposure reconstruction (biomonitoring and reverse dosimetry). United States Environmental Protection Agency. May 24, 2023. https://www.epa.gov/expobox/exposure-assessment-tools-approaches-exposure-reconstruction-biomonitoring-and-reverse
92. Yearby R, Clark B, Figueroa JF. Structural racism in historical and modern US health care policy: study examines structural racism in historical and modern US health care policy. *Health Aff*. 2022;41(2):187–194. doi:10.1377/hlthaff.2021.01466
93. Braveman PA, Arkin E, Proctor D, Kauh T, Holm N. Systemic and structural racism: definitions, examples, health damages, and approaches to dismantling: study examines definitions, examples, health damages, and dismantling systemic and structural racism. *Health Aff*. 2022;41(2):171–178. doi:10.1377/hlthaff.2021.01394
94. Bronson, E. What is medical racism? July 21, 2020. https://www.ywcaworks.org/blogs/firesteel/what-medical-racism
95. Rees M. Racism in healthcare: what you need to know. Medical News Today. 2020. https://www.medicalnewstoday.com/articles/racism-in-healthcare
96. Washington HA. *Medical Apartheid: The Dark History of Medical Experimentation on Black Americans from Colonial Times to the Present*. Doubleday Book; 2006.
97. Taylor D. *Toxic Communities*. New York University Press; 2014.
98. Smedley BD, Stith AY, Nelson AR. *Unequal Treatment: Confronting Racial and Ethnic Disparities in Health Care*. National Academies Press; 2003. doi:10.17226/12875
99. McFarling U. 20 years ago, a landmark report spotlighted systemic racism in medicine. Why has so little changed? February 23, 2022. https://www.statnews.com/2022/02/23/landmark-report-systemic-racism-medicine-so-little-has-changed/
100. Strand NH, Mariano ER, Goree JH, et al. Racism in pain medicine: we can and should do more. *Mayo Clin Proc*. 2021;96(6):1394–1400. doi:10.1016/j.mayocp.2021.02.030
101. Tello M. Racism and discrimination in health care: providers and patients. Harvard Health Blog. January 16, 2017:12. https://www.health.harvard.edu/blog/racism-discrimination-health-care-providers-patients-2017011611015
102. Feldman S, Jeffries A, Garcia-Garcia M. The data behind racism in healthcare. Ipsos. April 7, 2022. https://www.ipsos.com/en-us/knowledge/society/The-Data-Behind-Racism-in-Healthcare
103. St. Catherine University. Racial discrimination in healthcare: how structural racism affects healthcare. June 15, 2021. https://www.stkate.edu/academics/healthcare-degrees/racism-in-healthcare
104. Racism and health. Centers for Disease Control and Prevention. 2021. Updated September 18, 2023. https://www.cdc.gov/minorityhealth/racism-disparities/index.html
105. Rothstein R. *The Color of Law: A Forgotten History of How Our Government Segregated America*. Liveright Publishing; 2017.
106. Ortega RP. Teeth record pneumonia-and racism. *Science*. 2022;378(6619):459–461. doi:10.1126/science.adf6049
107. Serafini K, Coyer C, Speights JB, et al. Racism as experienced by physicians of color in the health care setting. *Fam Med*. 2020;52(4):282–287. doi:10.22454/FamMed.2020.384384
108. Ducharme J. U.S. Medical schools are struggling to overcome centuries of racism in health care. August 30, 2022. https://time.com/6208309/racism-us-medical-schools-kaiser-permanente/
109. Sustainability Solutions for Health Care. Practice Greenhealth. Accessed date June 18, 2024. https://practicegreenhealth.org/
110. Health Care Without Harm. https://noharm-uscanada.org/
111. Asmerom B, Legha RK, Mabeza RM, Nuñez V. An abolitionist approach to antiracist medical education. *AMA J Ethics*. 2022;24(3):194–200. Home. Accessed date June 18, 2024. doi:10.1001/amajethics.2022.194
112. van Diggele C, Roberts C, Burgess A, Mellis C. Interprofessional education: tips for design and implementation. *BMC Med Educ*. 2020;20(suppl 2):455. doi:10.1186/s12909-020-02286-z
113. Kromm JN, Frattaroli S, Vernick JS, Teret SP. Public health advocacy in the courts: opportunities for public health professionals. *Public Health Rep*. 2009;124(6):889–894. doi:10.1177/003335490912400618

114. Alliance of Nurses for Healthy Environments. Home. Accessed date June 18, 2024. https://envirn.org/
115. Macpherson CC, Wynia M. Should health professionals speak up to reduce the health risks of climate change? *AMA J Ethics*. 2017;19(12):1202–1210. doi:10.1001/journalofethics.2017.19.12.msoc1-1712
116. Sathyanarayana S, Focareta J, Dailey T, Buchanan S. Environmental exposures: how to counsel preconception and prenatal patients in the clinical setting. *Am J Obstet Gynecol*. 2012;207(6):463–470. doi:10.1016/j.ajog.2012.02.004
117. Di Renzo GC, Conry JA, Blake J, et al. International Federation of Gynecology and Obstetrics opinion on reproductive health impacts of exposure to toxic environmental chemicals. *Int J Gynaecol Obstet*. 2015;131(3):219–225. doi:10.1016/j.ijgo.2015.09.002
118. ACOG Committee Opinion No 575. Exposure to toxic environmental agents. *Fertil Steril*. 2013;100(4):931–934. doi:10.1016/j.fertnstert.2013.08.043
119. Goldman RH, Wylie BJ. Occupational and environmental risks to reproduction in females: specific exposures and impact. In: Wilkins-Haug L, Eckler K, eds. *UpToDate*. Wolters Kluwer; 2023. https://www.uptodate.com/contents/occupational-and-environmental-risks-to-reproduction-in-females-specific-exposures-and-impact
120. Goldman RH, Wylie BJ. Overview of occupational and environmental risks to reproduction in females. In: Wilkins-Haug L, Eckler K, eds. *UpToDate*. Wolters Kluwer; 2023. https://www.uptodate.com/contents/overview-of-occupational-and-environmental-risks-to-reproduction-in-females

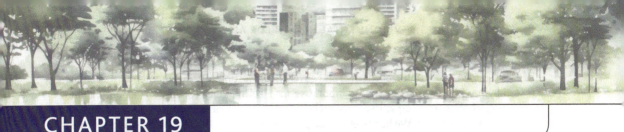

CHAPTER 19

Organizing for Environmental Health and Justice: Lessons From #StopGeneralIron

Jim Bloyd

With interviews with Olga Bautista, Wesley Epplin, Cheryl Johnson, Gina Ramirez, Óscar Sanchez, and Sophia Simon-Ortiz

LEARNING OBJECTIVES

- Explain the basics of community organizing for health.
- Examine the role of power in community organizing and how imbalances in power contribute to environmental injustice.
- Describe the events of the #StopGeneralIron campaign as an example of community organizing for health.
- Hear lessons directly from community organizers who led the #StopGeneralIron campaign in Chicago's Southeast Side.
- Examine the role of the local and federal government in protecting environmental health.
- Illustrate how historical and recent land use, permitting, zoning, or development decisions have the potential to promote environmental health or perpetuate environmental injustice.

KEY TERMS

- community engagement
- community organizing
- community power
- cumulative impact
- environmental racism
- power
- structural racism

"... millionaires and billionaires aren't used to losing. So I think that they're feeling it now. That is not enough if you can have organized money, but we have organized people. And in this case, enough organized people to win, to prevent this relocation."

— Olga Bautista, Organizer, Southeast Environmental Task Force

AUTHOR'S NOTE

"We're probably going to lose. It's a done deal."

This was the common refrain I heard from community organizers throughout 2020 and 2021 in the fight to #StopGeneralIron, an environmental justice campaign led by residents of the Southeast Side of Chicago. What was their goal? To advocate that the health department deny a permit that would allow a metal recycling facility to relocate to their already overburdened community. Simply put, they wanted clean air to breathe.

About 12 months into the COVID-19 pandemic, the mayor and public health department opposed the residents' requests. The *health department*. I had spent decades working toward

(continued)

health equity in community, academic, and government settings. At this moment, I was embarrassed by my field. As part of the Collaborative for Health Equity (CHE) Cook County, I knew our group of physicians, organizers, researchers, public health practitioners, and policy experts needed to join this fight. We had been working toward reducing structural racism and improving health equity in the region for years, and that is exactly what this was an opportunity to do.

Organizers had been mobilizing for a while and momentum was building. They were about to hold a hunger strike that would last 30 days. As the weeks and months unfolded, we at CHE Cook County joined hundreds of people in the public health and healthcare community and even high school students protesting and marching in sleet and rain. Many of us were mad about this terrible public health violation. I was energized and even hopeful about a collective effort to #StopGeneralIron.

In writing this chapter to understand the events of this campaign, I knew it was critical to hear from the voices of those Chicagoans from the Southeast Side who organized for environmental health and justice. Throughout, you will read several one-on-one interviews with these leaders for whom I am grateful and hold deep respect.

However, this chapter is written mostly by me—a cis-gender White male who has lived primarily in the western suburbs of Chicago, Illinois, and focused on health equity throughout his 30-year career in public health practice. I attempt to tell a story about courageous people organizing for a healthy neighborhood, about community power beating corporate power, and about the limits of governmental public health departments to fulfill their commitments to health equity. Admittedly, I am also limited by my own lived experience, perspective, and privilege.

In the end, you will see it wasn't a done deal, in fact. Organizers did win, and it was a milestone victory for environmental public health too. As Jobin-Leeds and AgitArte write in their book, *When We Fight, We Win*, "winning requires a 'we,' a community, a group, an organization. And transformative change, in the face of powerful forces, requires a fight."[1(pxvii)]

Editor's note: Jim Bloyd is Coordinator, Collaborative for Health Equity Cook County.

OVERVIEW

In 2018, the City of Chicago announced that the metal recycling operation known as General Iron would be relocated by its parent company the Reserve Management Group (RMG). Notorious for polluting a wealthy and gentrified North Side Lincoln Park neighborhood, General Iron planned to move to a new location about 15 miles south of Chicago's downtown area.[2] The operation, eventually rebranded as Southside Recycling, was to be located in the Calumet River Industrial Corridor, an area already overburdened by polluting industries, whose residents are primarily working-class Black and Brown Chicagoans. Like with most permitting, the industry proposal was expected to go through.

In response, neighborhood residents of the proposed location on the Southeast Side organized an uphill fight for clean air. They formed local alliances with public-health justice activists and launched the Stop General Iron campaign (known by its hashtags #StopGeneralIron and #DenythePermit). Against all odds, they were victorious: On February 18, 2022, the Chicago Department of Public Health (CDPH) Commissioner Dr. Allison Arwady informed the corporation that "CDPH hereby denies the permit."

The details of these events are the basis for this final chapter, which allows for an introduction to the concept of community organizing. **Community organizing** is:

> the process of building power through involving a constituency [specific groups of people] in identifying problems they share and the solutions to those problems that they desire; identifying the people and the structures that can make solutions possible; enlisting those targets in the effort through negotiation and using confrontation and pressure when needed; and building an institution that is democratically controlled by the constituency that can develop the capacity to take on further problems and that embodies the will and the power of that constituency.[3(p2)]

Alongside science and policy, community organizing is vital for ensuring environmental health and justice. Community organizers use skills in policy and media advocacy and a wide range of tactics in an effort to shift **power** and create lasting change. For instance, community organizers might:

- advocate to elect policy makers who are likely to promote environmental justice (EJ),
- rally communities to comment on major government decisions that affect environmental health,
- call for increased funding and enforcement to hold polluters accountable, or
- support communities harmed by environmental injustice.

After a brief introduction to community organizing, this chapter gives a detailed account of #StopGeneralIron. It begins with some history of environmental injustice in Chicago, followed by a detailed account of the goals, key players (allies, opponents, and decision makers), and tactics of the campaign. We hear directly from several organizers of the #StopGeneralIron campaign, including Olga Bautista, Wesley Epplin, Gina Ramirez, Óscar Sanchez, and Sophia Simon-Ortiz about the realities of this work. As the final chapter in this book, this case example shows the importance of listening to those harmed by cumulative environmental impacts if we are to ensure environmental health for all.

COMMUNITY ORGANIZING FOR HEALTH

There are many strategies for achieving health equity, and community organizing is a powerful approach in which communities mobilize to influence policy. (See Chapter 4, "Environmental Health Policies and Protections: Successes and Failures," for a reminder of what policies are and how they are different from programs.) Of course, communities are not a monolith with one single voice. They are made up of people with diverse perspectives, but with a particular feature that brings them together. That might be a shared geography, a shared identity, shared politics or values, or a shared interest or hobby, for instance.

Community organizing entails developing campaigns in the context of larger social movements using various tactics. #StopGeneralIron is an example of a campaign within the larger fight for EJ that intersects with civil rights, labor, and other movements. With regard to how organizing generally happens, there are a wide range of tactics. There are commonly known tactics such as petitions, town halls or listening sessions, door-to-door canvassing, and meetings with elected officials. There are direct action tactics such as rallies, protests, sit-ins, or other demonstrations. There are economic strategies, such as strikes or boycotts of specific businesses, for instance. There are creative tactics, such as art installations, among many others. There is also media advocacy, which uses social media and the traditional press to set narratives about a specific issue. Many of these tactics were used by #StopGeneralIron leaders to raise awareness among the general public, gain and engage allies, and direct attention on decision makers, encouraging them to stop the permit.

There are many models, theories, and frameworks for how to organize, and community organizing actually has deep roots in Chicago, as it is notably associated with the work of Saul Alinsky. Alinsky defined a community-organizing approach that shifted power to marginalized communities to challenge systemic inequalities, which he documented in his book, *Rules for Radicals*. He founded the Industrial Areas Foundation in Chicago in 1940, which became a central hub for training organizers and initiating grassroots movements. Of course, there are countless other historical and contemporary organizers we can learn from, each with different approaches for how to effect change.

A FEW ORGANIZERS TO KNOW

Cesar Chavez was a prominent American labor leader and civil rights activist who cofounded the National Farm Workers Association, later renamed the United Farm Workers. He is best known for his efforts in organizing and advocating for the rights of agricultural workers, particularly farmworkers, and leading nonviolent protests and boycotts to improve their working conditions.

(continued)

> **Winona LaDuke** is an American environmentalist, activist, writer, and two-time Green Party vice-presidential candidate known for her advocacy work on behalf of Indigenous rights, sustainable development, and environmental issues. She is a member of the Anishinaabe Tribe and has been a prominent figure in advocating for Indigenous sovereignty and environmental justice (EJ).
>
> **Grace Lee Boggs** was a prominent American philosopher, writer, and activist. She was known for her lifelong work in civil rights, feminism, labor rights, and EJ. Boggs was a key figure in the African American civil rights movement, advocating for social change, and she cofounded Detroit's influential activist organization, Detroit Summer.
>
> **Wangari Maathai** was a Kenyan environmentalist, political activist, and Nobel laureate. She founded the Green Belt Movement, an environmental organization that focused on tree planting, conservation, and women's rights. Maathai was the first African woman to receive the Nobel Peace Prize in 2004 for her contributions to sustainable development, democracy, and peace.
>
> **Nemonte Nenquimo** is an Indigenous Waorani leader from the Ecuadorian Amazon and a prominent environmental and Indigenous rights activist. She played a pivotal role in the landmark legal victory for Indigenous rights in Ecuador when the Waorani community won a lawsuit against the government, protecting half a million acres of rainforest from oil drilling in 2019.

In this chapter, we think about the #StopGeneralIron campaign using Jamila Michener's model of power for health justice, in which she describes two key ways that organizing engages with power: building power and breaking power.[4] *Building power* refers to the increasing political capacity of people who are the most harmed by health injustice, while *breaking power* involves dismantling the structures that maintain health inequities. Michener explains that community members can build power through community organizing, which often entails building coalitions and negotiating with institutions (like city government or health departments). She explains that breaking power entails profit minimization, regulation and enforcement, and institutional negotiation. We apply this framework to #StopGeneralIron later in the chapter.

HISTORY OF ENVIRONMENTAL INJUSTICE ON CHICAGO'S SOUTHEAST SIDE

Today's residents of Chicago's Southeast Side who occupy the Calumet Region are not the first to fight for a vision of civil and human rights and protection of the land. The racialized health inequities in Chicago and the struggle for health justice by people in neighborhoods along the Calumet River is a contemporary part of the U.S. legacy of colonialism, settler-colonialism, and slavery.[5] The Chicago region is Native American land, where the Miami, Potawatomi, Odawa, and Ojibwa people lived alongside each other for millennia and still do.[6]

In recent memory, the fight to #StopGeneralIron is not the only challenge that local community members have faced.[7] For decades, People for Community Recovery (PCR) has been fighting many more such threats and shaping a vision for a better life in the Calumet Region. Founded in 1982 by Hazel Johnson, a "mother of the Environmental Justice Movement," and her daughter Cheryl, PCR has "wage[d] the environmental justice war on multiple fronts and secure[d] key victories for Altgeld [Gardens public housing] residents: extending water and sewage service, a new health clinic, asbestos and PCB [polychlorinated biphenyl] removal, lead abatement, and a moratorium on new or expanded landfills in Chicago."[8(para5)] In just the past decade or so, PCR and many others on the Southeast Side have also worked to defeat a coal gasification plant, a police shooting range, new landfills, and the storage of tons of pet coke—a by-product of oil refining.

Chicago has long been known as one of the most racially segregated cities in the United States,[9] and the resulting economic and health inequities are clear. Lincoln Park has a median income 2.3 times greater than the City of Chicago as a whole, and 2.6 times, 2.6 times, 4 times, and 7.6 times greater than the median household income of the Hegewisch, East Side, South Deering, and Riverdale neighborhoods, respectively. In the wealthier Lincoln Park neighborhood, almost 80% of the population is White. In the Southeast, Riverdale, which includes

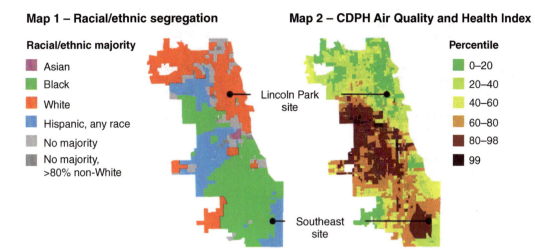

FIGURE 19.1. Maps of Chicago showing segregation (Map 1) and the CDPH Air Quality and Health Index (Map 2) near General Iron's Lincoln Park site and the proposed Southeast site.
The Air Quality and Health Index is a combination of several factors assigned to each block group, including many demographic variables, cancer risk, respiratory health, low birth weight, and much more. The Southeast site's 80th–98th percentile indicates air quality and health that is worse than at least 79% of the city.
CDPH, Chicago Department of Public Health.
Source: Gaige J, U.S. Department of Housing and Urban Development. Letter of findings of noncompliance with Title VI and Section 109 *Southeast Environmental Task Force, et al. v. City of Chicago* Case No. 05-20-0419-6/8/9. July 19, 2022. https://drive.google.com/file/d/1bZdRItk3iovsTwCX-rrmPEoYUAyq8fVl/view

Altgeld Gardens, is 95% Black; the East Side is over 87% Hispanic or Latino; South Deering is 64% Black and 30% Hispanic or Latino; and Hegewisch is 52% Hispanic or Latino, 40% White, and 7% Black. The inequities are also illustrated by various mapping tools that visually communicate cumulative impacts (see Chapter 8, "Mapping Environmental Health and Justice Issues," for a review), such as the Agency for Toxic Substances and Disease Registry's social vulnerability index (SVI) that calculates an index using various factors, including socioeconomic status, access to healthcare, transportation, and housing. According to the tool, the community next to General Iron's (now RMG's) proposed site is among the most vulnerable.[10(p18)]

Given all of these factors, it is unsurprising that residents of the Southeast Side have higher self-reported experiences of asthma, heart disease, and cancer than Chicago residents overall, according to the Chicago Department of Public Health (Figure 19.1).[10(p16)] Further, in 2021, Meleah Geertsma of the Natural Resources Defense Council noted, "The Southeast Side, like other low-income communities of color in Chicago, including those bearing heavy pollution burdens, has been disproportionately affected by the current COVID-19 respiratory pandemic."[11(p9)] This follows a national trend in which communities already overburdened with environmental exposures were among the hardest hit by COVID-19.[12]

#STOPGENERALIRON: THE FIGHT BEGINS

As shown in Figure 19.2, conversations about moving General Iron formally began in 2016, implicating multiple mayors, public health commissioners, industry representatives, and many other government leaders over the course of events. The planning to move the scrap-metal shredder began under Mayor Rahm Emanuel, who served from 2011 to 2019, and continued under Mayor Lori Lightfoot, who served from 2019 to 2023. Also notable, former 10th Ward Alderperson Susan Sadlowski Garza, the local elected representative who represented the area where the General Iron operation was set to move to, came out as a strong supporter of the project, much to the disappointment of EJ organizers.

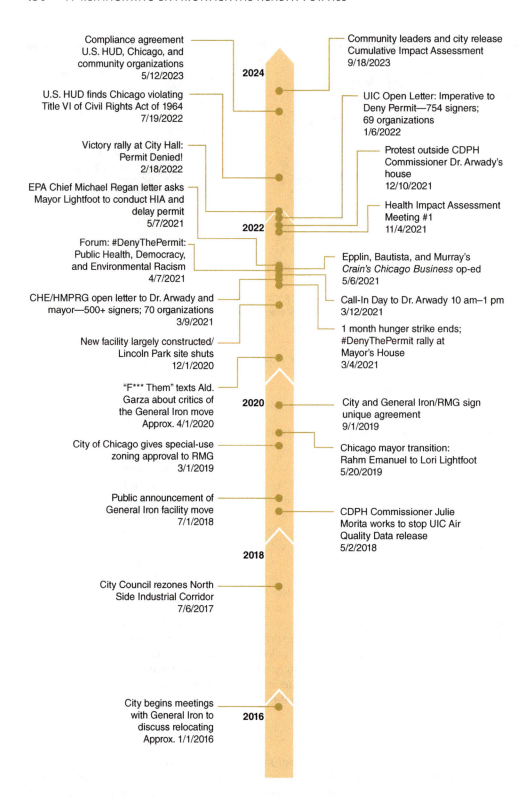

FIGURE 19.2. Abbreviated timeline of events in the struggle to #StopGeneralIron.
CDPH, Chicago Department of Public Health; CHE, Collaborative for Health Equity; EPA, Environmental Protection Agency; HIA, Health Impact Assessment; HMPRG, Health and Medicine Policy Research Group; HUD, Department of Housing and Urban Development; RMG, Reserve Management Group; UIC, International Union of Railways.

Two CDPH Commissioners provided leadership during this time as well, including Dr. Julie Morita from 1999 to 2019 and Dr. Allison Arwady from 2020 to 2023. CDPH Commissioners have numerous responsibilities, including overseeing hundreds of employees, various programs, and overall strategic planning, as well as ensuring agency practices promoted anti-racism and health equity. With regard to environmental issues related to General Iron, CDPH is responsible for facility inspection and permitting, air-quality management with the Illinois Environmental Protection Agency (EPA), and hazardous waste cleanup, among other duties.

Environmental advocates were concerned with CDPH's response to the General Iron proposal. Emails obtained by Michael Hawthorne of the Chicago Tribune showed that, in 2018, Commissioner Morita worked together with Planning Commissioner David Reifman in an apparent attempt to stop the air-monitoring data collected by University of Illinois Chicago researchers around the General Iron site in Lincoln Park from being released to the public.[13] In an email exchange with Commissioner Reifman on May 2, 2018, Dr. Morita wrote, "The researcher is very connected to the environmental advocacy groups and is not someone I can reason with . . . You may need to engage the [UIC] Chancellor if you want this to be stopped."[13(p2)] City leaders likely knew the data would show the harmful exposures associated with the General Iron facility and preferred to keep that information hidden.

Additionally, the Labkon family, which owned General Iron before selling a majority of it to RMG in 2019, sought to sell a plot of land that was now part of a revitalized stretch of the Chicago River.[14] With the City supporting the move of General Iron away from Lincoln Park, a plan was also in place to build a multibillion-dollar, high-end housing development, called Lincoln Yards. Many were critical that the city was subsidizing massive redevelopment for the wealthy White Lincoln Park neighborhood. A report by the nonprofit Chicago United for Equity spelled it out: The city was steering polluters to the Southeast Side, spending over $1 billion dollars for bridges and other infrastructure and increasing property taxes that would likely go to wealthy real estate developers.[15(p40)]

ORGANIZING TACTICS USED IN THE #STOPGENERALIRON EFFORTS

Meanwhile local organizers including Olga Bautista, Gina Ramirez, and Óscar Sanchez, as well as many others in the organizations and neighborhoods they represented, started launching a campaign. Several of their organizing tactics for #StopGeneralIron are described below, including media advocacy and legal action. Key events highlighted in Figure 19.2 include:

- a month-long hunger strike by activists;
- a letter-writing campaign to indicate solidarity;
  - a letter from Collaborative for Health Equity (CHE) Cook County and the Health and Medicine Policy Research Group (HMPRG), which marked the beginning of nongovernmental public health solidarity with Southeast Siders to #StopGeneralIron
  - a letter from University of Illinois School of Public Health, signed by the Dean and hundreds of public health professionals, health workers, elected officials, and other organizations, calling on Mayor Lori Lightfoot, Dr. Allison Arwady, and Candace Moore (Chicago's Chief Equity Officer) to deny the permit
- a protest and march outside Commissioner Arwady's house led by George Washington High School students (whose school was two blocks from the proposed site); and
- a victory rally on a cold February 18, 2022.

MEDIA ADVOCACY

Social media is a powerful organizing tool that helped #StopGeneralIron leaders to reach more people, make calls to action, and hold government officials publicly accountable. Table 19.1 describes the theme and text accompanying nine tweets used in a planned *social media storm* on November 30, 2021. Such storms are strategically planned bursts of posting by those leading and supporting the campaign (Figure 19.3).

TABLE 19.1. #STOPGENERALIRON SOCIAL MEDIA STORM—NOVEMBER 30, 2021

MAIN THEME	MAIN TEXT OF SOCIAL MEDIA GRAPHICS
Leaders must prioritize racial equity.	According to the Government Alliance on Race and Equity: "Leadership matters—transforming our systems towards greater racial equity requires consistent and courageous leadership. We recognize the importance of formal and informal leadership. We support formal leadership working to advance racial equity, as well as the development of emerging leadership."
Environmental racism requires robust action.	Lung health requires more than smoke-free policies. Chicagoans need freedom from environmental racism. We've seen enough data.
This permit decision was nationally significant.	The Stop General Iron campaign has national significance. Will it be more of the same environmental racism, or will this decision mark the beginning of a new era of environmental justice? The choice is clear. We've seen enough data. Deny the permit. Stop General Iron.
Chicago leaders must follow their own health-equity goals.	Don't violate Chicago's public health and air-quality plans. (The plans that you wrote.) Healthy Chicago 2025 says: "Communities disproportionately burdened by pollution . . . can expect a future 'ideal state' in which they 'Breathe clean air free of harmful pollutants.'"
City and health department officials are accountable for racial equity.	Failure to deny the permit would worsen environmental racism. Chicago City government has the authority to deny the permit. The Chicago Dept. of Public Health has committed to health equity. CDPH & City Government have responsibilities for public health. City Government has stated commitment to racial equity. Deny the permit! Stop General Iron!
City and health department officials are accountable for racial equity.	Because you keep saying your administration is all about equity. And we're holding you to it.
City and health department officials are accountable for racial equity.	CDPH Chicago Department of Public health [logo] Because it's the Chicago Department of Public Health NOT the Chicago Department of Public Harm.
Chicago leaders must pursue their own health-equity goals.	[image of page 20 Chart in "Healthy Chicago 2025 Closing Our Life Expectancy Gap"] @ChicagosMayor & @ChiPublicHealth should follow the public health plan that they wrote & published, *Healthy Chicago 2025*.
Chicago leaders must pursue their own health-equity goals.	[Marked up excerpt p46 graphic in "Healthy Chicago 2025 Closing Our Life Expectancy Gap"] @ChicagosMayor & @ChiPublicHealth Follow your assessment and plan, #HealthyChicago2025. #HealthEquity "will require fundamental changes" AND antiracist systems.

Each post named Mayor Lightfoot and Commissioner Arwady, and used the hashtags #StopGeneralIron, #DenyThePermit, or both. Graphics from the posts are described in brackets. Graphics from *Healthy Chicago 2025: Closing Our Life Expectancy Gap 2020–2025* can be accessed in the report itself: www.chicago.gov/content/dam/city/depts/cdph/CDPH/HC2025_917_FINAL.pdf. Also see examples of post graphics in Figure 19.3.
CDPH, Chicago Department of Public Health.

Advocates strategically partnered to develop op-eds. One such op-ed, opposing the relocation plan, was published in Crain's Chicago Business on May 6, 2021.[16] The article, coauthored by Olga Bautista, Wesley Epplin, and Dr. Linda Rae Murray, referred to the move of the metal shredder as "a textbook case of environmental racism,"[16(para3)] a central theme in the #StopGeneralIron movement. Olga Bautista is a Southeast Side resident and organizer with the Southeast Environmental Task Force, and was recognized as one of the ten most powerful leaders in Chicago[17] in 2022 by Axios Chicago. Wesley Epplin is the Policy Director of the Health and Medicine Policy Research Group. Dr. Linda Rae Murray is a renowned physician and leader

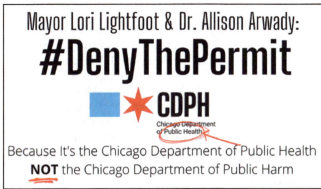

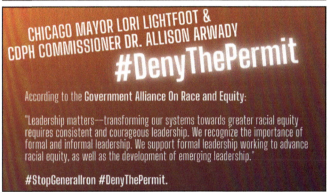

FIGURE 19.3. Examples of two social media graphics used in the November 30, 2021, Twitter storm by the Collaborative for Health Equity Cook County and the Health and Medicine Policy Research Group.

in the national and international public health community, having served as President of the American Public Health Association and in leadership positions in the public health departments of both Chicago and Cook County, Illinois. These three authors represented diverse but aligned interests working to stop the permit process. The joint authorship of the article highlighted the unity between the neighborhood-based EJ community and the community of nongovernmental public health workers.

> **IN OTHER WORDS: SOCIAL MEDIA STRATEGY**
>
> Be strategic when developing your own media advocacy campaign, whether drafting social media graphics or writing an op-ed. How will you frame the issue? How will you own the narrative in the media? Consider using some of these strategies:
>
> - Use authentic voices, and make sure that those most affected are able to tell their own story.
> - Include compelling visuals.
> - Relate to your audience with your ask or demands. For instance, will the issue impact their pocketbooks? Their community? Their children's health? Why should they care?
> - Use "social math." Translate data in a way that is compelling and understandable. For instance, you might make stark, ironic, or familiar statements or comparisons like: Did you know that in the United States, on average, it takes over 1,800 gallons of water to produce one pound of beef compared to less than 50 gallons to produce one pound of vegetables?
>
> We are living in a time where there is so much information available online. How do you push through the clutter and get decision makers to think about your issue differently? Check out the work of the Berkeley Media Studies Group (www.bmsg.org/) to learn more about media advocacy and advance your skills.

LEGAL STRATEGIES

An important strategy to #StopGeneralIron was a legal one. Lawyers interested in public health issues contributed to the cause by representing Southeast Side organizations in a formal complaint[18] to the U.S. Department of Housing and Urban Development (HUD) on August 12, 2020. "We filed this complaint because this move is only one example among decades of unfair zoning and land-use practices that discriminate against Black and Latino residents while benefiting White neighborhoods that have seen their home values soar,"[19(para9)] wrote organizer Gina Ramirez of the Center for Policy Advocacy in a blog post[19] on the one-year anniversary of filing the complaint. The complaint claimed the move was a violation of Section 109 of the Title VI, which is a section of the Civil Rights Act of 1964, a landmark piece of U.S. legislation that prohibits discrimination on the basis of race, color, or national origin in programs and activities that receive federal financial assistance.

On July 19, 2022, the HUD sent a "Letter of Findings"[20] that found the City was violating the civil rights of Chicagoans across the entire city:

> . . . the City discriminated on the basis of race and national origin in violation of Title VI and Section 109 by causing and facilitating the relocation of a large metal recycling facility from a majority White neighborhood to a majority Black and Hispanic neighborhood, and through a broader policy of constraining industrial and other polluting land uses to majority Black and Hispanic areas and relocating polluting facilities from predominantly White areas.[20(p2)]

Because the federal government does not provide funds to cities that discriminate against people of color, over 300 million dollars that funded 13 city departments was at risk.

PROTESTS AND HUNGER STRIKES

The hunger strike of February 2021 was seen as a last-ditch effort by many to protest the relocation plan, after trying several other tactics. Three people started the hunger strike, and others joined them, including George Washington High School teachers and students and a local official. Yesenia Chavez, one of the first hunger strikers from United Neighbors of the 10th Ward, described their inclusive organizing approach:

> A big focus of ours was to uplift voices that weren't heard. To have parents included that wouldn't always take the mic; to have students included, to have someone that's taking care of their elderly parent that's connected to an oxygen tank, that you wouldn't usually see on the news, but their voice in our community should still be respected . . . And I think that approach led to a lot of our success.[21(para52)]

CRYSTAL VANCE GUERRA, cofounder of Bridges//Puentes, a Southeast Side collective rooted in social justice, supported the hunger strikers by coordinating medics and commented on the shift in strategy:

> We had already done petitions, we had already done peaceful marches, we had already done marches at Lori Lightfoot's house, we had already done all these things. We needed something. And that something was the hunger strike.[21(para23)]

Hunger striker Jade Mazon recalled that volunteer medics from two groups, the Chicago Action Medical and the Black-led Ujimaa Medics, helped her keep her children fed during her strike so that she could rest. In a *Southside Weekly* news report[21] Mazon said:

> I was already well aware of the stakes, well aware of the potential for further destruction, further pollution in my community. . . . I am older. I am not in the best health. But this is one thing that I could do for my community. And I don't regret it at all. . . . When we were kids, we didn't know that we deserved better. That was never a question for us.[21(paras12,14)]

The hunger strike ended with a rally near Mayor Lightfoot's home because she had agreed to work with residents but had yet to call for stopping the relocation or denying the permit.

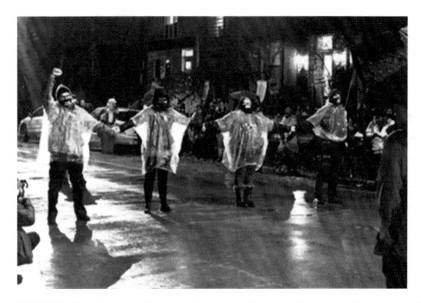

FIGURE 19.4. Four residents and organizers from the Southeast Side engaged in civil disobedience in front of Chicago Department of Public Health Commissioner Arwady's house in Lincoln Park, December 10, 2022.
Source: Isaia Sarju @isaiasarju.

On December 10, 2021, a peaceful march and protest was held in front of Commissioner Arwady's house in Lincoln Park, ironically the neighborhood General Iron was planning to leave. Despite the very cold rain, George Washington High School students made passionate statements calling for Commissioner Arwady to deny the final permit. One sign read "Dear Santa, All we want this year is Clean Air" in hand-printed letters on a glitter poster background. Chicago police arrested four protesters after they linked arms and moved into the street, blocking traffic in civil disobedience, as about 150 people chanted from the sidewalks (Figure 19.4).

#STOPGENERALIRON: PERMIT DENIED

Amid the organizing efforts, the campaign had gained attention from national leaders. In early May 2021, the news broke[22] that the top Federal EPA Administrator Michael S. Regan contacted Mayor Lightfoot, and the City subsequently paused the process of issuing the final permit in order to first conduct a Health Impact Assessment (HIA; HIAs are covered in more detail in Chapter 14, "Healthy Communities for All"). In the letter to the Mayor, Administrator Regan described how the current condition in the Southeast Side epitomized environmental injustice that resulted from decades of harmful actions. His letter described a list of the environmental threats to the health of residents.[23] In response, Mayor Lightfoot agreed to halt the approval process of the final permit. CDPH began carrying out an HIA that would entail consideration of environmental exposure and health data to inform the decision about General Iron. Although this news was seemingly good, many worried that the HIA would be used to pursue the city's agenda and dismiss the cumulative impacts and lived experiences of Southeast Side residents.

Months passed. Three community engagement sessions were held as part of an eight-month HIA process. Finally, after a multiyear organizing campaign, on February 18, 2022, Mayor Lightfoot's Office formally denied RMG's operating permit. It was an uphill fight that most people thought would be lost.

Of course, advocates continue to track the situation closely, as the larger battle for environmental health and justice persists. The city's new leadership must uphold a voluntary compliance agreement that Mayor Lightfoot signed with the HUD to reform its planning, zoning, and land-use practices that were deemed discriminatory. RMG continues to pursue the permit, appealing the decision in city court and winning in June 2023. As of the end of 2023, city leadership had not granted RMG a permit in light of this decision.

#STOPGENERALIRON: BUILDING AND BREAKING POWER

As sociologist Jason Beckfield puts it, "power and health go together."[24(p18)] In 2022, the National Academy of Medicine reported on a roundtable exploring power and public health practice. They reported that public health workers are generally comfortable engaging communities but less so in recognizing and addressing underlying power dynamics. One well-known framework for thinking about these dynamics is Arnstein's Ladder of Citizen Participation[25] and an updated version by Lifsay and Morgan.[26] Arnstein's Ladder is a conceptual framework that illustrates various levels of public participation in decision-making processes. The ladder consists of eight rungs or levels, ranging from tokenism to genuine community power, showcasing the different degrees of engagement that people can have in public decision-making. Lifshay and Morgan provided an adapted version of this framework in their Ladder of Community Participation in Health with seven rungs. Their framework ranges from: (1) Health Department Leads, (2) Informing and Educating, (3) Limited Community Consulting, (4) Comprehensive Consultation, (5) Communities Bridging by Sharing Health Department Information and Resources, (6) Power-Sharing, and (7) Community Leads. Rarely do agencies move to power-sharing or authentic community leadership.

As introduced earlier, a useful way to describe the organizing work done by the residents and their allies as part of #StopGeneralIron is through the *struggle for power* model described by Jamila Michener with examples in Figure 19.5.

BUILDING POWER

Building power first requires community organizing. #StopGeneralIron is a clear example of community organizing, or the process of building power through involving specific groups of people in identifying problems they share and the solutions to those problems that they desire. The interviews at the end of this chapter with community organizers Olga Bautista, Gina Ramirez, and Óscar Sanchez provide accounts of organizers working to build power in the fight for EJ. Community organizing is often strategic, sometimes messy, and always iterative. As seen in the case of #StopGeneralIron, it can involve a wide range of strategies, including public forums, media advocacy, and direct-action protests. These strategies often included stories about residents' personal experiences with pollution-related health effects and called attention to the responsibility of officials like Mayor Lightfoot and Commissioner Arwady to protect public health. Hundreds of people also worked together, participating in solidarity fasts in support of the hunger strike, which captured the attention of local and national media and was arguably a turning point in the organizing campaign.

Second, building power involves developing coalitions and alliances to strengthen relationships and align with others who are interested in the same issues. George Washington High School teachers joined as allies, as they understood firsthand the health and social needs of their students, the disinvestment in their local school building, and the threats to student health posed by a potential polluter nearby. Organizers welcomed offers from local public-health justice activists and experts through the local groups, CHE Cook County and HMPRG. Another strategic partnership was formed with the School of Public Health at the University of Illinois Chicago, which had a track record of providing scientific expertise to residents. Frequent meetings were also held with other EJ organizations at the local, state, and federal level to coordinate strategy and unify responses to city officials.

The third element of power building is strategic negotiation. In this case, organizers held local, state, and national political institutions accountable. Legally, RMG's individual permit

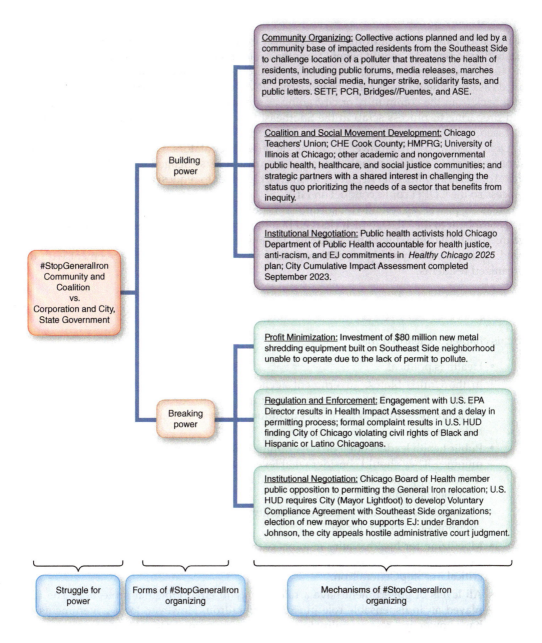

FIGURE 19.5. Michener's struggle for power applied to the #StopGeneralIron campaign.
ASE, Alliance for the SouthEast; CHE, Collaborative for Health Equity; EJ, environmental justice; EPA, Environmental Protection Agency; HMPRG, Health and Medicine Policy Research Group; HUD, Department of Housing and Urban Development; PCR, People for Community Recovery; SETF, Southeast Environmental Task Force.

may have met all the necessary requirements for approval. However, organizers highlighted that approving the permit would perpetuate environmentally racist decision-making within the larger system and among leaders. The CHE Cook County and HMPRG team also pressured Commissioner Arwady to uphold the ethics of public health and to fulfill the agency's commitment to health equity. Thanks to the HUD decision and city efforts to conduct a cumulative impact assessment in September 2023, there may be opportunities to sustain changes in land use, zoning, permitting, enforcement, and infrastructure planning.[27]

BREAKING POWER

In the case of #StopGeneralIron, breaking power meant minimizing profits for RMG and real estate developers who would benefit from their relocation. Organizing work entailed removing the economic incentive for corporate entities to use Black and Brown Chicago neighborhoods as dumping grounds for toxic industries. RMG expected to proceed without significant pushback from the community or city, going as far as completing construction of the facility and preparing to process scrap in the Southeast Side even before the health risks had been assessed.

Organizers also broke power in calling on federal regulators. Local ordinances were not strong enough to address cumulative impacts, so organizers engaged the EPA, with the result that Administrator Michael Regan wrote Mayor Lightfoot to request a pause in the permitting process so the CDPH could conduct an HIA.

Breaking power also entailed institutional negotiations. In this instance, there was the formal complaint to the HUD, which charged that the city was violating the civil rights of Chicagoans. The HUD agreed with the residents, and at the risk of losing tens of millions in federal funding, required Mayor Lightfoot to negotiate a voluntary compliance agreement with the organized residents.

MAIN TAKEAWAYS

In this chapter, we learned that:

- Health is political.
- In the United States, government agencies regularly commit to advancing health equity and racial justice. However, they may fail to correct harms from past policy decisions or withstand the power of influential corporations that challenge this commitment.
- Public health leaders often do not examine power dynamics when working with communities. They should consider what level of the Ladder of Community Participation in Health applies to their interactions, and if there are opportunities for power sharing or authentic community leadership.
- Alongside science and policy, community organizing is vital in efforts to achieving environmental health for all.
- Mobilizing for health equity requires partnerships. For instance, the relationship between public health workers and activists that existed independently of CDPH was critical in #StopGeneralIron.
- All levels of government have a role to play in environmental protection. The EPA played an indispensable role in #StopGeneralIron. However, local governments do have power and responsibility to address environmental racism too.

SUMMARY

This chapter describes the story of the #StopGeneralIron campaign and underscores the invaluable role of community organizers in the field of environmental health. The metal recycling operation was notorious for polluting in a wealthy North Side Chicago neighborhood, and if history were to repeat itself, it would be allowed to move to the less affluent and predominantly Black and Brown Southeast Side. In the United States, city governments and agencies, like the city of Chicago and the CDPH, may intend to promote health equity and racial justice. Nevertheless, without a redistribution of power to those on the frontlines, our systems often invite and enable powerful corporations to undermine these commitments.

INTERVIEWS WITH #STOPGENERALIRON ORGANIZERS

CHERYL JOHNSON
On Environmental Justice, Executive Director, People for Community Recovery

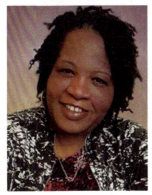

Cheryl Johnson, Executive Director of People for Community Recovery and a long-time EJ organizer in Altgeld Gardens, described the origins of what she described as a "classic example with General Iron on the North Side:"[28]

This is in Lincoln Park, a scrap yard, that they wanted to get rid of, because they want to build this big, multibillion dollar [Lincoln Yards] investment over there. So they hurried up and made an agreement for [General Iron] to relocate on the far South Side of Chicago. Before they even moved they had an explosion there. They had so many violations, they were not in compliance with the permits that allowed them to operate, but still the City of Chicago allowed them to relocate to a Hispanic, Black area. So we're saying that, if they're practicing bad in an affluent area, how do you think they're going to practice in a poor and Black, Brown neighborhood? So this is what we're talking about. And, the South Side of Chicago has always been the home for polluters for many, many years, who usually align themselves with our elected politicians who allow them to come into our community . . . and then when it comes to inspections, "We don't have enough inspectors."[29]

Cheryl Johnson is the daughter of Hazel Johnson, the "mother of environmental justice," who coined the term "the toxic donut" in describing how Altgeld Gardens is surrounded by a ring of toxic emitters and landfills. She described how she thinks about the nature of EJ:

Just imagine environmental justice is the umbrella. The spokes within this umbrella are the inadequate housing, poor food sources, poor education, poor health, and so on. Now tell me if this umbrella would be operable if any of those spokes were broken. That umbrella is not going to be operable for us. So we have to improve, we have to stabilize those spokes, in order to have that functional umbrella. So that's how I try to get people to see if any of those spokes are broken, then we will have a poor environment.[30]

ÓSCAR SANCHEZ
Organizer; Hunger Striker; Interviewed January 11, 2023, by Jim Bloyd

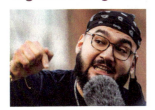

Q: You referred to your parents. Let me ask you a bit about yourself.

A: My father migrated here from Zacatecas, Mexico, at a young age. And he moved here to the Southeast Side. My mom has been working since middle school and high school. When she was young, she would work at a local church after school to be able to make ends meet. For her it's always been like "How do we provide?" In my childhood we were very poor. At one point in my life, we lived across the street from the BP oil refinery. We moved around third grade to the Hegwisch neighborhood on the Southeast Side of Chicago. I'm a 2015 alumnus from George Washington High School. We were always volunteering in the church. I was one of the youth leaders, and I still carry those values about what it means to love people. I also take values from some of my favorite leaders like James Baldwin: "if I love you I'm going to let you be aware of the harm you're doing and the harm that's being done to you."

---

* The publisher thanks the various organizations for sharing photos of our interviewees: Chicago Public Library, Colin Boyle/Block Club Chicago, Natural Resources Defense Council, and Southeast Environmental Task Force.

I think it's important to talk about what youth went through because it really broadens perspective about what violence is and what safety is. For them beginning their journey as young organizers, I would say this, we're always meant to organize. At a playground, when someone falls and hurts themselves and starts crying, other children crowd around that child. They look for an adult or somebody that can help. We're meant to help others, and that's the way I break it down for youth. It's easy to organize when you want to empower them and let them know.

Q: How did youth get involved in the Stop General Iron fight?

A: They were looking to remove police officers, school resource officers (SROs), after the uprisings because of the murder of George Floyd. And people were becoming more understanding of intersectionality between racism and how race impacts their livelihood. They were defining what safety looked like for their schools and then that led up to the fight of what does it look like to have a safe environment. You know we have gun violence, but for many of them it's also facing health impacts or respiratory issues: We are in a respiratory pandemic. Then it came to having another metal-shredding company coming here from the North Side to the Southeast Side, being a dumping site for the city. So going from safety and schools, to what does a safe environment look like for us?

Q: What is organizing?

A: Organizing for me, is someone who is a mobilizer, but also a facilitator of relationships. I might not be the answer for some of the roles that need to be played and seeing who fits these roles, who needs to be giving a testimony, who should be speaking at a press conference, who should be the one talking to our neighbors about certain issues, who are the experts when it comes to mental health, or previously incarcerated individuals, criminal justice reform. I think it's really about mobilizing people and facilitating relationships across different intersectionalities.

Q: What was your involvement with #StopGeneralIron?

A: I want to say it started in probably 2018. It was just short conversations that I had with Peggy Salazar, the executive Director for the Southeast Environmental Task Force (SETF) at the time. I became acquainted with SETF through Yesenia Balcazar, another amazing organizer and researcher. That was around the time we started the Southeast Youth Alliance (SYA). I worked with SETF. We did air quality monitoring with the local George Washington High School. In early 2020, we were being impacted by the pandemic; all of us were scared. Community members who are parents were crying, saying "What are we going to do?" So we developed this mutual aid network. From there we kind of stabilized things, making sure we had volunteers at food pantries, and creating information sessions where later on we'd do vaccination sites and testing sites. In all of which I was one of the main organizers. And then there was the murder of George Floyd. The SYA and a lot of those partners from the southeast response collective like SETF, and other organizations like Alliance for the SouthEast (ASE) responded by having our own marches. One of the largest protests here in South Chicago had over 500 community members coming out on Commercial Avenue. And it's crazy to be risky like this [in a pandemic]. We created relationships, more partnerships. Then there was the conversation of General Iron, and the lack of communication of what our 10th Ward Alderwoman Susan Sadlowski Garza was doing.

So we protested. From there we did more protests and information sessions and then town hall meetings. It built up to a 30-day hunger strike and then, a whole year later, to the final denial of the permit. For me it's, like when we talk about this experience, when I look back, it's such a long experience. However, you don't feel it when you're constantly in that crisis mode, like we have one more day, okay, we have another day. It's constantly, "How are we addressing this?" every single day.

"Hunger striker" is a traumatic title. I'm owning it more now, but it's very traumatic. We had to go on a 30-day hunger strike to be heard by the city of Chicago, to prevent this from happening. If we didn't go on a hunger strike, what would've happened? That's something I want people to truly understand. Nobody should have to go to those extremes. I think that's where, when we talk to people afterward it's like, "Oh, you're amazing." It's like, I suffered. I'll say that again, I suffered. I'm holding a title of suffering and people don't understand the repercussions that had on my health. Afterward I still was eating the same things but like, a little bit different. It takes a toll on your health.

Q: What do you think about the Health Impact Assessment process?

A: It felt like déjà vu: It was like the community meeting sessions that we had a year before. It felt just replicated: "What is your input?" "What is the health risk?" And even the fact that they allowed workers from RMG to attend these meetings, because of course they're going to have a bias in this. What are truly the health implications when it comes to this new facility? And it's not over with General Iron. It's also the zoning practices. It's not just about having this metal-shredding company come in: It's about the other metal-shredding companies already here, and how we have to create new zoning to eliminate the zoning we currently have. This fight isn't over. We found out recently from a January 6 article by Brett Chase in the *Sun-Times*[31] that in a court case going on now she [Alderwoman Garza] actually gave [General Iron] unreleased internal information that the city was going to issue a permit. So we see all along how she hasn't been for our community and has actively been working against us.

GINA RAMIREZ

Senior Advisor, Southeast Environmental Task Force; Midwest Outreach Manager, Natural Resources Defense Council; Interviewed November 22, 2022, by Jim Bloyd

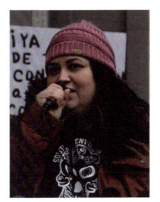

Q: What is your role?

A: I never heard of NRDC (Natural Resources Defense Council) before they came to my neighborhood in 2013. On the ground organizing stuff, I do that in my Southeast Environmental Task Force capacity where I am the Senior Advisor.

Q: Most people seemed to think General Iron would win.

A: I was also very convinced that General Iron would operate. Because the company was so confident. They built an $80-million facility without even having the final permits. All the odds were in the favor of the industry. Mayor Lori Lightfoot was at ribbon cuttings for General Iron, and Alderwoman Garza was fully supportive of General Iron. But I think the timing of the pandemic, the racial uprisings, and aggressive community organizing . . . came together and put a spotlight on environmental racism. Chicago is no stranger to racism. It's the most segregated city in the United States. The concentration of industry on the south and west sides is a new form of that redlining.

Q: What was your narrative?

A: The narrative was: "What isn't good enough for the North Side is not good enough for the Southside." Kind of that tale-of-two-cities narrative. We even had an art project that showed a North and South Side disparity with children, and the girl is wearing a gas mask. We used our NRDC map that showed the red zones are on the Southeast Side of Chicago where low-income communities of color are—that imagery. And social media: Our hashtags #StopGeneralIron, #DenyThePermit, were really impactful as well.

Q: How did you use Twitter (now known as X)?

A: Twitter was really popular because elected officials look at that more and are more prone to get embarrassed. A few times I would call out some senators, like "Why haven't you said anything about this?" And they would always immediately email me, and then want a meeting. So I ended up meeting with Senator Robert Peters after I tweeted at him. And Congressman Chuy Garcia after I tweeted at him.

Q: How do you explain the position of 10th Ward Alderwoman Susan Garza?

A: I grew up a block away from Ald. Susan Garza. She was a school counselor at Jane Addams and very well known in the neighborhood. 'Was a strong environmental justice advocate for the PetCoke fight.

We were at a town hall for an environmental justice meeting on manganese, a neurotoxin in our soil. Sue Garza came up to me and Olga [Bautista] and a few others and said, "We have a problem. I just heard from [Planning and Development] Commissioner [David] Reifman that General Iron wants to set up shop across the street from George Washington High School." And she was saying like "they're bullying me, we can't let this happen." And we were like "We have your back. We fought off the Koch brothers, we can fight off General Iron." And she was like, "okay, okay." But then she started having side conversations and private tours. She changed her narrative and kind of kept the community activists in the dark and was flip-flopping on the issue, telling us one thing, and telling industry the other . . . That delayed a lot of our advocacy for a year. The first initial permit that General Iron had to get was through a City board, Zoning Board of Appeals. That's like the very first step they had to take, and Sue Garza forgot to send the email for us to show up and testify to appeal it. And she didn't show up. We called her and said, "Hey, if you were serious about stopping this thing you should show up." She's like "I'm busy," so I knew then where she stood. I was so disappointed. I was so disappointed because she had been such a great ally, for the neighborhood, for years.

General Iron promised their 80 employees a job. They were going to simply relocate with their employees and maybe five other positions would be open. Why are we always pitting environmentalists and labor against each other? And these industry jobs that talk about recycling—that's green washing. I mean there are clean jobs. But you see a lot of companies saying they are "sustainable" and "state of the art." General Iron used all those words; it's just green washing.

The youth led a lot of this campaign. The high school students said, "Hey I don't want to be breathing in metal scraps across the street when I am at gym or at practicing for football." They really have a different vision for what the community looks like and were telling their elders that's not gonna fly anymore. They met on weekends, after school, organizing protests, doing artwork, marching to the alderwoman's house. They were working with chaperones, teachers, and other youth to organize a protest outside of the mayor's office. And they started an environmental justice club at George Washington High School. Trinity Colón is such an amazing speaker, just so wise beyond her years. She was featured in *Teen Vogue*.[32] There's a new generation of leaders. And the teachers are so supportive at Washington. Chuck Stark was one of the hunger strikers, and Lauren Bianchi is a very amazing organizer. There's so many amazing teachers that support their interest in social justice and environmental justice.

Q: How can people work in solidarity with EJ organizers?

A: I think uplifting and helping community activists . . . anecdotally we know what's going wrong in our neighborhood, we know our family members who have ailments and things like that. But you're not going to get heard at City Council and get legislation passed unless you have data. We knew that the South and West Sides were the most polluted in Chicago, but it wasn't until NRDC came in and, with the scientists, took the environmental justice screening tool and revamped it to show what we're saying is correct.

We've seen firsthand how Chicago Department of Public Health doesn't care about our neighborhoods, because they were ready to allow another facility to set up shop here, knowing that we have some of the worst air quality in the state, that we have some of the worst asthma rates, knowing that asthma vans are outside of our Chicago public schools on a monthly basis.

Q: What is happening with HUD finding that the city violated the civil rights of Chicago residents?

A: They [the city of Chicago] are at risk of losing over $100 million. For years they were saying that they were not willing to negotiate, that they had done nothing wrong, that they did not help to facilitate this move. Then this summer they switched gears. It's still at the negotiating table. We are so lucky to have our cadre of legal attorneys; as RMG would say, it definitely changed the game. There's never been a successful HUD complaint in the environmental sphere, ever. And we also filed a complaint against the Illinois EPA. That's also under negotiation as well. The Department of Justice is investigating that.

My son is 8. He's been breathing toxic air. I would love for the air quality here to be better. We sacrificed so many years of our life. But I really wish that the city would fast track this process of negotiation because of all the work we had to do to say, "You did something wrong, so fix it, and fast." We're not the only sacrifice zone in the United States. There is the cumulative burden of pollution in Detroit, Texas, and Louisiana. We need to be looking at this nationwide."

I think that genuine advocacy really tugged at the heartstrings of everyone. It really created a social movement, particularly the hunger strike. At the height of the pandemic we weren't vaccinated yet. People were risking their lives in both ways. We called on solidarity hunger strikes and over the course of those 30 days, 300 folks and organizations signed on to 1-day hunger strikes. It was like this social movement in Chicago for those 30 days. People were just . . . we just felt so loved.

OLGA BAUTISTA

Executive Director, Southeast Environmental Task Force; Interviewed November 22, 2022, by Jim Bloyd

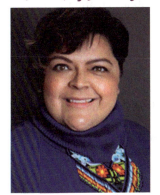

Q: What do you do at Southeast Environmental Task Force?

A: The Southeast Environmental Task Force has been around for about 30 years. Our mission area is the Calumet Region. A lot of the campaigns in recent years have been focused around the industrial corridor and the Calumet River right smack in the middle of the Southeast Side neighborhood on the South Side of Chicago.

Q: How do some of your organizing ideas and practices get reflected in the fight to #StopGeneralIron?

A: One thing that has been fundamental to organizing, since I've been involved with the Southeast Environmental Task Force, around environmental justice, is using the pedagogy of education like Paolo Freire's *Pedagogy of the Oppressed*. People come with their own lives, experience, and perspectives, and hopes, and traumas that are unique, that are their own. What we do in the work is come in with eyes wide open to learn what people are experiencing. To see if it's what we are experiencing. Where there's alignment, where there's an idea for a path forward that includes everybody, that is decided on in a very collective way. That's been really great for organizing because it builds a lot of trust with the folks that we are organizing with.

Q: One of the things that was so impactful to me was the participation at almost every event I went to, was leaders who are youth. And how did that come about?

A: The Stop General Iron campaign was happening in a really volatile time, during a very scary time for the whole world. There was a global pandemic. There were racial uprisings around the murder of George Floyd. The issues of race were very front and center. And students at George Washington High School had not met each other, had not met their teachers in person. They had been working 100% remote because of the pandemic.

And they still were able to organize a campaign to remove armed police officers from their school. It was hard fought. When they realized that they could indeed make decisions, demands, and win them, they didn't want to stop there. At that time, Óscar Sanchez, who was one of the hunger strikers in the Stop General Iron campaign, was a community youth organizer and was helping shepherd this activism, this energy.

When the campaign to remove their SRO's was won, the students unanimously voted to take that momentum and bring it to the Stop General Iron campaign. When they came, it was a moment where we had no more tricks up our sleeves and didn't know what we were going to do. A lot of us also needed to isolate, practice social distancing, because we were at higher risk, were older or had preexisting conditions like asthma. When we were approached by the youth, it was the answer that we needed. We got out of the way. We let them lead.

Q: It was not one person, like you said, you have the wisdom and the strength, the collective process.

A: We had meetings with organizations who were calling and asking, "How can we support?" Groups included the Sierra Club, the People's Lobby, United Working Families, and the Illinois Environmental Council. We would have our meetings with the community, with the youth, and everybody, and then we would let them know how to support those efforts by writing letters, attending protests, doing phone calls, and participating in Twitter storms. It was a combination of these young folks that were local, but also young folks that were part of these other organizations who were very tech savvy, very quick to turn a demand into a twitter storm. It was a combination of things. I think the big part was that we had to be vulnerable and say, "We don't know what to do next." And [the youth] were ready. There were so many leaders, young and old, multigenerational, multiethnic leaders, that any one of us could have left and this would've still kept going. My organization had full-time staff, ASE had full-time staff, but then there were smaller organizations and newer organizations like the Southeast Youth Alliance, or Bridges//Puentes. Trust was there, but it was about creating processes rooted in equity.

Q: What do you make of the support for General Iron by Alderwoman Garza?

A: I can only talk about what I observed, what I saw through the FOIAs [Freedom of Information Act requests] and emails that were going back and forth. Sue Garza let us know that this [proposal to relocate General Iron] was happening at a meeting that the EPA, CDPH, and others had. She told us, "Before you leave, come and talk to me in the side room." Fifteen of us came back there, some of our attorneys were with us and she said [City Department of Planning and Development] "Commissioner [David L.] Reifman is forcing us to accept this, the relocation of General Iron to our neighborhood. I need your help." We all sat and listened to her, and she cried. She said she was being bullied. So then we started working on the campaign, and what we saw later, through the FOIAs, was that she was under a lot of pressure by Commissioner Reifman. In one of those emails she essentially gave up the fight. I think she wanted to be on the winning side. She didn't think that we would be able to stop it and decided to jump ship. I don't know--that's what we saw happen. I think there's a lot of very powerful players involved. We have ships that come here from all over the world. There's so much money to be made. There's this logistical hub that happens to be the home of thousands, 50,000 residents. And also natural areas, migratory birds, all of these things exist here all at the same time. So I'm not surprised that there was that kind of pressure.

Q: What would you say would be important to pass along about this win?

A: If I look back and see all the work that the founder of this organization, Maryann Burns, did and all the people who came after her . . . there's been a lot of campaigns. There was a plan to bring an airport here, raze houses. There was a plan to expand the landfills. There was a plan to expand the CTA [Chicago Transit Authority] hub on 103rd St. And that was going to encroach on natural spaces. And all these campaigns were hard won, hard-fought. But winning I think is something else. Winning for me is justice: All the people [who] have been exposed for generations now being able to make that right, repair harm that's been caused, that's winning to me. I think what we're doing is holding the line. I don't think we're winning. I think we'll be winning when it's not a very far possibility to get a green new school for George Washington High School and George Washington Elementary School. That's a way to repair harm that's been caused to a community. To reinvest. We know that the safest communities in the world are the ones that have access to healthcare, the ones that have access to public transportation, the ones that have access to good quality food, and that there's jobs available. So that for me would be winning.

WESLEY EPPLIN, MPH POLICY DIRECTOR, HEALTH AND MEDICINE POLICY RESEARCH GROUP
SOPHIA SIMON-ORTIZ, MPH

Interviewed February 2023 by Jim Bloyd

Q: Why is organizing needed for advancing health equity?

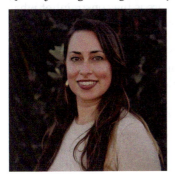

Sophia: Organizing is often left out of conversations within what we understand to be official "public health" spaces. I think it's so important to understand that the work of social justice organizers is also public health work! Organizing is about building collective power across a base of people with shared interests, to change and have say over lived conditions. Our work and that of folks working to change unequal and unjust conditions—organizers--are deeply intertwined.

We in the health sector have to focus on addressing (really, redressing) decades and centuries of these harms and their present day manifestations, which we see embodied—literally—in health inequities today.

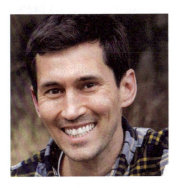

Wesley: I agree with so much of that . . . Health workers' personal and professional interests in and commitments to people's health generally, and health equity, in particular, provide a strong impetus to use one of the best tools we have to advance these, which is organizing to build power to demand the conditions that support health equity, what some colleagues and I have been calling "health organizing."

There are millions of health workers in the United States alone, so there is a massive opportunity for health workers of all types—community, public health, and healthcare—to organize politically to support communities' demands for justice

Q: What is the role of people working in the health sector in supporting social justice movements and campaigns?

Wesley: A 2010 World Health Organization discussion paper on the social determinants of health noted that, "The central role of power in the understanding of social pathways and mechanisms means that tackling the social determinants of health inequities is a political process that engages both the agency of disadvantaged communities and the responsibility of the state."[33] Health workers can help hold the government accountable for human rights and a just society.

It isn't just individual health workers, but also our public health and healthcare institutions—some of which have considerable political power—that can and should be much bolder in supporting social justice movements.

Sophia: To me, the unique role and power of our health sector is also a combination of leveraging the power of a health frame and narrative, combined with putting to use our particular access to data/information and institutions. A health frame is universally resonant and offers a window into illustrating the connections between injustices and their impact on health.

Q: What are some of the most significant barriers to health workers' and institutions' involvement in campaigns?

Sophia: Sometimes It originates from the notion that health-sector practice has to remain "neutral" to be regarded as rigorous and scientifically sound. But, as the late progressive historian Howard Zinn put it, "You can't be neutral on a moving train." I think, we need to really face the question head on: to whom are we accountable and whose interests do we center in our work?

There are real limits put on advocacy engagement for governmental workers, but sometimes the perceived limits are higher than they truly are, especially what can be done in one's personal time. Through the organizing network I help run, Public Health Awakened, we support our members to engage in local and national organizing "with their public health hats on," as we like to say—leveraging and engaging their expertise and health framing to support campaigns. A lot of members participate in our work as their individual selves, but some also engage their workplaces, which we encourage too where possible. Connecting through organizing is the best antidote to the fear and isolation that often drives hesitation to act more boldly.

Wesley: I'll add that funding for this work is often a barrier. There is the constraint of what foundations are willing to fund. Very often, funders have narrow interests, and often don't focus on campaigns, movement and power building, or changing unjust systems. Some funders may be deterred by more radical positions—a related barrier. Some of these barriers can be overcome by getting creative with funding, working the organizing into whatever course of work an organization does, and more foundations could become more creative and brave.

Q: How is organizing in the health sector different from health advocacy?

Wesley: Health organizing may be considered a new term for an old concept. Here's my working definition: "*Health organizing* develops a base of health workers with relationships, skills, leadership capacity, and resources, to build power and movement for health equity in order to support the demands for justice and related strategy put forward by communities who face oppression. Health organizing multiplies the power and influence of individual health workers by assembling these ingredients into coordinated strategic action and in support of ongoing community organizing. Health organizing can at times include prompting health institutions to use their power and influence to support community organizing efforts."

Health advocacy, which has its place and importance, tends to be led by health advocates often without direction from a directly impacted community. Health advocacy tends to focus on advancing particular policy changes but not on concurrently building power and a base of people to take on more organizing and movement growth.

Sophia: Part of my personal inspiration for organizing in the health field was my grandfather actually—he was a family medicine physician originally from Puerto Rico who became involved with the United Farm Workers union organizing in Arizona after witnessing the many health struggles his patients faced, the majority of whom were farmworkers. He testified at the state and federal levels for policy changes in working conditions, including the successful ban on the hand-held hoe, a tool that forced people to bend over really low all day.

Q: One of the key principles of equity-focused work is that those who are most directly impacted by a given inequity are leading efforts for necessary changes. What is the role of those who are not most directly affected in supporting social justice campaigns?

Sophia: Many of us now working and studying in health fields are ourselves from communities who have been targeted by oppressive structures and actions—something I don't often see named when we talk about health worker organizing with a false binary of "health worker" and "impacted communities." We all are members of the fabric of our communities. It's also important to share openly and build from strengths and leverage them toward the collective goals. This is solidarity in practice—leveraging power, resources, and knowledge for a collective purpose of confronting and addressing injustices. Ultimately, we are all impacted and harmed through the experience of living within these structures of harm and denials of power. White supremacy is a confining thing; it is based on dehumanization, as are all other systems of oppression. There's a quote often shared to illustrate this concept of deep solidarity which is, "If you have come to help me, then you are wasting your time. But if you have come because your liberation is bound up with mine, then let us work together."

Wesley: Yes. The concepts of "joint struggle," and solidarity are so essential to health organizing. I also agree wholeheartedly that the false dichotomy between "health workers" and "the community" is something we have to counter, because it separates health workers as if they're not community members themselves—it makes health workers seem disinterested and unaffected This Martin Luther King Jr. quote comes to mind here: "Injustice anywhere is a threat to justice everywhere. We are caught in an inescapable network of mutuality, tied in a single garment of destiny. Whatever affects one directly, affects all indirectly." One of the related frameworks I've been interested in is intersectional solidarity, which involves, among other things, recognizing and including intersectionality-marginalized social groups within active coalitions, working across individual- and group-identity differences, and negotiating power asymmetries.

END-OF-CHAPTER RESOURCES

DISCUSSION QUESTIONS

1. List all of the tactics #StopGeneralIron activists used. Which ones do you think were most effective and why? If you were leading the campaign, are there any other tactics you might have tried?
2. As sociologist Jason Beckfield says, "power and health go together."[25(p18)] What does he mean? Why is this important to understand when working toward environmental health and justice?
3. How did public health workers engage in #StopGeneralIron? What role do you think public health practitioners should play in community organizing for health?
4. Reflect on some of the lessons from the interviews in this chapter. What lessons might you carry into your own work now or in the future?

LEARNING ACTIVITIES

THE TIME IS NOW

Are you involved in any organizing campaigns? Research environmental organizations working on issues you care about—chemicals in everyday products, farmworker rights, permit decisions in your own community, or others. Analyze their campaigns. What is their policy goal? What tactics are they using? Are there ways you can get involved?

IN REAL LIFE

Learn to power map! A power map is a visual tool or diagram used to illustrate and analyze the relationships, influences, and power dynamics among various individuals, groups, organizations, or institutions within a specific context. It helps to identify who holds power, their relationships, and the degree of influence they wield over decisions or outcomes.

Pick an issue you care about—improving workers' rights, reducing pollution in your community, or advancing climate change programs in your state for instance. Name a specific campaign goal and begin adding all of the players. Who has decision-making power? Who can influence them? Who is undecided, but might be persuaded to support your effort? Try to name 8 to 10 specific people.

AMOUNT OF POWER		CAMPAIGN GOAL:		
High ↑	Decision maker			
	Major influencer			
	Can get attention			
↓ Low	Not on radar			
		Supporters	Undecided	Opponents

A robust set of instructor resources designed to supplement this text is located at http://connect.springerpub.com/content/book/978-0-8261-8353-8. Qualifying instructors may request access by emailing textbook@springerpub.com.

REFERENCES

1. Jobin-Leeds G, AgitArte. *When We Fight, We Win: Twenty-First-Century Social Movements and the Activists That Are Transforming Our World.* Kindle ed. The New Press; 2016.
2. Anderson J. An end to sacrifice zoning in Chicago. *Public Interest Law Rep.* 2022;28(1):10. 2016. https://lawecommons.luc.edu/pilr/vol28/iss1/3
3. Beckwith D, Lopez C. Community organizing: people power from the grassroots. Center for Community Change. 1997. Accessed July 11, 2024. https://www.participatorymethods.org/resource/community-organizing-people-power-grassroots
4. Michener J. Health justice through the lens of power. *J Law Med Ethics.* 2022;50(4):656–662. doi:10.1017/jme.2023.5
5. Krieger N. Structural racism, health inequities, and the two-edged sword of data: structural problems require structural solutions. *Front Public Health.* 2021;9:655447. doi:10.3389/fpubh.2021.655447 P3.
6. The Field Museum of Chicago, Miami Tribe of Oklahoma, Pokagon Band of Potawatomi. Journey through Calumet. ArcGIS StoryMaps. December 8, 2022. https://storymaps.arcgis.com/stories/8c8443f52a16469f8b46c03b4cd7b044
7. Lydersen K. First it was Detroit, now "PetKoch" piling up in Chicago. Energy News Network. October 14, 2013. http://energynews.us/2013/10/14/first-it-was-detroit-now-petkoch-piling-up-in-chicago/
8. Hazel M. Johnson's legacy. People for Community Recovery. 2023. Accessed June 17, 2024. https://www.peopleforcommunityrecovery.org/our-story/legacy
9. Benjamins MR, De Maio FG, eds. *Unequal Cities: Structural Racism and the Death Gap in America's Largest Cities.* Johns Hopkins University Press; 2023.
10. Chicago Department of Public Health. Health impact assessment. February 2022. https://www.chicago.gov/content/dam/city/sites/rgm-expansion/documents/RMG_RecyclingPermit_HealthImpactAssessment_Feb2022.pdf
11. Geertsma M. Comments submitted to commissioner Arwady and US EPA region V commissioner shore on CDPH EJ analysis for proposed Chicago metal shredding operation. Unpublished. 2021. https://5dd873fa-79ee-41a2-90f9-3c9e504d4026.usrfiles.com/ugd/5dd873_94c36c2f85a547ceae0b732374996041.pdf
12. Commodore S, Hernandez A, Sharma S. Lessons from COVID-19 for addressing air pollution health inequities: time to act. *Environ Justice.* Published online July 11, 2022. doi:10.1089/env.2022.0004
13. Hawthorne M. Five Julie Morita emails 2018. *Chicago Tribune.* 2020. https://www.documentcloud.org/documents/6772921-2018-5-Julie-Morita-Emails.html
14. Chase B. General Iron's Lincoln Park land will be cleared, possibly for sale. *Chicago Sun-Times.* November 10, 2022. https://chicago.suntimes.com/2022/11/10/23451965/general-irons-lincoln-park-land-cleared-possible-sale
15. Chicago United for Equity. Racial Equity Impact Assessment. 2021. https://www.chicago.gov/content/dam/city/depts/doh/qap/qap_2021/draft_reia_qap.pdf
16. Epplin W, Bautista O, Murray LR. Why Lightfoot and her public health chief should deny this permit. *Crain's Chicago Business.* May 6, 2021. https://www.checookcounty.org/_files/ugd/5dd873_4ccb997610f44351bfdc278d3a305d18.pdf
17. Eng M, Kaufmann J. 10 of Chicago's most powerful people in 2022. Axios Chicago. December 10, 2022. https://www.axios.com/local/chicago/2022/12/10/power-players-chicago-pritzker-chance-parker-ewing
18. People for Community Recovery, Chicago South East Side Coalition to Ban Petcoke, Southeast Environmental Task Force. Housing Discrimination Complaint, *Southeast Environmental Task Force, et al. V. City of Chicago, et al.*, Inquiry No.: 623101, HUD File No.: 05-20-01-0419-8, Title VI Case No.: 05-20-0419-6, Section 109 Case No.: 05—20—0419-9. 2020. Accessed June 17, 2024. https://www.hud.gov/sites/dfiles/Main/documents/Signed_VCA_Chicago.pdf

19. Ramirez G. One year after Chicago EJ civil rights complaint. NRDC. August 18, 2021. https://www.nrdc.org/experts/gina-ramirez/one-year-after-chicago-ej-civil-rights-complaint
20. Gaige J, US Department of Housing and Urban Development. Letter of findings of noncompliance with Title VI and Section 109 *Southeast Environmental Task Force, et al. v. City of Chicago* Case No. 05-20-0419-6/8/9. July 19, 2022. https://drive.google.com/file/d/1bZdRItk3iovsTwCX-rrmPEoYUAyq8fVl/view
21. Jay C, Sayles A, Stovicek O, Vaughn B, City Bureau. Stories and lessons from inside the Stop General Iron hunger strike. *South Side Weekly*. November 11, 2021. https://southsideweekly.com/stories-and-lessons-from-inside-the-general-iron-hunger-strike/
22. Chase B. Lightfoot halts General Iron permit after pressure from Biden's EPA chief. *Chicago Sun-Times*. May 7, 2021. https://chicago.suntimes.com/2021/5/7/22425285/general-iron-joe-biden-epa-lori-lightfoot-permit-southeast-side
23. Reagan M. USA Environmental Protection Agency Administrator Michael S. Regan Letter to City of Chicago Mayor Lori Lightfoot. May 7, 2021. https://www.epa.gov/system/files/documents/2022-02/letter-to-mayor-lightfoot-5.7.21.pdf
24. Beckfield J. *Political Sociology and the People's Health*. Oxford University Press; 2018.
25. Arnstein SR. A ladder of citizen participation. *J Am Plan Assoc*. 1969;35(4):216–224. doi:10.1080/01944366908977225
26. *Community Organizing and Community Building for Health and Social Equity*. 4th ed. Rutgers University Press. https://www.rutgersuniversitypress.org/community-organizing-and-community-building-for-health-and-social-equity-4th-edition/9781978824744/
27. Chicago Department of Public Health. Chicago's cumulative impact assessment. City of Chicago. 2023. https://www.chicago.gov/content/city/en/depts/cdph/supp_info/Environment/cumulative-impact-assessment.html
28. Johnson C. Everything is public health podcast: climate change [YouTube]. September 15, 2021. https://www.youtube.com/watch?v=nlFbDPk9xpM (quote at 16:20)
29. Johnson C. Everything is public health podcast: climate change [YouTube]. September 15, 2021. https://www.youtube.com/watch?v=nlFbDPk9xpM (quote at 17:44)
30. Johnson, C. Everything is public health podcast: climate change [YouTube]. September 15, 2021. https://www.youtube.com/watch?v=nlFbDPk9xpM (quote at 38:35)
31. Chase B. General Iron owner says 'smoking gun' from Ald. Susan Garza shows City Hall wrongly denied permit. *Chicago Sun-Times*. January 6, 2023. https://chicago.suntimes.com/2023/1/5/23541576/general-iron-owner-says-smoking-gun-from-ald-garza-shows-permit-was-wrongly-denied
32. Colón TA, Miller G. Environmental racism in Chicago will be made worse by General Iron facility. *Teen Vogue*. March 24, 2021. https://www.teenvogue.com/story/environmental-racism-chicago-southeast-side-protest
33. A conceptual framework for action on the social determinants of health. https://www.who.int/publications/i/item/9789241500852

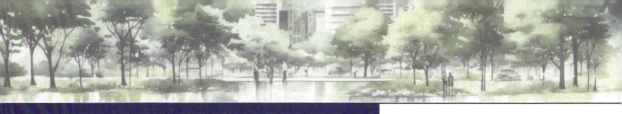

GLOSSARY OF KEY TERMS

Absorption, distribution, metabolism, and elimination (ADME): The process by which external agents (e.g., chemicals, biological toxins, toxicants, pharmaceuticals) come into the body and are eventually eliminated.

Advocacy: Includes any action that speaks in favor of, recommends, argues for a cause for, supports or defends, or pleads on behalf of others.

Air pollution: The modification and contamination of indoor or outdoor environments by any physical, chemical, or biological agent in the air that interferes with human health.

Allostatic load: The cumulative burden of chronic stress and life events over the course of one's life.

Ambient air pollution: Substances present in the outdoor air that can harm human health and the environment or cause property damage. They typically originate from various sources like industrial processes, vehicle emissions, natural events, and residential activities.

Amendment: A change or addition designed to improve a text, a piece of legislation, a contract, and so forth.

Anti-racist research: A research approach that considers and addresses racial disparities and injustices (e.g., the impact of race and racism on environmental exposures, health outcomes, and policies), aiming to dismantle systemic racism affecting marginalized communities. This research prioritizes equity and justice and encourages researchers to critically evaluate their biases and structural inequities in their work.

Built environment: Comprises the physical structures engineered and designed by people, including buildings, neighborhoods, streets, parks, and transportation systems.

Cancer cluster: Occurs when a specific geographic area or population experiences a higher-than-expected number of cancer cases in a specific timeframe.

Cascading failure: A crisis in a system of interconnected parts in which the failure of one or more parts brings about the failure of additional parts, potentially leading to system collapse.

Child-protective policies: Protecting children's rights and their best interests, placing the child as the first priority when dealing with all policy development.

Children's environmental health: The study of possible environmental causes of children's illnesses and disorders, as well as the prevention and treatment of illness.

Circular economy: A concept that seeks to create an economy that practically eliminates waste while also minimizing the demand for raw materials.

Climate and health adaptation: Involves actions to minimize the health impacts of climate change, focusing on enhancing resilience and reducing vulnerability to climate-related hazards.

Climate change: The broad range of long-term shifts in temperatures and weather patterns that are happening to our planet, mainly due to human activities.

Climate gentrification: A process in which investment in climate change adaptation strategies (e.g., increased green space) displaces low-wealth communities and communities of color in ways that may worsen health and economic inequities.

Climate justice: A principle that emphasizes the ethical and equitable considerations in addressing climate change. It seeks to rectify the disproportionate impact of climate change on marginalized and vulnerable populations, advocating for a fair distribution of environmental benefits and burdens. This approach integrates social justice with climate action, ensuring inclusive and equitable solutions.

Climate mitigation: Efforts aimed at reducing or preventing the emission of greenhouse gases to slow the pace of global warming. It encompasses strategies such as enhancing energy efficiency, transitioning to renewable energy sources, and promoting sustainable land-use practices. Mitigation is crucial for limiting long-term climate change impacts on environmental health.

Climate resilience: Climate resilience is the capacity of individuals, communities, and systems to anticipate, prepare for, respond to, and recover from the effects of climate change, thereby minimizing damage and disruption. It involves adaptive measures that enhance the ability to withstand and bounce back from climate-related hazards, ensuring sustained environmental health and well-being.

Climate vulnerability: Refers to the degree to which a system is susceptible to, or unable to cope with, adverse effects of climate change, including climate variability and extremes. It is a function of the character, magnitude, and rate of climate change and the system's sensitivity, exposure, and adaptive capacity, impacting environmental health outcomes.

Co-governance: A collaborative decision-making process that involves multiple partners, including government entities, communities, and private sectors, in the management of environmental resources and policies. This approach aims to enhance inclusivity, accountability, and effectiveness by leveraging diverse perspectives and expertise to address complex environmental health challenges.

Cohort study: A type of study that follows a set of participants over time.

Collective continuance: "A community's aptitude for being adaptive in ways sufficient for the livelihoods of its members to flourish into the future."[1(p601)]

Commercial determinants of health: A complementary determinants of health framework that considers the role of the private sector in influencing health.

Community benefits agreement (CBA): A contract between a developer and a community group that stipulates the benefits a community will receive in association with a new development project. CBAs aim to ensure that local projects offer direct advantages to the local population, such as employment opportunities, housing, and environmental improvements, and foster sustainable and equitable development.

Community engagement: Community engagement refers to meaningful opportunities for community members to take part in processes, provide knowledge, and share in leadership roles in community activities and governance.[2]

Community organizing: Community organizing refers to community members working together to address a systemic issue that affects them in a collective way. It is a way for oppressed and marginalized communities to build people power and counter the immense power that larger institutions and corporations may have in decision-making about issues that affect communities.

Community power: Community power is a potentially impactful outcome of community organizing, and means that community members have the infrastructure, teamwork, and accountability to push back against entities who may have interests that are different from those of its own community members.

Community resilience: An ecological concept often used in disaster preparedness to describe the ability of a system to maintain its normal patterns of functioning in the face of a significant disturbance. Note: The "normal patterns of functioning" of the system may not be ideal or equitable.

Community science: The collaborative effort between scientists and nonprofessional volunteers from the community to collect, analyze, and use data on local environmental conditions. This approach democratizes science, empowering communities to participate in research that informs policy and addresses local environmental health issues, enhancing engagement and outcomes.

Community-based participatory research (CBPR): A research approach that involves a collective, reflective, and systematic inquiry in which researchers and community partners engage equitably in all steps of the research process.

Community-owned and -managed research: A participatory research approach in which the community leads and controls the research process, from design to dissemination. It empowers communities to address their own environmental health concerns, ensuring that research is relevant, ethical, and aligned with community interests, fostering local capacity and actionable outcomes.

Comprehensive or general plan: "The general plan is the official statement of a municipal legislative body which sets forth its major policies concerning desirable future physical development. The published general plan document must include a single, unified physical design for the community, and it must attempt to clarify the relationships between physical development policies and social and economic goals."[3(p18)]

Consent agreement: A court order with terms agreed or consented to by all parties; it is made by a judge and not usually negotiated between parties.

Cumulative exposures: Past and/or present exposure (including relevant background exposure) of an entity or person to multiple environmental stressors.

Cumulative impacts: The combined effects of both chemical and nonchemical stressors on health, well-being, and quality of life. They include both current and lifelong exposures that affect individuals, communities, or defined populations. The distribution of these stressors plays a crucial role, as it encompasses both direct and indirect effects on people by impacting resources and the environment. By considering cumulative impacts, we can better understand the vulnerability or resilience of a community.

Cumulative risk: The combination of different environmental stressors and exposures that can increase the likelihood of negative health outcomes.

Data aggregation: The process of summarizing data by a geographic unit, such as aggregating asthma rates by census tracts or health districts.

Data justice: Involves issues related to data privacy, access, and control, as well as data residency and data sovereignty.

Data residency: Refers to where data are stored and used.

Data sovereignty: Refers to who controls the data, which can be affected by laws in the country where the study occurs.

Developmental origins of health and disease (DOHaD): Established theory positing that environment and conditions (nutrition, chemical, social, etc.) early in life affect the risk for adverse health outcomes later in life.

Disaster risk: Likelihood and scale of harm caused by a disaster's impacts. Structural disparities based on race, class, and other factors can worsen risk.

Disaster risk reduction: A set of ongoing societal actions that, taken together, lower disaster risk and losses across all economic, physical, social, cultural, and environmental aspects of society.

Disaster swarm: A mass of chronic and acute crisis blending ecosystem harm, physical violence, and disparities with rapid impacts that lead to further harm.

Disinfection by-products (DBP): Hazardous chemicals created when some types of disinfectants react with organic matter in water.

Ecosystem: A biological community of organisms that can provide essential resources such as clean air and water, food, and shelter. Healthy ecosystems can regulate the environment by purifying air, breaking down waste, and adapting to change. Humans are an integral part of ecosystems and can affect them in positive and negative ways.

Ecosystem services: All of the benefits, which can include food, water, and raw materials, that humans get from ecosystems.

Endocrine disruption: Chemicals harming the regulation of hormones.

Energy burden: The percentage of a household's income that is spent on energy-related expenses, such as electricity and heating.

Energy democracy: A system where individuals and communities can participate in decision-making processes related to energy production, distribution, and consumption to ensure equitable access, local empowerment, and environmental sustainability in the energy sector.

Energy justice: The idea that the costs of energy—including the health costs and benefits of energy production and use—are fairly distributed among populations.

Energy poverty: A condition in which a household spends more than 6% of its income on utility bills.

Energy Use Intensity (EUI): Energy use per square foot of home.

Environmental health: A core branch of public health that examines the interaction between people and their environment. It investigates how environmental factors, such as air and water quality and climate change, impact human health in various settings including where we live, work, learn, play, and pray. The field aims to reduce harmful exposures, manage risks, and ensure that all communities have access to healthy environments that promote well-being.

Environmental health disparities: The unequal distribution of environmental risks and benefits, often along racial and socioeconomic lines.

Environmental justice (EJ): The fair treatment and meaningful involvement of all people regardless of race, color, national origin, or income with respect to the development, implementation, and enforcement of environmental laws, regulations, and policies.

Environmental medicine: Integration of environmental health and medicine; a clinical practice that involves identifying and providing care for individuals who have been exposed to chemical and physical dangers within their residences, surroundings, and work environments, which may include contaminated soil, water, and air.

Environmental policy: Composed of specific government actions that affect or attempt to affect environmental quality or natural resources use and reduce harmful pollution emissions.

Environmental public health: The discipline that focuses on the study and management of environmental factors affecting human health and well-being. It encompasses the assessment, prevention, and control of environmental risks to health, including air and water quality, toxic substances, and climate change impacts, aiming to promote healthier environments and communities.

Environmental racism: The institutional rules, regulations, and policies, or government and/or corporate decisions, that deliberately target certain communities for locally undesirable land uses and limited or no enforcement of zoning and environmental laws, resulting in communities being disproportionately exposed to toxic and hazardous waste on the basis of race.

Epidemiology: The study (scientific, systematic, and data driven) of the distribution (frequency, pattern) and determinants (causes, risk factors) of health outcomes in specified populations. The method used to find the relationships between environmental exposures and health outcomes or cofactors across a population. Cofactors are anything that can contribute to disease like enzymes or blood pressure.

Epigenetics: The study of modifications to DNA and chromatin that regulate how genes work. Epigenetic modifications do not change the DNA (genetic) sequence. They can be heritable across cell divisions, but they are also responsive to the environment.

Epistemic justice: The opportunity for all to participate in knowledge production and dissemination. Epistemic justice calls for the valuing of diverse forms and sources of knowledge.

Ergonomics: Focuses on engineering products used by humans in such a way as to meet humans' physical and psychological needs.

Executive order: Written instrument through which a President can issue directives to the executive branch agencies and offices to shape policy without requiring Congressional approval. They are often utilized in cases that may benefit from public awareness or be subject to heightened scrutiny. They must be published in the Federal Register.

Exposome: The totality of exposures an individual person encounters over their life span, including chemical exposures, food, social stressors, the built environment, and behavioral factors.

Exposure: When a person comes into contact with chemical or nonchemical stressors that can potentially affect human health. These can be acute (short-term) or chronic (long-term or ongoing) and include physical, chemical, biological, or radiological agents or psychosocial stressors.

Exposure assessment: The process of determining or evaluating the extent to which individuals or populations come into contact with a particular substance, agent, or hazard. It involves identifying, measuring, and characterizing potential sources of exposure to understand the potential risks to human health or the environment.

False solutions: Those solutions that do not actually address the problem at hand substantially but deceive people into believing that they do, while at the same time triggering other serious problems.

Federal Register: The official daily publication for rules, proposed rules, and notices of federal agencies' and organizations' actions and decisions, as well as executive orders and other presidential documents, published by the Office of the Federal Register, National Archives.

Fenceline communities: Neighborhoods and populations living directly adjacent to industrial facilities, such as factories, chemical plants, or refineries. These communities often experience higher levels of exposure to pollution and environmental hazards owing to their proximity to these industrial sites.

Food: Any nutritious substance that is consumed or, in the case of plants, absorbed.

Food apartheid: Systemic disparities in access to healthy and nutritious food based on race, socioeconomic status, and geographic location.

Food safety: Refers to the conditions and practices that preserve the quality of food to prevent contamination and foodborne illness.

Food security: Refers to the ability for people to always have access to adequate amounts of food that is nutritious.

Food sovereignty: Refers to a food system in which the people who produce, distribute, and consume food also control the means and policies of food production and distribution.

Food system: An interconnected process of food production, distribution, consumption, and waste management, influenced by the environment, agriculture, infrastructure, official policies, the economy, social justice, and culture.

Foodborne outbreak: An incident in which two or more persons experience a similar illness after ingestion of a common food, and epidemiologic analysis implicates the food as the source.

Gentrification: The Urban Displacement Project defines *gentrification* as "a process of neighborhood change that includes economic change in a historically disinvested neighborhood—by means of real estate investment and new higher-income residents moving in—as well as demographic change—not only in terms of income level, but also in terms of changes in the education level or racial make-up of residents."[4]

Geographic information science (GISc): The field of spatial data and analysis that includes geographic information systems (GIS), remotely sensed images from satellites, global positioning systems (GPS), photogrammetry, geostatistics, cartography, artificial intelligence, data management, geospatial analysis, spatial modeling, mapping, and data visualization.

Harmful algal blooms: The rapid growths of algae in water bodies, usually due to excess nutrients like nitrogen and phosphorus. These blooms can discolor the water and disrupt ecosystems. They can produce cyanotoxins, which are harmful to human and animal health, as well as to the economic health of coastal communities reliant on tourism or recreational activities.

Health Impact Assessment (HIA): A process used to identify how a project, policy, or program might influence health. HIA uses a combination of procedures, methods, and tools to systematically judge the potential, and sometimes unintended, effects of a proposed project, plan, or policy on the health of a population and the distribution of those effects within the population.

Health in All Policies (HiAP): An approach to public policies across sectors that systematically takes into account the health implications of decisions to improve population health and health equity.

Hyperlocal data: Highly detailed information collected at a very fine geographic scale, typically focusing on specific communities or neighborhoods. In environmental health, it enables precise analysis of local environmental conditions, health outcomes, and exposures, facilitating targeted interventions and policies that address the unique needs and challenges of specific areas.

Immediate harm: Direct, visible consequence from a disaster, such as mortality and housing destruction.

Implicit bias: The unconscious attitudes or stereotypes that affect our understanding, actions, and decisions in an involuntary manner. In environmental health, recognizing and addressing implicit bias is crucial for ensuring equitable research, policy making, and health interventions that do not perpetuate disparities or prejudice against certain groups or communities.

Incinerators: Facilities that burn waste in a furnace at high temperatures and are sometimes used to produce heat or electricity.

Indigenization: Working to value Indigenous perspectives in policies and daily practices.

Industrial hygiene: A field that seeks to identify, measure, and control harmful exposures in the workplace.

Infrastructure: Infrastructure in environmental health refers to the fundamental physical and organizational structures needed for the operation of a society, including water and sewage systems, transportation, energy supply, and healthcare facilities. It plays a critical role in determining public health outcomes by influencing environmental conditions and access to health services.

Intersectionality: The ways in which different marginalized identities can intersect, causing unique and compounding experiences of discrimination or oppression.

Just transition: An approach to transitioning the energy industry from fossil fuels to alternative sources, prioritizing workers' rights, fostering economic opportunities for communities, and emphasizing sustainability amid climate justice.

Land use: The management and modification of natural environments or wilderness into built environments such as settlements and seminatural habitats. In environmental health, land use applies to how the allocation, development, and management of land resources impact human health, including the effects on air and water quality, exposure to hazards, and access to green spaces.

Landfill: A site designated for the burial of solid waste.

Legislation: The act of a governmental body in making or passing a law or laws.

Life cycle impact assessment: A method used to evaluate and quantify the environmental and health impacts associated with the entire life cycle of various energy sources—from the extraction of raw materials to the manufacturing, transportation, operation, and disposal or recycling of energy by-products.

Life-course exposure: The accumulation of environmental health risks and pollutants over the course of one's life.

Lobbying: In regard to public policy and legislation, the act of lawfully attempting to influence the actions, policies, or decisions of government officials.

Low-dose exposures: The theory that certain chemicals can cause a significant biological reaction at very low dose exposures.

Mental health: A person's condition with regard to their psychological and emotional well-being.

Microplastics (MPs): Tiny plastic particles less than 5 millimeters in diameter, resulting from the degradation of larger plastic products or released as small particles. In environmental health, microplastics are a concern due to their persistence in ecosystems, potential for bioaccumulation, and implications for human health through ingestion and exposure to toxins.

Mindful muddling: Disaster response that is adaptable and flexible, balancing urgency and deliberate consideration of response options. It often entails decentralizing decision-making authority across entities or levels rather than centralizing command and control.[5]

Occupational epidemiology: Assesses the distribution and determinants of work-related injuries, illnesses, and fatalities.

Occupational hazards: Factors at the workplace that may cause disease, injury, or other harms to physical or mental health. Different examples include safety, biological, and psychosocial hazards.

Occupational health: The branch of public health concerned with promoting and maintaining the highest degree of physical, mental, and social well-being of workers in all occupations.

Occupational health and safety: A field of expertise focused on illness and injury prevention and regulation in the workplace.

One Health: A collaborative approach in which many disciplines work together with a goal of improving health while recognizing the interconnectedness of people, animals, plants, and the environment. The One Health framework aligns with environmental health efforts to navigate food systems, land use, and global climate change.

Ordinance: Legislation enacted by a municipal authority.

Participatory geographic information systems (PGIS): Mapping initiatives that include opportunities for local community members to share local knowledge, offer contextual information about spatial data, and interact with or use data to enhance public involvement in policy making and planning.

Pediatric environmental medicine: A specialized medical field that focuses on the prevention, diagnosis, and treatment of illnesses due to preconception, prenatal, perinatal, and childhood exposures to environmental hazards.

Per- and polyfluoroalkyl substances (PFAS): PFAS are a group of human-made chemicals used in various industrial applications and consumer products for their water-, grease-, and stain-resistance properties. In environmental health, PFAS are concerning because of their persistence in the environment, bioaccumulation in wildlife and humans, and potential links to adverse health effects.

Planetary Health: A transdisciplinary field that emphasizes the interconnections between human health and the health of the planet and recognizes that human well-being is closely connected to sustainability, biodiversity, and ecosystem health. Planetary Health requires systems thinking in recognizing that everything is connected and as our environment changes, so does our health.

Political determinants of health: A complementary determinants of health framework that considers the role of policies and politics in influencing health.

Power: The ability of individuals or groups to influence decisions, shape policies, and create change that aligns with their interests, needs, or goals.

The precautionary principle: Describes the responsibility of environmental scientists to protect public health even in the absence of concrete proof of adverse health outcomes. For example: If there is the possibility that some chemical might harm human, animal, or plant life, then according to the precautionary principle, that chemical should not be used or approved for sale and use.

Prenatal and early-life exposures: The effects of environmental health risks and pollutants during pregnancy and early childhood on future health and disease risk.

Preparedness cycle: A traditional disaster-response model that includes mitigation, preparedness, response, and recovery; offers the false sense that all disasters have a clear "before" and "after."

Presidential memoranda: Similar to executive orders, they are routine executive decisions and determinations that direct agencies to perform duties consistent with the law or implement laws that are presidential priorities. However, presidential memoranda are not required to be published in the Federal Register.

Public health: What we as a society do collectively to ensure the conditions for people to be healthy.

Public health disaster: An impact that overwhelms a social system, whatever the cause, and hurts the underlying structures that support human health and flourishing.

Public policy: A course of government action (e.g., laws, regulations, executive orders) in response to social problems.

Public Water Commons: The conceptual and practical framework of managing water resources as a shared public good accessible to all. It emphasizes collective stewardship and equitable access to clean water for health, livelihoods, and ecosystems, challenging privatization and ensuring that water is preserved and managed sustainably for future generations.

Redlining: Redlining is the practice of denying people access to credit because of where they live, even if they are personally qualified for loans. Redlining maps were created by the Home Owners' Loan Corporation in the 1930s and were used to guide investment and disinvestment in communities. The red color on the maps, labeled "hazardous," were areas occupied by residents of color.

Reference maps: Maps we use to find our way, such as a road map or a navigational map for air or sea.

Regulatory science: The science of developing new tools, standards, and approaches to assess the safety, efficacy, quality, and performance of all regulated products.

Reproductive environmental health: A branch of public health that explores how environmental factors impact human reproductive health, from fertility to pregnancy outcomes, and the health of both mothers and infants.

Risk: The chance of harmful effects to human health or to ecological systems from exposure to an environmental stressor.

Risk assessment: A process of identifying potential hazards and analyzing what could happen if an exposure occurred.

Risk communication: According to the U.S. Environmental Protection Agency, "[r]isk communication is communication intended to supply audience members with the information they need to make informed, independent judgements about risks to health, safety, and the environment."[6(para2)]

Rule: Also known as a regulation. Refers to policy making for executive and independent agencies of the federal government; an agency cannot issue a rule unless authorized by law.

Sacrifice zones: Communities, often communities of color or low wealth, where industrial development, waste disposal, and other polluting industries are concentrated to avoid pollution in predominantly higher income, White communities.

Sensitive receptors: Specific populations or environments that are particularly vulnerable to adverse effects from pollutants, noise, or other environmental hazards.

Shared or joint-use agreement: A shared or joint-use agreement in environmental health is a formal arrangement between multiple parties, such as governments, organizations, or communities, to collaborate on addressing environmental health issues. It outlines the mutual responsibilities, resource sharing, and goals aimed at improving public health outcomes through cooperative efforts and shared decision-making processes.

Social determinants of health (SDOH): Conditions in the environments where people are born, live, learn, work, play, worship, and age that affect their health, functioning, and quality-of-life outcomes.

Stressors: Pollutants that cause negative impacts to human health and/or the environment.

Structural determinants of health: The overarching socioeconomic, cultural, and policy contexts that shape individuals' living conditions and health outcomes. They include factors such as income distribution, social policies, political systems, and economic policies, which determine access to resources, opportunities, and services essential for maintaining and improving health.

Structural harm: Negative consequences against the social determinants of health caused or catalyzed by a disaster impact, such as economic breakdowns.

Structural racism: The ways in which societal institutions, systems, and structures perpetuate racial discrimination and disparities, often systematically disadvantaging certain racial or ethnic groups while privileging others.

Structural violence: Refers to the harms inflicted on individuals or populations by social structures and institutions that perpetuate inequality, exclusion, and injustice. In environmental health, it manifests through policies and practices that disproportionately expose marginalized communities to environmental hazards and health risks, denying them equitable access to resources and protections.

Sustainable Development Goals (SDGs): As defined by the United Nations, a collection of 17 global objectives that serve as "the blueprint to achieve a better and more sustainable future for all. They address the global challenges we face, including those related to poverty, inequality, climate change, environmental degradation, peace, and justice."[7(para1)]

Syndemic: A synergistic epidemic in which two or more ills (e.g., racism, COVID-19, police brutality, climate change) affect each other and worsen impacts.

Systems thinking: A holistic approach that views problems and solutions as interconnected pieces of a larger system. In environmental health, systems thinking involves understanding the complex interactions between various environmental factors and their cumulative impact on human health.

10 Essential Public Health Services: As defined by the Centers for Disease Control and Prevention, they "provide a framework for public health and promote the health of all people in all communities. To achieve equity, these services were revised in 2020 . . . [to] actively promote policies, systems, and overall community conditions that enable optimal health for all."[8(para1)]

Thematic maps: Maps used to display the distribution of one or more specific variables that are aggregated by a geographic unit (such as a country, state, county, census tract, community district, health district, or postal code).

Toxicant: A toxicant is a toxic substance introduced to the environment, such as a pesticide. Includes the negative by-products of energy production, such as heavy metals, particulate air pollution, radioactive waste, CO_2, and noise.

Toxicology: The study of the adverse effects of chemical, physical, or biological agents on living organisms and the ecosystem, including the prevention and amelioration of these effects.

Toxin: A poison made by certain bacteria, plants, or animals.

Unequal risk: Describes how historically marginalized populations, such as Black, Brown, and Indigenous communities or lower wealth communities, are more likely to be exposed to multiple and higher levels of environmental risks over time.

Urban heat island effect: Describes the phenomenon wherein urban areas experience higher temperatures than their rural surroundings due to human activities. This is caused by the absorption and reradiation of heat by buildings, roads, and other infrastructure. It exacerbates heat-related illnesses and contributes to increased energy consumption and air pollution levels.

Vulnerability analysis: The systematic examination of the susceptibility of a population or ecosystem to harm from environmental hazards. It assesses the extent to which climate change, pollution, and other environmental factors can impact health, considering factors like sensitivity, exposure, and adaptive capacity to identify and mitigate risks.

Vulnerability index: An index used to measure how exposed a population is to multiple hazards or adverse health outcomes at once. A social vulnerability index, the most common type, measures potential negative exposures from social, economic, and natural stressors.

Waste: Any material, chemical, or substance that is disposed of or discarded for no further use.

Waste colonialism: The practice of shipping of waste from high-wealth countries to lower wealth nations.

Waste hierarchy: The guiding principle behind waste management that prioritizes waste reduction (at the source) over reuse, which is preferred to recycling, and that considers waste disposal as the last option.

Water stress: The level of pressure that human activities exert over natural freshwater resources, indicating the environmental sustainability of the use of water resources. A measure of how much freshwater is being withdrawn by all economic activities, compared to the total renewable freshwater resources available.

Weatherization: Housing modifications that improve the building envelope to retain healthy air quality and temperature.

Weatherization Assistance Program (WAP): A federal program that provides weatherization services for low-wealth households.

White supremacy: A sociopolitical ideology that holds White people as superior to people of other racial backgrounds, aiming to maintain and enforce racial hierarchies and privileges. In environmental health, it manifests in systemic inequalities, wherein marginalized communities disproportionately bear environmental risks and have limited access to health-promoting resources.

Windows of susceptibility: Specific periods of time when people are most susceptible to the effects of environmental exposures. These are usually critical stages of development or physiological change (e.g., prenatal, early childhood, adolescence, late adulthood).

Zero waste: A system that seeks to incrementally eliminate waste by following the principles of the waste hierarchy.

Zoning: The legislative process of dividing land into zones within which various uses and developments are permitted or prohibited. In environmental health, zoning is used to separate incompatible land uses, protect residential areas from environmental hazards, and ensure that development aligns with public health and safety objectives.

REFERENCES

1. Dotson K, Whyte K. Environmental justice, unknowability and unqualified affectability. *Ethics Environ*. 2013;18(2):55-79. doi:10.2979/ethicsenviro.18.2.55
2. Stakeholder Participation Working Group of the 2010 HIA in the Americas Workshop. Guidance and best practices for stakeholder participation in Health Impact Assessments, version 1.0. October 2011.
3. Kent TJ Jr. *The Urban General Plan*. American Planning Association; 1990.
4. Chapple K, Thomas T, Zuk M. What are gentrification and displacement: Gentrification explained [Video]. Urban Displacement Project; 2021. https://www.urbandisplacement.org/about/what-are-gentrification-and-displacement (quote at 0:20)
5. Kendra JM, Wachtendorf T. *American Dunkirk: The Waterborne Evacuation of Manhattan on 9/11*. Temple University Press; 2016.
6. Learn about risk communication. U.S. Environmental Protection Agency. Updated March 26, 2024. https://www.epa.gov/risk-communication/learn-about-risk-communication
7. Take action for the Sustainable Development Goals. United Nations. Accessed June 17, 2024. https://www.un.org/sustainabledevelopment/sustainable-development-goals
8. Environmental health and the 10 Essential Services. Centers for Disease Control and Prevention, National Center for Environmental Health. August 15, 2023. Updated February 22, 2024. https://www.cdc.gov/environmental-health-services/php/10-essential-services

INDEX

absorption, distribution, metabolism, and elimination (ADME), 144, 145
acute radiation syndrome, 377
ADME. *See* absorption, distribution, metabolism, and elimination
advocacy, 76, 202, 386, 402, 466
Affordable Care Act, 426–427
Agency for Toxic Substances and Disease Registry (ATSDR), 178, 436
agency staff and regulatory science, 77
agouti mice, studies with, 147–148
agroecology, 277–278, 285
air monitoring networks, designing and developing, 227, 228
air pollutants, 47–48, 50, 80
air pollution, 214, 403
   basics of, 216–218
   Clean Air Act (CAA), 221–224
   climate change and, 298, 300–301
   cumulative air pollution exposures and, 224–226
   environmental justice and, 226–229
   health and, 218–221
   history of, 215
   from power plants, 201
   sources of, 214–215
air quality, 44, 54, 327–328
air quality disparities (Los Angeles, California), case study, 25
Airs, Waters, and Places (Hippocrates), 215
air sensors. *See* sensors, low-cost
air toxics, 222
Alabama Sustainable Agriculture Network (ASAN), 283
Alaska Department of Environmental Conservation, 60
Alinsky, Saul, 447
Alliance of Nurses for Healthy Environments, 432, 434
allostatic load, 126
ambient air pollutants, 217–218
   sources of, 218
amendment, 74, 80, 82
American Community Survey, 201

American Dunkirk (Kendra and Wachtendorf), 347, 361
American Housing Survey, 201
American Institute of Certified Planners, 332
American Medical Association, 434
American Planning Association, 332
American Psychological Association, 432
American Public Health Association (APHA), 4, 15, 16, 17, 393, 397
   Addressing Environmental Justice to Achieve Health Equity, 17, 409
   Center for Climate Health and Equity, 413
   Children's Environmental Health Committee, 413
   Protecting Children's Environmental Health Policy Statement, 410
   Protecting the Health of Children A National Snapshot of Environmental Health Services Report, 406
American Steel and Wire Plant, 215
analytical epidemiology, 149
Anishinaabe Medicine Wheel, 31
antibiotic resistance, 279–280
   spreading of, 280
anti-racism, 98, 111, 409, 451
   anti-oppression and, 36, 37–38
   environmental racism and, 109
   healthcare and, 432–433
   research, 109–110
APHA. *See* American Public Health Association
Apsáalooke Nation public drinking water (Montana), case study, 256–257
Apsáalooke Water and Wastewater Authority (AWWWA), 256
aquaponic systems, 284
ArcGIS software, 183
Arkana chemical plant (Crosby, Texas), 13
Arnstein's Ladder of Citizen Participation, 35, 333, 456
arsenic, 245, 375
Art of Commenting, The (Mullin), 77
Arwady, Allison, 446, 455, 457

ASAN. *See* Alabama Sustainable Agriculture Network
asbestos, 245
    in Libby (Montana), 381–382
assistance versus affordability (water), 259
asthma, screening for, 422–423
Atlanta's watershed, pollution in (case study), 129–130
ATSDR. *See* Agency for Toxic Substances and Disease Registry
attribute data, 166
AWWWA. *See* Apsáalooke Water and Wastewater Authority

Basel Convention, 74
Bautista, Olga, 445, 452, 456, 463–464
Beauty Inside Out Campaign, 127
Belmont Report, 101
BenMAP software, 201
benzene, 374–375
Bhopal Gas Tragedy, 215
bias, 150–151
    types of, 151
big data and analytics, integration of, 14
BIL. *See* Bipartisan Infrastructure Law
biological hazards, 141, 376
biomarkers, 263
biomass burning, 194
biomonitoring, 133
    with communities, 263
bioretention garden, 261
biosolids, 307
bioswales, 61
Bipartisan Infrastructure Law (BIL)/Investment and Jobs Act (IIJA), 79, 87, 203, 244, 260
BIPOC. *See* Black, Indigenous, and People of Color
bisphenol A (BPA), 132, 148, 157, 401
Black Feminist Thought, 157
Black, Indigenous, and People of Color (BIPOC), 176, 430–431
black lung disease, 383
blood-borne pathogens, 376
Blue Greenway Taskforce, 35
body burden, 133
Boggs, Grace Lee, 448
Bonilla, Yarimar, 345
BPA. *See* bisphenol A (BPA)
Bradford Hill criteria, 150
breaking power, notion of, 448, 458
Break the Cycle of Health Disparities program, 409
Breathe Free Detroit campaign, 301
bromate, 247
building power, notion of, 448, 456–457
built environment, 321
    by design, 322–327
    for equity, reimagining, 334–336
    and health, pathways between, 327–331
Bullard, Robert D., 33, 175
Bureau of Labor Statistics, 373
    Census of Fatal Occupational Injuries, 373
    Survey of Occupational Injuries and Illnesses, 373

CAA. *See* Clean Air Act
CAFOs. *See* Concentrated Animal Feeding Operations
California, 258, 312, 401, 402
California Air Resources Board (CARB), 88
CalPUFF dispersion model, 201
Campaign for Healthier Solutions, 402
Cancer Alley petrochemical production (Louisiana), case study, 328–329
cancer and environmental health, in United States, case study, 423
cancer cluster, 14
CAP. *See* Climate Action Plan
Capacity Building Through Effective Meaningful Engagement (EPA), 35
CAPs. *See* Charleston Area Pollution Prevention Partnership
CARB. *See* California Air Resources Board
carbon monoxide (CO), 218, 374
Carpal-Tunnel Syndrome, 426
cascading failures, 344
case-control study, 153, 154
case series study, 153, 154
case studies
    air quality disparities (Los Angeles, California), 25
    Apsáalooke Nation public drinking water (Montana), 256–257
    Cancer Alley petrochemical production (Louisiana), 328–329
    chemical management regulations, United States versus European Union, 82–83
    Chicago Heat Wave of 1995 (Chicago, Illinois), 45
    childhood cancer and environmental health, 423
    Children & Nature Network, 401
    cobalt mining, exposures for artisanal miners (Democratic Republic of Congo), 197–198

community-based participatory research, cervical cancer screenings (Santa Clara County, California), 155–156
Community Health Effects of Industrial Hog Operations study (North Carolina), 107
Dearborn health department (Dearborn, Michigan), 36–37
Detroit trash-to-energy incinerator (Detroit, Michigan), 301
Detroit water crisis (Detroit, Michigan), 261–262
Dust Bowl (Great Plains region), 274–275
Elm Playlot and Pogo Park, joint-use agreement (Richmond, California), 325–326
energy burdens and energy injustice (Michigan), 201–202
environmental health in clinical case studies, 426
Environmental Justice for All Act (EJ4AA), 87
Environmental Justice Radar, public participation geographic information systems (Charleston, South Carolina), 183
flame-retardants chemicals and children's clothing, 402–403
Flint water crisis (Flint, Michigan), 349–350
food deserts (Texas), 276–277
healthy food access, environmental justice (New York City, New York), 170
heat wave, downstream impacts (Seattle, Washington), 352
Hurricane Maria (Puerto Rico), 346–347
Indigenous communities and climate change (Alaska), 60
Indigenous rights, Yucca Mountain (Nevada), 308
International Labor Organization (India), 391
intersectionality and environmental injustice in beauty products, 127
Love Canal disaster (Niagara Falls, New York), 304–305
National Institute of Environmental Health Sciences Worker Training Program, 388–389
"Occupational Groups and Environmental Justice" study (the Bronx, New York), 179–180
Out of Gas, In With Justice pilot study (New York City, New York), 217
Pueblo Food Experience (Tewa Pueblo, New Mexico), 282–283
radiation hazards and nuclear weapons waste in Indigenous communities, 142–143
sewage pollution and discriminatory policies (Atlanta, Georgia), 129–130
Toms River water supply (Toms River, New Jersey), 13–14
train derailment (East Palestine, Ohio), 10–11
West End Revitalization Association (Mebane, North Carolina), 107–108
case study, 153, 154
CBAs. *See* community benefit agreements
CBPR. *See* community-based participatory research
CCC. *See* Civilian Conservation Corps
CCT. *See* Concerned Citizens of Tillery
CDC. *See* Centers for Disease Control and Prevention
CDR. *See* community-driven research
CEHN. *See* Children's Environmental Health Network
CEJST. *See* Climate and Economic Justice Screening Tool
cement kilns, 299, 305
CEnR. *See* community-engaged research
Center for Health, Environment, and Justice, 302
Centers for Disease Control and Prevention (CDC), 9, 31, 99, 142, 280, 353, 359, 401, 430
  Agency for Toxic Substances and Disease Registry (ATSDR), 178
  Environmental Health Training in Emergency Response (EHTER), 354
  Ethical Guidance for Public Health Emergency Preparedness and Response, 358
  Foodborne Disease Outbreak Surveillance System (FDOSS), 281
CERCLA. *See* Comprehensive Environmental Response, Compensation, and Liability Act
cervical cancer screening increase, among Vietnamese American women, case study, 155–156
Charleston Area Pollution Prevention Partnership (CAPs), 183
Chavez, Cesar, 447
Chavez, Yesenia, 454
CHEIHO. *See* Community Health Effects of Industrial Hog Operations study
chemical hazard, 118, 141, 374–375

chemical management regulations, United States versus European Union (case study), 82–83
Chemical Safety and Hazard Investigation Board report, 13
chemicals and health, 12–13
Chesapeake Bay Open Data Portal, 262
Chicago Heat Wave of 1995 (Chicago, Illinois), case study, 45
childhood cancer and environmental health, case study, 423
child-protective policies, 406
Children & Nature Network, case study, 401
children, climate change impact on, 50
children's environmental health, 397–398
    critical competencies in, 409, 410
    critical exposures and, 400–404
    environmental health inequities and, 407–408
    environmental justice and, 408–411
    inequities addressing in, 408–409
    related policies, 405–407
    state of, 398–400
Children's Environmental Health and Disease Prevention Research Centers, 405
Children's Environmental Health Network (CEHN), 406
    Blueprint for Protecting Children's Environmental Health, 409
    Children's Environmental Health Day, 409
Children's Health Protection Advisory Committee, 405
Chile, 219
chlorite, 247
choropleth maps, 180
chromium, 245
CIRBs. *See* Community Institutional Review Boards
circular economy, 310
citizen science, 106
City of Chicago, 446, 448
Civilian Conservation Corps (CCC), 275
Civil Rights Act, 330, 454
Clean Air Act (CAA), 27, 35, 80–81, 221–224, 300
    enforcement of, 223–224
    regulatory air pollution monitoring and community air monitoring and, 224
CleanAirNow, 228
Clean Energy for Low-Income Communities Accelerator, 203
Clean Water Act (CWA), 35, 78–79, 244, 251, 253
Climate Action Plan (CAP), 58

climate adaptation
    to current reality, 59–61
    support, through healthcare, 61–62
Climate and Economic Justice Screening Tool (CEJST), 181
Climate and Health Lesson Plan for Grades 9–12 Toolkit, 413
Climate and Youth Education Toolkit, 413
climate change, 12, 43–44
    adaptation and, 59–61
    air pollution and, 298, 300–301
    built environment and, 327
    communication about, 62–63
    critical exposures for children and, 403–404
    environmental disruption and, 237
    impact on health, 44–49
    impact on vulnerability, 49–53
    in medical education, 432
    mitigation, for healthier lives, 58–59
    public health disasters and, 351
    tackling, within healthcare, 431–432
    water cycle and, 236–238
climate equity, 57
Climate Generation, 64
climate gentrification, 177
climate justice
    meaning of, 57
    pillars of, 57
Climate Justice Alliance, 204
Climate Leadership and Community Protection Act (New York), 217
climate resilience, 57
Climate Risk Index, 413
ClimateRx, 432
clinical trials, 151–152
CO. *See* carbon monoxide
Coal Mine Safety and Health Act, 383
cobalt mining, exposures for artisanal miners (Democratic Republic of Congo), case study, 197–198
Code of Hammurabi, 3
co-governance, 333, 335
cohort study, 153–154
cold exposure, risks from, 378
Collaborative for Health Equity (CHE) Cook County, 446
collective continuance, 360
colorism, 127
combined selection–information bias, 151
commercial determinants of health, 12
communities
    definition of, 322
    working with, 34–35
communities of color, 408

climate change impact on, 51
community-academic partnership, 106
community-based participatory research (CBPR), 105, 155–156
   cervical cancer screenings (Santa Clara County, California), case study, 155–156
   definition of, 106
community benefit agreements (CBAs), 322
community benefits agreements (CBAs), 333–334
community directed policies, 228
community-driven research (CDR), 105
community-engaged research (CEnR), 105
community engagement, 333, 335
Community Health Effects of Industrial Hog Operations (CHEIHO) study (North Carolina), case study, 107
community health workers and environmental health, 433
Community Institutional Review Boards (CIRBs), 101
community organizing, 34, 446–447
   for health, 447–448, 466
community-owned and -managed research (COMR), 106, 107–108
community power, 228, 446, 456
Community Preventive Services Task Force, 409
community resilience frameworks, 358
community science, 227
community survivance, 285
community trails, 152
complete streets, 334
Comprehensive Environmental Response, Compensation, and Liability Act (CERCLA; Superfund), 84, 388
comprehensive/general plan, 229, 323
COMR. *See* community-owned and -managed research
Concentrated Animal Feeding Operations (CAFOs), 279, 284
Concerned Citizens of St. John Parish, 328
Concerned Citizens of Tillery (CCT), 107
consent agreement, 82
construction and demolition debris, 306–307
Consumer Confidence Report, 239, 265
Consumer Product Safety Commission (CPSC), 131
Cooper, Christian, 325
COP. *See* United Nations Conference of Parties
copper, 245
corrective action, 303
correlation and causation, comparison of, 150

COVID-19 pandemic, 98, 99, 110, 281, 306, 354, 376, 383, 385, 390, 430
CPSC. *See* Consumer Product Safety Commission
CRA. *See* cumulative risk assessment
crisis epistemology, 356
crisis response, 355–356
Crisis Standards of Care, 358
critical exposures, for children
   air, water, and food and, 403
   chemicals in daily environment and, 401–403
   climate change and, 403–404
   settings and surroundings and, 400–401
cross-sectional study, 153, 154
cumulative air pollution exposures, 224–226
cumulative impacts, 9, 33, 224–225, 329
   laws, in select states, 225–226
cumulative risk, 14, 118
cumulative risk assessment (CRA), 123–125, 128, 129, 131, 133–134, 179, 248
CWA. *See* Clean Water Act
cyanotoxins, 250–251

data aggregation, 171
data justice, 102, 103
data residency, 103
data sovereignty, 103
DBCFSN. *See* Detroit Black Community Food Sovereignty Network
DBPs. *See* disinfection by-products
DDT. *See* dichlorodiphenyltrichloroethane
Dearborn health department (Dearborn, Michigan), case study, 36–37
Deep South Center for Environmental Justice, 328
defined contribution plans, implication of, 384
Demand–Control model, 376, 377
Democratic Republic of Congo, 219
   cobalt mining, exposures for artisanal miners, case study, 197–198
De Morbis Artificum Diatriba (Dissertation on Workers' Diseases) (Ramazzini), 379
Department of Health and Human Services, 27, 330, 383
Department of Justice (DOJ), 330
DES. *See* diethylstilbestrol
descriptive epidemiology, 149
desert ecosystems, 282
Detroit, 260
Detroit Black Community Food Sovereignty Network (DBCFSN), 283

Detroit Community-Academic Urban Research Center, 106
Detroit Food Commons, 283
Detroit trash-to-energy incinerator (Detroit, Michigan), case study, 301
Detroit Water and Sewerage Department, 261
Detroit water crisis (Detroit, Michigan), case study, 261–262
developmental origins of health and disease (DOHaD), 146–148
dichlorodiphenyltrichloroethane (DDT), 220–221
diethylstilbestrol (DES), 97–98
disaster, 344–346. *See also* public health disasters
  cascading, 349
  climate change impacts and, 351
  harms, specific, 348
  managing, 352–359
  typology of, 348
disaster preparedness cycle, 356–358
disaster risk, 346, 350
disaster risk reduction frameworks, 359
disaster swarm, 346, 352, 359–361
disease mapping, 163–164. *See also* geographic information science (GISc)
disinfection by-products (DBPs), 239, 247, 249
disinformation, 33, 110
disparate siting and exposures, impacts of, 176–178
distributed energy resource management systems, 204
distributive justice, 102
DOHaD. *See* developmental origins of health and disease
DOJ. *See* Department of Justice
Donora Smog, 215
Donora Zinc Works, 215
doorstep epidemiology, 107
dose-response assessment, 122
dose-response curves and toxicology, 145–146
drought, 47, 55, 237
dry lab, 151
DTE Energy, 201
Du Bois, W. E. B., 23
Dumping in Dixie (Bullard), 175
Dust Bowl (Great Plains region), case study, 274–275

Earthjustice, 328
eco-anxiety, 46, 48
Eco-Healthy Child Care® (EHCC), 406
ecological fallacy, 171

ecological studies, 154–155
ecology, 128
Ecology Center, 301
eco-paralysis, 46, 48
ecosystems, 4
ecosystem services, 272, 284
ECWTP. *See* Environmental Careers Worker Training Program
Effort–Reward Imbalance Model, 376
EHCC. *See* Eco-Healthy Child Care®
Eigg Electric Grid, 204
EJ. *See* environmental justice
EJ4AA. *See* Environmental Justice for All Act
EJI. *See* Environmental Justice Index
electrification, 204–205
Elm Playlot Action Committee (EPAC), 326
Elm Playlot and Pogo Park, joint-use agreement (Richmond, California), case study, 325–326
Emergency Food Assistance Program, 274
emergency management cycle, 344, 345
Emergency Management Performance Grant (EMPG) program, 357
Emergency Operations Centers (EOCs), 356
Emergency Planning and Community Right-to-Know Act (EPCRA), 175
EMPG. *See* Emergency Management Performance Grant program
endocrine disruption, 8–9
energy and health, 193–194
  electrification and, 204–205
  energy extraction impacts and, 197
  equities of, 198–202
  past and present, 194–198
  transitioning to renewable energy, 203–204
  weatherization and, 205–206
energy burden, 198
energy burdens and energy injustice (Michigan), case study, 201–202
energy democracy, 204
energy justice, 193
  in Southeast Michigan, case study, 201–202
energy poverty, 198
energy use and climate change mitigation, 58
Energy Use Intensity, 201
enforcement, significance of, 330
Environmental and Climate Justice Block Grants, 86
environmental burden index, 178
Environmental Careers Worker Training Program (ECWTP), 389
environmental hazards, 279
  types of, 141–142

environmental health. *See also individual entries*
  anti-racist healthcare and, 432–433
  community health workers and, 433
  current scenario of, 8–13
  disparities, 24–26
  essential services and fundamental activities, 27–31
  history of, 5–8
  inequities, 53–56
  inequities, in clinical practice, 429–431
  intersectionality and, 126
  life-course exposure and, 125
  policy, 130–132, 156–157
  in practice, 24, 26–30, 112–113, 185–186, 364, 436–437
  public health and, 353–355
  science and policy, 14
  socio-ecological model application to, 128–129
  tracking, 32–34
  working in, 15–16
environmental health in clinical case studies, 426
Environmental Health Playbook, 26
environmental health risks
  meaning and significance of, 118–120
  racism and, 119–120
  traditional assessment of, 121–123
environmental health science, 97–98
  as accessible and actionable, 110–111
  environmental justice and, 104–111
  science and environmental justice and, 101–104
  science and society and, 99–101
environmental justice (EJ), 98
  air pollution and, 219–221
  anti-racism and anti-oppression in practice and, 37–38
  community resilience and, 358
  crisis response and, 356
  disaster risk reduction frameworks and, 359
  Health in All Policies (HiAP) and, 36–37
  occupational and residential (the Bronx, New York), case study, 179–180
  occupational health and, 386–391
  preparedness cycle and, 358
  science and, 101–104
  working toward, 16–18, 57–63, 88, 104–111, 132–134, 157–158, 180–184, 203–207, 226–229, 258–262, 283–285, 309–313, 331–336, 408–411, 431–434
"Environmental Justice, Science, and Public Health" (Wing), 101

Environmental Justice for All Act (EJ4AA), 86
  case study, 87
Environmental Justice Index (EJI), 178–179
Environmental Justice Movement, 17
Environmental Justice Radar
  public participation geographic information systems (Charleston, South Carolina), case study, 183
environmental measures, 154
environmental medicine, 419
environmental pediatrics, 421–423
  environmental health history and, 422–423
environmental policy making, in United States, 75–77
environmental precision medicine, 433–434
Environmental Protection Agency (EPA), 19, 20, 25, 27, 33, 57, 60, 77, 79, 81, 82, 83, 107, 121, 132, 133, 207, 221–222, 223, 239, 265, 302, 303, 306–307, 350, 397, 405, 429
  Contaminant Candidate List 5 (CCL5), 239
  EJScreen, 178
  Green Book, 82
  National Primary Drinking Water Regulation list, 239, 245–247
environmental public health, 23
environmental racism, 8, 25, 109, 157, 182, 328, 350
environmental signals, 263
environmental toxicology, types of, 149–151
environmental variables, 263
EOCs. *See* Emergency Operations Centers
EPA. *See* Environmental Protection Agency
EPAC. *See* Elm Playlot Action Committee
EPCRA. *See* Emergency Planning and Community Right-to-Know Act
epidemiologic triangulation, 153, 154
epidemiology, 141
  studies, 149–151
epigenetics and DOHaD, 146–148
epigenome, 147, 148, 424
epistemic exclusion, 104
epistemic justice, 103, 104
Epplin, Wesley, 452, 465–467
equity
  co-governance models, Health in All Policies and tools for, 332–334
  equality and justice and, 331–332
  and justice, in disaster management, 355
ergonomic hazards, 377
ergonomics, 379
ESDA. *See* exploratory spatial data analysis
e-waste, 294
exclusionary zoning, 323

executive orders, 73, 76, 175, 405, 408
    for environmental health and justice, 83–85
experimental studies, 151–152, 153
exploratory spatial data analysis (ESDA), 166–167
exposome, 9, 419
    totality of exposures and, 143
exposure assessment, 122–123
exposure misclassification, 151
exposure to disease, pathway from, 143–144
extreme heat, 45, 54
    and energy outages, combination of, 196–197
extreme weather, 46, 54

factory farms. *See* Concentrated Animal Feeding Operations (CAFOs)
Fairfax County Public Schools (Virginia), 401
Fair Housing Act, 323
Fair Share Criteria, 175
false solutions, 88
FANN. *See* Food Access and Nutrition Network
Farm Bill, 83, 84, 274, 275, 286
fate and transport models. *See* source pathway models
FDA. *See* Food and Drug Administration
FECA. *See* Federal Employee's Compensation Act
Federal-Aid Highway Act, 323
Federal Emergency Management Agency (FEMA), 357, 359
Federal Employee's Compensation Act (FECA), 427
federal environmental health protections, 77–83
Federal Food, Drug, and Cosmetic Act, 274
federalism, 26–27
Federal Mine Safety and Health Act, 383
Federal Register, 77, 90
Federal Remediation and Relocation Plan, 329
federal water laws (United States), 244
FEMA. *See* Federal Emergency Management Agency
fenceline communities, 30, 33, 36, 223, 226, 228
fetal undernutrition, 146
Fifth National Climate Assessment, 58, 327
First National People of Color Environmental Leadership Summit, 17–18

flame-retardants chemicals and children's clothing, case study, 402–403
Flint water crisis (Michigan), 80, 140, 239
    case study, 349–350
flooding, 46, 55, 79, 237
flood risks, near hazardous facilities, 177
flourishing, idea of, 16
Flowering Tree Permaculture Institute, 282
Flowers, Catherine Coleman, 329, 330
fluoride, 246
food, 272
    and food policy, history of, 273–275
Food Access and Nutrition Network (FANN), 277
food and agricultural waste, 307
Food and Drug Administration (FDA), 273, 281
    Coordinated Outbreak Response and Evaluation (CORE) Network, 281
food apartheid, 170, 276, 279
foodborne outbreaks, 281
food deserts, 276
    in Texas, case study, 276–277
food environments, 326–327
Food Quality Protection Act (FQPA), 84
Food Safety Modernization Act, 274
food security, 276–277
food sovereignty, 277, 282, 283
food system, 272–273
    climate change mitigation and, 59
    environmental justice and, 283–285
    industrialized versus regenerative, 278–283
Foote, Eunice Newton, 12
formaldehyde, 375
Formosa Plastics, 328
fossil fuel
    burning of, 217
    related air pollution, 44, 329
FQPA. *See* Food Quality Protection Act
FrameWorks Institute, 16
Fresh Banana Leaves (Hernandez), 104
Fresh Food Financing Initiative, 327

GAO. *See* U.S. General Accounting Office
gender and sex, comparison of, 158
General Iron, 446
gentrification, 177, 324
geographic extent, 170
geographic information science (GISc), 164–165, 262
    environmental health policies with spatial considerations and, 174–175

in Environmental Justice Movement, 165–166
  geographic data units in, 172
  limitations of, 173–174
  maps and data in, 166–168
  research design of, 170–171
  spatial methods in, 168
  working of, 166–174
geographic information systems (GIS), 164
George Mason Center for Climate Communication, 62
Get2Green program, 401
GIS. *See* geographic information systems
GISc. *See* geographic information science
Global Health Security Index, 357
global measures, 154
global stormwater infrastructure (GSI), 260
Good Neighbor provision, of CAA, 81
Google Maps, 183
Gordie Howe International Bridge crossing, 78
grassroots organizations, 76, 181, 262, 327, 328
grasstops organizations, 76
Great Lakes Environmental Law Center, 201
Great Smog, 215
green bank, 73
Green Belt Movement, 448
Green Carts Program, 327
green gentrification, 177
greenhouse gasses, 44
Green Revolution, 278
green spaces, 61, 330–331
  parks and, 325
Green Zones, 335
groundwater, 236, 254
  contamination, 297–298
  treatment plants, 239
GSI. *See* global stormwater infrastructure
Guerra, Crystal Vance, 454
gynecological research, on enslaved Black women and immigrants, 99

HAA5. *See* haloacetic acids
HABs. *See* harmful algal blooms
haloacetic acids (HAA5), 247
Hamilton, Alice, 140, 372
harmful algal blooms (HABs), 250–251
Harris County (Texas), 401
Hawks Nest Tunnel disaster (West Virginia), 371
hazard mapping, 228
hazardous waste incinerators, 299, 305
hazardous waste landfills, 297

HDI. *See* Human Development Index
health adaptation and climate change, 59
healthcare, 419–420
  environmental health inequities in clinical practice and, 429–431
  environmental justice and, 431–434
  environmental pediatrics and, 421–423
  occupational health and, 420–421
  policy, and environmental health, 426–429
  prenatal, and environmental health, 423–426
healthcare professionals, as advocates, 434
Health Care Without Harm, 432
Health Impact Assessments (HIAs), 57–58, 133, 322, 333, 461
Health in All Policies (HiAP), 36–37, 333
health policies and protections, 72–73
  environmental policy making in United States and, 75–77
  executive orders and, 83–85
  federal environmental health protections and, 77–83
  global environmental policy making and, 73–75
  infrastructure and economic legislation and, 85–88
healthy communities, for all, 321–322
  air quality and, 327–328
  built environment by design and, 322–327
  climate change and, 327
  environmental justice and, 331–336
  injury and, 330
  mental health and, 330–331
  water and, 329
Healthy Corner Store Initiative, 277
healthy food access, environmental justice (New York City, New York), case study, 170
Healthy Food Access Portal, 287
Healthy Food Financing Initiative, 277
Healthy Housing Standard, 411
heat-related illness, 378
heat stroke and climate change, 45
heat wave, downstream impacts (Seattle, Washington), case study, 352
hermeneutical injustice, 104
HiAP. *See* Health in All Policies
HIAs. *See* Health Impact Assessments
Hierarchy of Controls, 380
highways, construction of, 323–324
Ho-Chunk Nation, 31
HOLC. *See* Home Owners' Loan Corporation
Home Owners' Loan Corporation (HOLC), 25, 176, 181, 199, 200

Honor the Earth, 308
Hooker Chemical and Plastics Corporation, 304
hopeful pessimism, 362–363, 364
housing affordability, 324
housing insecurity, climate change impact on, 53
How to Talk About Climate Change So People Will Listen (Hayhoe), 12
HUD. *See* U.S. Department of Housing and Urban Development
Human Development Index (HDI), 358
human health, 214, 220. *See also individual entries*
    environmental disruption and climate change impacting, 237
Human Rights Watch, 328
Hurricane Harvey, 13
Hurricane Katrina, 355
Hurricane Maria, 344, 345
    in Puerto Rico, case study, 346–347
Hvrvnrvcukwv Ueki-honecv Farm (Hummingbird Springs Farm), 283

IAP2. *See* International Association of Public Participation
ICS. *See* Incident Command System
IIJA. *See* Infrastructure Investment and Jobs Act; Bipartisan Infrastructure Law
Illinois Environmental Protection Agency public notice, 223
ILO. *See* International Labor Organization
immediate harm, 348
immunotoxicology, 263
implicit bias, 99–100
incidence, 148
Incident Command System (ICS), 356, 361
incinerators, 298–301
    air pollution and climate change and, 300–301
    anatomy of, 299
    facility, site map of, 300
    types of, 299
inclusionary zoning, 334
Indian Civil Rights Act, 30
Indian Health Care Improvement Act, 30
Indian Health Service (IHS), 30
Indian Self-Determination and Education Assistance Act, 30
Indigenous communities and climate change (Alaska), case study, 60
Indigenous communities, climate change impact on, 51–52
Indigenous health and uranium mining, in United States, 142–143
Indigenous Peoples Network, 308
Indigenous rights, Yucca Mountain (Nevada), case study, 308
Indigenous sovereignty, 283
indoor air pollutants, 216–217
indoor environments, 324–325
industrial and organizational psychology, 379
Industrial Areas Foundation, 447
industrial food system, 278–281
industrial hygiene, 379
industrial waste landfills, 297
industrial water contamination, books and movies about, 251
infectious diseases, and water, 237
Inflation Reduction Act (IRA), 86, 203
infodemic, 33, 110
information bias, 151
information layers, in GIS, 167
infrastructure and economic legislation, as environmental policy, 85–88
Infrastructure Investment and Jobs Act (IIJA). *See* Bipartisan Infrastructure Law (BIL)
Institutional Review Boards (IRBs), 101
integrated pest management (IPM), 406–407, 411
Integrated Resource Plans (IRPs), 209
intergenerational justice, 17
Intergovernmental Panel on Climate Change (IPCC), 351
International Alliance of Waste Pickers, 311
International Association of Public Participation (IAP2), 35, 333
International Labor Organization (ILO), 373
    in India, case study, 391
International Ladies Garment Workers Union, 371
International Property Maintenance Code, 335
interprofessional education (IPE), 433
intersectionality, 126
    application to environmental injustice of beauty, case study, 127
Interstate Commerce Clause, 381
ionizing radiation, 377
IPCC. *See* Intergovernmental Panel on Climate Change
IPE. *See* interprofessional education
IPM. *See* integrated pest management
IRA. *See* Inflation Reduction Act

IRBs. *See* Institutional Review Boards
IRPs. *See* Integrated Resource Plans

Jackson water crisis, 79
Jefferson Park incident, 25
Jemez Principles for Democratic Organizing and the Environmental Justice Principles, 109
Jim Crow laws, 24, 325
job insecurity and precarity, 376
Johnson, Cheryl, 459
Johnson, Hazel, 448
joint-use or shared agreements, 335
Judith River Nitrogen Project, 259
Judith Watershed, 259
justice, types of, 102–104
Justice40 Initiative, 181, 331
just transition, 204

Kaiser Family Foundation, 355
Kaiser Permanente, 431, 432
King, Martin Luther, Jr., 17, 466
Kyoto Protocol, 74

labor unions and worker centers, 390–391
LaDuke, Winona, 448
LA Live, 333–334
Landfill Directive (European Union), 312
landfills, 296–298
    air pollution and climate change and, 298
    anatomy of, 297
    groundwater and contamination and, 297–298
    structures, failures of, 298
    types and locations of, 292, 296–297
land use, 323
land-use regression, 179
Land Worker Mother model, 157
language justice, 103, 390
La Via Campesina, 277
lead (Pb), 139–140, 152, 218, 246, 260, 400, 422, 425
legislation, 76
Lemery, Jay, 434
lethal dose and lethal concentration, 146
LGBTQIA2S+, climate change impact on, 53
life-course approach, 117
life-course exposure, 125
life cycle impact assessment, 196

Life Lab program, 401
Lightfoot, Mayor Lori, 455, 456, 458
limit of detection (LOD), 146
LOD. *See* limit of detection
LOEL. *See* lowest-observed-effect limit
Los Angeles Black Worker Center, 389
Los Angeles County
    Department of Public Health, 58
    Sustainability Office, 58
Louisiana Bucket Brigade, 181, 328
Louisiana Department of Environmental Quality, 181
Louisiana Tumor Registry, 328
Love Canal disaster, 388
    case study, 304–305
lowest-observed-effect limit (LOEL), 146

Maathai, Wangari, 448
manganese, 246
mapping, 133. *See also* geographic information science (GISc)
    ethical considerations of, 183–184
    public and community-driven, 181–183
    tools of, 181–183, 185–186, 187
mapping patterns, of environmental health inequities
    disparate siting and exposures and impacts, 176–178
    history of, 175–176
    vulnerability indices and, 178–179
maps, as simple data visualizations, 180
Marwah, Harleen, 434
MATS. *See* Mercury Air Toxics Standards
MAUP. *See* modifiable areal unit problem
maximum contaminant level (MCL), 245
maximum contaminant level goal (MCLG), 245
mayor–council systems, 27
Mazon, Jade, 454
MCL. *See* maximum contaminant level
MCLG. *See* maximum contaminant level goal
media, for sharing environmental health science, 111
media advocacy, 451–453
median lethal dose (25% and 50%), 146
Medicaid, 422
medical education, climate change in, 432
medical racism, 430–431
medical waste, 306
Medical Waste Tracking Act, 306
MEJC. *See* Michigan Environmental Justice Coalition

Memphis Sanitation Strike, 17, 309
mental health, 48
  and built environment, 330–331
  burdens, 52, 53
  children's health, 246, 260
  and climate change, 44, 46–49, 53, 61, 62, 403
  and droughts, 237
  and green space, 9, 325, 327, 330
  and housing affordability, 324
  and inequities, 404–405
  negative effects, 295
  and occupational stress, 376
  and paid parental leave, 383
  and psychosocial harm, 414
mercury, 246
Mercury Air Toxics Standards (MATS), 84
mercury in fish, 428
metagenomics, 262–263
Methane Rule, 84
methyl bromide, 222
Metropolitan Alliance of Connected Communities, 103
Michener's struggle for power, 457
Michigan Department of Transportation, 78
Michigan Environmental Justice Coalition (MEJC), 201
microplastics, 251
mindful muddling, 361
mine safety, 383
mining and health hazards, 197–198
misinformation, 33
modifiable areal unit problem (MAUP), 171, 173
Montreal Protocol, 74
morbidity, 148
mortality, 148
MSW. *See* municipal solid waste
municipal solid waste (MSW)
  generation and management, 294
  incinerators, 293, 299
  landfills, 296
Murray, Linda Rae, 452
mutual aid, in disasters, 361

NAAQS. *See* National Ambient Air Quality Standards
NATECH. *See* Natural Hazards Triggering Technological Disasters
National Academies of Sciences, Engineering, and Medicine, 154
National Academy of Medicine, 456
National Academy of Sciences, 401
National Ambient Air Quality Standards (NAAQS), 27, 72, 80, 81, 221, 222, 225

National Center for Healthy Housing (NCHH), 409
National Commission for the Protection of Human Subjects of Biomedical and Behavioral Research, 101
National Congress of American Indians (NCAI), 103
National Council for Environmental Health and Equity, 16
National Environmental Coalition of Native Americans, 308
National Environmental Health Association (NEHA), 4, 432
National Environmental Policy Act (NEPA), 77–78
National Health and Nutrition Examination Surveys (NHANES), 423
National Healthy Housing Standard, 335
National Institute for Occupational Safety and Health (NIOSH), 372, 375, 378, 380, 421
National Institute of Environmental Health Sciences (NIEHS), 397, 405
  Worker Training Program, case study, 388–389
National Labor Relations Act (NLRA), 371, 382
National Labor Relations Board (NLRB), 390
National League for Nursing, 432
National Map Viewer, 262
National Oceanic and Atmospheric Administration, 60
National People of Color Environmental Leadership Summit, 346
National Pollution Discharge Elimination System (NPDES), 79
National Research Act, 101
National Research Council, 125, 301–302
"National Roadway Safety Strategy, The," 335
Native Land Digital, 164
natural gas, 197
Natural Hazards Triggering Technological Disasters (NATECH), 13
Navajo WaterGIS, 262
NCAI. *See* National Congress of American Indians
NCEJN. *See* North Carolina Environmental Justice Network
NEHA. *See* National Environmental Health Association
Nenquimo, Nemonte, 448
NEPA. *See* National Environmental Policy Act

network analysis, 170
New Deal, 371
New Jersey Department of Environmental Protection, 88
The New Jim Crow, 24
New York City
   electric vehicles in, 205
   healthy foods access in, case study, 170
New York City Pandemic Response Institute, 361
NHANES. *See* National Health and Nutrition Examination Surveys
NIEHS. *See* National Institute of Environmental Health Sciences
NIOSH. *See* National Institute for Occupational Safety and Health
nitrate, 246, 259
nitrogen oxides (NO$_x$), 218
NLRA. *See* National Labor Relations Act
NLRB. *See* National Labor Relations Board
NOAEL. *See* no observed-adverse-effect limit
NOEL. *See* no observed-effect limit
noise hazards, 378
nonchemical hazard, 118–119
nonionizing radiation, 377
nonuniformity of space, 171
no observed-adverse-effect limit (NOAEL), 146
no observed-effect limit (NOEL), 146
normal time and disaster time, 361–363
norovirus, 280
North Carolina Environmental Justice Network (NCEJN), 107
NO$_x$. *See* nitrogen oxides
NPDES. *See* National Pollution Discharge Elimination System
nuclear toxicology, 142–143
Nuclear Waste Policy Act (NWPA), 308
nuclear-weapons states (NWS), 142
NWPA. *See* Nuclear Waste Policy Act
NWS. *See* nuclear-weapons states

O$_3$. *See* ozone
observational studies, 153–155
occupational epidemiology, 379
"Occupational Groups and Environmental Justice" study (the Bronx, New York City), case study, 179–180
occupational groups, climate change impact on, 52
occupational health, 369, 420
   early leaders in, 372
   environmental justice and, 386–391

history of, 370–372, 421
inequities of, 383–386
occupational hazards and, 372–380
regulation of, 380–383
and safety protections, advancing, 386–387
Occupational Injury and Illness Classification System (OIICS), 373
occupational medicine, 379
Occupational Safety and Health (OSH) Act, 310, 372, 381
   General Duty Clause, 381
Occupational Safety and Health Administration (OSHA), 372, 374, 375, 386–387, 427, 436
Office of Workers' Compensation programs, 420
Ogoniland (Southern Nigeria), 198
OIICS. *See* Occupational Injury and Illness Classification System
older adults, climate change impact on, 50
One Health, 9–10, 283–284
ordinance, 72, 88
organic waste, 311
OSHA. *See* Occupational Safety and Health Administration
OSH Act. *See* Occupational Safety and Health Act
outdoor air pollutants. *See* ambient air pollutants
Out of Gas, In With Justice pilot study (New York City, New York), case study, 217
ozone (O$_3$), 218

Pap testing, 155, 156
PAR. *See* participatory action research
parasitic resilience, 359
parental leave, paid, 383
Paris Agreement, 73–74, 75
parks and green spaces, 325
participatory action research (PAR), 105
participatory geographic information systems (PGIS), 106, 181
participatory research, 105–106
   definition of, 105
particulate matter (PM, PM$_{2.5}$, PM$_{10}$), 47–48, 80, 81, 176, 194, 215, 216, 218, 221–222
Patel, Lisa, 434
Pb. *See* lead
PCR. *See* People for Community Recovery
Pearl River flood, 79
Pediatric Environmental Health, 422
Pediatric Environmental Health Specialty Units (PEHSUs), 405, 423, 436

PEHSUs. *See* Pediatric Environmental Health Specialty Units
PELs. *See* permissible exposure limits
People for Community Recovery (PCR), 448
people with disabilities, climate change impact on, 52
per- and polyfluoroalkyl substances (PFAS), 118, 140, 247, 248–249, 403, 423, 425
Perkins, Frances, 371
permissible exposure limits (PELs), 375, 427
Perry, Robert, 164
Personal Responsibility and Work Opportunity Act (PRWORA), 429
pesticides, 249–250, 400
PFAS. *See* per-and polyfluoroalkyl substances
PGIS. *See* participatory geographic information systems
pharmaceuticals, 250
PHE. *See* public health emergency
photovoice and videovoice, 106
phthalates, 125, 131
Planetary Health Alliance, 432
Planetary Health framework, 9, 10
plastics, in waste systems, 312
PM, $PM_{2.5}$, and PM_{10}. *See* particulate matter
Pogo Park, 326
point source, 79
political determinants of health, 12
polluter pays principle, 309
polycultures, 282
population health and environmental epidemiology, 148–156
Porter Ranch incident, 25
power
  co-governance, 332–334
  community data, 225
  community frameworks, 35
  community organizing and #StopGeneralIron, 446–448, 454, 455–456, 465–467
  electricity in communities, 206–207
  energy extraction, 197
  government, separation of powers, 75
  imbalances, 100
  power map, 467
  research, decolonizing and anti-racism, 104, 109
Practice Greenhealth network, 432
precautionary principle, 14, 83, 132, 228
precision medicine, 433–434
preexisting illness, climate change impact on, 51
pregnant people, climate change impact on, 50

prenatal and early-life exposures to chemicals, 148
prenatal healthcare, 423–426
  environmental health history and, 425–426
preparedness, domains of, 353
preparedness cycle, 356–357
Prescriptions (Rx) for Prevention program, 422
presidential memoranda, 76
prevalence, 148
primary research, 150
private water supplies, 242–244
private wells, 255–256
privatization, 253, 311
procedural justice, 103
prophylactic use of antibiotics, 279
prospective cohorts, 154
prospective studies, 168
proximity principle, 309
PRWORA. *See* Personal Responsibility and Work Opportunity Act
psychosocial harm, 141
psychosocial hazards, 376–377
psychoterratic syndromes, 46
public and community-driven mapping, 181–183
public comments, 77
Public Health Awakened, 466
Public Health Core Values, 15
public health data, translating, 148–149
public health disasters, 346
  classic definitions of, 347–349
  managing, 352–359
  readiness model, nonlinear, 362
  redefining, 351
public health emergency (PHE), 356
Public Health Emergency Preparedness Program, 353
Public Health Service Act, 356
public notices and air quality permit applications, 222–223
public participation GIS (PPGIS). *See* participatory geographic information systems
public transportation, 324
Public Utilities Commission Resolution, 88
Public Utility/Service Commission, 209
public water supplies, 251–257
  issues and challenges in, 253–257
Pueblo Food Experience (Tewa Pueblo, New Mexico), case study, 282–283
Pure Food and Drug Act, 273, 274
PureGro Company, 220
Purple Air, Inc., 183

QGIS software, 183
QSAR. *See* quantitative structure-activity relationship modeling
quantitative structure-activity relationship (QSAR) modeling, 133

racially restrictive covenants, 176
racially restrictive zoning, 176
racial segregation, 25
racism, 157
   environmental, 8, 25, 157, 182, 328, 350
   health disparities and, 100
   medical, 430–431
   structural, 8, 24, 38, 119–120, 199, 322, 334, 336
   systemic, 26, 84, 107, 119, 150, 261, 279, 328, 430
Racism that Upends the Cradle report, 408
Radiation Exposure Compensation Act (RECA), 142
radiation hazards, 377
radiation hazards and nuclear weapons waste in Indigenous communities, case study, 142–143
radioactive waste, 307
radiological and radioactive hazards, 141–142
radium 226 and radium 228, 247
Radium Girls, 378
Ramazzini, Bernardino, 379
Ramirez, Gina, 454, 456, 461–463
randomized controlled trials (RCTs), 152
RCRA. *See* Resource Conservation and Recovery Act
RCTs. *See* randomized controlled trials
REACH. *See* Registration, Evaluation, Authorization, and Restriction of Chemicals
RECA. *See* Radiation Exposure Compensation Act
recall bias, 154
recommended exposure limits (RELs), 375
redlining, 25, 51, 119, 158, 176, 199, 220, 279, 323
reference man standard, 157
reference maps, 168
Regan, Michael S., 455, 458
regenerative food systems, 281–282
   principles for, 285
   regenerative farming practices in desert and, 282
Regional Transmission Organizations (RTOs), 207
Registration, Evaluation, Authorization, and Restriction of Chemicals (REACH), 82–83

regulatory science, 77, 157
reliability, of study, 151
RELs. *See* recommended exposure limits
renewable energy, transitioning to, 203–204
reproductive environmental health, 419, 424
Request for Information (RFI), 27
research decolonization, 104
Residential Energy Consumption Survey, 201
resolution, 170
Resource Conservation and Recovery Act (RCRA), 84, 302, 303, 305, 306
retrospective cohorts, 154
retrospective studies, 168
rezoning, 328
RFI. *See* Request for Information
Right-to-Know laws, for workers, 388
right to work, 382
RISE St. James, 328
risk, 14, 117–118, 119
risk assessment, 121, 131, 168, 248, 430. *See also* cumulative risk assessment
   federal agencies and, 131
   steps in, 122–123
risk communication, 427–429
   message map for, 428
Robert T. Stafford Disaster Relief and Emergency Assistance Act. *See* Stafford Act
Roe v. Wade, overturning of, 383
RTOs. *See* Regional Transmission Organizations
rule, 75, 77, 81
Rules for Radicals (Alinsky), 447
rural communities, climate change impact on, 52
rural public water supplies, 255

sacrifice zones, 86, 309
Safe Drinking Water Act (SDWA), 79–80, 244, 245, 350
safe public drinking water (Detroit, Michigan), case study, 261–262
Safe Routes to School, 334
Safe Streets and Roads for All Grant Program, 335
Safe System Approach, 335
safety engineering, 380
safety hazards, 373–374, 420
Sanchez, Óscar, 456, 459–461
Santa Barbara Channelkeeper Stream Team Data Portal, 262
Santa Cruz City Schools (California), 401
Sarfaty, Mona, 434

Save Barnegat Bay, 13
science and policy, intersection of, 102, 221–222
SDGs. *See* Sustainable Development Goals
SDOH. *See* social determinants of health
SDWA. *See* Safe Drinking Water Act
sea level rise, 46–47, 55
SEATOR. *See* Southeast Alaska Tribal Ocean Research
secondary research, 150
seed selection and preservation, in desert ecosystems, 282
selection bias, 151
selenium, 246
Sendai Framework for Disaster Risk Reduction, 359
Sendai Hazard Definitions and Classifications Review, 347
Seneca, 215
sensitive receptors, 222
sensitivity, of study, 151
sensors, low-cost, 224, 225
sensor technologies, synoptics, and remote sensing, 263
SES. *See* socioeconomic status
Seven Generations Principles, 31
sewage and sewage sludge, 307
sewage pollution and discriminatory policies (Atlanta, Georgia), case study, 129–130
sex and gender, comparison of, 158
shared or joint-use agreements, 335
shutoffs, water, 258
sick leave, paid, 383
silvopasture, 284
Sims, J. Marion, 99
Six Cities study, 221
SNAP. *See* Supplemental Nutrition Assistance Program
social and physical environment, 11–12
social cohesion, 331
social determinants of health (SDOH), 11, 53, 54–56, 251, 346, 354–355, 359, 402
work as, 383–384
social-ecological model, application of, 128–129
social ecology, 128
social vulnerability, 178
social vulnerability indices (SVIs), 178
socioeconomic status (SES), 384
Soil Conservation Act, 275
solar and wind power, 197
solastalgia, 46, 48
Soot Rule, 81
source pathway models, 168

Southeast Alaska Tribal Ocean Research (SEATOR), 60
Southwest Detroit Community Benefits Coalition, 78
So$_x$. *See* sulfur oxides
Spark School Park Program, 401
spatial analysis, 167
spatial autocorrelation, 171
spatial statistics, issues unique to, 171, 173
spatial data, 166
Special Supplemental Nutrition Program for Women, Infants, and Children (WIC), 336
special wastes, categories of, 305–308
specificity, of study, 151
Stafford Act, 356, 357
#StopGeneralIron campaign, 279, 445–447
breaking power and, 458
building power and, 456–457
community organizing for health and, 447–448
environmental injustice history on Chicago's Southeast Side and, 448–449
fight of, 449–451
legal strategies to, 454
media advocacy on, 451–453
organizing tactics in, 451–455
permit denied in support of, 455–456
protests and hunger strikes and, 454–455
StoryMaps, 181, 182, 183
stress, occupational, 376
stressor, 14, 117, 118, 121, 132, 133
structural determinants of health, 24, 37
structural harm, 348, 349
structural justice, 103
structural racism, 8, 24, 38, 119–120, 199, 322, 334, 336
structural violence, 98
structural vulnerabilities, 179
subsistence resources, and water, 237
sulfur oxides (So$_x$), 218
Sunshine Project, 328
Superfund program, 176, 297, 305, 309, 324, 382, 388–389. *See also* Comprehensive Environmental Response, Compensation, and Liability Act (CERCLA; Superfund)
Supplemental Nutrition Assistance Program (SNAP), 274, 276, 336
surface water, 254
treatment plants, 239
surveillance, 32, 60, 61
survivance, 285
sustainability, 278, 283

Sustainable Development Goals (SDGs), 73, 74, 203, 258
SVIs. *See* social vulnerability indices
Swentzell, Roxanne, 282
Sympathetic State, The (Dauber), 355
syndemic, 98, 408
systemic racism, 26, 84, 107, 119, 150, 261, 279, 328, 430
systems thinking, 352–353

Taft–Hartley Act, 382
Task Force on Environmental Health Risks and Safety Risks to Children, 405
technology equity, 390
temperature hazards, 378
tent theory, 157
testimonial injustice, 104
Tewa Women United organization, 157
Texas Department of Agriculture, 277
Texas food deserts, case study, 276–277
thallium, 246
thematic maps, 168
    types of, 169
"three-sisters" method, 282
Toms River water supply (Toms River, New Jersey), case study, 13–14
total trihalomethanes (TTHMs), 247
Total Worker Health® (TWH), 386, 387
toxicants, 12, 141, 195, 196
toxic donut, 459
toxicology, 380
    and epidemiology, to understand environmental hazards, 140–148
Toxic Release Inventory (TRI), 19, 174, 175
Toxic Substances Control Act (TSCA), 81–82, 132, 402
Toxic Tides program, 177
Toxic Wastes and Race at Twenty, 176
Toxic Wastes and Race in the United States, 165, 176, 309
toxin, 141
traffic-related air pollution (TRAP), 218
train derailment (East Palestine, Ohio), case study, 10–11
training and education, for workers, 387–389
transportation planning, 323–324
TRAP. *See* traffic-related air pollution
TRI. *See* Toxic Release Inventory
Triangle Shirtwaist Factory fire (New York City), 370
Tribal public water supplies, 255
Tribes and Tribal communities, 30–31
trust, building, 110
Trust for Public Land analysis, 325

TSCA. *See* Toxic Substances Control Act
TTHMs. *See* total trihalomethanes
Tuskegee Syphilis Study, 99
TWH. *See* Total Worker Health®

UCC. *See* United Church of Christ
uncertainty, communicating, 110
UNEP. *See* United Nations Environment Programme
unequal risk, 118, 128, 129, 131
    assessment of, 123–125
UNESCO. *See* United Nations Educational, Scientific and Cultural Organization
unethical medical and public health research, 379
    ethical oversight, 101
    historical examples of, 99, 152, 155
UNFCCC. *See* United Nations Framework Convention on Climate Change
UNICEF, 413
United Church of Christ (UCC)
    Commission on Racial Justice, 165
    Toxic Wastes and Race, 165, 176, 309
    Toxic Wastes and Race at Twenty, 176
United Nations Conference of Parties (COP), 73, 75
United Nations Educational, Scientific and Cultural Organization (UNESCO), 104
United Nations Environmental Law, 73
United Nations Environment Programme (UNEP), 73, 198
United Nations Framework Convention on Climate Change (UNFCCC), 73, 74
United Neighbors of the 10th Ward, 454
United States and European Union regulations, comparison of, 82–83
unit of analysis, 170
Universal Declaration of Human Rights, 385
University of California Center for Climate Justice, 57
up-zoning, 334
uranium, 247
urban and regional planning, for climate change mitigation, 58
urban heat island effect, 43
U.S. Atomic Energy Commission, 142
U.S. Census Bureau, 420
U.S. Congress, 77
U.S. Constitution, 75
USDA. *See* U.S. Department of Agriculture
U.S. Department of Agriculture (USDA), 83, 275, 281, 287
U.S. Department of Housing and Urban Development (HUD), 454

U.S. Department of Labor, 420
U.S. Department of Transportation, 78
U.S. General Accounting Office (GAO), 165
U.S. Geological Survey (USGS), 248, 250, 255, 263
U.S. Global Change Research Program, 47
USGS. *See* U.S. Geological Survey

validity, of study, 151
Valley of the Drums, 388
vector changes, 48, 56
vermiculite, 381–382
VGI. *See* volunteered geographic information
videovoice and photovoice, 106
Vision Zero, 334–335
VOCs. *See* volatile organic compounds
volatile organic compounds (VOCs), 250, 400
volunteered geographic information (VGI), 181
vulnerability analyses, 354
vulnerability, child, 399–400
vulnerability indices, 178–179
vulnerable communities, 170

WAP. *See* Weatherization Assistance Program
Ward Transformer Company (Raleigh, North Carolina), 17
waste, 291–293
  environmental justice and, 309–313
  health impacts of, 295–296
  hierarchy, 310
  incinerators and, 298–301
  landfills and, 296–298
  management life cycle, 296
  management systems, principles to improve, 309–310
  policy, in United States, 303
  researching, and environmental health and justice impacts, 301–302
  system, regulating, 302–308
  and waste management, in United States, 293–295
  zero, 310–313
Waste: One Woman's Fight Against America's Dirty Secret (Flowers), 329
waste colonialism, 294–295, 313
Waste Framework Directive (European Union), 312
wastewater treatment, 239–242
  system of, 240–241

water, 235–236
  access, ensuring, 258–259
  built environment and, 329
  as commons, and public trust, 254
  contamination, reducing, 259–262
  cycle, and climate change, 236–238
  environmental justice and, 258–262
  and health, interactions between, 238
  human right to, and global water challenges, 257–258
  as property right, 254
  public, and wastewater treatment, 238–244
  research methods and technologies for, 262–263
  supplies, laws and regulations of, 244–251
  supplies, public, 251–257
waterborne pathogens, 241–242
water diversion systems, 282
water stress, 238, 257, 258
water table, 236
WE ACT. *See* West Harlem Environmental Action for Environmental Justice
weatherization, 200
  energy efficiency improvement through, 205–206
  nonenergy benefits of, 206
Weatherization Assistance Program (WAP), 205
wells and septic systems, 242–244
WERA. *See* West End Revitalization Association
West End Revitalization Association (WERA), case study, 107–108
West Harlem Environmental Action for Environmental Justice (WE ACT), 127, 217, 409
We the People of Detroit (WPD), 261
  Community Research Collective, 262
wet lab, 151
When We Fight, We Win (Jobin-Leeds and AgitArte), 446
White Earth Nation, 31
Whitehall Study, 384
White supremacy, 24, 37
WHO. *See* World Health Organization
WIC. *See* Special Supplemental Nutrition Program for Women, Infants, and Children
wildfires, 47–48, 56
Wilson, Brenda, 107
Wilson, Omega, 107
Wing, Steve, 101, 107, 113

work
- -related health inequities, 384–386
- as a social determinant of health, 383–384
- socioeconomic status and health and, 384

workers, of color, 384–385
workers' compensation, 382
Workers' Compensation program, 420
Worker Training Program, National Institute of Environmental Health Sciences, 389
work organization hazards, 378
workplace hazard, 420
workplace standards, 381
Works Progress Administration (WPA), 275
World Bank, 351
World Food Summit, 276
World Health Organization (WHO), 4, 50, 214, 216, 306, 397
- International Agency for Research on Cancer, 250

WPA. *See* Works Progress Administration
WPD. *See* We the People of Detroit

Yale Program on Climate Change Communication, 62
Yucca Mountain, fight for Indigenous rights at (case study), 308
Yuma region (Arizona), 280

Zack, Naomi, 358
zero waste, 310
- beyond city limits, 312–313
- cities and, 311–312
- worker empowerment through, 310–311
- Zero Waste Hierarchy, 310

ZIP code and genetic code, 26
zoning, 327, 334, 336
- exclusionary, 323
- inclusionary, 334
- land use and, 323
- racially restrictive, 176

zoonotic diseases, 48